Industrial Applications of Marine Biopolymers

Industrial Applications of Marine Biopolymers

Edited by

P.N. Sudha

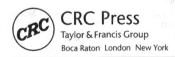

CRC Press
Taylor & Francis Group
Boca Raton London New York

CRC Press is an imprint of the
Taylor & Francis Group, an **informa** business

CRC Press
Taylor & Francis Group
6000 Broken Sound Parkway NW, Suite 300
Boca Raton, FL 33487-2742

First issued in paperback 2022

ISBN-13: 978-1-498-73148-5 (hbk)
ISBN-13: 978-1-03-233959-7 (pbk)
DOI: 10.4324/9781315313535

Library of Congress Cataloging-in-Publication Data

Names: Sudha, P.N. (Parappurath Narayanan)
Title: Industrial applications of marine biopolymers / [edited by] P.N. Sudha.
Description: Boca Raton : CRC Press, [2017] | Includes bibliographical references and index.
Identifiers: LCCN 2016055788 | ISBN 9781498731485 (hardback : alk. paper) | ISBN 9781315313535 (ebook)
Subjects: LCSH: Biopolymers--Industrial applications. | Marine resources.
Classification: LCC TP248.65.P62 I5275 2017 | DDC 333.91/64--dc23
LC record available at https://lccn.loc.gov/2016055788

Visit the Taylor & Francis Web site at
http://www.taylorandfrancis.com

and the CRC Press Web site at
http://www.crcpress.com

Dedication

Dedicated to my guides Dr. Manley Backyavathy and Dr. V.R. Vijayaraghavan, and my dear family members.

Contents

SECTION III Biomedical Applications of the Marine Biopolymers

SECTION IV Industrial Wastewater Treatment Applications of the Biopolymers

Editor

Dr. P.N. Sudha is presently working as a Principal at DKM College for Women (Autonomus), affiliated to Thiruvalluvar University, Vellore, Tamilnadu, India. She obtained her Doctoral degree in Chemistry–Biology Interdisciplinary Science from Madras University. She is a fellow of International Congress of Chemistry and Environment, and National Environmentalists Association. Her name was included in *Marquis Who's Who in the World* (2011). Her research interests are polymer chemistry, environmental chemistry, bioremediation, and photochemistry. She has authored 11 books and 13 book chapters. She is a life member of Asian Chitin Chitosan Society. She is a coeditor and reviewer of international journals. Her immense experience in research is the key asset for the development of research among the young women researchers under the rural area. She expanded her research fields up to the use to biomaterials such as chitin and chitosan for biomedical application. She has undertaken projects funded by University Grants Commission, New Delhi, India, Department of Science and Technology, New Delhi, India, Tamil Nadu State Council for Science and Technology, Chennai, India, and Ministry of Human Resource Development, Government of India, New Delhi, India. She has guided 40 PhD scholars and 50 MPhil scholars. She has published 160 research articles in journals mainly on the wastewater treatment and biomedical applications of chitin and chitosan.

Contributors

Masoud Abbaszadeh
Institute of Biological Sciences
Faculty of Science
University of Malaya
Kuala Lumpur, Malaysia

Mohaddeseh Adel
Institute for Biological Sciences
Faculty of Science
University of Malaya
Kuala Lumpur, Malaysia

Bakrudeen Ali Ahmed Abdul
Institute for Biological Sciences
Faculty of Science
University of Malaya
Kuala Lumpur, Malaysia

P. Angelin Vinodhini
PG and Research Department of
  Chemistry
D.K.M. College for Women
Thiruvalluvar University
Vellore, India

Sukumaran Anil
Dental Biomaterials Research Chair
King Saud University
Riyadh, Saudi Arabia

K. Arunkumar
Department of Plant Science
School of Biological Sciences
Central University of Kerala
Kerala, India

Anish Babu
Department of Pathology
Stephenson Cancer Center
University of Oklahoma Health
  Sciences Center
Oklahoma City, Oklahoma

Mohamed E.I. Badawy
Department of Pesticide Chemistry and
  Technology
Faculty of Agriculture
Alexandria University
Alexandria, Egypt

Ill-Min Chung
Department of Applied Bioscience
College of Life and Environmental
  Science
Konkuk University
Seoul, South Korea

Armando C. Duarte
Department of Chemistry
Centre for Environmental and Marine
  Studies
University of Aveiro
Aveiro, Portugal

Kranti Kiran Reddy Ealla
Department of Oral Pathology
MNR Dental College and Hospital
Sangareddy, India

Ana Cristina Freitas
Department of Chemistry
Centre for Environmental and Marine
  Studies
University of Aveiro
Aveiro, Portugal

and

ISEIT/Viseu
Instituto Piaget
Viseu, Portugal

Arijit Gandhi
Department of Quality Assurance
Albert David Limited
Mumbai, India

T. Gomathi
PG and Research Department of
  Chemistry
DKM College for Women
Thiruvalluvar University
Vellore, Tamil Nadu, India

Sairengpuii Hnamte
Department of Microbiology
School of Life Sciences
Pondicherry University
Pondicherry, India

Nazma Inamdar
Government College of Pharmacy
Aurangabad, Maharashtra, India

Sougata Jana
Department of Pharmaceutics
Gupta College of Technological
  Sciences
Asansol, West Bengal, India

Subrata Jana
Department of Chemistry
Vishwavidyalaya Engineering
  College
Sarguja University
Ambikapur, Chhattisgarh, India

Pongphen Jitareerat
Postharvest Technology Division
School of Bioresources and
  Technology
King Mongkut's University of
  Technology
Bangkok, Thailand

K. Kamala
Center for Environmental Nuclear
  Research
SRM University
Chennai, Tamil Nadu, India

J. Annie Kamala Florence
Department of Chemistry
Voorhees College
Vellore, Tamil Nadu, India

A. Kamaludeen
Department of Chemistry
College of Science
King Saud University
Riyadh, Saudi Arabia

Pegah Karimi
Institute for Biological Sciences
Faculty of Science
University of Malaya
Kuala Lumpur, Malaysia

Se-Kwon Kim
Department of Marine-Bio
  Convergence Science
Marine Bioprocess Research Center
Pukyong National University
Busan, South Korea

Kalyan Kumar Sen
Department of Pharmaceutics
Gupta College of Technological
  Sciences
Asansol, West Bengal, India

Srinivasan Latha
PG and Research Department of
  Chemistry
DKM College for Women
Thiruvalluvar University
Vellore, Tamil Nadu, India

Baboucarr Lowe
Department of Marine-Bio
  Convergence Science
Marine Bioprocess Research Center
Pukyong National University
Busan, South Korea

Ana L.P. Marques
3B's Research Group—Biomaterials,
    Biodegradables, and Biomimetics
The University of Minho
European Institute of Excellence
    on Tissue Engineering and
    Regenerative Medicine
Barco, Portugal

and

ICVS/3B's- PT Government
    Associated Laboratory
Braga, Portugal

A. Meera Moydeen
Department of Chemistry
College of Science
King Saud University
Riyadh, Saudi Arabia

V.K. Mourya
Government College of Pharmacy
Aurangabad, Maharashtra, India

R. Nithya
PG and Research Department of
    Chemistry
DKM College for Women
Thiruvalluvar University
Vellore, Tamil Nadu, India

Leonel Pereira
Marine and Environmental Sciences
    Center/Institute of Marine Research
Department of Life Sciences
Faculty of Sciences and Technology
University of Coimbra
Coimbra, Portugal

P. Supriya Prasad
PG and Research Department of
    Chemistry
DKM College for Women
Thiruvalluvar University
Vellore, Tamil Nadu, India

Entsar I. Rabea
Department of Plant Protection
Faculty of Agriculture
Damanhour University
Damanhur, Egypt

Paulo Ribeiro-Claro
Department of Chemistry
CICECO—Aveiro Institute of Materials
University of Aveiro
Aveiro, Portugal

Govindasamy Rajakumar
Department of Applied Bioscience
College of Life and Environmental
    Science
Konkuk University
Seoul, South Korea

R. Rajaram
Department of Marine Science
Bharathidasan University
Tiruchirapalli, Tamil Nadu, India

Barur R. Rajeshkumar
Division of Cardiovascular Medicine
Department of Medicine
University of Massachusetts Medical
    School
Worcester, Massachusetts

T. Rajeshwari
Department of Biotechnology
DKM College for Women
Vellore, Tamil Nadu, India

Rajagopal Ramesh
Department of Pathology
Stephenson Cancer Center
and
Graduate Program in Biomedical Sciences
University of Oklahoma Health
    Sciences Center
Oklahoma City, Oklahoma

Rui L. Reis
3B's Research
  Group—Biomaterials,
  Biodegradables, and Biomimetics
University of Minho
European Institute of Excellence on
  Tissue Engineering and Regenerative
  Medicine
Barco, Portugal

and

ICVS/3B's- PT Government Associated
  Laboratory
Braga, Portugal

Maximas H. Rose
Department of Chemistry
Manonmaniam Sundaranar
  University
Tirunelveli, Tamil Nadu, India

Chandrani Roy
Department of Pharmaceutics
Gupta College of Technological
  Sciences
Asansol, West Bengal, India

K. Sangeetha
PG and Research Department of
  Chemistry
DKM College for Women
Thiruvalluvar University
Vellore, Tamil Nadu, India

M. Saranya
Department of Chemistry
DKM College for Women
Thiruvalluvar University
Vellore, Tamil Nadu, India

G. Saraswathi
Department of Chemistry
Government College of Engineering,
  Bargur
Bargur, Tamil Nadu, India

Busi Siddhardha
Department of Microbiology
School of Life Sciences
Pondicherry University
Pondicherry, India

Tiago H. Silva
3B's Research Group—Biomaterials,
  Biodegradables, and Biomimetics
University of Minho
Department of Polymer Engineering
Braga, Portugal

P. Sivaperumal
Center for Environmental Nuclear
  Research
SRM University
Chennai, Tamil Nadu, India

Fabiana Soares
Department of Life Sciences
Faculty of Sciences and Technology
Marine and Environmental Sciences
  Center/Institute of Marine Research
University of Coimbra
Coimbra, Portugal

P.N. Sudha
PG and Research Department of
  Chemistry
DKM College for Women
Thiruvalluvar University
Vellore, Tamil Nadu, India

Apiradee Uthairatanakij
Postharvest Technology Division
School of Bioresources and Technology
King Mongkut's University of Technology
Bangkok, Thailand

Jayachandran Venkatesan
Department of Marine-Bio
  Convergence Science
Marine Bioprocess Research Center
Pukyong National University
Busan, South Korea

K. Vijayalakshmi
PG and Research Department of
Chemistry
DKM College for Women
Thiruvalluvar University
Vellore, Tamil Nadu, India

J. Vinoth
PG and Research Department of
Chemistry
DKM College for Women
Thiruvalluvar University
Vellore, Tamil Nadu, India

Section I

Isolation and Physicochemical Characterization of Marine Biopolymers

1 Introduction to Marine Biopolymers

P.N. Sudha, K. Sangeetha, and T. Gomathi

CONTENTS

1.1   INTRODUCTION

Biopolymers are a diverse and versatile class of materials that have potential applications in virtually all sectors of the economy. Marine biopolymers are polymers that are produced by biological systems such as microorganisms, insects, cramps, and shrimps in the marine environment. Some biopolymers can directly replace synthetically derived materials in traditional applications, whereas others possess unique properties that could open up a range of new commercial opportunities. Marine biopolymers are being developed for use as medical materials, packaging, cosmetics, food additives, clothing fabrics, water treatment chemicals, industrial plastics, absorbents, biosensors, and even data storage elements.

In this chapter, some of the important marine biopolymers are discussed with their properties and applications.

1.2   CHITIN

Chitin, a polysaccharide, is one of the most ubiquitous polymers found in nature. Chitin or poly-β-(1→4)-N-acetyl-D-glucosamine is a natural marine biopolymer synthesized by an enormous number of living organisms (Rinaudo 2006), and it belongs to the most abundant natural polymers after cellulose (Singla and Chawla 2001; Tangpasuthadol et al. 2003).

Chitin occurs naturally in three polymeric forms known as α-, β-, and γ-chitin (Blackwell 1973; Rudall and Kenchington 1973). Chitin and its most important deriv- ative, chitosan, have a number of useful physical and chemical properties, including high strength, biodegradability, and nontoxicity (Khan et al. 2002).

1.3   SOURCES OF CHITIN

Chitin is widely available from a variety of sources, among which the principal source is shellfish waste such as shrimps, crabs, and crawfish (Allan and Hadwiger 1979). It is also present naturally in a few species of fungi. Studies of Ashford and coworkers (1977) demonstrated that chitin represents 14%–27% and 13%–15% of the dry weight of shrimp and crab processing wastes, respectively.

1.4 PROPERTIES OF CHITIN

1.4.1 COLOR AND APPEARANCE

Chitin is a nitrogenous polysaccharide (Figure 1.1), which is colorless to half white, hard, and inelastic (Kurita 2001).

1.4.2 SOLUBILITY

Chitin is insoluble in water and most organic solvents. The hydrogen bonding in chitin is responsible for its poor solubility nature. To overcome the problem of solubility, the derivatives of chitin are generally prepared and used. Chitin is soluble in dimethylacetamide containing 5% lithium chloride (LiCl) (Rutherford and Austin 1978) and fluorinated solvents such as hexafluoroisopropanol and hexafluoroacetone (Capozza 1975).

1.4.3 MOLECULAR WEIGHT

The molecular weight of native chitin is usually >1,000,000 Da (Li et al. 1992). The general methods used to determine the molecular weight of chitin are viscometry, light scattering, or gel permeation chromatography (Hasegawa et al. 1993).

1.4.4 DEGREE OF DEACETYLATION

The degrees of deacetylation in chitin usually range from 5% to 15%. Chitin is generally crystalline in nature, and the degree of crystallinity is a function of the degree of deacetylation (Rathke 1993). The degree of deacetylation affects the chemical, physical, and biological properties of chitosan, such as adsorption, covalent linking, and encapsulation (Puvvada et al. 2012).

1.4.5 PROCESSABILITY

Chitin can easily be processed into gels, beads, powders, fibers, membranes, cotton, flakes, sponges, colloids, films, and spins.

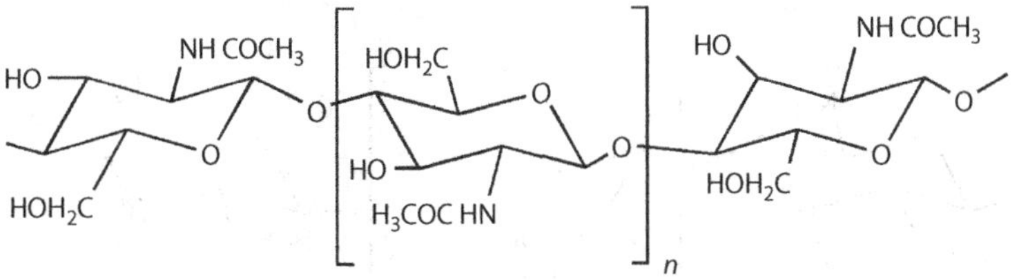

FIGURE 1.1   Structure of chitin.

1.5 APPLICATION OF CHITIN

1.5.1 PAPER AND TEXTILE INDUSTRY

In paper manufacturing, the addition of 1% chitin by weight greatly increases the strength of paper fibers, particularly when wet. Thus, chitin has been incorporated into diapers, shopping bags, and paper towels. Derivatives of chitin impart antistatic and soil repellent characteristics to the textile. Chitin can be used in printing and finishing processes.

1.5.2 AGRICULTURE

Chitin and its derivatives are used in agriculture to regulate the plant growth and development. It is used as an inducer for various crops such as rice (Hernández et al. 2007), tomato (Jin et al. 2005), peanut, and apple (Backman et al. 1994).

1.6 CHITOSAN

Chitosan is a modified natural carbohydrate polymer prepared by the partial N-deacetylation of the crustacean-derived natural biopolymer chitin (Sanford 1992). It is a heteropolymer consisting of β (1-4) 2-acetamido-2-deoxy-β-D-glucopyranose N-acetylglucosamine) and 2-amino-2-deoxy-β-D-glucopyranose (D-glucosamine) units, randomly or block distributed throughout the biopolymer. It is inexpensive and possesses the important physiological properties such as biocompatible, biodegradable, nonallergenic, and nontoxic for mammals (Sugimoto et al. 1988) (Figure 1.2).

1.7 PROPERTIES OF CHITOSAN

1.7.1 COLOR AND APPEARANCE

Chitosan powder is quite flabby in nature and its color varies from pale yellow to white.

1.7.2 WATER BINDING CAPACITY AND FAT BINDING CAPACITY

The water uptake capacity of chitosan was significantly greater than that of cellulose and chitin (Knorr 1982). The water binding capacity of chitosan ranges between

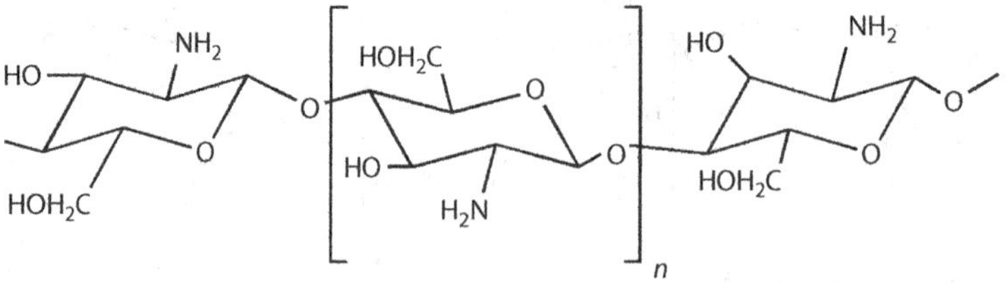

FIGURE 1.2 Structure of chitosan.

581% and 1150% with an average of 702% (Rout 2001). The process of decoloration also causes a decrease in the water binding capacity of chitosan.

1.7.3 MOLECULAR WEIGHT

The physicochemical properties, which include viscosity, solubility, adsorption on solids, elasticity, and tear strength, are dependent on the molecular weight of the polymer concerned (Khan et al. 2002). The molecular weight of chitosan can also influence the crystal size and morphological character of the film prepared using chitosan. It was also evident that the crystallinity of membrane increased with a decrease in chitosan molecular weight (Khan et al. 2002).

Depending on the source and preparation procedure, the average molecular weight of chitosan may range from 50 to 1000 kDa (Francis and Matthew 2000), 3.8 to 2000 kDa (Sinha et al. 2004), or 50 to 2000 kDa (Chenite et al. 2001). The low-molecular-weight chitosan has a greater inhibitory effect on phytopathogens than the high-molecular-weight chitosan (Hirano and Nagao 1989).

1.7.4 VISCOSITY

Viscosity is an important factor to influence the molecular weight of chitosan. Higher molecular-weight chitosan generally renders highly viscous solutions, which was undesirable for handling in industrial applications. Lower viscosity chitosan facilitates easy handling and is generally preferable. Viscosity of chitosan is considerably affected by physical (grinding, heating, autoclaving, and ultrasonication) and chemical (ozone) treatments, thereby decreasing its viscosity with an increase in treatment time and temperature (No et al. 1999).

The smaller size of particles (1 mm) generally produces highly viscous chitosan solution (Bough et al. 1978). However, in contrast, Lusena and Rose (1953) reported that the size of chitin particle within the range of 0.841–0.177 mm had no effect on the viscosity of the chitosan solutions.

1.7.5 SOLUBILITY

Chitosan is normally insoluble in water and most common organic solvents (e.g., dimethyl sulfoxide [DMSO], dimethylformamide [DMF], N-methyl-2-pyrrolidone [NMP], organic alcohols, and pyridine). The insolubility of chitosan in aqueous and organic solvents is a result of its crystalline structure, which is attributed to extensive intramolecular and intermolecular hydrogen bonding between the chains and the sheets, respectively (Yui et al. 1994). Chitosan solubility is enhanced by changing the pH value. Chitosan is soluble in dilute organic acidic solutions where the pH is <6.5 (e.g., formic, acetic, pyruvic, 10% citric and lactic acid) (Hayes et al. 1977; Kumar 2000).

1.7.6 ANTIMICROBIAL PROPERTIES

The antimicrobial properties of chitosan depend on its molecular weight and the type of bacterium. Many recent studies revealed that chitosan is effective in inhibiting the growth of bacteria. Chitosan shows stronger bactericidal effects for gram-positive bacteria than for gram-negative bacteria in the presence of 0.1% chitosan (No et al. 2002). Higher antibacterial activity of chitosan at lower pH suggests that the addition of chitosan to acidic foods will enhance its effectiveness as a natural preservative.

1.8 APPLICATIONS OF CHITOSAN

Chitosan is a versatile biopolymer, and therefore, its derivatives have shown various functional properties, which make them possible to be used in novel applications including food, cosmetics, biomedicine, agriculture, environmental protection, wastewater management, and fiber industries (Bhavani and Dutta 1999; Sridhari and Dutta 2000; Dutta et al. 2002).

1.8.1 BIOMEDICINE

Due to their high tensile strength and suitable permeability, chitosan membranes are widely used as artificial kidneys (Domard 2003; Dutta et al. 2002). Chitosans are used to prepare microspheres for oral and intranasal delivery. They possess antacid and antiulcer activities, which prevent drug irritation in the stomach (Muzzarelli 1996). Chitosan is a hemostatic agent, and due to its hemostatic property, it is used in the treatment of wounds in the form of sponges and bandages.

The high N-amino content in chitosan increases its attracting ability, which helps to reduce cholesterol and triglyceride blood plasma levels, which contribute to control obesity and cardiovascular disease (Muzzarelli 1983).

Chitosan has been used as an antibacterial and antifungal agent. The cationic amino groups of chitosan probably bind to the anionic group of microorganisms and fungi, such as *Escherichia coli, Fusarium oxysporum, Alternaria arbusti, Helminthosporium papulosum*, and *Aspergillus nidulans* resulting in growth inhibition (Leuba and Stossel 1985; Sudarshan et al. 1992). Chitosan and its derivatives act as antioxidants by scavenging oxygen radicals such as hydroxyl, superoxide, and alkyl and highly stable 2,2-diphenyl-1-picrylhydrazyl (DPPH) radicals tested *in vitro* (Park et al. 2003).

1.8.2 WASTEWATER TREATMENT

Chitosan has been used for about three decades in water purification process. When chitosan is spread over oil spills, it holds the oil mass together making it easier to clean up the spill. Water purification plants throughout the world use chitosan to remove oils, grease, heavy metals, and fine particulate matter that cause turbidity in wastewater streams (Sridhari and Dutta 2000). Chitosan also undergoes chelation with metal ions (Kurita et al. 1979; Sashiwa et al. 2002) and radioisotopes for the prevention of water pollution (Muzzarelli 1977). The removal of heavy metal ions by chitosan through chelation has received much attention (Ge and Huang 2010).

Chitosan is an important additive in the filtration process. Sand filtration apparently can remove up to 50% of the turbidity alone, whereas the chitosan with sand filtration removes up to 99% of the turbidity. Chitosan has been used to precipitate caseins from bovine milk and cheese making (Woodmansey 2002).

1.8.3 COSMETICS

A cosmetic is defined as any substance to be placed in contact with various surface parts of the human body (e.g., epidermis, hair systems, nails, lips, and external genital organs), or with teeth and the mucous membranes of the oral cavity with a view exclusively or principally to perfume them, protect them, and keep them in good condition, to change their appearance, or to correct body odors (Duke et al. 2012).

The high moisture retention and film-forming characteristics of chitosan have resulted in a number of applications in the cosmetics and personal care area.

Chitosan has different molecular weights and degrees of deacetylation, which is tailored for use in different cosmetic fields such as skin care, deodorants, and hair care (Dutta et al. 2002). The film-forming ability of chitosan assists in imparting a pleasant feeling of smoothness to the skin and in protecting it from adverse environmental conditions. Chitosan is used in sunscreen formulations as it significantly increases the water resistance. The chitosan film improves the adhesion of the ultraviolet filters and thus protected them against washing off.

1.8.4 FOOD INDUSTRY

In the food industry, it is used as a conservant, an emulsifier, a viscosity regulator, and a biologically active additive (Pillai et al. 2009). It is also used as a food packaging material because of its antimicrobial action (Ghaouth et al. 1991) and dietary fiber and a potential medicine against hypertension (Furda and Brine 1990). Chitosan and chitosan glutamate are used as a natural preservative for foods prone to fungal spoilage (Roller and Covill 1999).

1.8.5 PAPER INDUSTRY

In the paper industry, it is used for the production of high-quality paper that is stable for the external action and moisture (Pillai et al. 2009).

1.9 ALGINATES

Alginate is extracted mainly from brown seaweed and bacteria (Figure 1.3). It is a linear polysaccharide consisting of (1,4)-linked β-D-mannuronate (M) and its C-5 epimer α-L-guluronate (G). By partial acid hydrolysis, alginate was separated into three fractions (Haug 1964; Haug et al. 1966). Two of these contained almost homopolymeric blocks of consecutive G-residues (G-blocks) and consecutive M-residues (M-blocks), whereas the third fraction consisted of nearly equal proportions of both monomers of alternating M- and G-residues (MG-blocks) or randomly organized blocks (Grasdalen 1983) (Figure 1.4). Divalent cations such as Ca^{2+} and Mg^{2+} can bind the guluronic residues in adjacent alginate chains to form an egg-box structure (Grant et al. 1973; Smidsrod and Skjak-Braek 1990) and cause the gelation of aqueous alginate solutions. Monovalent ions such as Na^+ can also compete with calcium ions, thereby weakening the alginate gel (Le Roux et al. 1999) (Table 1.1).

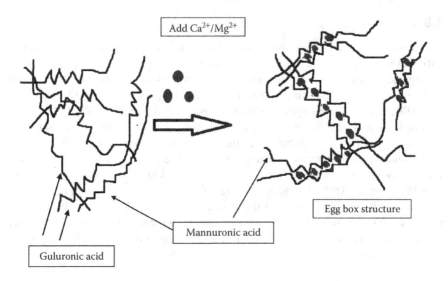

FIGURE 1.3 Structure of alginate.

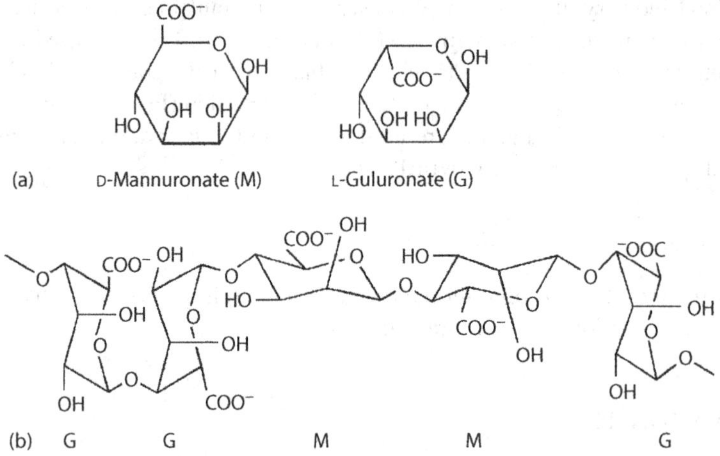

FIGURE 1.4 (a) Monomers of alginate. (b) Chemical structure of alginate.

TABLE 1.1
Some Potential Biomedical Application of Alginate-Encapsulated Cells

Cell Type	Treatment of	Reference
Adrenal chromaffin cells	Parkinson's disease	Aebischer et al. (1993)
Hepatocytes	Liver failure	Aebischer et al. (1993)
Parathyroid cells	Hypocalcemia	Aebischer et al. (1993)
Langerhans islets	Diabetes	Soon-shiong et al. (1993, 1994)
Genetically altered cells	Cancer	Read et al. (2000)

1.10 PROPERTIES OF ALGINATE

The physical properties of the alginate molecule were revealed mainly in the 1960s and the 1970s.

1.10.1 MOLECULAR WEIGHT AND POLYDISPERSITY

Alginates such as polysaaccharides, in general, are polydisperse with respect to molecular weight. The fraction M_w/M_n is called the polydispersity index. Polydispersity index values between 1.4 and 3.0 have been reported for commercial alginates and have been related to different types of preparation and purification processes (Mackie et al. 1980; Moe et al. 1995). The most common methods to calculate the molecular weight of alginate are intrinsic viscosity and light scattering measurements.

1.10.2 VISCOSITY

Viscosity is a function of the molecular weight of the biopolymer and its conformation in solution. Complete hydration of alginate is necessary to obtain the full functionality of the polymer. The viscosity of an alginate solution depends on the alginate concentration and the length of the alginate molecules, or the number of monomer units in the chains (i.e., average molecular weight), with longer chains resulting in higher viscosities at similar concentrations. Temperature defines the energetic state of any chemical molecule. Increasing temperature will result in a decrease in viscosity. As a general rule, temperature increases of 1°C lead to a viscosity drop of ~2.5% (Smidsrod and Draget 1996).

Aqueous solutions of alginates have shear-thinning characteristics, meaning that viscosity decreases as the shear rate, or stripped speed, increases. This property is known as pseudoplasticity or non-Newtonian flow.

1.10.3 SOLUBILITY

There are three important factors that influence the solubility of alginate: (1) pH of the solvent, (2) total ionic strength of the solute, and (3) hardness of the water. Alginates containing MG-block structure will precipitate at lower pH compared to the homogeneous polymeric G- and M-blocks.

1.10.4 GEL FORMATION

A gel is formed when the polymer gets cross-linked. It has the qualities of both solid and liquid. Alginates are soluble in cold water and develop into gels when exposed to calcium ions. They do not require heating and cooling processes to form a gel (Figure 1.5). Three basic components are used to form a typical alginate gel: (1) alginate, (2) calcium salt, and (3) sequestrant.

1.10.5 FILM FORMATION

Films formed using alginates in combination with a plasticizer are generally strong and flexible, and also provide a strong oxygen barrier. Alginates films can be either

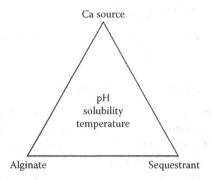

FIGURE 1.5 Factors influencing gel formation and properties.

soluble or insoluble. Soluble films of sodium alginate are made by casting and drying, whereas insoluble alginate films are produced by applying a layer of alginate solution followed by cross-linking with calcium salt and then drying.

1.11 APPLICATIONS OF ALGINATES

The alginate-based biomaterials are used in many applications, and new ones are being found all the time. Their uses range from applications in the food industry to wound dressings, medicines, tissue engineering, drug delivery, and dental impression materials (Table 1.2).

1.11.1 MEDICINE AND PHARMACY

Alginate gel cross-linked with calcium ions (Ca^{2+}) has been widely used for tissue engineering studies due to its low toxicity, biocompatibility, and spontaneous

TABLE 1.2

Applications of Different Types of Alginate

Types of Alginate	Brand Name	Main Applications
Alginic acid	Protacid	Anti-reflux tablets, natural disintegrant
Sodium alginate	Protanal	Anti-reflux suspensions, controlled release tablets, wound dressings, dental impression material, denture fixatives, viscosifier, encapsulations, films, foams
Magnesium alginate	Protanal	Anti-reflux suspensions for infants
Potassium alginate	Protanal	Dental impression material
Triethanolamine alginate	Protanal	Dental impression material
Propylene glycol alginate	Protanal ester	Suspending agent/stabilizer, plasticizer, binder, emulsifier

gelation (Paige et al. 1996; Wong et al. 2002; Masuda et al. 2003). Calcium alginate is used in wound dressings, and these dressings are particularly useful for slow healing wounds such as leg ulcers, which can continue to bleed and weep for a long time.

1.11.2 TEXTILE PRINTING

In textile printing, alginates are used as thickeners for the paste containing the dye. These pastes may be applied to the fabric by either screen or roller printing equipment. Alginates have become the important thickeners with the advent of reactive dyes. Textile printing accounts for about 50% of the global alginate market.

1.11.3 FOODS

Alginates are used as food additives to improve, modify, and stabilize the texture of foods. Alginate is a common food additive, E400. It is used as a thickener, a stabilizer, and a gelling agent. It is often found in ice cream, where it is used to thicken the product so that even if it melts, it does not drip too much. Sodium alginate is also used as a good thickener of jam, jellies, fruit fillings, chilli sauce, and tomato ketchup as the synergetic gelling between alginates high in guluronate and highly esterified pectins may be utilized (Toft et al. 1986).

1.12 AGAR

Agar is a phycocolloid extracted from a group of red-purple marine algae (Class Rhodophyceae) including *Gelidium*, *Pterocladia*, and *Gracilaria*. *Gelidium* is the preferred source for agars. Agar is a mixture of a neutral, dominating polysaccharide called *agarose* and a charged polymer called *agaropectin*. The agarose is composed of (1–4)-linked 3,6-anhydro-a-L-galactose alternating with (1–3)-linked b-D-galactose (Guiseley and Renn 1975).

Agar was first suggested for microbiological purposes in 1881 by Fannie Hesse. By the early 1900s, agar became the gelling agent of choice over gelatin because agar remains firm at growth temperatures for many pathogens. Agar is also generally resistant to a breakdown by bacterial enzymes. The use of agar in microbiological media significantly contributed to the advance of microbiology, paving the way for pure culture isolation and study (Figure 1.6).

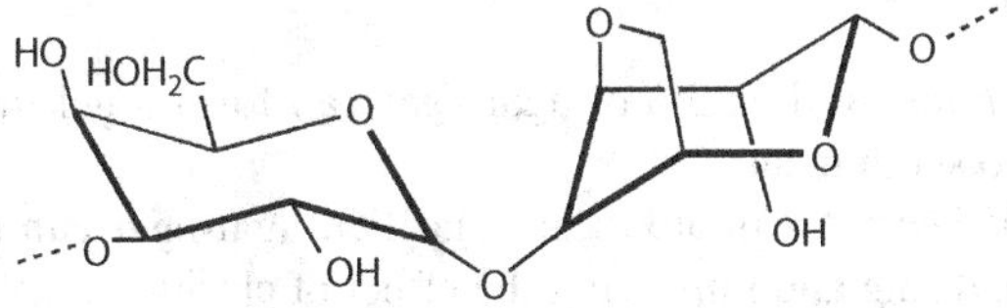

FIGURE 1.6   Structure of agar.

1.12.1 PROPERTIES OF AGAR

The properties of agar are as follows:

1. Agar can jellify or thicken products starting at 0.04%.
2. Agar is a gel at room temperature, remaining firm at temperatures as high as 65°C (Selby and Selby 1959).
3. Agar gels are stronger and firmer than gels obtained with other hydrocolloids.
4. Agar gels are formed without any addition of chemicals or organics.
5. Agar gels are formed independently of the pH or the contained solid matter.
6. Agar has a high gelation hysteresis.
7. Agar gels are thermoreversible.
8. Agar has an excellent resistance to enzymatic hydrolysis
9. Agar is compatible with proteins and other hydrocolloids.
10. Agar has a good flavor release.
11. Agar does not undergo any genetic modification.

1.12.2 APPLICATIONS OF AGAR

1.12.2.1 Medicine

The major application of agar is in the field of plant tissue culture. Agar as a culture medium is widely used for practically all pathogenic and nonpathogenic bacteria and fungi because it is not easy to metabolize and has a good gel firmness, elasticity, clarity, and stability (Guiseley and Renn 1975). On account of its high jellifying power and its vegetal origin, agar constitutes a natural nontoxic matrix for the formation of culture media in microbiology.

1.12.2.2 Food

Agar has been listed as generally recognized safe product by the United States Food and Drug Administration Ordinance. Agar can significantly change the quality of the food and improve food grade.

Beverage and food industry: Agar can also be used in the production of various beverages and food, for example, jelly, ice cream, bread, cake, and soft candy, and as a coagulator, a thickening agent, an emulsifier, and a stabilizer.

Fruit juice soft candy: The transparency and taste of soft candy will become better than others as long as the formula is added by 0.8%–1.5% of agar-agar.

Bread and cake: Owing to its water-holding function, adding proper agar-agar can prolong the storage time of bread and cake and improve the color and their taste.

Meat can and ham: Adding 2% of agar-agar can form a gel that can adhere effectively to scrap meat.

The clarifier of beer: As an auxilliary clarifier, agar-agar can accelerate the speed of clarifying and improving the effect of clarity.

1.13   CONCLUSION

Marine biopolymers are one among the most important natural sources and have high potential for providing novel types of polymeric material. They provide a great variety of applications, including medicine; virucidal, bactericidal, and fungicidal agents; and biocompatible and biomedical materials. Marine biopolymers are extensively used in all fields because they are ecofriendly, easily biodegradable, low cost, and easily available. Progress in this area is quite rapid as evidenced by a sharp increase in the number of papers and papers in the past decade.

REFERENCES

Aebischer, P., M. Goddard, P.A. Tresco. 1993. Cell encapsulation for the nervous system, in *Fundamentals of Animal Cell Encapsulation and Immobilization*, Ed., Goosen, M.F.A., pp. 197–224. Boca Raton, FL: CRC Press.

Allan, C.R. and L.A. Hadwiger. 1979. The fungicidal effect of chitosan on fungi of varying cell wall composition. *Exp. Mycol.* 3: 285–287.

Ashford, N.A., D. Hattis, A.E. Murray. 1977. Industrial prospects for chitin and protein from shellfish wastes, MIT Sea Grant Report MISG 77-3. Cambridge, MA: MIT.

Backman, P., R. Rodriguez-Kabana, N. Kokalis. 1994. Inventors, Auburn University, assignee. Method of controlling foliar microorganism populations. US Patent No. 5,288,488.

Bhavani, K.D. and P.K. Dutta. 1999. Physico-chemical adsorption properties on chitosan for dyehouse effluent. *Am. Dyestuff Rep.* 88: 53.

Blackwell, J. 1973. Chitin, in *Biopolymers*, Eds., Walton, A.G., Blackwell, J., pp. 474–489. New York: Academic Press.

Bough, W.A., W.L. Salter, A.C.M. Wu, B.E. Perkins. 1978. Influence of manufacturing variables on the characteristics and effectiveness of chitosan products. 1. Chemical composition, viscosity and molecular weight distribution of chitosan products. *Biotechnol. Bioeng.* 20: 1931.

Capozza, R.C. 1975. Enzymically decomposable bioerodible pharmaceutical carrier. German Patent No. 2,505,305.

Chenite, A., M. Buschmann, D. Wang, C. Chaput. 2001. Rheological characterization of thermogelling chitosan/glycerol phosphate solution. *Carbohydr. Polym.* 46: 39–47.

Domard, A. and M. Domard. 2003. Chitosan: Structure–properties relationship and biomedical applications, in *Polymeric Biomaterials*, Ed. Dumitriu, S., Second edition. New York: Marcel Dekker.

Duke, S.O., J. Lydon, W.C. Koskinen, T.B. Moorman, R.L. Chaney, R. Hammerschmidt. 2012. Glyphosate effects on plant mineral nutrition, crop rhizosphere microbiota, and plant disease in glyphosate-resistant crops. *J. Agric. Food Chem.* 60(42): 10375–10397.

Dutta, P.K., M.N.V. Ravikumar, J. Dutta. 2002. Chitin and chitosan for versatile applications. *JMS Polym. Rev.* C42: 307.

Francis Suh, J.K. and H.W.T. Matthew. 2000. Application of chitosan based polysaccharide biomaterials in cartilage tissue engineering: A review. *Biomaterials* 21: 2589–2598.

Furda, I. and C.J. Brine. 1990. *New Development in Dietary Fiber*. New York: Plenum Press.

Ge, H. and S. Huang. 2010. Microwave preparation and adsorption properties of EDTA-modified cross-linked chitosan. *J. Appl. Polym. Sci.* 115(1): 514–519.

Ghaouth, A.E., J. Arul, R. Ponnampalam, M. Boulet. 1991. Chitosan coating effect on storability and quality of fresh strawberries. *J. Food Sci.* 56: 1618–1620.

Grant, G.T., E.R. Morris, D.A. Rees, P.J.C. Smith, D. Thom. 1973. Biological interactions between polysaccharides and divalent cations-egg-box model. *Febs. Lett.* 32: 195–198.

Grasdalen, H. 1983. High-field 1H-N.M.R. spectroscopy of alginate: Sequential structure and linkage conformations. *Carbohydr. Res.* 118: 255–260.

Guiseley, K.B. and D.W. Renn. 1975. *Agarose: Purification, Properties, and Biomedical Applications*, pp. 1–34. Rockland, NY: Marine Colloids Division, FMC Corporation.

Hasegawa, M., A. Isogai, F. Onabe. 1993. Preparation of low-molecular-weight chitosan using phosphoric acid. *Carbohydr. Polym.* 20: 279–283.

Haug, A. 1964. Composition and properties of alginates, Thesis. Trondheim, Norway: Norwegian Institute of Technology.

Haug. A., B. Larsen, O. Smidsrod. 1966. A study of the constitution of alginic acid by partial hydrolysis. *Acta Chem. Scand.* 20: 183–190.

Hayes, E.R., D.H. Davies, V.G. Munroe. 1977. Organic solvent systems for chitosan, in *Proceedings of 1st International Conference on Chitin and Chitosan*, p. 103. Cambridge, MA: MIT Sea Grant Program.

Hernández, A.N., M. Hernández, M.G. Velásquez, M.G. Guerra, G.E. Melo. 2007. Actividad antifúngica del quitosano en el control de Rhizopus stolonifer (Ehreneb. FR.) Bullíy Mucor spp. *Rev. Mex. Fitopat.* 25: 109–113.

Hirano, S. and N. Nagao. 1989. Effects of chitosan, pectic acid, lysozyme and chitinase on the growth of several phytopathogens. *Agric. Biol. Chem.* 53: 3065–3066.

Jin, R.D., J. Suh, R.D. Park, Y.W. Kim, H.B. Krishnan, K. Kil Yong. 2005. Effect of chitin compost and broth on biological control of *Meloidogyne incognita* on tomato (*Lycopersicones culentum Mill*). *Nematology* 7(1): 125–32.

Khan, T.A., K. Peh, H.S. Cheng. 2002. Reporting degree of deacetylation values of chitosan: The influence of analytical methods. *J. Pharm. Pharm. Sci.* 5(3): 205–212.

Knorr, D. 1982. Functional properties of chitin and chitosan. *J. Food Sci.* 47: 593–595.

Kumar, M.N.V.R. 2000. A review of chitin and chitosan applications. *React. Funct. Polym.* 46: 1–27.

Kurita, K. 2001. Controlled functionalization of polysaccharide chitin. *Prog. Polym. Sci.* 26: 1921–1971.

Kurita, K., T. Takanori Sannan, Y. Yoshio Iwakura. 1979. Studies on chitin. VI. Binding on metal cations. *J. Appl. Polym. Sci.* 23: 511–515.

Le Roux, M.A., F. Guilak, L.A. Setton. 1999. Compressive and shear properties of alginate gel: Effects of sodium ions and alginate concentration. *J. Biomed. Mater. Res.* 47: 46–53.

Leuba, S. and P. Stossel. 1985. Chitosan and other polyamines: Antifungal activity and interaction with biological membranes, in *Chitin in Nature and Technology*, Eds., Muzzarelli, R.A.A., Jeuniaux, C., Gooday, C., p. 217. New York: Plenum Press.

Li, Q., E.T. Dunn, E.W. Grandmaison, M.F.A. Goosen. 1992. Applications and properties of chitosan. *J. Bioact. Compat. Pol.* 7: 370–397.

Lusena, C.V. and R.C. Rose. 1953. Preparation and viscosity of chitosans. *J. Fish. Res. Bd. Can.* 10(8): 521–522.

Mackie, W., R. Noy, D.B. Sellen. 1980. Solution properties of sodium alginate, *Biopolymers* 19: 1839–1860.

Masuda, K., R.L. Sah, M.J. Hejna, E.J. Thonar. 2003. A novel two-step method for the formation of tissue engineered cartilage by mature bovine chondrocytes: The alginate-recovered-chondrocyte (ARC) method. *J. Orthop. Res.* 21: 139–148.

Moe, S., K. Draget, G. Skjak-Braek, O. Smidsrod. 1995. Alginates, in *Food Polysaccharides and Their Applications*, Ed., Stephen, A.M., pp. 245–286. New York: Marcel Dekker.

Muzzarelli, R.A.A. 1977. *Chitin*. Oxford: Pergamon Press.

Muzzarelli, R.A.A. 1983. Chitin and its derivatives: New trends of applied research. *Carbohydr. Polym.* 3: 53–75.

Muzzarelli, R.A.A. 1996. Chitosan-based dietary foods. *Carbohydr. Polym.* 29(4): 309–316.

No, H.K., S.D. Kim, D.S. Kim, S.J. Kim, S.P. Meyers. 1999. Effect of physical and chemical treatments on chitosan viscosity. *J. Korean Soc. Chitin Chitosan* 4(4): 177–183.

No, H.K., N.Y. Park, S.H. Lee, S.P. Meyers. 2002. Antibacterial activity of chitosans and chitosan oligomers with different molecular weights. *Int. J. Food Microb.* 74: 65–72.

Paige, K.T., L.G. Cima, M.J. Yaremchuk, B.L. Schloo, J.P. Vacanti, C.A. Vacanti. 1996. De novo cartilage generation using calcium alginate-chondrocyte constructs. *Plast. Reconstr. Surg.* 97:168–178.

Park, P.J.J., Y. Je, S.K. Kim. 2003. Free radical scavenging activity of chitooligosaccharides by electron spins resonance spectrometry. *J. Agric. Food Chem.* 51: 4624–4627.

Pillai, C.K.S., W. Paul, C.P. Sharma. 2009. Chitin and chitosan polymers: Chemistry, solubility and fiber formation. *Prog. Polym. Sci.* 34: 641–678.

Puvvada Y.S., S. Vankayalapati, S. Sukhavasi. 2012. Extraction of chitin from chitosan from exoskeleton of shrimp for application in the pharmaceutical industry. *Inter. Curr. Pharm. J.* 1(9): 258–263.

Rathke, T. 1993. Determination of the degree of N-Deacteylation in chitin and chitosan as well as their monomer sugar ratios by near infrared spectroscopy. *J. Polym. Sci. Polym. Chem. Ed.* 31: 749–753.

Read, T.A., D.R. Sorensen, R. Mahesparan, P.O. Enger, R. Timpl, B.R. Olsen, M.H.B. Hjelstuen, O. Haraldseth, R. Bjerkevig. 2000. Local endostatin treatment of gliomass administered by microencapsulated producer cells. *Nature Biotechnol.* 19: 29–34.

Rinaudo, M. 2006. Chitin and chitosan: Properties and applications. *Prog. Polym. Sci.* 31: 603–632.

Roller, S. and N. Covill. 1999. The antifungal properties of chitosan in laboratory media and apple juice. *Int. J. Food Microbiol.* 47(1–2): 67–77.

Rout, S.K. 2001. *Physiochemical, Functional, and Spectroscopic Analysis of Crawfish Chitin and Chitosan as Affected by Process Modification.* Baton Rouge, LA: Dissertation Louisiana State University.

Rudall, K.M. and W. Kenchington. 1973. The chitin system. *Biol. Rev.* 40: 597–636.

Rutherford, F. and P.R. Austin. 1978. Marine chitin properties and solvents, in *Proceedings of the First International Conference Oil Chitin Chitosan*, Eds., Muzzarelli R.A.A., and Pariser E.R., pp. 182–192. Cambridge, MA: MIT.

Sanford, P.A. 1992. High purity chitosan and alginate: Preparation, analysis, and applications, front. *Carbohydr. Res.* 2: 250–269.

Sashiwa H., N. Kawasaki, A. Nakayama, E. Muraki, N. Yamamoto, H. Zhu, H. Nagano, Y. Omura, H. Saimoto, Y. Shigemasa. 2002. Chemical modification of chitosan. 13. 1 Synthesis of organosoluble, palladium adsorbable and biodegradable chitosan derivatives toward the chemical plating on plastics. *Biomacromolecules* 3: 1120–1125.

Selby, H.H. and T.A. Selby. 1959. Agar, in *Industrial Gums*, Ed., Whistler, R.L., p. 15. New York: Academic Press.

Sinha, V.R., A.K. Singla, S. Wadhawan, R. Kaushik, R. Kumria, K. Bansal, S. Dhawan. 2004. Chitosan microspheres as a potential carrier for drugs. *Int. J. Pharm.* 274: 1–33.

Singla, A.K. and M. Chawla. 2001. Chitosan: Some pharmaceutical and biological aspects—an update. *J. Pharm. Pharm.* 53: 1047–1067.

Smidsrod, O. and K.I. Draget. 1996. Chemistry and physical properties of alginates. *Carbohydr. Eur.* 14: 6–13.

Smidsrod, O. and G. Skjak-Braek. 1990. Alginate as immobilization matrix for cells. *TrendsBiotechnol.* 8: 71–78.

Soon-shiong, P., E. Feldman, R. Nelson, R. Heints, Q. Yao, T. Yao, N. Zheng et al. 1993. Long-term reversal of diabetes by the injection of immunoproctected islets. *Proc. Natl. Sci. USA* 90: 843–847.

Soon-shiong, P., R.E. Heintz, N. Merideth, Q.X. Yao, Z.W. Yao, T.L. Zheng, M. Murphy et al. 1994. Insulin independence in a type 1 diabetic patient after encapsulated islet transplantation. *Lancet* 343: 950–951.

Sridhari, T.R. and P.K. Dutta. 2000. Synthesis and characterization of maleilated chitosan for dye house effluent. *Ind. J. Chem. Tech.* 7: 198.

Sudarshan, N.R., D.G. Hoover, D. Knorr. 1992. Antibacterial action of chitosan. *Food Biotechnol.* 6: 257–272.

Sugimoto, M., M. Morimoto, H. Sashiwa, H. Saimoto, Y. Shigemasa. 1998. Preparation and characterization of water-soluble chitin and chitosan derivatives. *Carbohydr. Polym.* 36(1): 49–59.

Tangpasuthadol, V., N. Pongchaisirikul, V.P. Hoven. 2003. Surface modification of chitosan films. Effects of hydrophobicity on protein adsorption. *Carbohydr. Res.* 338: 937–942.

Toft, K., H. Grasdalen, O. Smidsrod. 1986. Synergistic gelation of alginates and pectins, *ACS Symp. Ser.* 310: 117–132.

Woodmansey, A. 2002. Chitosan Treatment of Sediment Laden Water - Washington State I-90 Issaquah Project. (Highway Engineer). Federal Highway Administration. U.S. Department of Transportation.

Wong, M., M. Siegrist, V. Gaschen, Y. Park, W. Graber, D. Studer. 2002. Collagen fibrillogenesis by chondrocytes in alginate. *Tissue Eng.* 8: 979–987.

Yui, T., K. Imada, K. Okuyama, Y. Obata, K. Suzuki, K. Ogawa. 1994. Molecular and crystal structure of the anhydrous form of CS. *Macromolecules* 27: 7601–7605.

2 Extraction, Isolation, and Characterization of Alginate

K. Arunkumar

CONTENTS

2.1   INTRODUCTION

Phycocolloids are high-molecular-weight polysaccharides composed mainly
of simple sugars extracted from both freshwater and marine algae. On analyzing
the marine polysaccharides, only the polysaccharides extracted from marine red
and brown algae—such as agar, carrageenan, and alginate—are economic and of
commercial significance. These water-soluble colloids are noncrystalline substances
exhibiting viscous and sticky properties in solution and are simply referred to as seaweed gum (Percival 1979; Lahaye and Robic 2007). They can be extracted with hot
water or alkaline solution and exhibit excellent gelling, stabilizing, and emulsifying properties with many applications in the food, pharmaceutical, cosmetic, and
biotechnology industries. Alginate is the major carbohydrate polymer among the
members of marine brown algae belonging to the class Phaeophyceae.

2.2   ALGINATE

Alginate (or algin) is a group of naturally occurring polysaccharides, which was
first described by the British chemist E.C.C. Stanford in 1881 (Chapman 1970)
while searching for useful products from a seaweed called Kelp. It occurs as a structural component in marine brown algae (Phaeophyceae) and is not found in land
plants (Sime 1990). The Phaeophyceae members are commonly called brown seaweeds that are exclusively found in marine waters consisting mainly of water (90%)
and polysaccharides (alginates, cellulose, laminarins, and fucoidans). Other components include proteins, free mannitol, minerals such as iodine and arsenic (inorganic and organic), polyphenols, peptides, fatty compounds, and various pigments
(Torres et al. 2007). The carbohydrates present in brown seaweeds are (1) mannitol,
a sugar alcohol; (2) laminarin, a β-1,3-linked glucan that also contains mannitol;
(3) alginate, which is composed of mannuronic and guluronic acids; and (4) fucoidan, a sulfated fucan that contains other sugars such as fucose, galactose, xylose,
and uronic acid (Percival and Dowel 1967). Quantitatively, the major structural
polysaccharide of the brown seaweeds is alginic acid reaching up to 40% of the dry
weight (Moe et al. 1995). Alginate content on a dry weight basis in some brown seaweeds is recorded as 22%–30% in *Ascophylum nodosum*, 25%–44% in *Laminaria
digitata* fronds, 35%–47% in *L. digitata* stipes, 17%–33% in *L. hyperborea* fronds,
25%–38% in *L. hyperborea* stipes (Rinaudo 2007), and 17%–45% in *Sargassum* spp.
(Chapman and Chapman 1980; Fourest and Volesky 1996). Alginate in brown algae
occurs as gels containing sodium, calcium, strontium, magnesium, and barium ions
(Haug and Smidsrod 1967). It is a polysaccharide consisting of unbranched chains
comprising blocks of contiguous β-1,4-linked D-mannuronic acid and blocks of
contiguous α-1,4-linked L-guluronic acid. The average lengths of the blocks are

about 20 units, and these are interspersed with a statistical mixture of the two acids (Haug and Smidsrod 1967). The proportions of the two acids vary from species to species and from different parts of the same seaweed (Haug et al. 1974). Alginates are used as thickening agents in the food industry and as binders, gelling agents, and wound absorbents in the pharmaceutical industry. (Torres et al. 2007).

In addition, alginates are present as capsular polysaccharides in soil bacteria. The function of alginates in algae is thought to be primarily skeletal, with the gel located in the cell walls and intercellular matrix conferring the strength and flexibility necessary to withstand the force of the water in which the seaweed grows (Johnson et al. 1997).

In seaweeds, algin is extracted as a mixed salt of sodium and/or potassium, calcium, and magnesium. The exact composition varies with algal species. Since Stanford discovered algin, the name has been applied to a number of substances, for example, alginic acid and all alginates, derived from alginic acid. The extraction process is based on the conversion of an insoluble mixture of alginic acid salts of the cell wall in a soluble salt (alginate), which is appropriate for water polysaccharide derived from several genera of brown algae (e.g., mixed Fucales and Laminariales) that are utilized as raw materials by commercial alginate producers; these include *Macrocystis*, *Laminaria*, *Lessonia*, *Ascophyllum*, *Alaria*, *Ecklonia*, *Eisenia*, *Nereocystis*, *Sargassum*, *Cystoseira*, and *Fucus*, with *Macrocystis pyrifera* and *Ascophyllum nodosum* being the principal sources of the world's alginate supply. The intercellular mucilage in these seaweeds has been regarded as the principal site of algin, although it has also been found to occur in the cell walls.

2.3 CHEMICAL STRUCTURE OF ALGINATE

Alginate is a salt of alginic acid, which is a linear polysaccharide, composed of (1–4)-β-D-mannuronic acid and its C-5-epimer α-L-guluronic acid (Pereira et al. 2009). Usually, this linear copolymer is composed of two monomeric units: D-mannuronic acid and L-guluronic acid (Fischer and Dorfel 1955). They are organized in a block-wise fashion as polymannuronic acid (MM blocks), polyguluronic acid (GG blocks), and heteropolymeric sequences containing both mannuronic and guluronic acids (MG blocks) (Haug et al. 1974). The proportions of these three polymer segments (MM, GG, and MG blocks) in alginic acid extracted from different brown algae vary widely (Glicksman 1987). The ratio of D-mannuronic acid and L-guluronic acid components and their sequence predetermine the properties observed for alginates extracted from different seaweed sources (Haug et al. 1967; Clare 1993).

Alginate is found in plants as salts of different metals, primarily sodium and calcium, in the intercellular regions and cell walls. Its biological functions in seaweeds are of structural and ion exchange type. Alginate enriched in polymannuronic acid is found in young cell wall tissue and/or intercellular regions, whereas polyguluronic-rich alginate is found in the cell wall (Haug et al. 1969) having a high affinity for Ca^{2+}, which is mainly responsible for gel strength. Alginate polymer is synthesized in the cytoplasm and then transported to the cell surface (Abe et al. 1973).

2.4 ISOLATION OF ALGINATE

As alginic acid exists in the seaweeds as an insoluble mixed salt, it is necessary to convert it into its soluble salt forms such as sodium or potassium (Clare 1993). The alginate was made alternately insoluble and soluble in solvent by ion-exchange reactions to separate out from the other constituents of alga. (Percival and McDowell 1967). As large molecules have to diffuse out from the plant tissues, the seaweed is preferably reduced to small particles as a preliminary step. Therefore, the first step is to mill and wash the seaweed. Alginate isolation is essentially an ion-exchange process, and alginate is brought into solution as sodium alginate by treating it with a strong alkali (McHugh 1987; Sime 1990). There are several methods to separate the alginate from other soluble substances from the crude alginate extract solution. For example, addition of alcohol (Haug and Smidsrod 1967) would precipitate out sodium alginate. Adding a solution of calcium chloride with good stirring precipitate out calcium alginate, whereas adding hydrochloric acid precipitate out alginic acid (Percival and McDowell 1967).

2.4.1 SOURCE AND EXTRACTION

The source of alginate extraction mainly relies on various species of brown seaweeds such as *Ascophyllum, Laminaria, Lessonia, Macrocystis, Ecklonia, Nereocystis, Undaria, Sargassum, Turbinaria,* and *Durvillea* (Lahaye 1991; Istinii et al. 1994). The extraction of alginate is employed by mild acid treatments that remove undesirable compounds and transform cell wall alginate into alginic acid. The alginic acid is recovered as a soluble sodium form by neutralizing with sodium carbonate or sodium hydroxide. The insoluble residue is removed by filtration, flotation, or centrifugation, and the soluble alginate is precipitated by conversion into alginic acid or calcium/sodium alginate. The alginic acid is then converted into the required counter ion by neutralization with appropriate hydroxides and the calcium alginate is converted into alginic acid and then neutralized as mentioned previously. The difference in the alginate recovery process depends on the source and structure constituents of alginate (McHugh 1987).

2.4.2 METHOD OF EXTRACTION

Sodium alginate extraction was carried out according to the works of Nishigawa (1985). Using this method, a dried sample weighing 10 g was chopped into small pieces and treated with 500 mL of 0.2 N sulfuric acid and kept in a slow shaker overnight at room temperature in order to remove the acid-soluble salts. The mixture was filtered through nylon and washed with 50–100 mL distilled water and filtered again. The residue was extracted with 500 mL of 1% sodium carbonate solution by shaking overnight at room temperature. The sample was diluted with 1 L distilled water before filtration and then filtered through nylon. In order to recover the alginate extract, 50 mL of 0.1%–0.2% NaCl was added to the filtrate and the solution was stirred. The filtrate was then added to ethanol (two times of filtrate volume) in small volumes by continuously stirring with a glass rod. The stringy precipitate attaches itself to the glass rod. The precipitate was washed with ethanol and dried in an oven at 50°C for 24 hours. In order to bleach the alginate, the samples were treated with formaldehyde solution (0.1%–0.4%) for 3–5 hours at room temperature and then washed with water before acid pretreatment (McHugh 1987).

2.4.3 EXTRACTION OF SODIUM ALGINATE

Sodium alginate was extracted according to the procedure of Calumpong et al. (1999). Collected sample of brown seaweeds was collected from the intertidal and subtidal regions of the coasts and cleaned by washing with seawater followed by tap water and then dried depending on your requirement and stored in aerated bags in a shaded and ventilated site. The dried sample weighing 25 g was soaked in 800 mL of 2% formaldehyde for 24 hour at room temperature, washed with water, and then 0.2 M HCl (800 mL) was added and left for 24 hour, and again washed with water. Then the sample was extracted with 2% sodium carbonate for 3 hour at 100°C. The soluble fraction was collected by centrifugation (10,000g, 30 minutes) and polysaccharides were precipitated by three volumes of 95% ethanol. Sodium alginate collected was washed twice with 100 mL of acetone, dried at 65°C, and dissolved in 100 mL of distilled water. It was then precipitated again with ethanol (v/3v) and dried at 65°C.

2.4.4 COMMERCIAL METHODS

Two basic methods, Green's cold process and Le Gloahec–Herter process (Green 1936; Le Gloahec and Herter 1938; Chapman 1970), are available for commercial extraction of alginate from seaweeds. A commercially available, water-soluble alginate includes sodium, potassium, ammonium, calcium, and mixed ammonium–calcium salts of alginic acid, propylene glycol alginate, and alginic acid (Cottrell and Kovacs 1980). Depending on the salts present, its physical properties may vary.

2.5 ALGINATE PRODUCTION

Although the total number of brown seaweed species was estimated to be 997 (FAO 1985), many of them are not used as commercial sources of algin owing to their thin thallus, harvesting difficulties, or processing problems (McNeely and Pettitt 1973). The commercial seaweeds commonly processed are the species of *Laminaria*, *Macrocystis*, *Ecklonia*, *Lessonia*, *Ascophyllum*, and *Sargassum*.

2.6 MOLECULAR WEIGHT

The molecular weight of alginic acid varies depending upon its mode of preparation and algal source. Normally, sodium alginate ranges from 35,000 to 1,500,000 Da (Haug and Smidsrod 1967). The molecular weight distributions are influenced by the method of extraction and the species (Morris 1998). They can have implications for the uses of alginate, as low-molecular-weight alginates with fragments containing only short G-blocks may not take part in gel-network formation and consequently do not contribute to the gel strength (Smidsrod and Haug 1968; Moe et al. 1995).

2.7   CHEMICAL COMPOSITION OF ALGINATE

2.7.1   ALGINATE CONTENT

The alginate content extracted from the seaweed sample was measured by the phenol–sulfuric acid method (Dubois et al. 1956) as described in the following text:

A 0.5 mL sample solution was vortex-mixed with 0.5 mL of 5% phenol in water. After addition of 2.5 mL concentrated sulfuric acid rapidly from a glass dispenser, the mixture was vortex-mixed and allowed to stand for 30 minutes at room temperature. The amount of sugar was measured by reading the absorbance at 490 nm. A calibration curve was made by using a commercial alginate with different viscosities at different concentrations.

2.7.2   MOISTURE CONTENT

The moisture content of all seaweed samples was determined by an LP 16 infrared (IR) moisture analyzer (Mettler, Greifensee, Switzerland) by heating the samples with IR radiation at a wavelength between 2 and 3.5 μm.

2.7.3   CRUDE PROTEIN CONTENT

Alginate weighing 2 mg was transferred to an aluminum capsule, which was then compressed into a dice by forceps. The compressed aluminum dice was transferred into an autosampler of a CHNS/O Elemental Analyzer (PerkinElmer 2400, Sheffield, UK) to determine the nitrogen content of the sample at 970°C by combustion. The crude protein content was calculated by multiplying the nitrogen content with a factor of 6.25.

2.7.4   ASH CONTENT

Alginate sample was weighed into a preweighed porcelain crucible and placed in a temperature-controlled furnace preheated to 525°C. This temperature was maintained for 24 hours and the crucible was cooled in a desiccator. The amount of ash in the sample was determined gravimetrically (AOAC 1996).

2.7.5   MONOSACCHARIDE COMPOSITION

2.7.5.1   Acid Depolymerization

Samples including whole seaweed and its alginate extracts were subjected to acid hydrolysis for the determination of sugar composition. A 15 mg sample was hydrolyzed with 0.7 mL 12 M sulfuric acid at 35°C for 1 hour with stirring. The hydrolysate was diluted to 2 M with 3.5 mL of distilled water and heated in a boiling water bath with shaking for 1 hour. The hydrolysate was then cooled to room temperature.

2.7.5.2   Neutral and Amino Sugar Derivatization

A 3 mL hydrolysate was used to prepare alditol acetates of the neutral and amino sugars according to the method described by Blakeney et al. (1983) with the rest of the hydrolysate reserved for uronic acid determination. Beta-D-allose (1 mg/mL) was added as an internal standard into the sugar hydrolysate. Concentrated ammonia (12 M) was then added to neutralize the hydrolysate followed by 5 μL octan-1-ol to prevent foaming. Freshly prepared sodium boron tetrahydride (200 mg/mL; 0.2 mL) was added to the neutralized hydrolysate, and the mixture was kept at 40°C for 30 minutes. The hydrolysate was reduced by adding sodium borontetrahydride, and 0.1 mL glacial acetic acid was added to stop the reaction. Acetic acid anhydride (2.0 mL) was then added together with a catalyst, 1-methylimidazole (0.3 mL), and the acetylation was preceded at room temperature for 10 minutes. Distilled water (5.0 mL) was added to decompose the excess acetic acid anhydride. Dichloromethane (1.0 mL) was added, and the mixture was vortex-mixed and allowed to stand for 10 minutes for phase separation. Although the top aqueous layer was removed, the bottom organic layer was washed with distilled water (2 × 2 mL) and dried with anhydrous sodium sulfate and stored in a vial at −20°C before gas chromatography (GC) analysis.

2.7.5.3   Determination of Neutral Sugars by Gas Chromatography

Alditol acetates of the neutral sugars were quantified by an HP6890 gas chromatography (GMI, Ramsey, MN) using an Alltech DB-225 capillary column (15 mm × 0.25 mm internal diameter, 0.25 mm film thickness) with the following oven temperature program: initial temperature of 180°C followed by an increase of 4°C/minute to 220°C for 30 minutes. The injector and detector temperatures were maintained at 270°C and the injection sample volume was 2 μL, the carrier gas was helium, and was detected by flame ionization.

Individual sugars were corrected for losses during hydrolysis and derivatization and for the response of the GC detector. The values for monosaccharides were expressed as polysaccharide residues (anhydrosugars) by multiplying the amounts of pentoses and deoxypentoses by a factor of 0.88 and hexoses by a factor of 0.90.

2.7.5.4   Uronic Acid Content

The uronic acid content was determined colorimetrically according to the Official Methods of Analysis (AOAC 1996). An aliquot of hydrolysate (0.3 mL) was added to a sodium chloride/boric acid solution (0.3 mL, dissolving 2 g sodium chloride and 3 g boric acid in 100 mL water), and the mixture was vortex-mixed. Concentrated sulfuric acid (5 mL) was added to the mixture followed by vortex-mixing, and the mixture was kept at 70°C for 40 minutes. After cooling the mixture to room temperature, dimethyphenol (0.2 mL, dissolving 0.1 g 3, 5-dimethyphenol in 100 mL glacial acetic acid) was added. The mixture was vortex-mixed and stood at room temperature for 10 minutes. A blank (2 M sulfuric acid) and galacturonic acid standards (10, 50, 100, 200, and 500 μg/mL) were treated similarly. The absorbances of the sample solutions at 400 and 450 nm against the blank were measured. The reading at 400 nm was subtracted from 450 nm to correct the interference from hexoses.

2.7.5.5   Uronic Acid Block Composition

2.7.5.5.1   MG-, MM-, and GG-Block Determination

The different uronic acid blocks of alginate were determined according to the method of Haug et al. (1974) with modifications. Partial hydrolysis was carried out by suspending 0.1 g of purified alginate in 10 mL of 0.3 M hydrochloric acid at 100°C for 2 hours. The suspension was cooled to room temperature and centrifuged (2665g, 15 minutes). The supernatant consisted mainly of blocks with an alternating sequence of mannuronic and guluronic acid residues (MG blocks). The amount of MG blocks was determined by the phenol–sulfuric acid method (Dubois et al. 1956). The residue was suspended in 0.1 M sodium chloride and dissolved by neutralization with 0.2 M sodium hydroxide. The solution was then adjusted to pH 2.8–3.0 with 0.1 M hydrochloric acid for precipitation, and the mixture was diluted to 10 mL with 0.1 M sodium chloride. The precipitate recovered by centrifugation (2665g, 15 minutes) was redissolved in 0.1 M sodium hydroxide and diluted to 10 mL with 0.1 M sodium chloride. The precipitate and supernatant consisted of homopolymeric blocks of guluronic acid residues (GG blocks) and mannuronic acid (MM blocks), respectively.

The amounts of MM and GG blocks were determined by the phenol–sulfuric acid method (Dubois et al. 1956) similar to the MG blocks, using the alginate standard MG, MM, and GG blocks extracted from *Laminaria hyperhorea*.

2.7.5.5.2   M/G Ratio Determination
Based on the values of MG-, MM-, and GG-block composition obtained as described previously, the M/G ratio was calculated from the MM and GG blocks, assuming that the alternating MG blocks have an M/G ratio of 1.0 (Haug et al. 1974). The M/G ratio was calculated as follows:

$$\frac{MM \times 2 + MG}{GG \times 2 + MG}$$

where MM, GG, and MG were the percentages of MM, GG, and MG blocks obtained, respectively.

2.7.5.5.3   Phenol–Sulfuric Acid Method
As described in Section 2.7.5.5.2, the amount of sugar was measured by reading the absorbance at 490 nm using the standard MG, MM, and GG blocks extracted from the selected brown seaweed sample (Dubois et al. 1956).

2.7.6   Physicochemical Properties of Alginate

2.7.6.1   Viscosity

2.7.6.1.1   Ostwald Viscometer
The viscosity of dilute alginate solution was measured using an Ostwald capillary viscometer (NSIC Ltd, New Delhi, India) (No. 200, capacity 50 mL) fitted in a 25°C water bath. A 15% of the alginate sample was dissolved in 0.1 M sodium chloride with mechanical stirring, and the solution was filtered through a Whatman 40 ashless filter paper (Wipro GE Healthcare Pvt. Ltd., Chennai, India). A volume of 15 mL of alginate stock solution was used for viscosity measurement. Viscosity data at different alginate concentrations were obtained by diluting the above stock solution with sodium chloride to give 1.0% and 0.5% solutions. The concentration

of the alginate stock solution was determined by the phenol–sulfuric acid method using commercial alginate as a standard.

The intrinsic viscosity [η] is defined as the specific viscosity (η_{sp}) at zero concentration, and the specific viscosity (η_{sp}) was obtained by comparing the flow rate (in seconds) of test solutions with that of the ultrapure water, carried out using the same viscometer and under similar experimental conditions.

η_{sp} = (flow rate of sample solution/flow rate of ultrapure water) − 1

The relationship of η_{sp} and [η] is described in the Huggins equation:

$$\frac{\eta_{sp}}{c} = \left[\eta\right] + k\left[\eta\right]^2 c$$

where:

k is the Huggins coefficient

c is the concentration of the solution

The Huggins equation showed that η_{sp}/c is positively correlated with c. By plotting η_{sp}/c versus c, which is known as the Huggins plot, the intrinsic viscosity [η] was obtained from extrapolation of the above plot to zero concentration.

2.7.6.1.2 Molecular Weight

2.7.6.1.2.1 *From Intrinsic Viscosity* The intrinsic viscosity of alginate was used as a means of estimating the molecular weight (Haug and Smidsrod 1967). The relationship between the intrinsic viscosity and the weight average molecular weight (Mw) of the alginate samples in 0.1 M sodium chloride can be represented approximately (Smidsrod 1970; Matsumoto and Mashiko 1990) by the following equation:

$$\left[\eta\right] = 2.0 \times 10^{-5} Mw^{1.0}$$

where [η] is expressed 100 mL/g (note that [η] is not a *viscosity* at all, as it has units of reciprocal concentration which is in mL/g, rather than Pa s or Poise) (Ross-Murphy 1995).

2.7.6.1.2.2 *Gel Permeation Chromatography–Laser Light Scattering* Gel permeation chromatography (GPC) combined with static laser light scattering (GPC–LLS) is a convenient method for the determination of true molecular weight and its distribution without the aid of standard samples. The measurements of alginate were performed on a multiangle laser light scattering (MALLS) instrument equipped with a He–Ne laser (λ = 632.8 nm) (DAWN® DSP, Wyatt Technology Co., CA) in an angular range from 49°C to 135°C at 25 ± 1°C. The DAWN DSP multiangle laser photometer mentioned previously combined with a peristaltic pump p 100 equipped with a TSK-GEL G6000 PWXL column (7.8 mm × 300 mm) and a differential refractive index detector (RI-150) at 25°C. The eluent used was 0.5 M NaCl solution with a flow rate of 1.0 mL/minute. The refractive index increments (*dn/dc*) were measured with a double-beam differential refractometer (DRM-1020,

Otsuka Electronics Co., Osaka, Japan) at 633 nm and at 25°C. The polysaccharide solutions were dialyzed against the eluent for 72 hours. The value of a specific refractive index increment dn/dc in 0.5 M NaCl solution was determined to be 0.133 cm^3 g^{-1}. All the solutions used were filtered with a sand filter, and then 0.45 μm filter (Whatman, Scientific & Surgical Corporation, Mumbai, India). Astra software (Wyatt Technology Co., CA) was utilized for data acquisition and analysis. The weight average molecular weight (Mw) and the number average molecular weight (Mn) were calculated according to the GPC–LLS results (Ding et al. 1998).

2.7.7 FUNCTIONAL PROPERTIES OF ALGINATE

2.7.7.1 Emulsifying Activity and Emulsion Stability

The emulsifying activity (EA) and emulsion stability (ES) of the alginate samples were determined according to the method of Yasumatsu et al. (1972) with some modifications. A 100 mg of alginate sample was added to 10 mL distilled water in a 50 mL graduated centrifuge tube. The mixture was homogenized at 12,000 rpm for 30 seconds with a PT-3000 Homogenizer (Polytron, Kinematica AG, Luzern, Switzerland). A 10 mL corn oil was then added into the centrifuge tube, and the mixture was further homogenized at 12,000 rpm for 1 minute. The emulsion formed was centrifuged at 240g for 5 minutes. The EA was calculated from the ratio of the volume of the emulsion to the total volume of the initial materials expressed as a percentage.

For ES, the emulsions thus prepared were heated in a water bath at 80°C for 30 minutes and cooled to room temperature. The centrifuge tube was then further centrifuged at 240g for 5 minutes. The ES was calculated in the same way as the EA and was also expressed as a percentage.

2.7.7.2 Gel Formation

The method of gel preparation was modified from a commercial standard method (Kelco Co. Ltd., Shanghai, China) (Howell et al. 1998). Sodium alginate weighing 3 g was slowly dispersed in 200 mL distilled water with vigorous mixing for 10 minutes and allowed to stand for 1 hour to give a 1.5% stock solution. Each time 20 mL of this solution was used for gel preparation. Calcium chloride (0.4%, 4 mL) solution and gluconic acid lactone (0.1%, 2 mL) were added to the alginate solution (20 mL). The solutions were stirred gently for 2 minutes, and the gel was allowed to set in a labeled 100 mL beaker at 4°C overnight.

2.7.7.3 Gel Strength and Syneresis

The strength of the gels prepared as described in Section 2.2 was measured by a Texture Analyzer (TA-XT2i, Stable Micro Systems Ltd., Godalming, UK) with a cylindrical probe (P/0.5) at room temperature. The probe was penetrated into the alginate gel at a compression rate of 0.5 mm/second to a depth of 4 mm where the maximum force reading (i.e., the resistance to penetration) was obtained and translated as the *strength* (g) of the gel. This penetration method is an industrial standard method for gelatin gels (the Bloom test) (British Standard BS757).

Syneresis was measured as the final weight of the gel relative to the initial weight of the gel as determined by the total volume of the gelling solution (Draget et al. 1991).

This was simply done by placing the gel on a water absorbent paper at room temperature with a cover. Syneresis was measured and calculated by the following equation:

$$\frac{W_i - W_f}{W_i} \times 100 \%$$

where:
W_i is the initial weight of the gel
W_f is the final weight of the gel after drying

2.7.8 STRUCTURAL CHARACTERIZATION OF ALGINATE BY VIBRATIONAL SPECTROSCOPY

The main polysaccharide found in the studied brown seaweeds (Phaeophyceae) was alginate, a linear copolymer of mannuronic (M) and guluronic (G) acids. Different types of alginic acid present different proportions and/or different alternating patterns of guluronic (G) and mannuronic (M) units. The presence of these acids can be identified from their characteristic bands in the vibrational spectra; according to the work of Mackie (1971), these phycocolloids show two characteristic bands in IR spectra: 808 cm^{-1}, assigned to M units, and 787 cm^{-1}, assigned to G units. However, alginate specimens of *Lessonia* genus, assign both bands to G units. Filippov and Kohn (1974) proposed that M/G ratios of the different samples can be estimated from the ratio of absorbance of the bands at 1320 and 1290 cm^{-1} in FTIR spectra. According to Sakugawa et al. (2004) the M/G concentration ratio characterizing a certain alginate sample can be inferred from the relative intensity ratio of the two bands 1030/1080 cm^{-1}, in calcium alginate and 1019/1025 cm^{-1}, in manganese alginate. They further suggested that the absorbance at 1030 cm^{-1} directly reflects the change of mannurate concentration of calcium alginate and the 1025 cm^{-1} is attributed to the OH bending of guluronate (Sakugawa et al. 2004).

Alginate M/G ratio was tentatively estimated from the 1030/1080 cm^{-1} band ratio in IR spectra, suggesting higher values of mannuronic than guluronic acid blocks (M/GG > 1) in *Himanthalia elongata* (Pereira 2013). However, the Fourier transform infrared (FTIR) spectra of *Saccorhiza polyschides* show an intense broad band centered at 1025 cm^{-1}, indicating that the samples considered are particularly rich in guluronic acid. According to several works of the authors (Skriptsova et al. 2004; Torres et al. 2007; Sahayaraj et al. 2012; Pereira 2013), the spectrum of *Undaria pinnatifida* (old adult thallus) indicates that the relative amounts of both mannuronate and guluronate residues are similar.

The spectra presented by Pereira (2013), suggesting higher values of guluronic than mannuronic acid blocks in *Padina pavonica* and similar amounts of both mannuronate and guluronate residues in *Sargassum vulgare*, are in accordance with other published works (Skriptsova et al. 2004; Torres et al. 2007; Sahayaraj et al. 2012). Some brown algae, such as *S. polyschides* and *U. pinnatifida*, also exhibit a broad band around 1220–1260 cm^{-1}, assigned to the presence of sulfate ester groups (S=O), which is a characteristic component in fucoidan and sulfated polysaccharides other than alginate in brown seaweeds. *P. pavonica* and *S. vulgare* also exhibit a broad band in this region (around 1195–1237 cm^{-1} for *Padina* and 1210–1280 cm^{-1} for *Sargassum*) assigned to (S=O). However, *S. vulgare* contains a larger amount of fucoidan than *P. pavonica* (Pereira 2013). According to Camara et al. (2011), the characteristic sulfate absorptions were identified in the FTIR spectra of heterofucans: bands around 1239–1247 cm^{-1} for asymmetric S=O stretching vibration and bands around 1037–1071 cm^{-1} for symmetric C–O vibration associated with a C–O–SO$_3$ group. The peaks at 820–850 cm^{-1} were assigned to the bending vibration of C–O–S. However, *S. vulgare* and *P. pavonica* contain little amounts of laminaran (Nelson and Lewis 1974; Rioux et al. 2010; Jiao et al. 2011).

2.7.9 ALGINATE ANALYSIS BY FT-RAMAN

The most prominent FT-Raman band centered at 950 cm^{-1} is mainly due to the O–H deformation mode, whereas the band at 1400 cm^{-1}, strong in both FTIR and FT-Raman spectra, is ascribed to the deformation of the CH$_2$ groups. The C–O–C and C–OH stretching modes give rise to several close-lying bands in the spectral regions of 1250–1290 and 1000–1025 cm^{-1}, respectively (Sartori et al. 1997; Nivens et al. 2001).

Different types of alginate present different proportions and/or different alternating patterns of guluronic and mannuronic units. The presence of these acids can be identified from their characteristic bands. The guluronic units originate a band at ~1025 cm^{-1}, and the mannuronic units originate a band at ~1100 cm^{-1}. Thus, the guluronic/mannuronic concentration ratio, characterizing a certain alginate sample, can be inferred from the relative intensity ratio of the 1025 and 1100 cm^{-1} band (Sartori et al. 1997).

2.7.10 NUCLEAR MAGNETIC RESONANCE SPECTROSCOPY

Alginate is a linear polysaccharide containing 1,4-linked β-D-mannuronic (M) and α-L-guluronic (G) acid residues arranged in a nonregular, blockwise order along the chain (Figure 2.1). Polymannuronic acid is a flat ribbonlike chain, its molecular repeat is 10.35Å, and it contains two diequatorially (1e,4e)-linked β-D-mannuronic acid residues in the chair form (Atkins et al. 1973a). In contrast, polyguluronic acid contains two diaxially (1a,4a)-linked α-L-guluronic acid residues in the chair form, which produce a rodlike conformation with a molecular repeat of 8.7Å (Atkins et al. 1973b).

For nuclear magnetic resonance (NMR) study, special extraction methods can be adopted. For alkaline extraction of alginate, sample was extracted in a 2% solution of Na$_2$CO$_3$ according to a slight modification of the method of Percival and McDowell (1967). The extraction was carried out at 80°C instead of room temperature in order to reduce the viscosity (for NMR work) and ensure the complete extraction of

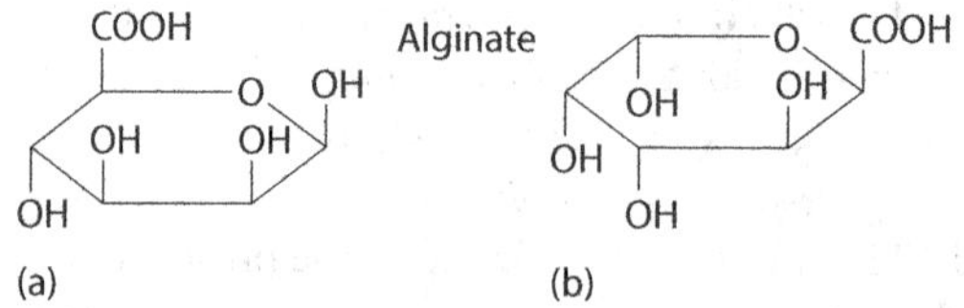

FIGURE 2.1   Monomers of alginate. (a) β-D-Mannuronic acid (b) α-L-Guluronic acid.

the alginate. In the presence of excess Na_2CO_3, the alginic acid was converted to Na alginate and was solubilized. The resulting Na alginate solution was separated from the solid phase by filtration. This step is followed by the precipitation of the alginic acid by the addition of dilute hydrochloric acid and conversion of the sodium salt to the insoluble acid (pH < 1.0). The alginic acid was pelleted by centrifugation and then washed with 95% aqueous solution prior to its conversion back to the sodium salt upon the addition of a concentrated sodium carbonate solution.

For neutral extraction, sample was extracted (Davis et al. 2003) three times in 0.2 N HCl prior to filtration and washing with water. The residue was resuspended in distilled water, and sufficient sodium hydroxide was added to neutralize the alginic acid and maintain the pH between 6.5 and 7.5. The suspension was gently stirred overnight and then filtered and extracted once more. All filtrates were pooled and sodium chloride was added to the solution to obtain a 1% (w/w) final concentration. An equal volume of ethanol was added to precipitate the alginate, which was then washed first with a 60% aqueous ethanol solution, then two times with ethanol, and three times with ethyl ether. The alginate was dried at 30°C–40°C. In contrast to the alkaline extraction, the standard neutral extraction yields viscous alginates and increases the time necessary for the preparation of the NMR samples by requiring an additional prehydrolysis step.

^{1}H NMR data on the composition of alginates extracted from whole and individual parts of *Sargassum* spp. are presented in Table 2.1 (Davis et al. 2003).

2.7.11　Matrix-Assisted Laser Desorption/Ionization Time-of-Flight Mass Spectrometry

Recently, matrix-assisted laser desorption/ionization time-of-flight mass spectrometry (MALDI-TOF MS) has been considered as a rapid and sensitive approach for obtaining the fingerprints of polysaccharides isolated (Hung et al. 2012; Gil et al. 2015). The spectra of alginate exhibit a distinct series of peaks with repetitive signal

TABLE 2.1
^{1}H NMR Data on the Composition of Alginates Extracted from Whole and Individual Parts of *Sargassum* spp.

Source	Composition, Fractions		Doublet Frequencies				M/G
	FM	FG	FMM	FMG	FGM	FGG	
S. fluitans, frond	0.13	0.87	0.02	0.11	0.11	0.76	0.15
S. fluitans, whole	0.16	0.84	0.13	0.03	0.03	0.81	0.19
S. fluitans, stipe	0.37	0.63	0.34	0.03	0.03	0.60	0.60
S. fluitans, bladder	0.41	0.59	0.37	0.03	0.03	0.56	0.69
S. siliquosum, frond	0.41	0.59	0.38	0.03	0.03	0.56	0.70
S. siliquosum, whole	0.42	0.58	0.41	0.01	0.01	0.57	0.72
S. siliquosum, stipe	0.48	0.52	0.46	0.03	0.03	0.49	0.94
S. siliquosum, bladder	0.42	0.58	0.41	0.01	0.01	0.57	0.72

patterns that are typical of polymers. It is noted that MALDI-TOF does not merely reflect the presence of a certain unit or moiety in an analyte. For example, similar to alginate, xanthan and gellan also contain uronic acid units in their structure. However, the chemical structure of xanthan and gellan differs from that of alginate as xanthan and gellan ionization occurred in the glucose residue (i.e., peak-to-peak signals 162 m/z) but not in the uronic acid (i.e., peak-to-peak difference of 176 m/z as observed in alginate), thus resulting in distinct MALDI-TOF MS spectra for these polysaccharides. This illustrates that although different polysaccharides share uronic acids in their structure, MALDI-TOF signals can differ as a result of differences in their chemical structure. Other polysaccharides containing uronic acids are of animal (mostly human) or plant origin (Garron and Cygler 2010), and MALDI-TOF MS signals of plant origin differ from alginate signals (Monge et al. 2007).

2.8 CONCLUSION

In this chapter, the major species of brown algae commercially utilized for alginate extraction and the chemical structure of alginate have been presented. Further, it states that various types of extraction of alginate isolation and its complete characterization using biochemical and spectroscopic tools have been compiled.

REFERENCES

Abe, K., T. Sakamoto, S.F. Sasaki, and K. Nisizawa. 1973. In vivo studies on the synthesis of alginic acid in *Ishige okamurai*. *Botaniea Marina* 16: 229–234.

AOAC. 1996. *Association Analytical Chemists of Official*, 16th edition. Washington, DC.

Atkins, E.D.T., I.A. Nieduszynski, W. Mackie, K.D. Parker, and E.E. Smolko. 1973a. Structural components of alginic acid. I. The crystalline structure of poly-β-D-mannuronic acid. Results of X-ray diffraction and polarized infrared studies. *Biopolymers* 12: 1865–1878.

Atkins, E.D.T., I.A. Nieduszynski, W. Mackie, K.D. Parker, and E.E. Smolko. 1973b. Structural components of alginic acid. II. The crystalline structure of poly-α-D-mannuronic acid. Results of X-ray diffraction and polarized Infrared studies. *Biopolymers* 12: 1879–1887.

Blakeney, A.B., P.J. Harris, R.J. Henry, and B.A. Stone. 1983. A simple and rapid preparation of alditol acetates for monosaccharide analysis. *Carbohydrate Research* 113: 291–299.

Camara, R.B.G., L.S. Costa, G.P. Fidelis, L.T.D.B. Nobre, N. Dantas-Santos, S.L. Cordeiro, M.S.S.P. Costa, L.G. Alves, and H.A.O. Rocha. 2011. Heterofucans from the brown seaweed *canistrocarpus cervicornis* with anticoagulant and antioxidant activities. *Marine Drugs* 9: 124–138.

Calumpong, H.P., A.P. Maypa, and M. Magbanua. 1999. Population and alginate yield and quality assessment of four sargassum species in Negros island, Central Phillipines. *Hydrobiologia* 398–399: 211–215.

Chapman, V.J. 1970. *Seaweeds and Their Uses*. 2nd edition. pp. 194–217. Methuen & Co: London.

Chapman, V.J., and D.J. Chapman. 1980. *Seaweeds and Their Uses*. Chapman & Hall: London.

Clare, K. 1993. Algin. In *Industrial Gums: Polysaccharides and Their Derivatives*. Whistler, R.L., and BeMiller, J.N. (Eds.) pp. 105–143. Academic Press: New York.

Cottrell, I.W., and P. Kovacs. 1980. Alginates. In *Handbook of Water-soluble Gums and Resins*. Davidson, R.L. (Ed.) pp. 1–43. McGraw-Hill: New York.

Davis, T.A., F. Llanes, B. Volesky, G. Diaz-Pulido, L. Mccook, and A. Mucci. 2003. ^{1}H-NMR study of Na alginates extracted from *Sargassum* spp. in relation to metal biosorption. *Applied Biochemistry and Biotechnology* 110: 75–90.

Ding, Q., S. Jiang, L. Zhang, and C. Wu. 1998. Laser light-scattering studies of pachyman. *Carbohydrate Research* 308: 339–343.

Draget, K.L., K. Ostgaard, and O. Smidsrod. 1991. Homogeneous alginate gels: A technical approach. *Carbohydrate Polymers* 14: 159–178.

Dubois, M., K.A. Gilles, J.K. Hamilton, P.A. Rebers, and F. Smith. 1956. Colorimetric method for determination of sugars and related substances. *Analytical Chemistry* 28: 350–356.

FAO. 1985. *Year Book of Fishery Statistics.* Vol. 60. FAO: Rome, Italy.

Filippov, M.P., and R. Kohn. 1974. Determination of composition of alginates by infra-red spectroscopic methods. *Chemické Zvesti* 28: 817.

Fischer, F.G., and H. Dorfel. 1955. Die polyuronsauren der braunalgen (Kohlenhydrate der Algen I). *Z. Physiological Chemistry* 302: 186.

Fourest, E., and B. Volesky. 1996. Contribution of sulfonate groups and alginate to heavy metal biosorption by the dry biomass of *Sargassum fluitans*. *Enviromental Science and Technology* 30: 277–282.

Garron, M.L., and M. Cygler. 2010. Structural and mechanistic classification of uronic acid-containing polysaccharide lyases. *Glycobiology* 20: 1547–1573.

Gil, G.G., L. Thomas, A.H. Emwas, P.N.L. Lens, and P.E. Saikaly. 2015. NMR and MALDI-TOF MS based characterization of exopolysaccharides in anaerobic microbial aggregates from full-scale reactors. *Scientific Reports* 5: 14316.

Glicksman, M. 1987. Utilization of seaweed hydrocolloids in the food industry. *Hydrobiologia* 151/152: 31–47.

Green, H.C. 1936. Process for making alinic acid and product. US Patent no. 2,036, 934.

Haug, A., and O. Smidsrod. 1967. Strontium-calcium selectivity of alginates. *Nature* 215: 757.

Haug, A., S. Myklestad, B. Larsen, and O. Smidsrød. 1967. Correlation between chemical structure and physical properties of alginates. *Acta Chemica Scandinavica* 21: 768–778.

Haug, A., B. Larsen, and E. Baadseth. 1969. Comparison of the constitution of alginates from different sources. *Proceedings of International Seaweed symposium* 6: 443–451.

Haug, A., B. Larsen, and O. Smidsrod. 1974. Uronic acid sequence in alginate from different sources. *Carbohydrate Research* 32: 217–225.

Howell, N., E. Bristow, E. Copeland, and G.L. Friedli. 1998. Interaction of deamidated soluble wheat protein with sodium alginate. *Food Hydrocolloids* 12: 317–324.

Hung, W.T., S.-H. Wang, Y.-T. Chen, H.-M. Yu, C.-H. Chen and W.-B. Yang. 2012. MALDI-TOF MS analysis of native and permethylated or benzimidazole-derivatized polysaccharides. *Molecules* 17: 4950–4961.

Istinii, S., M. Masao Ohno, and H. Kusunose. 1994. Methods of analysis for agar, carrageenan and alginate in seaweed. *Bulletin of Marine Science and Fisheries.* 14: 49–55.

Jiao, G.L., G.L. Yu, J.Z. Zhang, and H.S. Ewart. 2011. Chemical structures and bioactivities of sulfated polysaccharides from marine algae. *Marine Drugs* 9(2): 196–223.

Johnson, F.A., D.Q.M. Craig, and A.D. Mercer. 1997. Characterization of the block structure and molecular weight of sodium alginates. *Journal of Pharmaceutical Pharmacology* 49: 639–643.

Lahaye, M. 1991. Marine algae as sources of fibers: Determination of soluble and insoluble dietary fiber contents in some "sea vegetables." *Journal of the Science of Food and Agriculture* 54: 587–594.

Lahaye, M., and A. Robic. 2007. Structure and functional properties of ulvan, a polysaccharide from green seaweeds. *Biomacromolecules* 8: 1766–1774.

Le Gloahec, V.C.E., and J.R. Herter. 1938. Method of treating seaweeds. US Patent 2,128,551.

Mackie, W. 1971. Semi-quantitative estimation of composition of alginates by infra-red spectroscopy. *Carbohydrate Research* 20: 413–415.

Matsumoto, T., and K. Mashiko. 1990. Viscoelastic properties of alginate aqueous solutions in the presence of salts. *Biopolymers* 29: 707–1713.

McHugh, D.J. 1987. Production, the properties and uses of alginates. In *Production and Utilization of Products from Commercial Seaweeds*, pp. 58–115. FAO: Rome, Italy.

McNeely, W.H., and D.J. Pettitt. 1973. Algin. In *Industrial Gums: Polysaccharides and Their Derivatives*. Whistler, R.L. (Ed.) 2nd edition. pp. 49–81. Academic Press: New York.

Moe, S.T., K.I. Draget, G. Skjak-Braek, and O. Smidsrod. 1995. Alginates. In *Food Polysaccharides and Their Applications*. Stephen, A.M. (Ed.) pp. 245–284. Marcel Dekker: New York.

Monge, M.E., R.M. Negri, A.A. Kolender, and R. Erra-Balsells. 2007. Structural characterization of native high-methoxylated pectin using nuclear magnetic resonance spectroscopy and ultraviolet matrix-assisted laser desorption/ionization time-of-flight mass spectrometry. Comparative use of 2,5-dihydroxybenzoic acid and nor-harmane as UV-MALDI matrices. *Rapid Communication in Mass Spectrometry* 21: 2638–2646.

Morris, V.J. 1998. Gelation of polysaccharides. In *Functional Properties of Food Macromolecules*. Hill, S.E., Ledward, D.A., and Mitchell, J.R. (Eds.) 143–226. Aspen Publishers: Frederick, MD.

Nelson, T.E., and B.A. Lewis. 1974. Separation and characterization of the soluble and insoluble components of insoluble laminaran. *Carbohydrate Research* 33(1): 63–74.

Nishigawa, K. 1985. Extract method of alginic acid. In, *Research Methods of Algae*. Nishigawa, K. and Chthara, M. (Eds.) pp. 624–626.

Nivens, D.E., D.E. Ohman, J. Williamn, and M.J. Franklin. 2001. Role of alginate and its O-acetylation in formation of pseudomonas aeruginosa microcolonies and biofilms. *Journal of Bacteriology* 183: 1047–1057.

Percival, E. 1979. The polysaccharides of green, red and brown seaweeds: Their basic structure, biosynthesis and function. *British Phycological Journal* 14(2): 103–117.

Percival, E., and R.H. McDowell. 1967. *Chemistry and Enzymology of Marine Algal Polysaccharides*. pp. 99–126. Academic Press: London.

Pereira, L. 2013. Population studies and Carrageenan properties in eight Gigartinales (rhodophyta) from western coast of Portugal. *The Scientific World Journal* 2013: 11, Article ID 939830.

Pereira, L., A.T. Critchley, A.M. Amado, and P.J.A. Ribeiro-Claro. 2009. A comparative analysis of phycocolloids produced by underutilized versus industrially utilized carrageenophytes (Gigartinales, Rhodophyta). *Journal of Applied Phycology* 21: 599–605.

Rinaudo, M. 2007. Comprehensive glycoscience. In *Seaweed Polysaccharides*. Volume 2. Kamerling, J.P. (Ed.) Elsevier: Amsterdam, the Netherlands.

Rioux, L.E., S.L. Turgeon, and M. Beaulieu. 2010. Structural characterization of laminaran and galactofucan extracted from the brown seaweed Saccharina longicruris. *Phytochemistry* 71(13): 1586–1595.

Ross-Murphy, S.B. 1995. Rheology of boipolymer solutions and gels. In *New Physicochemical Techniques for the Characterization of Complex Food System*. Dickinson, E. (Ed.) pp. 139–156. Blackie Academic & Professional: London.

Sahayaraj, K., S. Rajesh, and J.M. Rathi. 2012. Silver nanoparticles biosynthesis using marine alga *Padina pavonica* (Linn.) and its microbicidal activity. *Digest Journal of Nanomaterials and Biostructures* 7: 1557–1567.

Sakugawa, K., A. Ikeda, A. Takemura, and H. Ono. 2004. Simplified method for estimation of composition of alginates by FTIR. *Journal of Applied Polymer Science* 93: 1372–1377.

Sartori, C., D.S. Finch, B. Ralph, and K. Gilding. 1997. Determination of the cation content of alginate thin films by FTIR spectroscopy. *Polymer* 38(1): 43–51.

Sime, W.J. 1990. Alginates. In *Food Gels*. Harris, P. (Ed.) pp. 53–78. Elsevier Applied Science: London.

Skriptsova, A., V. Khomenko, and I. Isakov. 2004. Seasonal changes in growth rate, morphology and alginate content in *Undaria pinnatifida* at the northern limit in the Sea of Japan (Russia). *Journal of Applied Phycology* 16(1): 17–21.

Smidsrod, O. 1970. Solution properties of alginate. *Carbohydrate Research* 13: 359–372.

Smidsrod, O., and A. Haug. 1968. The relative extension of alginates having different chemical composition. *Acta Chemica Scandinavica* 22: 797–810.

Torres, R.M., P.A.A. Sousa, E.A.T.S. Filho, D.F. Melo, J.P.A. Feitosa, R.C.M. de Paulab, and M.G.S. Lima. 2007. Extraction and physicochemical characterization of *Sargassum vulgare* alginate from Brazil. *Carbohydrate Research* 342: 2067–2074.

Yasumatsu, K., K. Sawada, S. Moritaka, and K. Ishii. 1972. Whipping and emulsifying properties of soybean products. *Agricultural and Biological Chemistry* 36: 719–727.

3 Extraction, Characterization, and Use of Carrageenans

Leonel Pereira, Fabiana Soares,
Ana Cristina Freitas, Armando C. Duarte,
and Paulo Ribeiro-Claro

CONTENTS

3.1 INTRODUCTION

Seaweeds have been utilized by mankind for several hundreds of years, directly for food, medicinal purposes, and agriculture fertilizers. Today, seaweed is used in many countries for very different purposes: directly as food; as a source of phycocolloid extraction; for extraction of compounds with antiviral, antibacterial, or antitumor activity; and as biofertilizers (Rudolph 2000; Wang et al. 2008; Pereira 2010a,b).

Seaweeds have attracted attention, as a possible renewable feedstock to biorefinery applications, for the production of multiple streams of commercial interest, including biofuels such as bioethanol and biogas (Sitompul et al. 2012; Hughes et al. 2013), particularly because they have considerable contents of carbohydrates. In this field, seaweeds have several advantages over terrestrial biomass, primarily because of their potentially high yields, no competition with food crops for the use of arable land and freshwater resources, and utilization of carbon dioxide as the only carbon input (Daroch et al. 2013).

The industry uses 7.5–8 million tons of wet seaweed annually (FAO 2004). This is harvested either from naturally grown (wild) seaweed or from open-water, cultivated (marine agronomy, farmed) crops (FAO 2010). Commercial harvesting occurs in ~35 countries, spread between the Northern and the Southern Hemisphere, in waters ranging from cold, through temperate, to tropical (FAO 2004).

The consumption and utilization of seaweed worldwide are associated with a myriad of products that generate nearly $8 billion per year (FAO 2010). Direct use as food has strong roots in the East Asia, whereas the West is more interested in thickeners and gelling properties of some polysaccharides extracted from seaweeds. The use of seaweeds for fertilizer and soil improvement was also well known in Europe, and both large brown algae and calcified red algae have been collected for this purpose (Guiry and Bluden 1991; Pereira 2010b).

Many seaweeds are receiving increased attention as a potential, renewable source for the food industry, as a feed for livestock, and as food directly (FAO 2010). Algae are a rich mine of health—vitamins and trace elements—and also offer a dizzying variety of flavors, fragrances, and textures. Algae are low in fat, an essential feature in weight loss diets. In addition, they are rich in dietary fiber, which may facilitate intestinal transit, lowering the rate of blood cholesterol and reducing certain diseases such as colon cancer (Pereira 2010a,b, 2011a).

Industrialized countries are currently increasing efforts regarding the manufacturing of high-value products derived from algae, because these contain chemical components (e.g., polysaccharides, proteins, lipids, and polyphenols) with a wide range of biological activities. Algal polysaccharides (phycocolloids), such as agar, alginates, and carrageenans, are produced in a large scale (Bixler and Porse 2011) and have a wide range of applications in food, pharmaceutical, and cosmetic industries.

Phycocolloids are very important in terms of their industrial commercialization. In fact, they had an estimated global value of approximately $1 billion in 2009 and represented more than half of the nonfood macroalgal market products (Bixler and Porse 2011; Lorbeer et al. 2013). European output of phycocolloids is estimated to have an annual wholesale value of approximately €130 million, which is 97.5% of the total for all algal products in Europe (Earons 1994). This huge production stems from the growing worldwide demand for phycocolloids, particularly for agar and carrageenan. Eight percent of the global agar and carrageenan production and 30% of the global alginate production are used in the food industry. Phycocolloids' popularity also arises from their low cost in production and nontoxic nature (Kim and Pangestuti 2015). For this reason, this chapter is focused on these seaweed-derived hydrocolloids, with special attention to carrageenan and its extraction, characterization, and applications.

3.2 BIOPOLYMERS DERIVED FROM MARINE ALGAE

3.2.1 MORPHOLOGY AND TAXONOMY OF SEAWEEDS (BRIEF INTRODUCTION)

Algae are photosynthetic aquatic organisms that can be small and single celled or large and have a multiplicity of cells. Due to their high morphological diversity and structure, algae can be divided into microalgae and macroalgae (marine seaweeds). Microalgae are unicellular or colonial organisms that can be found in oceans, lakes, rivers, and as in the bark of trees or on the side of buildings. They can also be found in desert and ice areas. However, seaweeds are larger algae, are visible to the human eye, and can grow more than 60 m in length (Kelp forests). Some seaweeds grow attached to surfaces that are bathed by water—underside of boats, ropes, or rock faces—whereas others grow attached themselves to the shell of crabs, or grow on the surfaces of other seaweeds. Some species such as *Sargassum* can be free-floating (Thomas 2002).

Marine seaweeds play an important role in the ecosystem. They are the primary producers in the oceans, and thus, they are crucial to life not only in the aquatic food webs but in the rest of the planet, because they are the original source of fossil carbon found in crude oil and natural gas, and have a contribution of 40%–50% on the total amount of oxygen in the atmosphere (Preisig and Andersen 2005; Kilinç et al. 2013).

Marine seaweeds, as well as land plants, belong to Domain Eukarya and Kingdom Plantae (red and green algae), and although their appearance may be similar to each other, marine seaweeds are much smaller and less structurally complex than plants (Graham and Wilcox 2000; Pereira 2009a); the brown algae belong to Kingdom Chromista (Pereira 2009a).

Seaweeds are divided into three main groups, according to their pigment composition and the way that their photosynthetic membranes are organized (Kilinç et al. 2013):

* Green algae—Phylum Chlorophyta—possess chlorophyll *a*, *b* and carotenoids. Chlorophyll *a* is the pigment responsible for their green color and appearance similar to land plants (Graham and Wilcox 2000). This pigment is essential for photosynthesis, which requires great amounts of light, and therefore, green seaweeds cannot be found at deep and shadowed places. It gives them an advantage, the ability to live higher up shore without competition from the red or brown seaweeds. Green seaweeds are found on both sandy and rocky beaches. Many can tolerate low salinity and will colonize areas where rivers meet the sea. Some green seaweeds such as *Codium* and *Ulva* (formerly *Enteromorpha*) are commonly used as food sources.
* Brown algae—Phylum Heterokontophyta or Ochrophyta—are often found on rocky intertidal shores. This group of algae includes species such as the giant kelp *Macrocystis* or the invasive alga *Sargassum*. The brown algae, as well as the green and red algae, can be used as food sources and can be consumed by humans as edible raw, dried, or cooked. Brown algae are also harvested for industrial and pharmaceutical uses (Chapman 2013; Kilinç et al. 2013).
* Red algae—Phylum Rhodophyta—have had a more diverse evolution than the green and brown algae. Many species cannot stand desiccation and dominate the intertidal rock pools. Others tolerate desiccation, such as the red alga *Porphyra* spp., which can often be seen stretched out like a dry black film over mussel beds on rocky beaches. Red algae exhibit a broad range of morphologies and simple anatomy, and display a wide array of life cycles. About 98% of the species are marine, 2% freshwater, and a few rare terrestrial/subaerial representatives (Gurgel and Lopez-Bautista 2007; Pereira 2012).

Some species such as *Gelidium* and *Gracilaria* are used in the manufacture of agar, and others, such as *Eucheuma* and *Kapaphycus alvarezzi*, are used in the production of carrageenan. The red alga *Porphyra*, also known as *Nori*, is commonly used in sushi all over the world. Worldwide about 221 species of algae are used: 125 Rhodophyta (red algae), 64 Phaeophyceae (brown algae), and 32 Chlorophyta (green algae). Of these, about 145 species are used (66%) directly in food: 79 Rhodophyta, 38 Phaeophyceae, and 28 Chlorophyta. In phycocolloid industry, 101 species are used: 41 alginophytes (algae that produce alginic acid), 33 agarophytes (algae producing agar), and 27 carrageenophytes (algae producing carrageenan). Other activities will use 24 species in traditional medicine; 25 species in agriculture, animal feed, and fertilizers; and about 12 species cultivated in *marine agronomy* (Zemke-White and Ohno 1999; Pereira et al. 2009b).

3.2.2 PHYCOCOLLOIDS

Phycocolloids are structural polysaccharides of high molecular weight found in the cell wall and intercellular spaces of freshwater and marine algae. They usually form colloidal solutions—an intermediate state between a solution and a suspension—which give these polysaccharides the ability to be used as thickeners, gelling agents, and stabilizers for suspensions and emulsions in diverse industries.

Phycocolloids possess a high number of functional roles in seaweeds. Some seaweeds grow attached to rocks in very turbulent waters, requiring maximum flexibility to survive, and these contain a higher amount of phycocolloids than those seaweeds growing in calm waters. The basis of phycocolloid properties relies on the nature and extent of intermolecular associations in ordered assemblies forming hydrated gel networks or on their interactions by entanglement of random coil polysaccharides (Stephen and Phillips 2010). Pyranose (five carbons and one oxygen) sugar rings (primary structure) are the main building units of phycocolloids, and these rings adopt in general the most energetically favorable chair conformations noted, $^4C_1$ or $^1C_4$, depending on the positions of C-4 and C-1. Notably, the gelling ability of phycocolloids depends on the overall shape enabled by the glycosidic linkage angles and the ability of the polysaccharides to form intra- and intermolecular physical linkages (hydrogen bonds, electrostatic interactions, and *van der Waals* interactions).

Sulfated galactans (e.g., agars and carrageenans) can be obtained from red algae, and alginates and other sulfated polysaccharides (e.g., laminaran and fucoidan) are obtained from brown algae. Phycocolloids are used in food industries as natural additives and have different European codes: E400 (alginic acid), E401 (sodium alginate), E402 (potassium alginate), E403 (ammonium alginate), E404 (calcium alginate), E405 (propylene glycol alginate), E406 (agar), E407 (carrageenan), and E407A (semirefined carrageenan (SRC) or processed *Eucheuma* seaweed) (Pereira et al. 2013a). Agar, alginates, and carrageenans are of the highest economic and commercial significance, because these polysaccharides exhibit high molecular weights, high viscosity, and excellent gelling, stabilizing, and emulsifying properties. They are extracted in fairly high amount from the algae. All these polysaccharides are water soluble and could be extracted with hot water or alkaline solution (Minghou 1990).

3.2.2.1 Alginates

Alginate is the term usually used for the salts of alginic acid, but it can also refer to all the derivatives of alginic and alginic acids itself; in some publications, the term *algin* is used instead of alginate. Chemically, alginates are linear copolymers of β-D-mannuronic acid (M) and α-L-guluronic acid (G) (1–4)-linked residues, arranged in either heteropolymeric (MG) and/or homopolymeric (M or G) blocks (see Figure 3.1) (Larsen et al. 2003; Pereira et al. 2003; Leal et al. 2008).

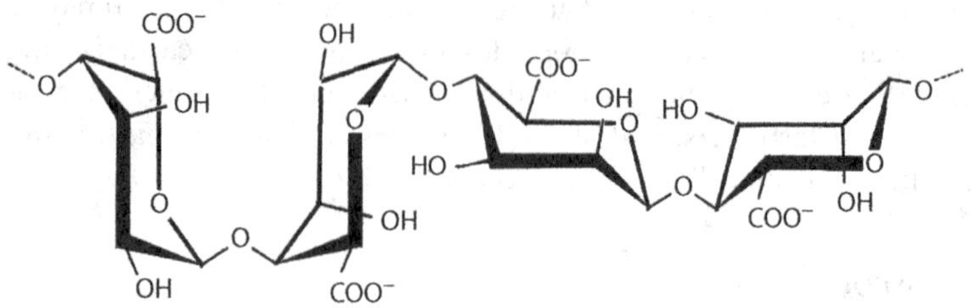

FIGURE 3.1 Idealized structure of the chemical units of alginic acid.

Alginic acid was discovered in 1883 by E.C.C. Stanford, a British pharmacist who called it algin. It is extracted as a mixed salt of sodium and/or potassium, calcium, and magnesium. Since Stanford discovered algin, the name has been applied to a number of substances, for example, alginic acid and all alginates, derived from alginic acid. The extraction process is based on the conversion of mixed insoluble salts of alginic acid of the cell wall into a soluble salt (alginate) which is appropriate for the water extraction (Lobban and Chapman 1988; Lahaye 2001). Alginic acid is present in the cell walls of brown seaweeds, where it is partially responsible for their flexibility.

In this context, brown seaweeds that grow in more turbulent conditions usually have higher alginate content than those that grow in calmer waters (McHugh 2003).

Although any brown seaweed could be used as a source of alginate, the actual chemical structure of the alginate varies from one genus to another, and similar variability is found in the properties of the alginate that is extracted from the seaweed. As the main applications of alginate are in thickening aqueous solutions and forming gels, its quality is judged on how well it performs in these uses (McHugh 2003).

Almost all extraction of alginates took place in Europe, the United States, and Japan 25–30 years ago. The major change in the alginate industry over the last decade has been the emergence of producers in China in the 1980s. Initially, production was limited to low-cost, low-quality alginate for the internal, industrial markets produced from the locally cultivated *Saccharina japonica*. By the 1990s, Chinese producers were competing in Western industrial markets to sell alginates, primarily based on low cost (Pereira 2011a).

A high-quality alginate forms strong gels and gives thick, aqueous solutions. A good raw material for alginate extraction should also give a high yield of alginate. Brown seaweeds that fulfill the above criteria are species of *Ascophyllum*, *Durvillaea*, *Ecklonia*, *Fucus*, *Laminaria*, *Lessonia*, *Macrocystis*, and *Sargassum*. However, *Sargassum* is only used when nothing else is available: its alginate is usually of borderline quality and the yield is also low (Draget et al. 2004; Pereira 2008).

The goal of the extraction process is to obtain dry, powdered, sodium alginate. The calcium and magnesium salts do not dissolve in water, but the sodium salt does. The rationale behind the extraction of alginate from the seaweed is to convert all the alginate salts into the sodium salt, dissolve this in water, and remove the seaweed residue by filtration (McHugh 2003).

Water-in-oil emulsions such as mayonnaise and salad dressings are less likely to separate into their original oil and water phases if thickened with alginate. Sodium alginate is not useful when the emulsion is acidic, because insoluble alginic acid forms; for these applications, propylene glycol alginate (PGA) is used because this is stable in mild acid conditions. Alginate improves the texture, body, and sheen of yogurt, but PGA is also used in the stabilization of milk proteins under acidic conditions, as found in some yogurts. Some fruit drinks have fruit pulp added, and it is preferable to keep this in suspension; addition of sodium alginate, or PGA in acidic conditions, can prevent sedimentation of the pulp and create foams. In chocolate milk, the cocoa can be kept in suspension by an alginate–phosphate mixture, although in this application it faces strong competition from carrageenan. Small amounts of alginate can thicken and stabilize whipped cream (Nussinovitch 1997; Onsoyen 1997).

Alginates have several commercial applications based on their thickening, gelling, emulsifier, and stabilizing properties. They are used in the food industry for improving the textural quality of numerous products such as salad dressing, ice cream, beer, jelly, and lactic drinks, but also in cosmetics, pharmaceutical, textile, and painting industries (Murata and Nakazoe 2001; Kim and Lee 2008; Pereira 2011a).

Moreover, due to their outstanding properties in terms of biocompatibility, biodegradability, non-antigenicity, and chelating abilities, the use of alginates is growing in a variety of biomedical applications (e.g., tissue engineering, drug delivery, and some formulations of preventing gastric reflux) (Lee and Mooneya 2012). The use of alginates and/or alginate derivatives as remedies for the treatment of gastritis and gastroduodenal ulcers is protected by patents in several countries (Pereira et al. 2009c). Also, numerous products of alginate-containing drugs, such as Gaviscon (Reckitt Benckiser, Inc., NJ), have been shown to effectively suppress postprandial (after eating) acidic refluxes, binding of bile acids, and duodenal ulcers in humans (Khotimchenko et al. 2011).

3.2.2.2 Agars

Agar is the phycocolloid of most ancient origin, and its name comes from Malaysia and means "red alga." Agar was, and still is, prepared and sold as an extract in solution (hot) or in gel form (cold), to be used promptly in areas near the factories (FAO 2010). The product was known as *Tokoroten*. Its industrialization as a dry and stable product began in the early eighteenth century, and since then, it has been called *Kanten*. Currently, agar–agar and agar are the most accepted worldwide terms. However, it is also called *Gelosa* in French- and Portuguese-speaking countries (Armisen and Galatas 1987; Minghou 1990; FAO 2010).

This polysaccharide is the dried hydrophilic, colloidal substance extracted commercially from certain marine algae of Phylum Rhodophyta. The most important commercial agarophyte genera are *Gelidium*, *Pterocladiella*, *Gelidiella*, and *Gracilaria*. Agar has also been found in species of *Ceramium*, *Phyllophora*, *Ahnfeltia*, *Campylaephora*, *Acanthopeltis*, and *Gracilariopsis* (Pereira et al. 2013a).

Agar consists of a mixture of at least two polysaccharides: agarose and agaropectin (Armisen and Galatas 2000). Typically, agarose is the predominant fraction of agar (50%–90%) (Araki 1937; Nussinovitch 1997) and is also responsible for its gelling properties (Nussinovitch 1997). It consists of high-molecular-weight polysaccharides composed of repeating units of $(1\rightarrow3)$-β-D-galactopyranosyl-$(1\rightarrow4)$-3,6-anhydro-α-L-galactopyranose (see Figure 3.2), although some variations can occur, depending on factors such as the species of seaweed, and environmental and seasonal conditions (Armisen and Galatas 2000). In turn, agaropectin is a less clearly defined, more complex polysaccharide of lower molecular weight than agarose, and it exhibits thickening

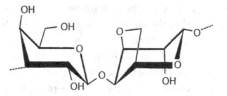

FIGURE 3.2 Idealized structure of the chemical units of agar.

properties (Armisen and Galatas 2000; Pereira 2011a). Its structure is essentially made up of alternating $(1\rightarrow3)$-β-D-galactopyranose and $(1\rightarrow4)$-3,6-anhydro-α-L-galactopyranose residues (Armisen and Galatas 2000; Qi et al. 2008).

Approximately 90% of the agar produced globally is intended for food applications. The origin of agar as a food ingredient was in Asia, where it has been consumed for several centuries (Pereira 2011a). Its extraordinary qualities as a thickening, stabilizing, and gelling agent make it an essential ingredient for preparing processed food such as fruit jellies, milk products, fruit pastilles, caramels, chewing gum, canned meat, soups, confectionery and baked goods, icing, and frozen and salted fish. Moreover, its satiating and gut-regulating characteristics make it an ideal fiber ingredient in the preparation of low-calorie food products (Armisen and Galatas 2000; Pereira 2011a; Pereira and Ribeiro-Claro 2014).

Agar has been classified as generally recognized as safe (GRAS) by the U.S. Food and Drug Administration, which has set maximum usage levels depending on particular applications. In the baked goods industry, the ability of agar gels to withstand high temperatures allows for its use as a stabilizer and thickener in pie fillings, icings, and meringues. Cakes, buns, and so on are often pre-packed in various kinds of modern wrapping materials and often stick to them, especially in hot weather; by reducing the quantity of water and adding some agar, a more stable, smoother, nonstick icing may be obtained (McHugh 2003; Pereira et al. 2009b). Some agars, especially those extracted from *Gracilaria chilensis*, can be used in confectionery with very high sugar content, such as fruit candies. These agars are said to be *sugar reactive* because the sugar (sucrose) increases the strength of the gel. As agar is tasteless, it does not interfere with the flavors of foodstuffs; this is in contrast to some of its competitive gums that require the addition of calcium or potassium salts to form gels. In Asian countries, it is a popular component of jellies; this has its origin in the early practice of boiling seaweed, straining it, and adding flavors to the liquid before it cooled and formed a jelly (McHugh 2003; Pereira 2011a).

Besides food applications, agar is fundamental in biotechnology studies, and is used in the preparation of inert, solidified culture media for bacteria, microalgae, fungi, and tissue culture. It is also used to obtain monoclonal antibodies, interferons, steroids, and alkaloids. The biotechnological applications of agar are increasing—it is essential for the separation of macromolecules by electrophoresis, chromatography, and DNA sequencing (Pereira 2008; Pereira 2010b).

3.2.2.3 Carrageenans

For several hundred years, carrageenan has been used as a thickening and stabilizing agent in food in Europe and Asia. In Europe, the use of carrageenan started more than 600 years ago in Ireland. In the village of Carraghen, on the south Irish coast, flans were made by cooking the so-called Irish moss (red seaweed species *Chondrus crispus*) in milk. The name carrageenin, as it was first called, was used for the first time in 1862 for the extract from *C. crispus* and was dedicated to this village (Tseng 1945). The name was later changed to carrageenan so as to comply with the -*an* suffix for the names of polysaccharides (Pereira et al. 2009c; Pereira 2011a). The extraction method was first described by Smith et al. in 1955 (van de Velde and de Ruiter 2002).

The Irish moss has been used in industry since the nineteenth century in the clarification of beer (Therkelsen 1993). The industrial extraction of carrageenan started in 1930 in New England, from *C. crispus* and *Mastocarpus stellatus* stalks, for the preparation of chocolate milk. The interruption of agar imports during World War II led to its replacement by carrageenan. This situation was the starting point of a booming industry (Ribier and Godineau 1984).

Fractionation of crude carrageenan extracts started in the early 1950s (Smith et al. 1955), resulting in the characterization of the different carrageenan types. A Greek prefix was introduced to identify the different carrageenans. In the same period, the molecular structure of carrageenans was determined (Oneill 1955a,b). The structure of 3,6-anhydro-D-galactose in kappa-carrageenan, as well as the type of linkages between galactose and anhydrogalactose rings, was determined.

Today, the industrial manufacture of carrageenan is no longer limited to extraction from *C. crispus*, and numerous red seaweed species (Gigartinales, Rhodophyta) are used. For a long period of time, these seaweeds have been harvested from naturally occurring populations. Seaweed farming started almost 200 years ago in Japan. Scientific information about the seaweed life cycles allowed artificial seeding in the 1950s. Today, lots of seaweed *taxa* are cultivated, lowering the pressure on naturally occurring populations (Critchley and Ohno 1998).

Carrageenans represent one of the major texturizing ingredients used by the food industry; they are natural ingredients, which have been used for decades in food applications and are GRAS.

Carrageenans are commercially important hydrophilic colloids, which occur as a matrix in numerous species of red seaweed (Stanley 1987). They are the third most important hydrocolloids in the food industry, after gelatin (animal origin) and starch (plant origin) (van de Velde and de Ruiter 2002). This phycocolloid has annual sales of more than $200 million and represents 15% of the world use of food hydrocolloids. The market for carrageenan has consistently grown at 5% per year, from 5,500 tons in 1970 up to 20,000 tons in 1995 (Bixler 1996). Shortages of carrageenan-producing seaweeds suddenly appeared in mid-2007, resulting in doubling of the price of carrageenans; this price increase was due to increased fuel costs and the weakness of US dollars (most seaweed polysaccharides are traded in US dollars). The reasons for shortages of the raw materials for processing are less certain: perhaps it is a combination of environmental factors, sudden increases in demand, particularly from China, and some market manipulation by farmers and traders. Most hydrocolloids are experiencing severe price movements (Pereira 2013b).

The modern industry of carrageenans dates from the 1940s where it was found to be the ideal stabilizer for the suspension of cocoa in chocolate milk. In the past few decades, due to their physical functional properties, such as gelling, thickening, emulsifying, and stabilizing abilities, carrageenans have been used in food industry to improve the texture of cottage cheese, puddings and dairy desserts, and the manufacture of sausages, patties, and low-fat hamburgers (van de Velde and de Ruiter 2002; van de Velde et al. 2004; Pereira et al. 2009b; Pereira and van de Velde 2011b; Li et al. 2014).

The most commonly used commercial carrageenans are extracted from *K. alvarezii* and *Eucheuma denticulatum* (McHugh 2003). Primarily wild-harvested genera such as *Chondrus*, *Furcellaria*, *Gigartina*, *Chondracanthus*, *Sarcothalia*, *Mazzaella*, *Iridaea*, *Mastocarpus*, and *Tichocarpus* are also mainly cultivated as carrageenan raw materials, and carrageenan-producing countries include Argentina, Canada, Chile, Denmark, France, Japan, Mexico, Morocco, Portugal, North Korea, South Korea, Spain, Russia, and the United States (Pereira et al. 2009c; Bixler and Porse 2011; Pereira 2013b).

As discussed previously, the original source of carrageenans was from the red sea-weed *C. crispus*, which continues to be used, but in limited quantities. *Betaphycus gelatinus* is used for the extraction of beta (β)-carrageenan. Some South American red algae used previously only in minor quantities have, more recently, received attention from carrageenan producers, as they seek to increase the diversification of raw materials in order to provide for the extraction of new carrageenan types with different physical functionalities and, therefore, increase the product development, which in turn stimulates the demand (McHugh 2003; Pereira 2011a). *Gigartina skottsbergii*, *Sarcothalia crispata*, and *Mazzaella laminarioides* are currently the most valuable species and all are harvested from natural populations in Chile and Peru. Large carrageenan processors have fuelled the development of *K. alvarezii* (commercial name *cottonii*) and *E. denticulatum* (commercial name *spinosum*) farming in several countries, including the Philippines, Indonesia, Malaysia, Tanzania, Kiribati, Fiji, Kenya, and Madagascar (McHugh 2003; Pereira 2011a). Indonesia has recently overtaken the Philippines as the world's largest producer of dried carrageenophytes biomass (Pereira 2011a).

3.3   CHEMICAL STRUCTURE OF CARRAGEENANS

The most common carrageenan types are traditionally identified by a letter of the Greek alphabet (see Table 3.1) (Craigie 1990; Chopin et al. 1999). The three most important commercial carrageenans are iota (ι)-, kappa (κ)-, and lambda (λ)-carrageenans, whose chemical names according to International Union of Pure and Applied Chemistry and to the letter code are 2,4′-disulfate (G4S-DA2S), carrageenose 4′-sulfate (G4S-DA), and carrageenose 2,6,2′-trisulfate (G2S-D2S,6S), respectively (van de Velde et al. 2002a).

Carrageenans are sulfated polysaccharides present in the cell walls of members of the Gigartinales (Pereira et al. 2007; Pereira et al. 2009c). Polysaccharides are carbohydrates that can be composed of only one kind of repeating monosaccharide, or formed by two or more different monomeric units (heteropolysaccharides; e.g., agar, alginate, carrageenan). The conformation of the polysaccharide chains depends not only on the pH and ionic strength of the medium but also on the temperature and the concentration of certain molecules. Polysaccharides are divided into two subtypes: anionic and cationic polysaccharides. Carrageenans are naturally occurring anionic sulfated linear polysaccharides (Prajapati et al. 2014).

The molecular chains of carrageenans have two fundamental characteristics: they are composed of a monomer—galactose—and a high proportion of sulfate esters ($-O-SO_3$), to which the negative charge is provided by the compound. Galactose (a), in aqueous solution, is capable of fixating a water molecule to the carbon1 (C_1),

TABLE 3.1

Different Types of Carrageenans

Carrageenan	G β-D-Galactose Units	D α-D-Galactose Units	Letter Code	
Kappa Family				
Kappa (κ)	4-Sulfate	3,6-Anhydro	G4S	DA
Iota (ι)	4-Sulfate	3,6-Anhydro 2-Sulfate	G4S	DA2S
Mu (μ)	4-Sulfate	6-Sulfate	G4S	D6S
Nu (ν)	4-Sulfate	2,6-Dissulfate	G4S	D2S6S
Omicron (o)	4-Sulfate	2-Sulfate	G4S	D2S
Lambda Family				
Lambda (λ)	2-Sulfate	2,6-Disulfate	G2S	D2S6S
Xi (ξ)	2-Sulfate	2-Sulfate	G2S	D2S
Theta (θ)	2-Sulfate	3,6-Anhydro 2-Sulfate	G2S	DA2S
Pi (π)	Pyruvate 2-Sulfate	2-Sulfate	GP, 2S	D2S
Beta Family				
Beta (β)	–	3,6-Anhydro	G	DA
Alpha (α)	–	3,6-Anhydro 2-Sulfate	G	DA2S
Gamma (γ)	–	6-Sulfate	G	D6S
Delta (δ)	–	2,6-Dissulfate	G	D2S6S
Omega Family				
Omega (ω)	6-Sulfate	3,6-Anhydro	G6S	DA
Psi (ψ)	6-Sulfate	6-Sulfate	G6S	D6S

Sources: Stortz, C.A., Cases, M.R., Cerezo, A.S., Red seaweed galactans, in *Techniques in Glycobiology*, Townsend, R.R., Hotchkiss, A.T. (eds.), New York, CRC Press, 1997, pp. 567–593; Amimi, A., Mouradi, A., Givernaud, T., Chiadmi, N., Lahaye, M., *Carbohydr. Res.*, 333, 271–279, 2001.

which leads to an unstable structure (b) that is self-cyclized in a pyranose form to form an oxygen bridge between C_1 and C_5 (c). The cyclization can occur in three different ways—in the form of β-D-galactopyranose (d), α-D-galactopyranose (e), or 3,6 anhydro-α-D-galactopyranose (f)—through an intermediate oxygen bridge between C_3 and C_6 of α-D-galactopyranose (Figure 3.3).

Both β-D-galactopyranose-α-D-galactopyranose (or β-D-galactopyranose-3,6-anhydro-α-D-galactopyranose) units bind through an intermediate oxygen bridge between the C_1 of β-D-galactopyranose and the C_4 of α-D-galactopyranose, in the form of a β-type link (or 3,6-anhydrogalactopyranose), with the release of a water molecule. The β-D-galactopyranose-α-D-galactopyranose (or β-D-galactopyranose-3,6-anhydro-α-D-galactopyranose) assembly constitutes a *dimer* or a *sequence*. The carrageenan chain is formed by a series of this type of sequences. One sequence is

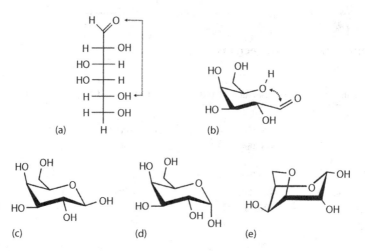

FIGURE 3.3 Carrageenans, basic chemical structure: (a) galactose (aldose form, Fisher projection); (b) idealized view of the cyclization of the molecule (pyranose ring formation through C1–O–C5); (c) β-D-galactopyranose; (d) α-D-galacto-pyranose; (e) 3,6 anhydro-α-D-galactopyranose.

linked to the next one through an oxygen bridge between the C_1 of one sequence and the C_3 of the next one, with the release of a water molecule (Figure 3.4), in the form of an α-type link (McCandless 1981; Perez et al. 1992).

Carrageenans are classified according to the degree of substitution that occurs on their free hydroxyl groups. Substitutions are generally either the addition of ester

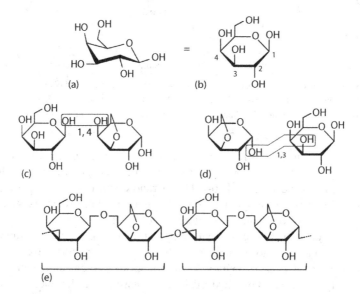

FIGURE 3.4 Carrageenan chain formation through 1,4 and 1,3 glycosidic bonds: (a) idealized structure and (b) identical Haworth projection, (c) 1,4 bonding, (d) 1,3 bonding, (e) chain of two 1,4 "dimers."

sulfate or the presence of the 3,6-anhydride residues (Campo et al. 2009; Nanaki et al. 2010). In addition to D-galactose and 3,6-anhydro-D-galactose as the main sugar residues and sulfate as the main substituent, other carbohydrate residues commonly exist in carrageenans, such as xylose, glucose, and uronic acids (Prajapati et al. 2014). Thus, the structure of the various types of carrageenans is defined by the number and position of sulfate groups, the presence of 3,6 anhydro-D-galactose, and the conformation of the pyranose ring (Chopin et al. 1999; Pereira 2013b).

3.3.1 MAIN INDUSTRIAL TYPES

Commercial carrageenans are usually classified into kappa (κ, G4S-DA), iota (ι, G4S-DA2S), and lambda (λ, G2S-D2S,6S) carrageenans (Pereira and van de Velde 2011b).

In 1954, Smith and Cook discovered that adding potassium chloride to a carrageenan solution resulted in the separation of two phases: one soluble and another insoluble. The solution of kappa-carrageenan leads, after heating, to the formation of a gel, whereas the lambda-carrageenan solution never allows the formation of an aqueous gel.

3.3.1.1 Lambda-Carrageenan

This carrageenan consists of a β-D-galactopyranose unit, with a sulfate group on C_2, and an α-D-galactopyranose unit, with a sulfate group on the C_2 and C_6, which leads to the formation of the following dimmer (G2S-D2S,6S). In a space representation, due to the carbon valence angle, each monomer takes a spatial *chair* arrangement (Figure 3.5).

The presence of three sulfate esters (–O–SO$_3$⁻) substitutions, which are responsible for the strong electronegativity of the dimmers, causes repulsion between the chains. However, the *zig-zag* spatial arrangement does not allow the helical structure formation. The chains of lambda-carrageenan remain scattered in water, whatever the cation that enters its constitution. This is the reason why lambda-carrageenan never forms a gel in aqueous solution, but increases its viscosity. This carrageenan is soluble at cold or low temperatures (15°C–20°C) (McCandless 1981; Perez et al. 1992).

3.3.1.2 Kappa-Carrageenan

The hydrolysis of kappa-carrageenan reveals the presence of β-D-galactopyranose-4-sulfate and 3,6-anhydro-α-D-galactopyranose (G4S-DA). In a space representation, each monomer takes a *chair* arrangement, and the sequence forms a helical structure (Figure 3.6).

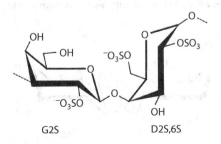

G2S   D2S,6S

FIGURE 3.5 Spatial representation of β-D-galactopyranose-2-sulfate-*O*-α-D-galactopyranose-2,6-sulfate (G2S-D2S,6S).

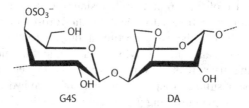

FIGURE 3.6 Spatial representation of β-D-galactopyranose-4-sulfate-*O*-3,6-anhydro-α-D-galactopyranose (G4S-DA).

The presence of an oxygen bridge (CH$_2$–O–C) between C$_3$ and C$_6$ of the 3,6-anhydro-D-galactopyranose constitutes an hydrophobic formation. This tendency is offset by the presence of radical OSO$_3^-$ of the β-D-galactopyranose. The chain of kappa-carrageenan arranges itself in the space in a sequence of helices. Each chain moves toward the next one to protect the hydrophobic groups from the water molecules. Consequently, kappa-carrageenans are capable of jellifying the solution where it is present under proper conditions (Figure 3.7) (McCandless 1981; Perez et al. 1992).

3.3.1.3 Iota-Carrageenan

Although kappa-carrageenan reveals the presence of β-D-galactopyranose-4-sulfate and 3,6-anhydrogalactopyranose units, iota-carrageenan reveals the presence of an additional sulfate ester substituted on the C$_2$ of 3,6-anhydrogalactopyranose (G4S-DA2S). The presence of two sulfated esters reduces the hydrophobic character of the carrageenan: the gel produced by this carrageenan is soft and has no syneresis (Figure 3.8) (McCandless 1981; Perez et al. 1992).

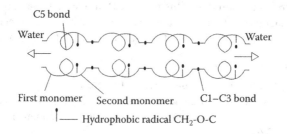

FIGURE 3.7 Arrangement of a chain of kappa-carrageenan in a sequence of helices.

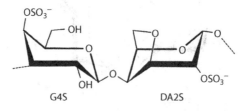

FIGURE 3.8 Spatial representation of β-D-galactopyranose-4-sulfate-*O*-3,6-anhydro-α-D-galactopyranose-2-sulfate (G4S-DA2S).

The different types of carrageenan are obtained from different species of the Gigartinales (Rhodophyta) (Pereira and van de Velde 2011b). Kappa-carrageenan is predominantly obtained by extraction from the cultivated, tropical seaweed *K. alvarezii*. *E. denticulatum* is the main species for the production of iota-carrageenan (Pereira et al. 2009c). Lambda-carrageenan is obtained from different species from the genera *Gigartina* and *Chondrus* (Van de Velde and de Ruiter 2002). Kappa- and iota-carrageenans have gelling properties, whereas lambda-carrageenan acts as a thickening agent (Prajapati et al. 2014). The kappa-carrageenan usually forms gels that are hard, strong, and brittle, whereas iota-carrageenan forms soft and weak gels.

3.3.2 OTHER TYPES

3.3.2.1 Beta-Carrageenan (G-DA)

This carrageenan is extracted from *B. gelatinus* and differs from kappa-carrageenan due to the absence of the radical sulfate ester OSO_3^- on the C_4 of β-D-galactopyranose. This absence emphasizes the hydrophobic character of the molecule, which results in the production of a harder gel, with a more pronounced syneresis than that of the kappa-carrageenan (Figure 3.9).

The spatial structure of iota- and beta-carrageenans is similar to that of kappa-carrageenan (helical chains). In the gelling process, the chains are closer in beta-carrageenan than in kappa-carrageenan, and are more elongated in iota-carrageenan (McCandless 1981; Perez et al. 1992).

3.3.3 INTRACELLULAR CARRAGEENANS (BIOLOGICAL PRECURSORS)

The study of carrageenophytes by nuclear magnetic resonance spectroscopy, the chemical modifications by the action of periodate, and the analysis by infrared (IR) spectroscopy revealed the existence, in algae, of other types of carrageenan whose chemical formula is related to the following:

Kappa-type: mu-carrageenan
Iota-type: nu-carrageenan
Beta-type: gamma-carrageenan
Theta-type: lambda-carrageenan

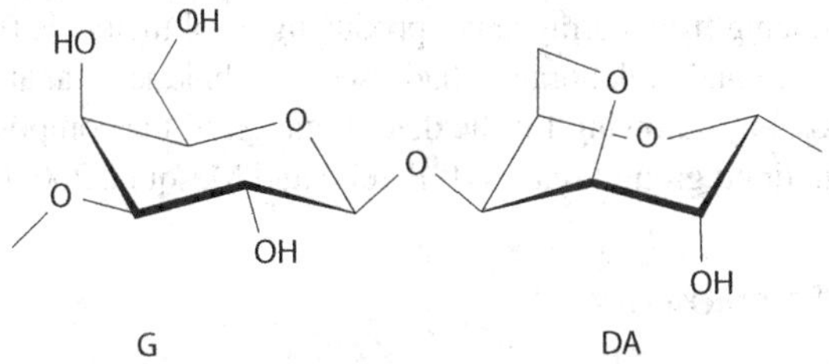

FIGURE 3.9 Spatial representation of beta-carrageenan (G-DA).

These carrageenans differ from the first ones because the second element of the sequence is found on the α-D-galactopyranose-6-sulfate and not on the 3,6-anhydrogalactopyranose, as seen on kappa-, iota-, and beta-carrageenans. The mu-, nu-, and gamma-carrageenans are the biological precursors of kappa-, iota-, and beta-carrageenans, respectively (see Table 3.2 and Figure 3.10). This transformation is the result of the absence of the ester sulfate group of C_6 and the formation of an oxygen bridge between C_3 and C_6. This *mutation* is caused, inside the cell, by the action of the enzyme sulfohydrolase or, externally, by an alkali extraction. Thus, it is not possible to find mu-, nu-, and gamma-carrageenans in solutions that resulted from alkali extractions.

It is possible to identify another type of carrageenan: the xi type (ξ-carrageenan). This carrageenan results from the metabolic evolution of the lambda-carrageenan (see Figure 3.11) and can be found either in the cell or in solutions that resulted from alkali extractions in a very small percentage (Pereira 2004).

3.4 SPECTROSCOPIC ANALYSIS (VIBRATIONAL SPECTROSCOPY)

The industrial applications of phycocolloids (alginates, agar, and carrageenans) are based on their particular properties to form gels in aqueous solution. However, the need for a more accurate identification of the natural composition of the polysaccharides produced by these seaweeds leads to the use of new spectroscopic techniques. With the combination of two spectroscopic techniques (Fourier transform IR-attenuated total reflectance [FTIR-ATR] and Fourier transform Raman [FT-Raman]), it is possible to identify the principal seaweed colloids in ground seaweed samples as in extracted material (Pereira et al. 2009d).

3.4.1 FTIR Spectroscopy

IR spectroscopy has been applied for many years in the characterization of sulfated polysaccharides from seaweeds, and it was, until recently, the most frequently used vibrational technique for studying the natural products (Matsuhiro 1996; Pereira et al. 2003). This technique presents three main advantages: it is fast, it is nonaggressive, and it requires small sample quantities (milligrams) (Pereira et al. 2003). However, conventional IR spectroscopy requires laborious procedures to obtain spectra with a good signal-to-noise ratio (Chopin and Whalen 1993). Thus, to overcome this limitation, an interferometric IR technique (associated with the Fourier transform algorithm), known as FTIR spectroscopy (Pereira et al. 2009d) was developed. FTIR spectroscopy is useful in distinguishing agar-producing from carrageenan-producing algal materials (Matsuhiro 1996). More recently, Pereira and collaborators had used a technique of analysis based on the FTIR-ATR spectroscopy, allowing for the determination of the composition of different phycocolloids from dried ground seaweed (Pereira and Mesquita 2004b; Pereira 2006).

3.4.2 Raman Spectroscopy

In contrast to FTIR-ATR spectroscopy, the application of traditional Raman spectroscopy was limited until recently, due to the need for an incident visible laser in dispersive

TABLE 3.2
Identification of the Different Types of Carrageenan by FTIR-ATR

Wave Number (cm^{-1})	Bridge (s)/Group (s)	Letter Code	Carrageenan Type							
			Kappa (κ)	Mu (μ)	Iota (ι)	Nu (ν)	Beta (β)	Theta (θ)	Lambda (λ)	Xi (ξ)
1240–1260	S=O of sulfate esters		++	++	++	+++	−	++	+++	++
1070	C–O of the 3,6-anhydrogalactose	DA	+	−	+	−	+	s	−	−
970–975	Galactose	G/D	+	s	+	s	+	+	−	−
930	C–O of the 3,6-anhydrogalactose	DA	+	−	+	−	+	+	−	−
905	C–O–SO$_3$ on C$_2$ of the 3,6-anhydrogalactose	DA2S	−	−	+	−	−	+	−	−
890–900	β-D-Non-sulfated galactose	G/D	−	−	−	−	+	−	−	−
867	C–O–SO$_3$ on C$_6$ of the galactose	G/D6S	−	+	−	+	−	−	+	−
845	C–O–SO$_3$ on C$_4$ of the galactose	G4S	+	+	+	+	−	−	−	−
825–830	C–O–SO$_3$ on C$_2$ of the galactose	G/D2S	−	−	−	+	+	+	+	n
815–820	C–O–SO$_3$ on C$_6$ of the galactose	G/D6S	−	+	−	+	−	−	+	−
805	C–O–SO$_3$ on C$_2$ of the 3,6-anhydrogalactose	DA2S	−	−	+	−	−	+	−	−

Sources: Pereira, L., Estudos em macroalgas carragenófitas (Gigartinales, Rhodophyceae) da costa portuguesa—Aspectos ecológicos, bioquímicos e citológicos. PhD Thesis, Universidade de Coimbra, Coimbra, Portugal, 293, 2004a; Pereira, L., Amado, A.M., Critchley, A.T., van de Velde, F., Ribeiro-Claro, P.J.A., *Food Hydrocol.*, 23, 1903–1909, 2009c; Pereira, L., Ribeiro-Claro, P.J., Chapter 7—Analysis by vibrational spectroscopy of seaweed with potential use in food, pharmaceutical and cosmetic industries, in *Marine Algae—Biodiversity, Taxonomy, Environmental Assessment and Biotechnology*, Leonel, P., João, M.N. (eds.). Boca Raton, FL, Science Publishers, an Imprint of CRC Press/Taylor & Francis Group, 2014, pp. 225–247.

Notes: (−), absent; (+), medium; (++), strong; (+++) very strong; (s), shoulder form peak; (n), narrow peak.

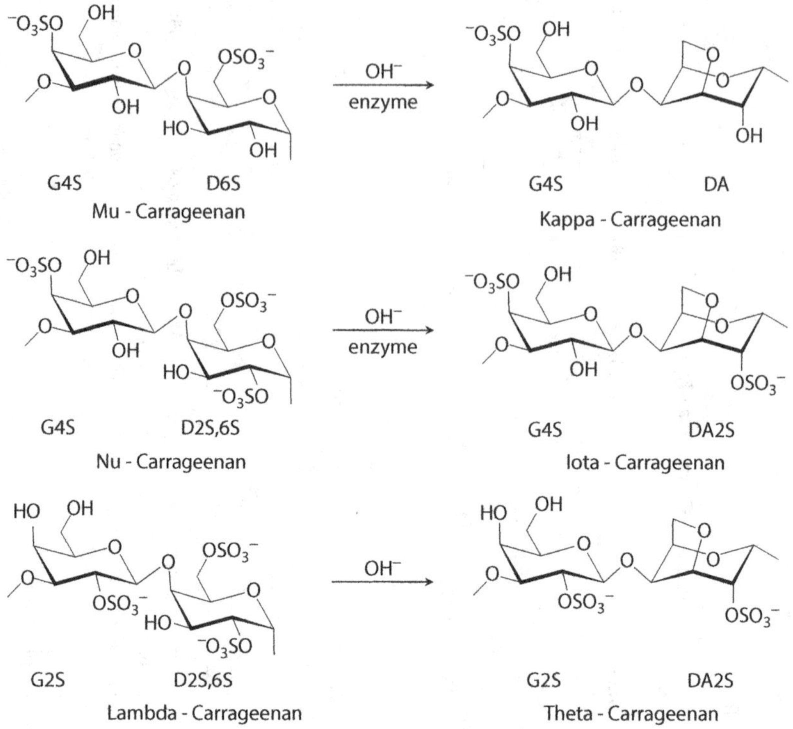

FIGURE 3.10 Biological precursors of kappa, iota and theta carrageenans. (Adapted from Pereira, L., Correia, F., Algas marinhas da costa Portuguesa—ecologia, biodiversidade e utilizações, Nota de Rodapé Edições, 2015.)

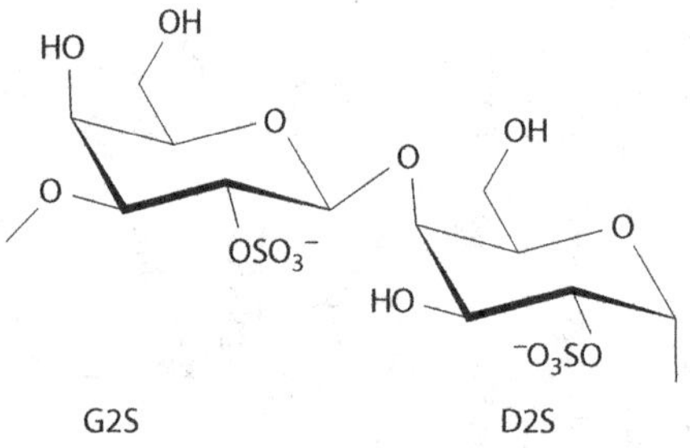

FIGURE 3.11 Spatial representation of xi-carrageenan (G2S-D2S).

spectrometers: the visible laser light often excites electronic transitions in biochemical samples, which can lead to either sample degradation or strong background signal from unwanted laser-induced fluorescence (Pereira et al. 2009d). Moreover, recording the spectra with good signal-to-noise ratio was often time consuming (Pereira et al. 2003). These limitations were greatly overcome through the development of near-IR FT-Raman spectroscopy, with which fluorescence, risk of sample destruction, and spectra recording time are greatly reduced (Matsuhiro 1996), whereas the spectral resolution and signal-to-noise ratio are enhanced (Pereira et al. 2003). Raman spectra are similar to IR, in the sense that both result from the interaction of light with molecular vibrations. However, as they rely on different physical processes (oscillating dipole moment for IR, polarizability change for Raman), the intensity of the vibrational modes is not the same in IR and Raman. In particular, certain low-intensity bands in FTIR appear clear in the Raman spectra, a fact that facilitates the identification of the different fractions present in the samples (Givernaud-Mouradi 1992). According to Pereira et al. (2003), FT-Raman spectra present, in general, better resolution than the IR spectra, allowing the assignment of a number of characteristic bands used in the identification of different types of carrageenans. In some cases, phycocolloids can be identified only with the use of Raman spectroscopy. For example, some variants of the family of lambda-carrageenan (xi and theta) can be easily identified by FT-Raman.

Tables 3.2 and 3.3 summarize the absorption peaks of the eight main carrageenan types by FTIR-ATR and FT-Raman spectroscopy, respectively.

3.5 SOURCES AND EXTRACTION METHODS OF CARRAGEENANS

Most of carrageenan is extracted from *K. alvarezii* and *E. denticulatum*. The original source of carrageenan was *C. crispus*, and this is still used to a limited extent. *Betaphycus gelatinum* is used for a particular type of carrageenan (beta-carrageenan). Some South American species that have previously been used to a limited extent are now gaining favor with carrageenan producers as they look for more diversification in the species available to them and the types of carrageenans that can be extracted. *G. skottsbergii*, *Sarcothalia crispate*, and *Mazzaella laminaroides* are currently the most valuable species, all collected from natural resources in Chile. Small quantities of *Chondracanthus canaliculatus* (formerly *Gigartina canaliculata*) are harvested in Mexico. *Hypnea musciformis* has been used in Brazil (McHugh 2003).

K. alvarezii and *E. denticulatum* were originally harvested from natural stocks growing in Indonesia and the Philippines. In the 1970s, cultivation began in both countries, and this now supplies most of these species, with only small quantities being collected from the wild. Cultivation has spread to other countries, most successfully in Tanzania (Zanzibar), Vietnam, and some of the Pacific Islands, such as those of Kiribati. Wild *B. gelatinum* is harvested mainly in Hainan Island, China, Taiwan Province of China, and the Philippines, and it is cultivated on Hainan Island. *C. crispus* is harvested for carrageenan production in Canada (Nova Scotia and Prince Edward Island), the United States (Maine and Massachusetts), and France (McHugh 2003).

3.5.1 Laboratory Extraction Methodology (Alkali Extraction)

The seaweed samples are rinsed in distilled freshwater to eliminate salt and debris from the thallus surface and dried to constant weight at 60°C for 24 hours minimum. The dried seaweeds are finely ground in order to render the samples uniform (Pereira 2004a, 2006). For the extraction, 2×1 g of seaweed (dry weight) is necessary. Before phycocolloid extraction, the ground dry material (1 g) is rehydrated and pretreated with a mixture of acetone/methanol (75 mL acetone and 75 mL methanol), at room temperature, for 12 hours, to eliminate the organo-soluble fraction (Zinoun and Cosson 1996).

TABLE 3.3
Identification of the Different Types of Carrageenan by FT-Raman

Wave Number (cm¹)	Bridge (s)/Group (s)	Letter Code	Kappa (κ)	Mu (μ)	Iota (ι)	Nu (ν)	Beta (β)	Theta (θ)	Lambda (λ)	Xi (ξ)
1240–1260	S=O of sulfate esters		++	++	++	+++	–	++	++	++
1075–1805	C–O of the 3,6-anhydrogalactose	DA	+++	–	+++	–	+	+	–	–
970–975	Galactose	G/D	+	+	s	s	+	+	–	–
925–935	C–O of the 3,6-anhydrogalactose	DA	+	–	+	–	+	+	–	–
905–907	C–O–SO$_3$ on C$_2$ of the 3,6-anhydrogalactose	DA2S	–	–	+	–	–	+	+	+
890–900	β-D-Non-sulfated galactose	G/D	–	–	–	–	+	–	–	–
867–871	C–O–SO$_3$ on C$_6$ of the galactose	G/D6S	–	s	–	+	–	–	+	–
845–850	C–O–SO$_3$ on C$_4$ of the galactose	G4S	++	+	++	+	–	–	+	+
825–830	C–O–SO$_3$ on C$_2$ of the galactose	G/D2S	–	–	–	+	–	+	+	–
815–825	C–O–SO$_3$ on C$_6$ of the galactose	G/D6S	–	s	–	s	–	–	+	+
804–808	C–O–SO$_3$ on C$_2$ of the 3,6-anhydrogalactose	DA2S	–	–	++	–	–	+	–	–

Sources: Pereira, L., Estudos em macroalgas carragenófitas (Gigartinales, Rhodophyceae) da costa portuguesa—Aspectos ecológicos, bioquímicos e citológicos. PhD Thesis, Universidade de Coimbra, Coimbra, Portugal, 293, 2004a; Pereira, L., Amado, A.M., Critchley, A.T., van de Velde, F., Ribeiro-Claro, P.J.A., *Food Hydrocol.*, 23, 1903–1909, 2009c; Pereira, L. Ribeiro-Claro, P.J., Chapter 7—Analysis by vibrational spectroscopy of seaweed with potential use in food, pharmaceutical and cosmetic industries, in *Marine Algae—Biodiversity, Taxonomy, Environmental Assessment and Biotechnology*, Leonel, P., João, M.N. (eds.), Boca Raton, FL, Science Publishers, an Imprint of CRC Press/Taylor & Francis Group, 2014, pp. 225–247.

Notes: (–), absent; (+), medium; (++), strong; (+++) very strong; (s), shoulder form peak.

The samples are then placed in a solution (150 mL/g) of NaOH (1 M) in a hot bath, at 80°C–85°C, for 3–4 hours, and neutralized to pH 6–8 with 0.3 M HCl (Pereira and Mesquita 2004b).

The solutions are hot filtered twice under vacuum through cloth and glass fiber filter. The extract is evaporated under vacuum to one-third of the initial volume. The carrageenan is precipitated by adding to the warm solution twice its volume of ethanol (96%). With a glass rod, the carrageenans are pulled out into a clean glass and are squeezed in order to drain the soaked liquid; 100 mL of absolute alcohol is added (12–24 hours). Finally, the alcohol is removed and the carrageenans are dried at 50°C–60°C for 24 hours (Pereira and Mesquita 2004b).

3.5.2 Industrial Methods

The extraction of carrageenans is mostly done by using dry seaweeds. However, first, it is necessary to determine the characteristics of the dried material: humidity, sand content, salts present, epiphytes, carrageenan content, and quality of the extract. These elements allow the adjustment of the extraction methods.

3.5.2.1 Classic Extraction

The first step is the depuration of the raw material. Seaweeds must be immersed in water and rinsed, in order to remove sand, shells, dead fish, and other foreign matter. During this step, there might be dissolution of a small part of the carrageenans, which is lost during washing. This can be overcome by given seaweeds a solution of calcium chloride, which makes carrageenan insoluble. After the first wash, seaweed color removal is made by the addition of sodium hypochlorite, which will be eliminated by a slight excess of sodium hydrogen sulfite (sodium bisulfite) (Genu 1985; Perez et al. 1992).

3.5.2.1.1 Extraction of Carrageenan Solution

Seaweeds are then immersed in an alkali solution of $CH_2(OH)_2$ or NaOH (0.1M) at a rate of 100 L/kg; plant material disintegrates progressively under the pressure of a pestle. A small quantity of soluble phosphate (about 1 kg per 10,000 L) is added in order to increase the carrageenan final yield. The alkali treatment is intended to *swallow* and soften the seaweeds so that they can be easily disaggregated. Moreover, the alkali treatment aims at converting α-D-galactopyranose-6-sulfate monomers into hydrophobic units of 3,6-anhydro-α-D-galactopyranose, which elevates the gel strength and the reactivity of carrageenans.

Lambda-carrageenan dissolves at low temperatures (15°C–20°C), whereas kappa- and iota-carrageenans are dissolved at higher temperatures (60°C–95°C). At higher temperatures, dissolutions of other polysaccharides can occur, such as starch and fluoride (Genu 1985; Perez et al. 1992).

3.5.2.1.2 Isolation of Carrageenan Solution

It is extremely difficult to separate a solution of carrageenans from small-sized solid particles. The method currently used by the extraction industries is filtration performed inside cylinders in a hot environment and under pressure. The mixture, to which diatomaceous ground was added previously, is then filtered through sackcloth. The resulting mixture contains 1%–2% carrageenans.

3.5.2.1.3   Isolation of Carrageenans

The main problem of the isolation of carrageenan is separating carrageenans from an aqueous mixture (1–2 g of carrageenan for each 48 g of water). Some manufacturers reduce the quantity of water by partial evaporation, passing the solution through hot cylinders, to achieve a carrageenan concentration of 4%. In most cases, the carrageenan solution is poured into a bowl of isopropyl alcohol. Carrageenans then precipitate in the form of whitish fibrous agglomerate. The isopropyl alcohol and the formed clots are then projected by a pump toward a vibrating sieve, which allows the alcohol to pass but retains the carrageenan clots; these are then subjected to a series of alcohol washes. At this time, the polysaccharide chain is extremely fragile.

Some producers submit the clot to centrifugation on a drying machine provided by big baskets; others, to obtain a better final quality, proceed to dehydration of the carrageenans pulp through low temperatures (0°C–5°C), or microwave.

The alcohol that is used during different stages of extraction is recovered and sent to a distillation column for its purification, although 10%–15% of alcohol is lost in each cycle of utilization.

The fibrous carrageenan clot is grounded into particles with size ranging from 80 to 270 µm, packed, and submitted to a control that verifies its composition and functional properties: humidity, purity, viscosity, and gel strength (Genu 1985; Perez et al. 1992).

3.5.2.2   Refined Carrageenan and SRC

There are two different methods of producing carrageenan based on different principles. In the original method—the only one used until the late 1970s to the early 1980s—the carrageenan is extracted from the seaweed into an aqueous solution, then the seaweed residue is removed by filtration and the carrageenan is recovered from the solution, eventually as a dry solid containing little else than carrageenan. This recovery process is difficult and expensive comparatively to the costs of the second method. In the second method, the carrageenan is never actually extracted from the seaweed. Rather the principle is to wash everything out of the seaweed that will dissolve in alkali and water, leaving the carrageenan and other insoluble matter behind. This insoluble residue, consisting largely of carrageenan and cellulose, is then dried and sold as Semi refined carrageenan (SRC). As the carrageenan does not need to be recovered from solution, the process is much shorter and cheaper (McHugh 2003).

3.5.2.2.1   Refined Carrageenan

Refined carrageenan is the original carrageenan, and until the late 1970s to the early 1980s, it was simply called carrageenan. It was first made from *C. crispus*, but now the process is applied to *K. alvarezii*, *E. denticulatum*, *G. skottsbergii*, and *S. crispata*.

The seaweed is washed to remove sand, salts, and other foreign matter. It is then heated with water containing an alkali, such as sodium hydroxide, for several hours, with the time depending on the seaweeds being extracted and determined by prior small-scale trials, or experience. Alkali is used because it causes a chemical change that leads to increased gel strength in the final product. In chemical terms, it removes some of the sulfate groups from the molecules and increases the formation of 3,6-anhydrogalatopyranose units: the more the latter, the better the gel strength. The seaweed that does not dissolve is removed by centrifugation or a coarse filtration, or a combination. The solution is then filtered again in a pressure filter using a filter aid that helps to prevent the filter cloth becoming blocked by fine, gelatinous particles. At this stage, the solution contains 1%–2% carrageenan, and this is usually concentrated to 2%–3% by vacuum distillation and ultrafiltration.

The processor now has a clear solution of carrageenan, and there are two methods for recovering it as a solid: an alcohol precipitation method and a gel method. An alcohol precipitation method can be used for any of the carrageenans. A gel method can be used for kappa-carrageenan only, and the gel can be dehydrated either by squeezing or by subjecting it to a freeze–thaw process.

In the alcohol method, isopropanol is added until all the carrageenan is precipitated as a fibrous coagulum that is then separated using a centrifuge or screen (a fine sieve). The coagulum is pressed to remove solvent and washed with more alcohol to dehydrate it further. It is then dried and milled to an appropriate particle size, 80 mesh or finer. For the process to be economic, the alcohol must be recovered, from both the liquids and the dryer, and recycled.

The gel method relies on the ability of kappa-carrageenan to form a gel with potassium salts. The gel may be formed in various ways. For the freeze–thaw process, it is convenient to form it as spaghetti-like pieces by forcing the carrageenan solution through fine holes into a potassium chloride solution. The fine *spaghetti* is collected and washed with more potassium chloride to remove more water, pressed to remove surplus liquid, and then frozen. When allowed to thaw, separation of water occurs by syneresis; the pieces are washed with more potassium chloride, chopped up, and dried in a hot air dryer. Inevitably, the product contains some potassium chloride. The alternative to freeze–thaw is to force water out of the gel by applying pressure to it, using similar equipment to that used for agar. After squeezing for several hours, the sheets of gel are chopped, dried in a hot air dryer, and milled to an appropriate particle size. Many agar processors are now using their equipment and similar techniques to produce kappa-carrageenan as well (McHugh 2003). Figure 3.12 summarizes the above processes.

3.5.2.2.2   Semi refined Carrageenan

SRC was the name given to the product first produced by the second method. This is the method in which the carrageenan is never actually extracted from the seaweed.

In the production of SRC, *K. alvarezii*, contained in a metal basket, is heated in an alkaline solution of potassium hydroxide for about 2 hours. The hydroxide part of the reagent penetrates the seaweed and reduces the amount of sulfate in the carrageenan, and increases the 3,6-anhydrogalactopyranose units so the gel strength of the carrageenan in the seaweed is improved. The potassium part of the reagent combines with the carrageenan in the seaweed to produce a gel, and this prevents the carrageenan from dissolving in the hot solution. However, any soluble protein, carbohydrate, and salts do dissolve and are removed when the solution is drained away from the seaweed. The residue, which still looks like seaweed, is washed several times to remove the alkali and anything else that will dissolve in the water. The alkali-treated

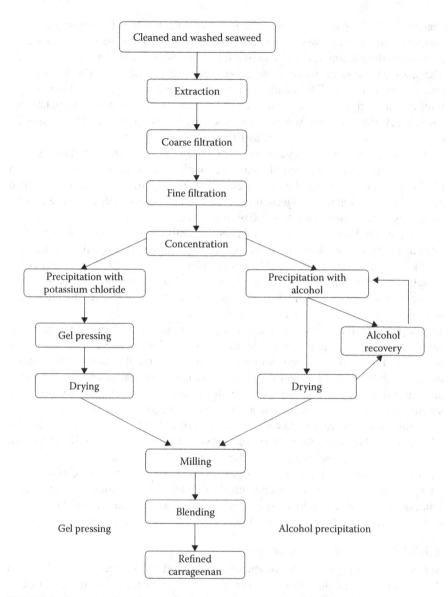

FIGURE 3.12 Flow chart for the production of refined carrageenan. (Adapted from Porse, H., Global seaweed market trends, In *Plenary presentation at XVIth International Seaweed Symposium*, Cebu City, the Philippines, 1998.)

seaweed is now laid out to dry. After approximately 2 days, it is chopped and fed into a mill for grinding to the powder that is sold as SRC or seaweed flour (McHugh 2003). This process is summarized in Figure 3.13.

K. alvarezii is used in this process because it contains mainly kappa-carrageenan, and this is the carrageenan that forms a gel with potassium salts. Iota-containing seaweeds can also be processed by this method, although the markets for

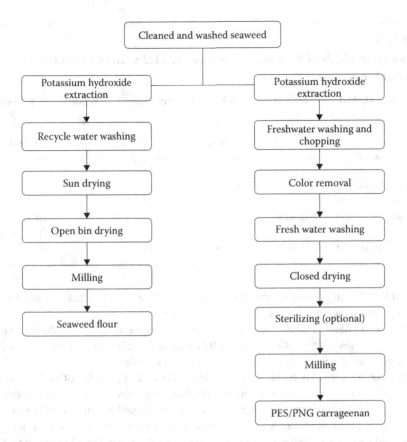

FIGURE 3.13 Flow chart for the production of seaweed flour. (Adapted from Bixler, H.J., *Hydrobiologia*, 326/327, 35–57, 1996.)

iota-carrageenan are significantly less than those for kappa-carrageenan. Lambda-carrageenans do not form gels with potassium and would therefore dissolve and be lost during the alkali treatment.

The simplicity of the process means the product is considerably cheaper than the refined carrageenan. There is no alcohol involved that must be recovered, no distillation equipment to purify alcohol, no equipment for making gels, no refrigeration to freeze the gels, nor any expensive devices to squeeze the water from the gel (McHugh 2003).

3.5.3 REFINED AND SEMIREFINED EXTRACTIONS OF *K. ALVAREZII* ON A LABORATORY SCALE

Both refined and semirefined extractions can be applied to *K. alvarezii*. Recently, Pereira and collaborators reproduced refined and semirefined extractions of *K. alvarezii* in laboratory (unpublished data). Production yields and FTIR-ATR spectra can be found in Table 3.4 and Figure 3.14, respectively.

TABLE 3.4
Production Yields of Refined and Semirefined Laboratory Extractions of *Kappaphycus alvarezii*

Extraction Method	Refined	Semirefined	Semirefined	Refined	Refined
Code	A	B	C	D	E
Alkali used	NaOH (1M)	8.5% KOH	0.5% KOH	–	NaOH (1M)
Temperature of bath (°C)	90	60	60	–	90
Length of extraction (hours)	3	1	1	–	3
Precipitation method	10% KCl	–	–	–	Ethanol precipitation
Yield (% dry weight)	95.8%	89.6%	86.2%	–	58.1%

Table 3.2 brings together the diagnosis for each of the absorption peaks of the eight main carrageenan types.

The broad band at 1240 cm⁻¹, observed in all spectra, is related to the stretching vibration modes of the S=O group. For this reason, its relative intensity is related to the content of the S=O esters group present in the sample.

In contrast with this band, which is always present in samples of sulfated polysaccharides, there are several vibrational band characteristics of carrageenans. For example, the absorption band at 930 cm⁻¹ is related to the vibrations of the 3,6-anhydrogalactose bridges and, therefore, can be found in the spectra of kappa-, iota-, and theta-carrageenans. In addition, the absorption band at 845 cm⁻¹, which is associated with the vibrations of $C_{(4)}$–O–SO$_3$ (a fragment of the sulfated galactose), is characteristic of the kappa, mu, iota, and nu spectra. However, the band at 805 cm⁻¹, which is associated with the vibrations of $C_{(2)}$–O–SO$_3$ (a fragment of sulfated 3,4-anhydrogalactose), can only be observed in iota- and theta-carrageenan spectra. Thus, the relative intensity of the 805 and 845 cm⁻¹ peaks (805/845 cm⁻¹ ratio) allows the determination of the iota/kappa ratio on hybrid carrageenans.

The FTIR-ATR of kappa-carrageenans (see Figure 3.14) shows a peak at 845 cm⁻¹, which is related to the presence of D-galactose-4-sulfate (G4S) and a strong peak at approximately 930 cm⁻¹, which indicates the presence of 3,6-anhydro-D-galactose (DA).

3.6 PHYSICOCHEMICAL CHARACTERISTICS OF CARRAGEENANS

The industrial interest and economic importance of carrageenans are due to their ability to increase the viscosity of solutions or to form thermo-reversible gels (Glicksman 1983). Cations play an essential role in controlling the gelation of these biopolymers (Heyraud et al. 1990; Zhang et al. 1994), and their physicochemical properties depend on the chemical structure and molecular weight (Rochas et al. 1990; Yermak and Khotimchenko 1997).

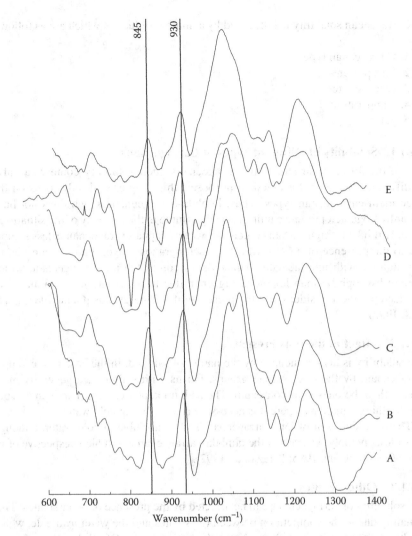

FIGURE 3.14 *Kappaphycus alvarezii* FTIR-ATR spectra of alkaline (KOH) extracted carrageenan (A), semi-refined-extracted 8.5% (B) and 2.5% (C), commercial sample from Sigma (D), and alkaline (NaOH)-extracted carrageenan (E) (unpublished original data).

3.6.1 Solubility

Carrageenans display the solubility characteristic of hydrophilic colloids: it is soluble in water and insoluble in most organic solvents. Alcohols and ketones, although water miscible, do not represent carrageenan solvents; however, they can be tolerated in a blend of carrageenan solutions above 40%.

Some very polar solvents, such as formamide and *N,N*-dimethylformamide, are tolerated when mixed with carrageenan solutions in high proportions. However, these solvents promote a clear swelling of the polymer (Genu 1985; Perez et al. 1992).

Carrageenan solubility is influenced by a number of factors which are as follows:

1. Carrageenan type
2. Ions present
3. Other solutes
4. Temperature
5. pH

3.6.1.1 Solubility of Different Types of Carrageenans

Due to the different structures of carrageenans, their solubility content can also be different. However, for practical purposes, this chapter will only focus on the three main carrageenan types. Thus, lambda-carrageenan, which does not have 3,6-anhydrogalactopyranose units, is easily soluble in the majority of the situations, but only if it has a high sulfate content. However, kappa-carrageenan is less soluble due to the presence of 3,6-anhydro-D-galactopyranose (hydrophobic units) on its constitution. With intermediate characteristics comes the iota-carrageenan, which is more hydrophilic than kappa-carrageenan due to the position of 3,6-anhydro-D-galactopyranose residues and the presence of sulfate groups (Genu 1985; Perez et al. 1992).

3.6.1.2 Effect of the Ions Present

The solubility is also influenced by the nature of salt and, in the case of the kappa-carrageenan, by the ester sulfate groups. Forms with sodium are generally more soluble than the ones with potassium. The sodium kappa-carrageenan is more suitable for those situations where it is necessary a solubility in cold water.

The potassium salt of iota-carrageenan is also insoluble in cold water, although it swallows notably. The salt of the lambda-carrageenan is soluble irrespective of its type of nature (Genu 1985; Perez et al. 1992).

3.6.1.3 Other Solutes

The solubility of carrageenans can be affected by the presence of other solutes. This is mainly due to the competition between the solutes and the water available, which results in a change in the polysaccharide hydration status. Of all the carrageenans, the kappa-type reveals to be more sensitive to the presence of solutes.

Organic salts are more effective in changing the hydration of carrageenans, particularly those whose cation is potassium: 1.5%–2% of potassium chloride is enough to prevent the dissolution of kappa-carrageenan, at room temperature; solutions of 4%–4.6% (or higher values) of sodium chloride have exactly the same effects.

The hydration of kappa-carrageenan is less affected in the presence of sucrose in concentrations equal to 50%; even for higher values, the presence of glycerol is required in large quantities for a significant effect to be observed.

In those cases where more than one solute is present, their combined effect in hydration is generally addictive and can be predicted by understanding their separated effects. For example, in the presence of large amounts of glycerol, solubility is greatly influenced by the presence of potassium ion residues.

The iota-carrageenan dissolves itself, after heating, in solutions with high concentrations of salt and can, therefore, promote gelling in situations where large amounts of salts automatically prevent the use of kappa-carrageenan (Genu 1985).

3.6.2 Dispersion

Although carrageenans are water-soluble polysaccharides, they do not disperse easily due to the formation of a membrane around each carrageenan particle, which leads to the formation of large agglomerates.

If a carrageenan is less soluble, it will disperse easily. For example, the potassium kappa-carrageenan (insoluble in cold water) disperses easier in cold water than the sodium kappa-carrageenan. All the factors that are able to reduce/increase the solubility of carrageenans have the opposite effect regarding their dispersion.

In most part of their applications, carrageenans need to be previously mixed with other ingredients, that is, sugar (1 part of carrageenan for 10 parts of sugar), in order to promote their dispersion. In some cases, carrageenans cannot be mixed with other ingredients; therefore, it is necessary to use a high-speed rotating mixer in order to break the agglomerates previously formed by the addition of carrageenan to water. The mechanical dispersion, through the aid of high-speed mixers, reduces approximately 3% the strength of the dispersion.

Although potassium and calcium carrageenans are less soluble (or insoluble), they are able to form viscous dispersions when in contact with water.

Carrageenans can be dissolved in hot water (60°C–75°C) and form solutions of 7%–8% (Genu 1985).

3.6.3 Reactions

3.6.3.1 Stability in Solution

Acid and oxidative agents can hydrolyze carrageenan solutions, leading to loss of their physical properties due to the cleavage of glycosidic bonds. Acid hydrolysis depends on the following factors:

- pH
- Temperature
- Period of time

In order to promote a reduction on the degradation, it is necessary to use high temperatures and short periods of time. In solution, carrageenans reveal a maximum stability at pH = 9; however, their hot processing cannot be possible at pH values below 3.5. At pH values equal or higher than 6, carrageenan solutions are stable, just like what happens in fish sterilization and in the manufacturing of meat products.

Acid hydrolysis takes place when the carrageenan is dissolved and the temperature and/or processing time are elevated. However, acid hydrolysis does not occur when carrageenans are present in the form of gel (Genu 1985).

3.6.3.2   Reaction with Other Electrically Charged Hydrocolloids

Carrageenans are sulfated galactans with strong negative charge all over the whole pH range found in food products.

They can interact with other electrically charged macromolecules such as proteins, in order to obtain variations regarding viscosity, gelling, stabilization, and precipitation. The result of the carrageenan/protein interaction depends on the pH value of the system and on the isoelectric point of the protein. For example, when carrageenan is mixed with gelatin on a system with a pH value higher than the isoelectric point of gelatin, carrageenan is able to promote the increase of the gel melting temperature without significantly influencing its texture (Genu 1985; Craigie 1990).

The structures of kappa- and iota-carrageenans are presented in the form of double helices that, when joined together, form a tridimensional molecular chain (see Figure 3.15). The structure of lambda-carrageenans does not allow the formation of double helices.

3.6.3.2.1   Gelation of Kappa- and Iota-Carrageenans

In the presence of cations with gelling properties, kappa- and iota-carrageenans are able to form thermo-reversible aqueous gels with concentrations equal or higher than 0.5%. The gel has properties of solids and liquids; thus, it presents a container arrangement but preserves the vapor pressure and the conductivity of the liquid that is made of. The rigidity and the melting and gelification temperatures of the kappa-carrageenan increase with increasing concentrations of potassium ions (Rees 1963; Smidsrod and Grasdalen 1984; Genu 1985; Perez et al. 1992).

In practice, the use of potassium chloride (to increase the consistence of the gel and change the gelification temperature) is limited due to the fact that it adds to the solution a *bitter* taste. The maximum content of potassium chloride that can be added to food products with a delicate flavor is 0.1%–0.2%. In salty foods, potassium chloride can be substituted by sodium chloride.

The most consistent kappa-carrageenan gel is produced in the presence of potassium and calcium ions. However, calcium ions turn the gel brittle, whereas in the presence of potassium ions, the gel becomes elastic, colorless, and cohesive.

The addition of great amounts of sodium ions disturbs the gelification of carrageenan and reduces the gel consistency, a fact that should be taken into account when dealing with gelled meat products, because it is common to add sodium chloride as an additive to these products.

The consistency, texture, and gelification temperature can be influenced by the presence of other solutes such as sucrose. This solute increases the gelification temperature and the melting point of the gel. The addition of sucrose involves the use of high temperatures so that the carrageenan can be dissolved; at this stage, if the pH is acid, there is a possibility of degradation. For this reason, in sucrose blends, the addition of acidic substances must be done as late as possible. In practice, it is not possible to use kappa-carrageenans in food products with sugar contents higher than 60% (Genu 1985).

Contrary to kappa-carrageenan, the iota-carrageenan gel reveals its most consistency in the presence of calcium ions. The resulting gel is elastic and cohesive, and does not exude water. Iota-carrageenan is the only type of carrageenan whose

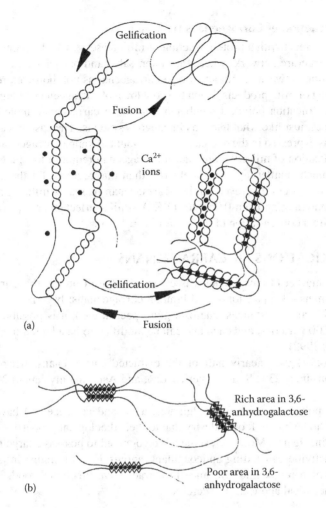

FIGURE 3.15 Jellification mechanism of carrageenans: (a) As soon as the temperature drops, the molecular chains regroup in pairs, linking up two by two, by the action of calcium ions. As soon as the temperature rises, starts the reverse process, fusion. (b) In the process of jellification, the carrageenan chains are placed so that the areas rich in hydrophobic radicals remain face to face. (Adapted from Pereira, L., Estudos em macroalgas carragenófitas [Gigartinales, Rhodophyceae] da costa portuguesa—Aspectos ecológicos, bioquímicos e citológicos. PhD Thesis, Universidade de Coimbra, Coimbra, Portugal, 293, 2004a.)

freeze–thaw process is stable, unlike what happens to kappa-carrageenan gel, as it forms a brittle gel with syneresis (exudes water) (Pereira 2004a).

3.6.3.3 Interaction with Other Gums

In situations where gelatin is traditionally preferred over carrageenans (particularly gelatin desserts), the industry introduced combinations of kappa-carrageenan with other gums in order to simulate the texture produced by gelatin (Pereira 2004a).

3.6.3.4   Reaction of Carrageenans with Milk

Carrageenans react with a protein fraction of milk (casein), which results in a tridimensional structure network, where the water, salts, and particles remain trapped. The interaction between casein and kappa-carrageenan is not, however, responsible for the gelling of milk products. Upon the cooldown of carrageenan (at temperatures below the gelification point), a number of sectors of carrageenan molecules form double helices, just like what happens in aqueous systems. The casein–carrageenan interaction is expressed in the decrease of the amount of kappa-carrageenan required for the gelification of milk: the amount of carrageenan required for the gelification of milk is much smaller (approximately 1/5) than that required for the gelification of an aqueous system. However, lambda-carrageenan increases milk viscosity with concentrations ranging from 0.05% to 0.1%. A similar effect in an aqueous system would require a concentration of 0.5%–1% (Genu 1985).

3.7   APPLICATIONS OF CARRAGEENANS

The global market of carrageenans is essentially based on the three main types of carrageenans—kappa-, iota-, and lambda-carrageenans; by mixing these with other colloids and substances (sucrose, guar, pectin, etc.), it is possible to create more than 200 varieties, and each one can be modified to be adapted to every need (Perez et al. 1992).

Europe (45%) uses nearly half of the extracted carrageenans, whereas North America consumes 23%, South America 12%, and Asia (mainly Japan) 20% (Perez et al. 1992).

Sulfated polysaccharides (e.g., alginates, agar, and carrageenan) have become valuable additives in the food industry due to their rheological properties as gelling and thickening agents. Moreover, some are recognized to possess a large number of biological activities, including anticoagulant, antiviral, and immune-inflammatory activities, which might find relevance in nutraceutical/functional food, cosmetics, and pharmaceutical applications (Pereira 2011a).

3.7.1   Industrial Applications of Carrageenans

3.7.1.1   Food Industry

Carrageenans are versatile as food additives, as they are capable of binding water, promoting gel formation, and acting as thickeners and stabilizing agents. They are used to gel, thicken, or suspend; therefore, they are used in emulsion stabilization, for syneresis control, and for bodying, binding, and dispersion (Pangestuti and Kim 2014).

The first mention of the use of carrageenans in food industry dates from the nineteenth century as they were used as a clarifying beer agent (Booth 1975). Since then, due to the extensive list of their properties and characteristics, the industry of dairy products has emerged and began spreading out.

Standardized carrageenans: Carrageenans are used in a wide diversity of products at concentrations ranging from 0.005% to 3%. The different types of standardized carrageenans are mainly used as gelling agents in aqueous and dairy systems.

Standardization can be obtained by combining different quantities of carrageenans and/or by combining them with an inert substance, such as sucrose or dextrose. The standardization of the mixture of carrageenans and other sugars is recognized and authorized by the European Union and by the Food and Agriculture Organization (FAO) of the United Nations and World Health Organization (WHO) on Food Additives (JECFA).

Due to its reactivity with milk, from which results a gel that is soft and pleasant to papillae, 52% of carrageenan applications referred to the dairy industry (milk industry and derivatives). In gelled milk desserts, the gelling agent that is commonly used is kappa-carrageenan due to its low cost: this carrageenan is generally used in the preparation of *powder flans*. As kappa-carrageenan reveals to be insufficient to maintain the jelly structure of *ready-to-eat* flans, sometimes it has to be combined with iota-carrageenan or with low methoxyl (LM) pectin. This way, it is possible to produce dairy desserts and flans without having to use eggs and flour (Morand et al. 1991).

Iota-carrageenan used in desserts offers the advantage of producing a gel structure comparable to that of gelatin but with a higher melting point. The desserts can then be commercialized in topical countries or in places without refrigeration systems. The stabilization of cocoa particles and chocolate milk fat suspensions can be achieved with the addition of 0.02%–0.03% of kappa-carrageenan. The control of its viscosity and stability can be obtained by the introduction of lambda-carrageenan.

Many products such as soy milk, chocolate and other flavored milks, dairy products, infant formulas, and nutritional supplement beverages rely on carrageenans for their uniform consistencies. A large number of dairy products, such as chocolate milk, milkshakes, flans, yogurts, acid desserts, and industrial ice creams, could not be made, packaged, and stored for long periods of time without these sulfated polysaccharides. Besides dairy products, carrageenans are also used in the preparation of powdered drinks and restructured products such as fruits, vegetables, sausages, fish, crustaceans, soups, and jams, and as wine- and beer- clarifying agent (Ribier and Godineau 1984; Genu 1985; Gayral and Cosson 1986; Morand et al. 1991; Perez et al. 1992; Jensen 1993; Tardieu 1993).

3.7.1.2 Cosmetics Industry

Extract of seaweed is often found on the list of ingredients on cosmetic packages, particularly in face, hand, and body creams or lotions. This usually refers to the use of alginate or carrageenan in the product. There appears to be no shortage of products with ingredients and claims linked to seaweeds: creams, face masks, shampoos, body gels, bath salts, and even a do-it-yourself body wrap kit (FAO 2010).

The cosmetics industry has been increasing the use of carrageenans in the production of lotions, creams, and perfumed gels. The ability of carrageenans to form fine films makes it a good hair conditioner. Carrageenans can also be used in the stabilization of tooth pastes. In this case, they compete directly with carboxymethyl cellulose; carrageenans are then preferred because they resist to enzymes that attack cellulosic colloids. Their capacity to form highly stable aqueous gels against enzymatic degradation makes them a unique emulsifying agent in this kind of pastes. Its structure allows, under these circumstances, the release of flavors and aroma during tooth brushing (Booth 1975; Stanley 1987; De Roeck-Holtzhauer 1991; Indergaard and Ostgaard 1991).

One of the most interesting carrageenan applications is on beauty creams, because the fast evaporation of the emulsion aqueous phase releases on the skin an oiled microfilm with medicinal and protecting properties (Blunden 1991).

3.7.1.3   Pharmaceutical and Biotechnological Applications

Approximately 78% of carrageenans are used in food industry; the remaining 22% are used in cosmetics industry, personal hygiene, pharmaceutical industry (about 10%), and medicine (Morand et al. 1991; Smidsrod and Christensen 1991).

In the pharmaceutical industry, carrageenans are used as laxatives and in the preparation of insoluble compounds. Due to their viscosity, these phycocolloids are used in the treatment of digestive tract ulcers; this is the result of the carrageenan/protein reaction: the difficulty in curing gastric ulcers is due to the fact that once the stomach wall is damaged, the pepsin (gastric enzyme that hydrolyzes proteins) also attacks the cells that form the wall. All of this is aggravated by the acidity of the gastric juice (García et al. 1993). The use of sodium carrageenan triggers two reactions:

1. The reaction of carrageenan/pepsin (positively charged protein at acidic pH), which leads to the neutralization of the enzyme
2. The reduction of gastric acid by the action of sodium

According to Dr. Alain Saury (1984), carrageenans can be used, internally, to treat enteritis, dysentery, diarrhea, chronic constipation, glandular deficiencies, obesity, weight loss, rickets, bronchitis, and pneumonia. Externally, it can be used to treat vaginitis, conjunctivitis, and blepharitis.

Due to the stiff nature of its gels, kappa-carrageenan has a significant application in biotechnology. Its capacity to form strong, colorless, and thermo-reversible gels in the presence of potassium salts makes kappa-carrageenan a possible gelling agent of enzymes and living cells: bacterial and yeast cells can be encapsulated and immobilized in small spheres. These small spheres can then be used, directly or indirectly (modified) in bioconversions (Renn 1990; Skjak-Broek and Martinsen 1991).

The possibility of using plant cells immobilized in carrageenans has been studied for the commercial production of secondary metabolites (Renn 1990). Some special carrageenans, which are able to chemically jellify without the addition of heat, can be used for bacterial growth on solid medium.

Carrageenans can also be used to preserve fish: Americans preserve fish inside fishing boats through the administration of antibiotics; the addition of carrageenans, before freezing, allows a better distribution of the antibiotics and, therefore, the increase of their effectiveness (Ribier and Godineau 1984).

Table 3.5 summarizes the applications of carrageenans and other phycocolloids (e.g., agar and alginates).

TABLE 3.5
Applications of Seaweed Phycocolloids

Use	Phycocolloid	Function
Food Additives		
Baked food	Agar kappa, iota, lambda	Improves quality and controlling moisture
Beer and wine	Alginate kappa	Promotes flocculation and sedimentation of suspended solids
Canned and processed meat	Alginate kappa	Holds the liquid inside the meat and texturing
Cheese	Kappa	Texturing
Chocolate milk	Kappa, lambda	Keeps the cocoa in suspension
Cold preparation puddings	Kappa, iota, lambda	Thickening and gelling
Condensed milk	Iota, lambda	Emulsifies
Dairy creams	Kappa, iota	Stabilizes the emulsion
Fillings for pies and cakes	Kappa	Gives body and texture
Frozen fish	Alginate	Adhesion and moisture retention
Gelled water-based desserts	Kappa + iota / Kappa + iota + CF	Gelling
Gums and sweets	Agar iota	Gelling, texturing
Hot preparation flans	Kappa, kappa + iota	Gelling and improving taste
Jelly tarts	Kappa	Gelling
Juices	Agar kappa, lambda	Viscosity, emulsifier
Low-calorie gelatins	Kappa + iota	Gelling
Milk ice cream	Kappa + GG, CF, X	Stabilizes the emulsion and prevents ice crystals formation
Milkshakes	Lambda	Stabilizes the emulsion
Salad dressings	Iota	Stabilizes the suspension
Sauces and condiments	Agar kappa	Thickens
Soymilk	Kappa + iota	Stabilizes the emulsion and improve taste
Cosmetics		
Shampoos	Alginate	Vitalization interface
Toothpaste	Carrageenan	Increase viscosity
Lotions	Alginate	Emulsification, elasticity, and skin firmness
Lipstick	Alginate	Elasticity, viscosity
Medicinal and Pharmaceutical Uses		
Dental mold	Alginate	Form retention
Laxatives	Alginate carrageenan	Indigestibility and lubrification
Tablets	Alginate carrageenan	Encapsulation
Metal poisoning	Carrageenan	Binds metal
HSV	Alginate	Inhibits virus
Industrial and Lab Uses		
Paints	Alginate	Viscosity and suspension glazing
Textiles	Agar, carrageenan	Sizing and glazing
Paper making	Alginate, agar, carrageenan	Viscosity and thickening

(Continued)

TABLE 3.5 (*Continued*)
Applications of Seaweed Phycocolloids

Use	Phycocolloid	Function
Analytical separation	Alginate, carrageenan	Gelling
Bacteriological media	Agar	Gelling
Electrophoresis gel	Agar, carrageenan	Gelling

Sources: van de Velde, F., de Ruiter, G.A., Carrageenan, in *Biopolymers: Polysaccharides II, Polysaccharides from Eukaryotes*, Vol. 6, Vandamme, E.J., Baets, S.D., Steinbèuchel, A. (eds.), Weinheim, Germany, Wiley-VCH, 2002, pp. 245–274; Dhargalkar, V.K., Pereira, N., *Sci. Cul.*, 71, 60–66, 2005; Pereira, L., Estudos em macroalgas carragenófitas (Gigartinales, Rhodophyceae) da costa portuguesa—Aspectos ecológicos, bioquímicos e citológicos. PhD Thesis, Universidade de Coimbra, Coimbra, Portugal, 293, 2004a; Pereira, L., As algas marinhas e respectivas utilidades. Monografias. Available online at: http://br.monografias.com/trabalhos913/algas-marinhas-utilidades/algas-marinhas-utilidades.pdf, 2008; Pereira, L., Ribeiro-Claro, P.J., Chapter 7—Analysis by vibrational spectroscopy of seaweed with potential use in food, pharmaceutical and cosmetic industries, in *Marine Algae—Biodiversity, Taxonomy, Environmental Assessment and Biotechnology*, Leonel, P., João, M.N. (eds.), Boca Raton, FL, Science Publishers, an Imprint of CRC Press/Taylor & Francis Group, 2014, pp. 225–247.

3.8 BIOLOGICAL ACTIVITIES OF CARRAGEENANS

In recent years, much attention has been focused on polysaccharides isolated from natural sources. During the last decade, numerous bioactive polysaccharides with interesting functional properties have been discovered from seaweeds. The biological features of the sulfated polysaccharides reported till now are antioxidant, antitumor, immunomodulatory, inflammation, anticoagulant, antiviral, antibacterial, and antilipemic (Patel 2012).

Many reports of anticoagulant activity and inhibited platelet aggregation of carrageenan exist (Hawkins and Leonard 1963; Kindness et al. 1979). Among the carrageenan types, lambda-carrageenan (primarily from *C. crispus*) has approximately twice the activity of unfractioned carrageenan and four times the activity of kappa-carrageenan (*K. alvarezii* and *E. denticulatum*). The most active carrageenan has approximately one-fifteenth the activity of heparin but the sulfated galactan from *Grateloupia indica* collected from Indian waters exhibited the anticoagulant activity as potent as heparin (Sen et al. 1994). The principal basis of the anticoagulant activity of carrageenan appeared to be an antithrombotic property. Lambda-carrageenan showed greater antithrombotic activity than kappa-carrageenan, probably due to its higher sulfate content, whereas the activity of the unfractionated material remained between the two.

Several studies have reported that carrageenans have an antiproliferative activity in cancer cell lines *in vitro* and an inhibitory activity of tumor growth in mice (Yuan et al. 2004; Zhou et al. 2004; Yuan et al. 2006; Zhou et al. 2006). In addition, they have an antimetastatic activity by blocking the interactions between cancer cells and the basement membrane, and inhibit tumor cell proliferation and tumor cell adhesion to various substrates, but their exact mechanisms of action are not yet completely understood. Yamamoto et al. (1986) reported that the oral administration of several seaweeds can cause a significant decrease in the incidence of carcinogenesis *in vivo*.

The antioxidant activity of carrageenans has been determined by various methods (Sokolova et al. 2011a; Yuan et al. 2005, 2006). In terms of inhibition of superoxide radical and hydroxyl radical formation, lambda-carrageenan has relatively stronger inhibitory activity compared with kappa- and iota-carrageenans (De Souza et al. 2007). Furthermore, it has also been demonstrated that carrageenans with lower molecular weights had better antioxidant activity (Sun et al. 2010). Souza et al. (2012) isolated a sulfated polysaccharide by aqueous extraction from the red seaweed *Gracilaria birdiae* and observed that the slimy substance exhibits moderate antioxidant properties as measured by DPPH free-radical scavenging effect. Barahona et al. (2011) evaluated the antioxidant capacity of sulfated galactans from red seaweed *G. skottsbergii* and *Schizymenia binderi*—commercial carrageenans—and reported that *S. binderi* exhibited the highest antioxidant capacity.

3.8.1 ANTICOAGULANT AND ANTITHROMBOTIC ACTIVITY

The review by Prajapati et al. (2014) on carrageenan indicates that many reports of the anticoagulant activity of carrageenan exist, describing that lambda-carrageenan has approximately twice the activity of unfractionated carrageenan and four times the activity from kappa-carrageenan, which could be related to the antithrombotic properties and, in turn, correlated with higher sulfate content. Amidolytic studies showed initially that the antithrombotic activity might be mediated via anti-thrombin-III (AT-III), the major mechanism by which heparin acts and carrageenans appeared to inhibit amidolysis of thrombin directly and via AT-III; however, no certainties were achieved in the studies reviewed by Prajapati et al. (2014) dated from 1963 to 1994 (Hawkins and Leonard 1963; Kindness et al. 1979, 1980a,b; Wunderwald et al. 1979; Sen et al. 1994).

More recent studies showed that linear sulfated galactans express the anticoagulant activity as a function of charge density but also depend on monosaccharide composition, number, position, and distribution of sulfate groups along galactan chain (Groth et al. 2009; Yermark et al. 2012). For example, no correlation between the anticoagulant activity of carrageenan and the amount of sulfates was observed by Yermark et al. (2012), indicating that the existence of sulfate groups is not enough to confer the anticoagulant activity, but factors such as the position and distribution of these groups along galactan chain may be determinant for the anticoagulant activity. Araújo et al. (2013) performed a selective sulfation of carrageenan and studied the influence of sulfate regiochemistry on the anticoagulant properties. According to these authors, the sulfation at C_2 of 3,6-anhydro-α-D-Galactopyranose and C_6 of α-D-Galactopyranose increased the anticoagulant activity. The evaluation of the anticoagulant properties of the major types of commercial carrageenans was studied by Silva et al. (2010), which reported that lambda-carrageenan (high sulfate) was the most potent anticoagulant with activated partial thromboplastin time (aPTT) of 240 s at 20 µg, whereas for kappa- (low sulfate) and iota-carrageenans, aPTT was 240 s and 132 s, respectively, but at 100 µg. Liang et al. (2014) studied the effects of the molecular weight of kappa-carrageenan and the sulfate substitution degree and position on the anticoagulant activity; the substitution position rather than the substitution degree of sulfate groups shows the biggest impact on the anticoagulant activity. According to these authors, lambda-carrageenan might have a stronger interaction with the blood cells resulting in prolonged blood coagulation, and the unit containing C-6 substituted sulfate groups, which displays longer clotting time in blood test, might have stronger interactions with the surface proteins on blood cells.

3.8.2   IMMUNOMODULATORY ACTIVITY

The ability of carrageenans to influence the cytokine production by human cells is greatly dependent on the concentration and structure of polysaccharides according to Yermark et al. (2012). These authors reported that (1) all types of carrageenans induced the secretion of anti-inflammatory interleukin (IL)-10 in a dose-dependent manner with a hybrid kappa/beta-carrageenan showing higher activity independent of the concentration and (2) lambda-carrageenan presented the higher activity in the synthesis of IL-6 at 100 μg/m. These differences, according to the authors, may be attributed to the less number of ester sulfate groups on the disaccharide chain of kappa/beta-carrageenan than other types of carrageenans and their hybrid structure. Therefore, the three main dissimilarities in the primary structure, such as the molar ratio of galactose to 3,6-anhydrogalactose, the number and position of the sulfate group in some α-D-galactose residues, and the regular or irregular (hybrid) structure of the carbohydrate chain of polysaccharides, may have the influence on the level of immunomodulation effects (Yermark et al. 2012). Achievements by Xu et al. (2012) showed that kappa-carrageenans have a role in the regulation of immune activity, protecting microglial cells from being activated by lipopolysaccharides (LPS) *in vitro* and that there was a positive relationship between the sulfate content of kappa-carrageenan and its protection function; kappa-carrageenan was able to inhibit the viability and content of nitric oxide (NO), tumor necrosis factor-alpha (TNF-α), and IL-10 released by LPS-activated microglial cell, whereas desulfated derivatives of kappa-carrageenan had much lower activity.

3.8.3   ANTITUMOR ACTIVITY

Liang et al. (2014) studied the effects of molecular weight of kappa-carrageenan and the sulfate substitution degree and position on growth inhibition of human umbilical vein endothelial cells (HUVECs):

1. kappa-carrageenan with high molecular weight inhibits HUVEC proliferation in a concentration-dependent manner—lower molecular weights had lower cytotoxicity effects;
2. the amount of sulfated groups influences the cell viability and the cytotoxicity might be increased with rising sulfate groups;
3. sulfated kappa-carrageenan also causes cell growth inhibition in a concentration-dependent manner (for concentrations lower than 100 μg/mL, no growth inhibition is observed), but iota-carrageenan exhibits no cytotoxicity and promotes the proliferation of HUVEC (for concentrations between 5 and 1000 μg/mL), indicating that the substitution on A2 may eliminate the cytotoxicity and benefit the cell growth.

According to Liang et al. (2014), the substitution position rather than the degree of substitution of the sulfate had the most significant effect on cell proliferation. According to Fedorov et al.'s (2013) review on anticancer and cancer preventive properties of marine polysaccharides, low-molecular-weight carrageenans and carrageenan oligosaccharides seem to be more promising cancer preventive agents than high-molecular-weight carrageenans. Several works with carrageenan oligosaccharides from red algae *Kappaphycus striatus* (formerly *Kappaphycus striatum*), *Chondrus ocellatus*, and *Champia feldmanni* showed antitumor effects; some of them potentiated the antitumor effect of 5-fluorouacil, a therapeutic agent (Yuan et al. 2005; Zhou et al. 2005; Hu et al. 2006; Yuan et al. 2006; Lins et al. 2009). More recently, Yuan et al. (2011) have studied the immunostimulatory and antitumor activity of different derivatives of kappa-carrageenan oligosaccharides from *K. striatum*; treatment with different kappa-carrageenan oligosaccharide derivatives resulted in an increase in tumor inhibition rate and macrophage phagocytosis and cellular immunity, especially on spleen lymphocyte proliferation—sulfated derivative at the dose 200 μg/g per day had the highest antitumor activity with 54% tumor weight inhibition and increase in the activity of nature killer cells up to 76% on S180-bearing mice. According to the results of Yuan et al. (2011), sulfation of carrageenan oligosaccharides can enhance their antitumor effect and boost their antitumor immunity.

Degraded carrageenan has long been known to cause concern because it can cause ulcerative colitis in rats and guinea pigs (Delahunty et al. 1987; Benard et al. 2010). According to Ariffin et al. (2014), the cytotoxicity of food-grade carrageenan prepared in acid and water to liver and intestine cells was still unclear. Therefore, these authors determined the cytotoxic effects of degraded and undegraded carrageenans on cancer and normal human intestinal and liver cell lines through exposition of Caco-2, FHs74 Int, HepG2, and Fa2N-4 cells to degraded and undegraded kappa- and iota-carrageenans. Degraded kappa-carrageenan inhibited cell proliferation in Caco-2, FHs 74 Int, HepG2, and Fa2n-4 cell lines, and the antiproliferative effect was related to apoptosis together with inactivation of cell proliferation genes as determined by morphological observation and molecular analysis. According to these authors, no cytotoxic effect was found in undegraded carrageenan toward normal and cancer intestine and liver cell lines. Jin et al. (2013) demonstrated the antitumor activity of degraded iota-carrageenan toward the osteosarcoma cell line.

The conjugation of antitumor and antiangiogenic activities is an interesting approach to the treatment of cancer. The formation of new blood vascular network from preexisting vessels designed as angiogenesis is considered critical to the growth and metastasis of tumors, and therefore, small molecules with the antiangiogenic activity are important for clinical trials of cancer. Yao et al. (2014) studied the antitumor and antiangiogenic activities of kappa-carrageenan oligosaccharides enzymatically obtained from kappa-carrageenans. A mixture of kappa-neocarrabiose-sulfate, kappa-neocarrahexaose-sulfate, and kappa-neocarraoctaose-sulfate (κOS) was tested, and the antitumor activity was observed using S180 xenograft tumor in Kunming mice models with an inhibiting activity for 200 mg/kg κOS, almost equivalent to positive control. κOS also exhibited the antiangiogenic activity because it was able to inhibit the proliferation, migration, and tube formation of ECV304 cells, which are the main steps of angiogenesis (Yao et al. 2014).

3.8.4 Antimicrobial Activity

There is an increasing interest in animal-pathogenic fungi, particularly in those species that are opportunistic pathogens in people whose immune systems have been compromised, either as a result of disease (e.g., sufferers of acquired immune deficiency syndrome) or as a consequence of immunosuppressive drug therapy (Tariq 1991). The search continues for naturally occurring compounds that may be used in the treatment of mycoses. Marine algae have received a lot of attention as potential sources of compounds possessing a wide range of biological activities, including the antimicrobial properties. The antimicrobial activities of numerous algae species have been tested and reported, presenting an extended spectrum of action against bacteria and fungi (Guedes et al. 2012).

Carrageenans are proved to have effects against some bacterial strains such as *Salmonella enteritidis*, *S. typhimurium*, *Vibrio mimicus*, *Aeromonas hydrophila*, *Escherichia coli*, *Listeria monocytogenes*, and *Staphylococcus aureus*. The growth of all the bacterial strains except *L. monocytogenes* was significantly inhibited by them, particularly by the iota-carrageenan. A growth inhibition experiment using *S. enteritidis* showed that the inhibitory effect of the carrageenans was not bactericidal but bacteriostatic. Removal of the sulfate residues eliminated the bacteriostatic effect of iota-carrageenan, suggesting that the sulfate residues in carrageenan play an essential role in this effect (Venugopal 2008). In 2014, Sebaaly et al. reported that carrageenans isolated from the red alga *Corallina* sp. exhibited the antibacterial activity against *Staphylococcus epidermidis*. IR spectroscopy showed that the isolated carrageenan was of lambda type.

Shanmughapriya et al. (2008) showed that extracts from *Gracilaria corticata* were found to be effective against *Pseudomonas aeruginosa* and *E. coli*. It was also effective against *Micrococcus luteus*, *Staphylococcus epidermidis* and *Enterococcus faecalis*.

In 2007, Salvador et al. evaluated the antifungal and antibacterial activities of 82 Iberian macroalgae (18 Chlorophyta, 25 Phaeophyceae, and 39 Rhodophyta) against three Gram-positive bacteria (*Bacillus subtilis*, *B. cereus*, *S. aureus*), two Gram-negative bacteria (*E. coli* and *P. aeruginosa*), and one yeast (*Candida albicans*). The bioactivity was analyzed from crude extracts of fresh and lyophilized samples. Of the seaweeds analyzed, 67% were active against at least one of the six test microorganisms. The highest percentage of active taxa was found in Phaeophyceae (84%), followed by Rhodophyta (67%) and Chlorophyta (44%). Nevertheless, red algae had both the highest values and the broadest spectrum of bioactivity. In particular, *Bonnemaisonia asparagoides*, *B. hamifera*, and *Asparagopsis armata* (and *Falkenbergia rufolanosa* phase) (Bonnemaisoniales) were the most active taxa. In this study, Ceramiales and Gigartinales had a noteworthy antimicrobial activity, and Bonnemaisoniales was the order that had the highest bioactivity.

In another study, extracts from 44 species of seaweed from Canary Islands (Spain) were screened for the production of antifungal and antibacterial compounds against a panel of Gram-negative and Gram-positive bacteria, mycobacterium, yeasts and fungi. A total of 28 species displayed the antibacterial activity, of which 6 also showed the antifungal activity. Regarding the antifungal activity, six of the species tested—*Asparagopsis taxiformis* (Rhodophyta), *Cymopolia barbata* (Chlorophyta), *Caulerpa prolifera* (Chlorophyta), *Dictyota* sp. (Phaeophyceae), *Ulva muscoides* (formerly *Enteromorpha muscoides*) (Chlorophyta), and *Osmundea hybrida* (Rhodophyta) presented the activity against the filamentous fungus *Aspergillus fumigatus*, and/or the yeasts *C. albicans* and *Saccharomyces cereviseae*. *A. taxiformis* and *C. barbata* were the species with the strongest activities against the broadest spectrum of target microorganisms. All the species with the antibacterial activity were active against Gram-positive bacteria (*S. aureus* and *B. subtilis*), whereas only two species, *A. taxiformis* and *O. hybrida*, were active against mycobacterium. Only one species—*A. taxiformis*—showed the activity against the whole panel of nine target microorganisms: *P. aeruginosa*, *Serratia marcescens*, *Enterococcus faecium*, *Mycobacterium smegmatis*, *S. aureus*, *B. subtilis*, *C. albicans*, *S. cereviseae*, and *A. fumigatus*. (Gonzalez del Val et al. 2001). Genovese et al. (2013) also showed that *A. taxiformis* has the antifungal activity against *A. fumigatus*, *A. terreus*, and *A. flavus*.

In 2011, Stein et al. reported that five species of the red alga *Laurencia* (Rhodophyta) showed the fungistatic (the lowest concentration of the agent that results in the maintenance or reduction of the inoculum) and/or fungicidal activity (the lowest concentration of the agent that results in no growth) against three strains of pathogenic fungi—*C. albicans*, *C. parapsilosis*, and *Cryptococcus neoformans*. Chloroform and methanol extracts of *Laurencia dendroidea* showed the fungistatic effects against *C. albicans*. Crude water extracts of the species showed a reasonable percentage of inhibition against *C. neoformans*; the chloroform extract of *L. catarinensis* proved to have a fungistatic effect against *C. parapsilosis*, and a fungicidal effect against *C. albicans* and *C. neoformans*; of all the extracts of *Laurencia intricata*, the chloroform extract was the most active; a fungistatic effect was observed for the methanol extract of *L. aldingensis* against the three pathogenic fungi. The hexane and chloroform extracts of this species had fungicidal effects against *C. parapsilosis*. The same extracts were fungistatic against *C. albicans* and *C. neoformans*. Thus, *L. aldingensis* appears to be a particularly interesting alga, showing an activity against all the three strains tested.

Tariq (1991) reported that extracts of *Dilsea carnosa*, *Laurencia pinnatifida*, *Odonthalia dentata*, and *Vertebrata lanosa* (formerly *Polysiphonia lanosa*) reduced the rate of colony extension in *Microsporum canis* and *Trichophyton verrucosum*, with seasonal variations in the levels of inhibitory activity.

3.8.5 Antiviral Activity

The potential antiviral activity of marine algal polysaccharides was first shown by Gerber et al. (1958), who observed that the polysaccharides extracted from *Gelidium robustum* (formerly *Gelidium cartilagineum*) (Rhodophyta) protected the embryonic eggs against influenza B or mumps virus. Many species of marine algae contain significant quantities of complex structural sulfated polysaccharides, which have been shown to inhibit the replication of enveloped viruses, including the members of the flavivirus, togavirus, arenavirus, rhabdovirus, orthopoxvirus, and herpesvirus families (Witvrouw and De Clercq 1997). Polysaccharides extracted from Rhodophyta have been shown to exhibit the antiviral activity against a wide spectrum of viruses, including the important human pathogenic agents such as human immunodeficiency virus (HIV), herpes simplex virus (HSV), vesicular stomatitis virus, and cytomegalovirus (Witvrouw and De Clercq 1997). The chemical structure, including the degree of sulfation, molecular weight, constituent sugars, conformation, and dynamic stereochemistry, determines the antiviral activity of algal sulfated polysaccharides (Lüscher-Mattli 2000; Damonte et al. 2004; Adhikari et al. 2006). In addition, both the degree of sulfation and the distribution of sulfate groups on the constituent polysaccharides play an important role in the antiviral activity of these sulfated polysaccharides. Algal polysaccharides with low degrees of sulfation are generally inactive against viruses (Damonte et al. 2004).

Marine polysaccharides can either inhibit the replication of virus through interfering viral life cycle or improve the host antiviral immune responses to accelerate the process of viral clearance. The life cycle of viruses differs greatly between species, but there are six basic stages in the life cycle of viruses: viral adsorption, viral penetration, uncoating of capsids, biosynthesis, viral assembly, and viral release. Marine polysaccharides can inhibit the viral life cycle at different stages or directly inactivate virions before virus infection. A specific antiviral mechanism of marine polysaccharides is commonly related to specific structure features of the polysaccharides and specific viral serotypes (Damonte et al. 2004).

Carrageenan might inhibit virus infection via direct actions on the virus surface by its negative charge (Wang et al. 2012). Several studies showed that carrageenan has a direct virucidal action on some enveloped viruses, which makes the viruses lose the ability to infect cells, thus effectively reducing the virus multiplication. Carlucci et al. (2002) found that lambda-type carrageenan could firmly bind to the HSV, leading to the inactivation of the HSV virion, thus inhibiting the replication of HSV. Their studies further suggest that carrageenan changes the structure of the glycoproteins gB and gC of HSV (Carlucci et al. 1999; Carlucci et al. 2002). Moreover, Harden et al. (2009) reported that carrageenan polysaccharides derived from red algae could directly inactivate HSV-2 at low concentrations. The virucidal activities increase with increased molecular weight of carrageenan polysaccharide up to 100 kDa, after which the virucidal activities level off. The direct virucidal actions of carrageenan may be due to the formation of a stable virion–carrageenan complex where binding is not reversible and hence the sites on the viral envelope required for virus attachment to host cells are occupied by the sulfated polysaccharide, which renders the virus unable to complete the subsequent infection process (Damonte et al. 2004).

Several studies have shown that carrageenan can mask the positive charge of host cell surfaces by the negative charge of its sulfate groups, so as to interfere with the adsorption process of viruses. Mazumder et al. (2002) obtained a high molecular weight sulfated galactan from red algae, and showed its antiviral activities against HSV 1 and 2 in bioassays, which is likely due to an inhibition of the initial viral attachment to the host cells. Carlucci et al. (1997, 1999) noted that lambda-carrageenan and partially cyclized mu/iota-carrageenan from G. skottsbergii have potent antiviral effects against different strains of HSV types 1 and 2 during the virus adsorption stage. They subsequently confirmed the firm binding of carrageenan to virus receptors on the host cell surface. Their studies demonstrate that lambda-carrageenan interferes with the adsorption process of the virus to the host cell surfaces.

Buck et al. (2006) found that carrageenan could directly bind to the HPV capsid, so as to inhibit not only the viral adsorption process but also the subsequent entry and uncoating process of the virus. They also found that the inhibition actions of carrageenan against HPV might be related to a mechanism that is independent of the heparan sulfate after viral adsorption. Moreover, Talarico et al. (2005, 2007a,b) reported that lambda- and iota-carrageenans could interfere with both dengue virus (DENV)-2 adsorption and internalization into host cells, and they are only effective if added together with the virus or shortly after infection. The mechanism of this inhibition action may be due to that although DENV virus can enter into host cell in the presence of carrageenans, its subsequent uncoating and releasing from endosomes may be interfered by the carrageenans. The inhibition action of iota-carrageenan on the uncoating process of DENV may be attributed to the direct interaction of carrageenans with the virus membrane glycoprotein E. Talarico et al. (2007a, 2011) also reported that iota-carrageenan could inhibit DENV replication in mammalian and mosquito cells, and the mode of action of iota-carrageenan in both cell types is strikingly different.

Yamada et al. (1997, 2000) reported that O-acylated carrageenan polysaccharides with different molecular weights had an increased anti-HIV activity by depolymerization and sulfation. Thus, the antiviral activities of carrageenan polysaccharides are associated with their molecular weights and the content of sulfates.

In conclusion, the antiviral activities of carrageenans are very broad, which can suppress the replication of both enveloped and nonenveloped viruses. The antiviral effects of carrageenans are closely related to the molecular weights and the degree of sulfation of them. Moreover, the inhibitory actions of carrageenans on different viruses are usually different, which are associated with the types of carrageenans, the virus serotypes, and the host cell itself (Damonte et al. 2004; Talarico et al. 2005).

3.8.6 OTHER BIOLOGICAL ACTIVITIES

In vitro antioxidant properties of lambda-, iks-, kappa/beta- and kappa/iota-carrageenans from Gigartinaceae and Tichocarpaceae families were studied by Sokolova et al. (2011b) through several *in vitro* tests. According to the authors, the antioxidant action of these different carrageenans against reactive oxygen/nitrogen species depends on several factors: polysaccharide concentration, presence of hydrophobic 3,6-anhydrogalactose unit, and amount and position of sulfate groups, and the oxidant agent—iks-carrageenan containing three sulfate groups per disaccharide unit and a 3,6-anhydrogalactose unit was among the most effective superoxide anion and nitric oxide scavenger. According to Sun et al. (2010), kappa-carrageenans with lower molecular weight had a higher antioxidant activity as scavengers of superoxide anions and hydroxyl radicals.

The antimutagenic activity of carrageenans was studied in cultured meristematic cells of *Allium cepa* (Nantes et al. 2014). The results showed that carrageenan is not mutagenic; rather, it has a significant chemopreventive potential that is mediated by both demutagenic and bio-antimutagenic activities. This study demonstrated that carrageenan could absorb agents that are toxic to DNA and inactivate them.

Carrageenan could also modulate the enzymes of the DNA repair system. Damage reduction ranged from 62.5% to 96.7%, reflecting the compound's high efficiency in preventing the type of mutagenic damage that may be associated with tumor development (Nantes et al. 2014).

3.9 FOOD ADDITIVE CARRAGEENAN AND ITS SAFETY

Carrageenan has been used as a safe additive in food industry and a pharmaceutical excipient (Li et al. 2014; Weiner 2014), but several questions about the safety of carrageenans have been raised since many years ago (Li et al. 2014). Watson (2008) published a review and analysis on public health and carrageenan regulation. The author discussed four cases of public controversies about carrageenan safety, which enable to contextualize the reader in relation to regulatory responses and their public health significance. According to Watson (2008), "it is concluded that current assessments of risk associated with carrageenan have in some contexts, failed to take into account the full spectrum of safety assessments that have been carried out and the maturing of food additive regulations thereby allowing a myth of risk to continue." More recent critical reviews on the use of carrageenan as a food additive were duly performed by Mckim (2014) who focused on *in vitro* studies, potential pitfalls, and implications for human health and safety, and by Weiner (2014) who focused on *in vivo* safety studies. The reading of these two papers is recommended for readers pursuing more knowledge and details in this topic. The authors of this chapter will only summarize the main lines about carrageenan safety and, in particular, the main worries arisen in recent years.

According to Mckim (2014), confusion over nomenclature, basic carrageenan chemistry, type of carrageenan tested, interspecies biology, and misinterpretation on both *in vivo* and *in vitro* data has resulted in the dissemination of incorrect information regarding the safety of carrageenan. For example, poligeenan that is produced by subjecting carrageenans to acid hydrolysis at low pH (±1.0) and high temperatures ($>80°C$) for a long period of time with molecular weights between 10,000 and 20,000 Da, it has no utility in the food sector. Poligeenan has been shown to be responsible for inflammatory responses in the intestine, and carrageenan has not shown to be broken down in the gastrointestinal tract to poligeenan by acid hydrolysis or microflora. Commercial carrageenan has a molecular weight ranging between 200,000 and 800,000 Da, and fragments with molecular weight range between 20,000 and 50,000 Da (Mckim, 2014). According to Weiner (2014), it is recognized by the research community that intact carrageenan is not degraded by gastrointestinal microflora to poligeenan because intestinal enzymes are not able to recognize the unique alternating α-(1–3) and β-(1–4) glycosidic bonds of carrageenan, and enzymes such as carrageenases and galactosidades are not present in the human gastrointestinal tract or microflora. Due to their high-molecular-weight structure and stability when bound to protein, carrageenans are not significantly absorbed and metabolized or do not significantly affect the absorption of nutrients. Doses up to 5% in the subchronic and chronic feeding studies in rodents did not induce any toxicological effects other than soft stools or diarrhea (a common effect caused by nondigestible high-molecular-weight compounds) neither produce intestinal ulceration (Weiner 2014).

According to the Joint Food and Agriculture Organization (FAO) of the United Nations and World Health Organization (WHO) on Food Additives (JECFA) (79th meeting, June 2014) regarding the use of carrageenan in infant formula and in formulas for special medical purposes intended for infants, this committee concluded that concentrations up to 1000 mg/L are not of concern. According to Weiner (2014), the use of carrageenan in infant formula has been shown to be safe in infant baboons (McGill et al. 1977), and its use in human infants at a level of 0.1% in formula has been demonstrated to be safe when administered for up to 112 days (Borsches et al. 2002).

REFERENCES

Adhikari, U., C.G. Mateu, K. Chattopadhyay, C.A. Pujol, E.B. Damonte, and B. Ray. 2006. Structure and antiviral activity of sulfated fucans from *Stoechospermum marginatum*. *Phytochemistry* 67: 1474–2482.

Amimi, A., A. Mouradi, T. Givernaud, N. Chiadmi, and M. Lahaye. 2001. Structural analysis of *Gigartina pistillata* carrageenans (Gigartinaceae, Rhodophyta). *Carbohydrate Research* 333(4): 271–279.

Aquino, R.S., C. Grativol, and P.A.S. Mourão. 2011. Rising from the sea: Correlations between sulphated polysaccharides and salinity in plants. *PLoS One* 6: e18862.

Araki, C.H. 1937. Acetylation of agar like substance of gelidium amansii. *Journal of the Chemical Society* 58: 1338–1350.

Araújo, C.A., M.D. Noseda, T.R. Cipriani, A.G. Gonçalves, M.E.R. Duarte, and D.R.B. Ducatti. 2013. Selective sulfation of carrageenans and the influence of sulfate regiochemistry on anticoagulant properties. *Carbohydrate Polymers* 91: 483–491.

Ariffin, S.H.Z., W.W. Yeen, I.Z.Z. Abidin, R.M.A. Wahab, Z.Z. Ariffin, and S. Senafi. 2014. Cytotoxicity effect of degraded and undegraded kappa and iota carrageenan in human intestine and liver cell lines. *BMC Complementary and Alternative Medicine* 14: 508.

Armisen, R. and F. Galatas. 1987. Chapter 1—Production, properties and uses of agar. In *Production and Utilization of Products from Commercial Seaweeds*, McHugh, D.J. (ed.). FAO Fisheries Technical Paper 288, Rome, Italy.

Armisen, R. and F. Galatas. 2000. Agar. In *Handbook of Hydrocolloids*, Phillips, G.O., Williams, P.A. (eds.). Boca Raton, FL: CRC Press, pp. 21–40.

Barahona, T., N.P. Chandía, M.V. Encinas, B. Matsuhiro, and E.A. Zuniga. 2011. Antioxidant capacity of sulfated polysaccharides from seaweeds. A kinetic approach. *Food Hydrocolloids* 25: 529–535.

Benard, C., A. Cultrone, C. Michel, C. Rosales, J. Segain, M. Lahaye, J. Galmiche, C. Cherbut, and H.M. Blottière. 2010. Degraded carrageenan causing colitis in rates induces TNF secretion and ICAM-1 upregulation in monocytes through NF-kB activation. *PLoS One* 5(1): e8666.

Bixler, H.J. 1996. Recent developments in manufacturing and marketing carrageenan. *Hydrobiologia* 326/327: 35–57.

Bixler, H.J. and H. Porse. 2011. A decade of change in the seaweed hydrocolloid industry. *Journal of Applied Phycology* 23: 321–335.

Blunden, G. 1991. Chapter 3—Agricultural uses of seaweeds and seaweed extracts. In *Seaweed, Resources in Europe. Uses and Potential*, Guiry, M.D. (ed.). Chichester: John Wiley & Sons, pp. 65–93.

Booth, E. 1975. Seaweeds in industry. In *Chemical Oceanography*, Vol 4, Riely, J.P., Skirrow, G. (eds.). New York: Academic Press, pp. 219–268.

Borsches, M.W., B. Barretr-Reis, G.E. Baggs, and T.A. William. 2002. Growth of healthy term infants fed a powdered casein hydrolysate-based formula (CHF). *FASEB Journal* 16: A66.

Buck, C.B., C.D. Thompson, J.N. Roberts, M. Muller, D.R. Lowy, and J.T. Schiller. 2006. Carrageenan is a potent inhibitor of papillomavirus infection. *PLOS Pathogens* 2, e69.

Campo, V.L., D.F. Kawano, D.B. da Silva, and I. Carvalho. 2009. Carrageenans: Biological properties, chemical modifications and structural analysis—A review. *Carbohydrate Polymers* 77: 167–180.

Carlucci, M.J., C.A. Pujol, M. Ciancia, M.D. Noseda, M.C. Matulewicz, E.B. Damonte, and A.S. Cerezo. 1997. Antiherpetic and anticoagulant properties of carrageenans from the red seaweed Gigartina skottsbergii and their cyclized derivatives: Correlation between structure and biological activity. *International Journal of Biological Macromolecules* 20: 97–105.

Carlucci, M.J., L.A. Scolaro, and E.B. Damonte. 1999. Inhibitory action of natural carrageenans on herpes simplex virus infection of mouse astrocytes. *Chemotheraphy* 45: 429–436.

Carlucci, M.J., L.A. Scolaro, and E.B. Damonte. 2002. Herpes simplex virus type 1 variants arising after selection with an antiviral carageenan: Lack of correlation between drug susceptibility and synphenotype. *Journal of Medical Virology* 68: 92–98.

Chapman, R.L. 2013. Algae: The world's most important "plants"—An introduction. *Mitigation Adaptation Strategies for Global Change* 8(1): 5–12.

Chopin, T., B.F. Kerin, and R. Mazerolle. 1999. Phycocolloid chemistry as taxonomic indicator of phylogeny in the Gigartinales, Rhodophyceae: A review and current developments using Fourier transform infrared diffuse reflectance spectroscopy. *Phycological Research* 47: 167–188.

Chopin, T. and E. Whalen. 1993. A new and rapid method for carrageenan identification by FTIR diffuse-reflectance spectroscopy directly on dried, ground algal material. *Carbohydrate Research* 246: 51–59.

Craigie, J.S. 1990. Cell walls. In *Biology of the Red Algae*, Cole, K.M., Sheath R.G. (eds.). Cambridge: Cambridge University Press, pp. 221–257.

Critchley, A.T. and M. Ohno. 1998. *Seaweed Resources of the World*. Yokosuka, Japan: Japan International Cooperation Agency, p. 431.

Damonte, E.B., M.C. Matulewicz, and A.S. Cerezo. 2004. Sulfated seaweed polysaccharides as antiviral agents. *Current Medicinal Chemistry* 11: 2399–2419.

Daroch, M., S. Geng, and G. Wang. 2013. Recent advances in liquid biofuel production from algal feedstocks. *Applied Energy* 102: 1371–1381.

Delahunty, T., L. Recher, and D. Hollander. 1987. Intestinal permeability changes in rodents: A possible mechanism for degraded carrageenan-induced colitis. *Food Chemistry and Toxicology* 25: 113–118.

De Roeck-Holtzhauer, Y. 1991. Chapter 4—Uses of seaweeds in cosmetics. In *Seaweed, Resources in Europe. Uses and Potential*, Guiry, M.D., Blunden, G. (eds.). Chichester: John Wiley & Sons, pp. 83–94.

De Souza, M.C.R., C.T. Marques, C.M.G. Dore, F.R.F. da Silva, H.A.O. Rocha, and E.L. Leite. 2007. Antioxidant activities of sulfated polysaccharides from brown and red seaweeds. *Journal of Applied Phycology* 19: 153–160.

Dhargalkar, V.K. and N. Pereira. 2005. Seaweeds: Promising plants of the millennium. *Science and Culture* 71: 60–66.

Draget, K.I., O. Smidsrød, and S. Skjåk-Broek. 2004. Alginates from algae. In *Biopolymers, Polysaccharides II: Polysaccharides from Eukaryotes*, vol. 6, Baets, S.D., Vandamme E., Steinbüchel, A. (eds.). Weinheim, Germany: Wiley, pp. 215–224.

Earons, G. 1994. Littoral seaweed resource management. A report prepared for the minch project by Environment & Resource Technology Ltd Prepared for the Web by Gavin Earons, IT Unit, Comhairle nan Eilean Siar, 37.

FAO. 2004. Highlights of special studies. In *The State of World Fisheries and Aquaculture*, FAO, Sofia.

FAO. 2010. The state of world fisheries and aquaculture. FAO, Rome, Italy, 197.

Fedorov, S.N., S.P. Ermakova, T.N. Zvyagintseva, and V.A. Stonik. 2013. Anticancer and cancer preventive properties of marine polysaccharides: Some results and prospects. *Marine Drugs* 11: 4876–4901.

García, I., R. Castroviel, and C. Neira. 1993. Las algas en galicia. Alimentacion y otros usos. Xunta de Galicia, 229.

Gayral, P. and J. Cosson. 1986. Connaitre et Reconnaitre les Algues Marines. Ouest-France: 38–44.

Genovese, G., S. Leitner, S.A. Minicante, and C. Lass-Florl. 2013. The Mediterranean red alga *Asparagopsis taxiformis* has antifungal activity against *aspergillus* species. *Mycoses* 56: 516–519.

Genu. 1985. Carrageenan. GENU, the Copenhagen Pectin Factory, Ltd., 19.

Gerber, P., J. Dutcher, E. Adams, and J. Sherman. 1958. Protective effect of seaweed extracts for chicken embryos infected with influenza virus B or mumps virus. *Proceedings of the Society for Experimental Biology and Medicine* 99: 590–593.

Givernaud-Mouradi, A. 1992. Recherches biologiques et biochimiques pour la production d'agarose chez Gelidium latifolium (Rhodophycées, Gálidiales). These de Doctorat D'État, Sciences, University de Caen, France, 351.

Glicksman, M. 1983. Red seaweed extracts. In *Food Hydrocolloids*, Vol. 2, Glicksman, M. (ed.). Boca Raton, FL: CRC Press, pp. 73–113.

Gonzalez del Val, A., G. Platas, A. Basilio, A. Cabello, J. Gorrochategui, I. Suay, F. Vicente, E. Portillo, M. Jimenez del Rio, G.C. Reina, and F. Pelaez. 2001. Screening of anti-microbial activities in red, green and brown macroalgae from Gran Canaria (Canary Islands, Spain). *International Microbiology—The Official Journal of the Spanish Society for Microbiology* 4: 35–40.

Graham, L.E. and L.W. Wilcox. 2000. *Algae.* Upper Saddle River, NJ: Prentice Hall, p. 640.

Groth, L., N. Grunewald, and A. Susanne. 2009. Pharmacological profiles of animal- and nonanimal-derived sulfated polysaccharides—Comparison of unfractionated heparin, rhe semisynthetic glucan sulphate PS3, and the sulfated polysaccharide fraction isolated from Delesseria sanguinea. *Glycobiology* 19: 408–410.

Guiry, M.D. and G. Blunden. 1991. *Seaweed Resources in Europe: Uses and Potential.* Chichester: John Wiley & Sons, p. 432.

Guiseley, K.B. 1989. Chemical and physical properties of algal polysaccharides used for cell immobilization. *Enzyme and Microbial Technology* 11: 706–716.

Guedes, E.A., M.A. Dos Santos Araújo, A.K. Souza, L.I. de Souza, L.D. de Barros LD, F.C. de Albuquerque Maranhão, and A.E. Santana. 2012. Antifungal activities of different extracts of marine macroalgae against dermatophytes and *Candida* species. *Mycopathologia* 174: 223–232.

Gurgel, C.F.D. and J. Lopez-Bautista. 2007. Red algae. In *Encyclopedia of Life Sciences.* Chichester, UK: John Wiley & Sons. doi:10.1002/9780470015902.a0000335.

Harden, E.A., R. Falshaw, S.M. Carnachan, E.R. Kern, and M.N. Prichard. 2009. Virucidal activity of polysaccharide extracts from four algal species against herpes simplex virus. *Antiviral Research* 83: 282–289.

Hawkins, W.W. and V.G. Leonard. 1963. Antithrombic activity of carrageenan in human blood. *Canadian Journal of Biochemistry and Physiology* 41(5): 1325–1327.

Heyraud, A., M. Rinaudo, and C. Rochas. 1990. Physical and chemical properties of phycocolloids. In *Introduction to Applied Phycology*, Akatsuka, I. (ed.). The Hague, the
Netherlands: SPB Academic Publishing BV, pp. 151–176.

Hu, X., X. Jiang, E. Aubree, P. Boulenguer, and A.T. Critchley. 2006. Preparation and in vivo
antitumor activity of kappa-carrageenan oligosaccharides. *Pharmacology Biology* 44:
646–650.

Hughes, A.D., K.D. Black, I. Campbell, J.J. Heymans, K.K. Orr, M.S. Stanley, and M.S.
Kelly. 2013. Comments on "Prospects for the use of macroalgae for fuel in Ireland and
UK: An overview of marine management issues". *Marine Policy* 38: 554–556.

Indergaard, M. and K. Ostgaard. 1991. Chapter 7—Polysaccharides for food and pharmaceutical uses. In *Seaweed, Resources in Europe. Uses and Potential*, Guiry, M.D.,
Blunden, G. (eds.). Chichester: John Wiley & Sons, pp. 169–183.

Jensen, A. 1993. Present and future needs for algae and algal products. *Hydrobiologia*
260/261: 15–23.

Jin, Z., Y.X. Han, and X.R. Han. 2013. Degraded iota-carrageenan can induce apoptosis in
human osteosarcoma cells via the Wnt/Beta-Catenin signaling pathway. *Nutrition and
Cancer* 65(1): 126–131.

Khotimchenko, Y.S., V.V. Kovalev, O.V. Savchenko, and O.A. Ziganshina. 2001. Physical-
chemical properties, physiological activity, and usage of alginates, the polysaccharides
of brown algae. *Russian Journal of Marine Biology* 1: 53–64.

Kilinç. B., S. Cirik, G. Turan, H. Tekogul, and E. Koru. 2013. Seaweeds for food and industrial applications. In *Food Industry*, Muzzalupo, I. (ed.). ISBN: 978-953-51-0911-2,
InTech, doi:10.5772/53172.

Kim, I.H. and J.H. Lee. 2008. Antimicrobial activities against methicillin resistant
Staphylococcus aureus from macroalgae. *Journal of Industrial Engineering Chemistry*
14: 568–572.

Kim, S.K. and R. Pangestuti. 2015. An overview of phycocolloids: The principal com-
mercial seaweed extracts. In *Marine Algae Extracts: Processes, Products, and
Applications*, vol. 2, Kim, S.K., Chojnacka, K. (eds.). Weinheim, Germany: Wiley-
VCH, pp. 319–331.

Kindness, G., F.B. Williamson, and W.F. Long. 1979. Effect of polyanetholesulphonic acid
and xylan sulphate on antithrombin III activity. *Biochemical and Biophysical Research
Communications* 13(88): 1062–1068.

Kindness, G., W.F. Long, and F.B. Williamson. 1980a. Anticoagulant effects of sulphated
polysaccharides in normal and antithrombin III-deficient plasmas. *British Journal of
Pharmacology* 69: 675–677.

Kindness, G., F.B. Williamson, and W.F. Long. 1980b. Involvement of antithrombin III in anticoagulant effects of sulphated polysaccharides. *Biochemical Society Transactions* 8:
82–83.

Lahaye, M. 2001. Chemistry and physico-chemistry of phycocolloids. *Cahiers de Biologie
Marine* 42(1–2): 137–157.

Larsen, B., D.M.S.A. Salem, M.A.E. Sallam, M.M. Mishrikey, and A.I. Beltagy. 2003.
Characterization of the alginates from algae harvested at the Egyptian red sea coast.
Carbohydrate Research 338: 2325–2336.

Leal, D., B. Matsuhiro, M. Rossi, and F. Caruso. 2008. FT-IR Spectra of alginic acid block
fractions in three species of brown seaweeds. *Carbohydrate Research* 343: 308–316.

Lee, K.Y. and D.J. Mooneya. 2012. Alginate: Properties and biomedical applications. *Progress
in Polymer Science* 37(1): 106–126.

Li, L., R. Ni, Y. Shao, and S. Mao. 2014. Carrageenan, and its applications in drug delivery.
Carbohydrate Polymers 103: 1–11.

Liang, W., X. Mao, X. Peng, and S. Tang. 2014. Effects of sulfate group in red seaweed polysa-
chraide anticoagulant activity and cytotoxicity. *Carbohydrate Polymers* 101: 776–785.

Lins, K.O., D.P. Bezerra, A.P. Alves, N.M. Alencar, M.W. Lima, V.M. Torres, W.R. Farias, C. Pessoa, M.O. de Moraes, and L.V. Costa-Lotufo. 2009. Antitumor properties of a sulfated polysaccharide from the red seaweed *Champia feldmannii* (Diaz-Pifferer). *Journal Applied Toxicology* 29: 20–26.

Lobban, C.S. and D.J. Chapman. 1988. Experimental phycology: A laboratory manual. *Phycological Society of America*. Cambridge: Cambridge University Press.

Lorbeer, A.J., R. Tham, and W. Zhang. 2013. Potential products from the highly diverse and endemic macroalgae of Southern Australia and pathways for their sustainable production. *Journal of Applied Phycology* 25(3): 717–732.

Lüscher-Mattli, M. 2000. Polyanions—A lost chance in the fight against HIV and other virus diseases? *Antiviral Chemistry and Chemotherapy* 11: 249–259.

Matsuhiro, B. 1996. Vibrational spectroscopy of seaweed galactans. *Hydrobiologia* 327: 481–489.

Mazumder, S., P.K. Ghosal, C.A. Pujol, M.J. Carlucci, E.B. Damonte, and B. Ray. 2002. Isolation, chemical investigation and antiviral activity of polysaccharides from *Gracilaria corticata* (Gracilariaceae, Rhodophyta). *International Journal of Biological Macromolecules* 31: 87–95.

McCandless, E.L. 1981. Chapter 16—Polysaccharides of the seaweeds. In *The Biology of Seaweeds*, Christopher S. Lobban and Michael J. Wynne (eds.). La Jolla, CA: Blackwel Scientific Publications, pp. 559–588.

McGill, Jr, H.C., C.A. McMahan, H.S. Wigodsky, and H. Sprinz. 1977. Carrageenan in formula and infant baboon development. *Gastroenterology* 73: 512–517.

McHugh, D.J. 2003. A guide to the seaweed industry. FAO, Fisheries Technical Paper 441: 73–90.

McKim, J.M. 2014. Food additive carrageenan: Part I: A critical review of carrageenan in vitro studies, potential pitfalls, and implications for human health and safety. *Critical Review in Toxicology* 44: 211–243.

Minghou, J. 1990. Processing and extraction of phycocolloids. In *Regional Workshop on the Culture and Utilization of Seaweeds*, Vol. II. FAO Technical Resource Papers. Cebu City: the Philippines.

Morand, P., B. Carpentier, R.H. Charlier, J. Mazé, M. Orlandini, B.A. Plukett, and J. Waart. 1991. Chapter 5—Bioconversion of seaweeds. In *Seaweed, Resources in Europe. Uses and Potential*, Guiry, M.D., Blunden, G. (eds.). Chichester: John Wiley & Sons, pp. 91–148.

Murata, M. and Nakazoe, J. 2001. Production and use of marine algae in Japan. *Japan Agricultural Research Quartery* 35: 281–290.

Nanaki, S., E. Karavas, L. Kalantzi, and D. Bikiaris. 2010. Miscibility study of carrageenan blends and evaluation of their effectiveness as sustained release carriers. *Carbohydrate Polymers* 79: 1157–1167.

Nantes, C.I., J.R. Pesarini, M.O. Mauro, A.C.D. Monreal, A.D. Ramires, and R.J. Oliveira. 2014. Evaluation of the antimutagenic activity and mode of action of carrageenan fiber in cultured meristematic cells of Allium cepa. *Genetics and Molecular Research* 13(4): 9523–9532.

Nussinovitch, A. 1997. *Hydrocolloid Applications: Gum Technology in the Food and Other Industries*. London: Chapman & Hall, p. 354.

Oneill, A.N. 1955a. 3,6-Anhydro-D-galactose as a constituent of κ-carrageenin. *Journal of the American Chemical Society* 77(10): 2837–2839.

Oneill, A.N. 1955b. Derivatives of 4-O-beta-D-galactopyranosyl-3,6-anhydro-D-galactose from κ-carrageenin. *Journal of the American Chemical Society* 77(23): 6324–6326.

Onsoyen, E. 1997. Alginates. In *Thickening and Gelling Agents for Food*, Imeson, A. (ed.). London: Blackie Academic and Professional, pp. 22–44.

Pangestuti, R., and Kim, S.K. 2014. Biological activities of carrageenan. *Advances in Food and Nutrition Research* 72: 113–124.

Patel, S. 2012. Therapeutic importance of sulfated polysaccharides from seaweeds: Updating the recent findings. *Biotech* 2(3): 171–185.

Pereira, L. 2004. Estudos em macroalgas carragenófitas (Gigartinales, Rhodophyceae) da costa portuguesa—Aspectos ecológicos, bioquímicos e citológicos. PhD Thesis, Universidade de Coimbra, Coimbra, Portugal, 293.

Pereira, L. 2006. Identification of phycocolloids by vibrational spectroscopy. In *World Seaweed Resources—An authoritative reference system*, Critchley, A.T., Ohno, M., Largo, D.B. (eds.). Wokingham: ETI Information Services Ltd. Hybrid Windows and Mac DVD-ROM; ISBN: 90-75000-80-4.

Pereira, L. 2008. As algas marinhas e respectivas utilidades. Monografias. Available online at: http://br.monografias.com/trabalhos913/algas-marinhas-utilidades/algas-marinhas-utilidades.pdf

Pereira, L. 2009a. Guia ilustrado das macroalgas—Conhecer e reconhecer algumas espécies da flora Portuguesa. Imprensa da Universidade de Coimbra, Coimbra, Portugal, 90.

Pereira, L. 2010a. Seaweed: An unsuspected gastronomic treasury. *Chaîne de Rôtisseurs Magazine* 2: 50.

Pereira, L. 2010b. Littoral of Viana do Castelo—Algae, uses in agriculture, gastronomy and food industry (Bilingual). Câmara Municipal de Viana do Castelo, Portugal, 68.

Pereira, L. 2011a. A review of the nutrient composition of selected edible seaweeds. In *Seaweed: Ecology, Nutrient Composition and Medicinal Uses*, Pomin, V.H. (ed.). New York: Nova Science Publishers Inc, pp. 15–47.

Pereira, L. 2012. Chapter 4—Cytological and cytochemical aspects in selected carrageenophytes (Gigartinales, Rhodophyta). In *Advances in Algal Cell Biology*, Heimann, K., Katsaros, C. (eds.). Berlin, Germany: De Gruyter, pp. 81–104.

Pereira, L. 2013b. Population studies and carrageenan properties in eight Gigartinales (Rhodophyta) from western coast of Portugal. *The Scientific World Journal* 2013: 11.

Pereira, L., A.M. Amado, A.T. Critchley, F. van de Velde, and P.J.A. Ribeiro-Claro. 2009c. Identification of selected seaweed polysaccharides (Phycocolloids) by vibrational spectroscopy (FTIR-ATR and FT-Raman). *Food Hydrocolloid* 23: 1903–1909.

Pereira, L., A.M. Amado, P.J.A. Ribeiro-Claro, and F. van de Velde. 2009d. Vibrational spectroscopy (FTIR-ATR and FT-RAMAN)—A rapid and useful tool for phycocolloid analysis, pp. 131–136. In *Proceedings of the Biodevices—International Conference on Biomedical Electronics and Devices, 2nd International Joint Conference on Biomedical Engineering Systems and Technologies—BIOSTEC*, Porto, Portugal, January 14–17. ISBN: 978-989-8111-72-2.

Pereira, L. and F. Correia. 2015. Algas marinhas da costa Portuguesa—ecologia, biodiversidade e utilizações. Nota de Rodapé Edições.

Pereira, L., A.T. Critchley, A.M. Amado, and P.J.A. Ribeiro-Claro. 2009b. A comparative analysis of phycocolloids produced by underutilized versus industrially utilized carrageenophytes (Gigartinales, Rhodophyta). *Journal of Applied Phycology* 21: 599–605.

Pereira, L., S.F. Gheda, and P.J.A. Ribeiro-Claro. 2013a. Analysis by vibrational spectroscopy of seaweed polysaccharides with potential use in food, pharmaceutical, and cosmetic industries. *International Journal of Carbohydrate Chemistry* vol. 2013: 7.

Pereira, L. and J.F. Mesquita. 2004b. Population studies and carrageenan properties of *Chondracanthus teedei* var. lusitanicus (Gigartinaceae, Rhodophyta). *Journal of Applied Phycology* 16: 369–383.

Pereira, L. and P.J. Ribeiro-Claro. 2014. Chapter 7—Analysis by vibrational spectroscopy of seaweed with potential use in food, pharmaceutical and cosmetic industries, In *Marine Algae—Biodiversity, Taxonomy, Environmental Assessment and Biotechnology*, Leonel, P., João, M.N. (eds.). Boca Raton, FL: Science Publishers, an Imprint of CRC Press/Taylor & Francis Group, pp. 225–247.

Pereira, L., A. Sousa, H. Coelho, A.M. Amado, and P.J.A. Ribeiro-Claro. 2003. Use of FTIR, FT-Raman and 13C-NMR spectroscopy for identification of some seaweed phycocolloids. *Biomolecular Engineering* 20: 223–228.

Pereira, L. and F. van de Velde. 2011b. Portuguese carrageenophytes: Carrageenan composition and geographic distribution of eight species (Gigartinales, Rhodophyta). *Carbohydrate Polymers* 84: 614–623.

Pereira, L., F. van de Velde, and J.F. Mesquita. 2007. Cytochemical studies on underutilized carrageenophytes (Gigartinales, Rhodophyta). *International Journal of Biology and Biomedical Engineering* 1(1): 1–5.

Perez, R., R. Kaas, F. Campello, S. Arbault, and O. BAarbaroux. 1992. La Culture dês algues marines dans le monde. IFREMER, Plouzane, France, 613.

Porse, H. 1998. Global seaweed market trends. In *Plenary Presentation at XVIth International Seaweed Symposium*, Cebu City: the Philippines.

Prajapati, V.D., P.M. Maheriya, G.K. Jani, and H.K. Solanki. 2014. Carrageenan: A natural seaweed polysaccharide and its applications. *Carbohydrate Polymers* 105: 97–112.

Preisig, H.R. and R.A Andersen. 2005. Chapter 1—Historical review of algal culturing techniques. In *Algal Culturing Techniques*, Andersen, R.A. (ed.). London: Elsevier, pp. 1–12.

Qi, H., D. Li, J. Zhang, L. Liu, and Q. Zhang. 2008. Study on extraction of agaropectin from *Gelidium amansii* and its anticoagulant activity. *Chinese Journal of Oceanology and Limnology* 26(2): 186–189.

Rees, D.A. 1963. The carrageenan system of polysaccharides. Part I. The relation between the kappa and lambda-components. *Journal of the Chemical Society* 340: 1821–1832.

Renn, D.W. 1990. Seaweeds and biotechnology—Inseparable companions. *Hydrobiologia* 204/205: 7–13.

Ribier, J. and J.C. Godineau. 1984. Les algues. La Maison Rustique, Flammarion, France, 15–26.

Rochas, C., M. Rinaudo, and S. Landry. 1990. Role of the molecular weight on the mechanical properties of kappa carrageenan gels. *Carbohydrate Polymers* 12: 255–266.

Rudolph, B. 2000. Seaweed products: Red algae of economic significance. In *Marine and Freshwater Products Handbook*, Martin, R.E., Carter, E.P., Davis, L.M., Flich, G.J. (eds.). Lancaster, PA: Technomic Publishing Company Inc., pp. 515–529.

Salvador, N., A.G. Goméz, L. Lavelli, and M.A. Ribera. 2007. Antimicrobial activity of Iberian macroalgae. *Scientia Marina* 71: 101–113.

Saury, A. 1984. A saúde pelas algas. Enciclopédia da Vida Prática—24. Editorial Notícias, Lisboa, Portugal, 157.

Sebaaly, C., S. Kassem, E. Grishina, H. Kanaan, A. Sweidan, M.S. Chmit, and H.M. Kanaan. 2014. Anticoagulant and antibacterial activities of polysaccharides of red algae *Corallina* collected from Lebanese coast. *Journal of Applied Pharmaceutical Science* 4(4): 30–37.

Sen, A.K., A.K. Das, N. Banerji, A.K. Siddhanta, K.H. Mody, B.K. Ramavat, V.D. Chauhan, J.R. Vedasiromoni, and D.K. Ganguly. 1994. A new sulfated polysaccharide with potent blood anti-coagulant activity from the red seaweed *Grateloupia indica*. *International Journal of Biological Macromolecules* 16: 279–280.

Shanmughapriya, S., J. Krishnaveni, J. Selvin, R. Gandhimathi, M. Arunkumar, T. Thangavelu, G.S. Kiran, and K. Natarajaseenivasan. 2008. Optimization of extracellular thermotolerant alkaline protease produced by marine *Roseobacter* sp. (MMD040). *Bioprocess and Biosystems Engineering* 31: 427–433.

Silva, F.R.F., C.M.P.G. Dore, C.T. Marques, M.S. Nascimento, N.M.B. Benevides, H.A.O. Rocha, S.F. Chavante, and E.L. Leite. 2010. Anticoagulant activity, paw edema and pleurisy induced carrageenan: Action of major types of commercial carrageenans. *Carbohydrate Polymers* 79: 26–33.

Sitompul, J.P., A. Bayu, T.H. Soerawidjaja, and H.W. Lee. 2012. Studies of biogas production from green seaweeds. *International Journal of Environmental and Bioenergy* 3(3): 132–144.

Skjak-Broek, G. and A. Martinsen. 1991. Chapter 9—Applications of some algal polysaccharides in biotechnology. In *Seaweed, Resources in Europe. Uses and Potential*, Guiry, M.D., Blunden, G. (eds.). Chichester: John Wiley & Sons, pp. 219–257.

Smidsrod, O. and H. Grasdalen, 1984. Polyelectrolytes from seaweeds. *Proceedings of International Seaweed Symposium* 11: 18–28.

Smidsrod, O. and B.E. Christensen. 1991. Chapter 8—Molecular structure and physical behavior of seaweed colloids as compared with microbial polysaccharides. In *Seaweed, Resources in Europe. Uses and Potential*, Guiry, M.D., Blunden, G. (eds.). Chichester: John Wiley & Sons, pp. 185–217.

Smith, D.B. and H.W. Cook. 1954. Physical studies on carrageenin and carrageenin fractions. *Archives of Biochemistry and Biophysics* 45: 232–233.

Smith, D.B., A.N. Oneill, and A.S. Perlin. 1955. Studies on the heterogeneity of carrageenin. *Canadian Journal of Chemistry* 33(8): 1352–1360.

Sokolova, E.V., A.O. Barabanova, R.N. Bogdanovich, V.A. Khomenko, Solov'eva and I.M. Yermak. 2011a. In vitro antioxidant properties of red algal polysaccharides. *Biomedicine & Prevention Nutrition* 1: 161–167.

Sokolova, E., A. Barabanova, V. Homenko, T. Solov'eva, R. Bogdanovich, and I. Yermak. 2011b. In vitro and ex vivo studies of antioxidant activity of carrageenans, sulfated polysaccharides from red algae. *Bulletin of Experimental Biology and Medicine* 150: 426–428.

Souza, B.W.S., M.A. Cerqueira, A.I. Bourbon, A.C. Pinheiro, J.T. Martins, J.A. Teixeira, M.A. Coimbra, and A.A. Vicente. 2012. Chemical characterization and antioxidant activity of sulfated polysaccharide from the red seaweed *Gracilaria birdiae*. *Food Hydrocolloids* 27: 287–292.

Stanley, N. 1987. Production, properties and uses of carrageenan. FAO Fisheries Technical Paper, 116–146.

Stein, E.M., D.X. Andreguetti, C.S. Rocha, M.T. Fujii, M.S. Baptista, P. Colepicolo, and G.L. Indig. 2011. Search for cytotoxic agents in multiple *Laurencia* complex seaweed species (Ceramiales, Rhodophyta) harvested from the Atlantic Ocean with emphasis on the Brazilian State of Espírito Santo. *Revista Brasileira de Farmacognosia* 21: 239–243.

Stephen, A.M. and G.O. Phillips. 2010. *Food Polysaccharides and Their Applications*. Boca Raton, FL: CRC Press. p. 743.

Stortz, C.A., M.R. Cases, and A.S. Cerezo. 1997. Red seaweed galactans. In *Techniques in Glycobiology*, Townsend, R.R., Hotchkiss, A.T. (eds.). New York: CRC Press, pp. 567–593.

Sun, T., H. Tao, J. Xie, S. Zhang, and X. Xu. 2010. Degradation and antioxidant activity of k-carrageenans. *Journal of Applied Polymer Science* 117: 194–199.

Talarico, L.B. and E.B. Damonte. 2007a. Interference in dengue virus adsorption and uncoating by carrageenans. *Virology* 363: 473–485.

Talarico, L.B., M.E.R. Duarte, R.G.M. Zibetti, M.D. Noseda, and E.B. Damonte. 2007b. An algal-derived DL-galactan hybrid is an efficient preventing agent for in vitro dengue virus infection. *Planta Medica* 73: 1464–1468.

Talarico, L.B., M.D. Noseda, D.R.B. Ducatti, M.E. Duarte, and E.B. Damonte. 2011. Differential inhibition of dengue virus infection in mammalian and mosquito cells by iota-carrageenan. *Journal of General Virology* 92: 1332–1342.

Talarico, L.B., C.A. Pujol, R.G. Zibetti, P.C. Faría, M.D. Noseda, M.E. Duarte, and E.B. Damonte. 2005. The antiviral activity of sulfated polysaccharides against dengue virus is dependent on virus serotype and host cell. *Antiviral Research* 66: 103–110.

Tardieu, V. 1993. Algas à moda da Bretagne. J. Libération. (CEVA). *Contacto* 26(5): 18–21.

Tariq, V.N. 1991. Antifungal activity in crude extracts of marine red algae. *Mycological Research* 95:1433–1440.

Therkelsen, G.H. 1993. Carrageenan. In *Industrial Gums: Polysaccharides and Their Derivatives*, Whistler, R.L., Bemiller, J.N. (eds.). San Diego, CA: Academic Press, pp. 145–180.

Thomas, D. 2002. *Seaweeds*. Washington, DC: Smithsonian Books. p. 96.

Tseng, C.K. 1945. The terminology of seaweed colloids. *Science* 101(2633): 597–602.

van de Velde, F. and G.A. de Ruiter. 2002. Carrageenan. In *Biopolymers: Polysaccharides II, Polysaccharides from Eukaryotes*, Vol. 6, Vandamme, E.J., Baets, S.D., Steinbèuchel, A. (eds.). Weinheim, Germany: Wiley-VCH, pp. 245–274.

van de Velde, F., S.H. Knutsen, A.I. Usov, H.S. Rollema, and A.S. Cerezo. 2002a. H-1 and C-13 high resolution NMR spectroscopy of carrageenans: Application in research and industry. *Trends in Food Science and Technology* 13(3): 73–92.

van de Velde, F., L. Pereira, and H.S. Rollema. 2004. The revised NMR chemical shift data of carrageenans. *Carbohydrate Research* 339: 2309–2313.

Venugopal, V. (ed.). 2008. *Marine Products for Healthcare: Functional and Bioactive Nutraceutical Compounds from the Ocean*. CRC Press: Boca Raton, FL.

Wang, H., E.V. Ooi, and P.O. Ang. 2008. Antiviral activities of extracts from Hong Kong seaweeds. *Journal of Zhejiang University Science* B9: 969–976.

Wang, W., P. Zhang, G.L. Yu, C.X. Li, C. Hao, X. Qi, L.J. Zhang, and H.S. Guan. 2012. Preparation and anti-influenza A virus activity of κ-carrageenan oligosaccharide and its sulphated derivatives. *Food Chemistry* 133: 880–888.

Watson, D.B. 2008. Public health and carrageenan regulation: A review and analysis. *Journal of Applied Phycology* 20(5): 505–513.

Weiner, M.L. 2014. Food additive carrageenan: Part II: A critical review of carrageenan in vivo safety studies. *Critical Review in Toxicology* 44: 244–269.

Witvrouw, M. and E. De Clercq. 1997. Sulfated polysaccharides extracted from sea algae as potential antiviral drugs. *General Pharmacology* 29: 497–511.

Wunderwald, P., W.J. Schrenk, and H. Port. 1979. Antithrombin BM from human plasma: An antithrombin binding moderately to heparin. *Thrombosis Research* 15: 49–60.

Xu, L., Z. Yao, H. Wu, F. Wang, and S. Zhang. 2012. The immune regulation of kappa-carrageenan oligosaccharide and its desulfated derivatives on LPS-activated microglial cells. *Neurochemistry International* 61: 689–696.

Yamada, T., A. Ogamo, T. Saito, H. Uchiyama, and Y. Nakagawa. 2000. Preparation of O-acylated low-molecular-weight carrageenans with potent anti-HIV activity and low anticoagulant effect. *Carbohydrate Polymers* 41: 115–120.

Yamada, T., A. Ogamo, T. Saito, J. Watanabe, H. Uchiyama, and Y. Nakagawa. 1997. Preparation and anti-HIV activity of low-molecular-weight carrageenans and their sulfated derivatives. *Carbohydrate Polymers* 32: 51–55.

Yamamoto, I., H. Maruyama, M. Takahashi, and K. Komiyama. 1986. The effect of dietary or intraperitoneally injected seaweed preparations on the growth of sarcoma-180 cells subcutaneously implanted into mice. *Cancer Letters* 30: 125–131.

Yao, Z., H. Hu, S. Zhang, and Y. Du. 2014. Enzymatic preparation of kappa-carrageenan oligosacharides and their anti-angiogenic activity. *Carbohydrate Polymers* 101: 359–367.

Yermak, I.M. and Y.S. Khotimchenko. 1997. Physical and chemical properties, applications, and biological activities of carrageenan, a polysaccharide of red algae. *Marine Biology* 23: 129–142.

Yermark, I.M., A.O. Barabanova, D.L. Aminin, V.N. Davydova, E. Sokolova, T.F. Solov'eva, Y.H. Kim, and K.S. Shin. 2012. Effects of structural peculiarities of carrageenan on their immunomodulatory and anticoagulant activities. *Carbohydrate Polymers* 87: 713–720.

Yuan, H., J. Song, X. Li, N. Li, and J. Dai. 2004. Immunomodulation and antitumor activity of κ-carrageenan oligosaccharides. *Pharmacological Research* 50: 47–53.

Yuan, H., J. Song, X. Li, N. Li, and J. Dai. 2006. Immunomodulation and antitumor activity of κ-carrageenan oligosaccharides. *Cancer Letters* 243: 228–234.

Yuan, H., J. Song, X. Li, N. Li, and S. Liu. 2011. Enhanced immunostimulator and anti-tumor activity of different derivatives of kappa-carrageenan oligosaccharides from Kappaphycus striatum. *Journal of Applied Phycology* 23: 59–65.

Yuan, H., W. Zhang, X. Li, X. Lu, N. Li, and X. Gao. 2005. Preparation and in vitro antioxidant activity of kappa-carrageenan oligosaccharides and their oversulfated, acetylated, and phosphorylated derivatives. *Carbohydrate Research* 340: 685–692.

Zemke-White, W.L. and M. Ohno. 1999. World seaweed utilisation: An end-of-century summary. *Journal of Applied Phycology* 11: 369–76.

Zhang, W., L. Piculell, S. Nilsson, and S.H. Knutsen. 1994. Cation specificity and cation binding to low sulfated carrageenans. *Carbohydrate Polymers* 23: 105–110.

Zinoun, M. and J. Cosson. 1996. Seasonal variation in growth and carrageenan content of *Calliblepharis jubata* (Rhodophyceae, Gigartinales) from the Normandy coast, France. *Journal of Applied Phycology* 8(1): 29–34.

Zhou, G., Y. Sun, H. Xin, Y. Zhang, Z. Li, and Z. Xu. 2004. In vivo antitumor and immunomodulation activities of different molecular weight lambda-carrageenans from *Chondrus ocellatus*. *Pharmacological Research* 50: 47–53.

Zhou, G., W. Sheng, W. Yao, and C. Wang. 2006. Effect of low molecular-carrageenan from *Chondrus ocellatus* on antitumor H-22 activity of 5-Fu. *Pharmacological Research* 53: 129–134.

Zhou, G., H. Xin, W. Sheng, Z. Li, and Z. Xu. 2005. In vivo growth-inhibition of S180 tumor by mixture of 5-Fu and low molecular lambda-carrageenan from *Chondrus ocellatus*. *Pharmacology Research* 51: 153–157.

4 Influence of Physico-Chemical Properties on the Potential Application of Marine Biopolymers

K. Sangeetha, P. Supriya Prasad,
K. Vijayalakshmi, and P.N. Sudha

CONTENTS

4.1   INTRODUCTION

4.1.1   MARINE BIOPOLYMERS

During the past 10 years, there has been an increasing interest in biodegradable polymers isolated from sources found in nature. The marine environment is rich in biodiversity with novel species of microorganisms and macroorganisms, which could serve as a source for a variety of novel products and processes.

4.1.2   NEED FOR MARINE BIOPOLYMER

Biopolymer is a term commonly used to refer to polymers biologically synthesized by nature. Polysaccharide is one such class of biopolymers, comprising simple monosaccharide (sugar) molecules connected by ether-type linkages to give high-molecular-weight polymers. Chitin and chitosan are unique and typical marine biomaterials, which have attracted the interest of many researchers of various disciplines. Chitin/chitosan and their modified derivatives find extensive applications in medicine, biomedical, agricultural, environmental, and industrial fields (Cheba 2011). In this work, we discuss in detail the marine biopolymers chitin and chitosan.

4.2   CHITIN AND CHITOSAN

Most of the naturally occurring polysaccharides, for instance, cellulose, dextran, pectin, alginic acid, agar, agarose, and carrageenans, are neutral or acidic in nature, whereas chitin and chitosan are the examples of highly basic polysaccharides (Kumar 2000).

4.2.1   OCCURRENCE AND SOURCES OF CHITIN

Chitin was first discovered in mushroom by French botanist Henri Braconnot in 1811. Odier named it as *chitine* from Greek, which means *tunic* or *coverage* (Domard 1996).

Chitin is the second abundant biopolymer that occurs in nature next to cellulose (Knorr 1984; Cauchie 2002; Dutta et al. 2002). It is a linear polysaccharide composed of β-(1-4)-poly-N-acetyl-D-glucosamine monomers (Muzzarelli 1977). The traditional source of chitin is crustacean shells, but the main chitin producers are mycelial fungi (Gamayurova et al. 1998). Newer sources for chitin production continue to be explored from fungi (Kuhlmann et al. 1999) and insect larvae (Struszczyk et al. 1999). In the native state, chitin occurs as ordered crystalline microfibrils that form structural components in the exoskeleton of arthropods or in the cell walls of fungi and yeast. It is also produced by a number of other living organisms in the lower plant and animal kingdoms. It has been estimated that tons of chitin are biosynthesized each year (Percot et al. 2003).

When the number of acetamido groups is >50% (more commonly 70%–90%), the biopolymer is termed chitin. In chitin terminology, the number of acetamido groups is termed as the degree of acetylation (DA). The nitrogen content in purified samples is <7% for chitin sample. Chitin is known to be nontoxic, odorless, biocompatible in animal tissues, and enzymatically biodegradable (Cooney et al. 2009). Its unique properties include polyoxy salt formation, ability to form films, chelation with metal ions, and optical structural characteristics (Kumar 2000). Chitin and its derivatives are used in various fields, such as agriculture, food preservation, drug delivery, tissue engineering, wastewater treatment, molecular imprinting, and cosmetics.

4.3 PHYSICOCHEMICAL PROPERTIES OF CHITIN

4.3.1 CHITIN CRYSTALLINITY

Chitin occurs naturally in three polymeric forms known as α-, β-, and γ-chitins (Rinaudo 2006) based on the differences in packing and the polarities of adjacent chains in successive sheets, which influence the crystal structure (Pillai et al. 2009; Hajji et al. 2014). α-Chitin is arranged in an antiparallel configuration, whereas β-chitin is organized in a parallel configuration (Tolaimate et al. 2003). The α- and β-chitins are differentiated by infrared spectroscopy and solid-state ^{13}C nuclear magnetic resonance spectroscopy (Tanner et al. 1990; Jang et al. 2004) for determination of the deacetylation degree (DD) of chitin and for control of purification conditions. However, the third polymeric form γ-chitin has a parallel and antiparallel structure, which is a combination of both α-chitin and β-chitin (Jang et al. 2004) (See Figure 4.1).

α-Chitin is the most abundant form found in nature, whereas β-chitin is more reactive (Kurita et al. 1994) and shows a higher affinity for solvents (Sannan et al. 1976). Both α-chitin and β-chitin are crystalline (Rinaudo 2006). On dissolution or extensive swelling, β-chitin converts into α-chitin (Rudall and Kenchington 1973). Another commonly used method to convert β-chitin into γ-chitin is by using alkaline treatment followed by flushing in water (Noishiki et al. 2003).

Chitin polymorphs are related to the diversity of their functions (Rudall and Kenchington 1973; Roberts et al. 1992a). α-Chitin is mainly found in organisms where extreme mechanical properties are required (hardness), and it is commonly associated with inorganic compounds (Ehrlich et al. 2010). β-Chitin is usually found in organisms where both flexibility and toughness are required (Roberts 1992b).

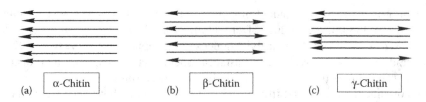

FIGURE 4.1 Schematic representation of the three polymorphic forms of chitin: (a) α-chitin, (b) β-chitin, and (c) γ-chitin.

4.3.2 COLOR AND APPEARANCE

Chitin is colorless to half white, hard, inelastic, nitrogenous polysaccharide (Kurita 2001). In its pure unmodified form, chitin is translucent, pliable, resilient, quite tough, and relatively inert.

4.3.3 DEGREE OF DEACETYLATION

Degree of deacetylation (DDA) refers to the removal of acetyl group from the chain and is determined by potentiometric titration using the formula DD% = 100 − DA%, where DA is the degree of acetylation (Zhang et al. 2011). The DDs in chitin usually range from 5% to 15%. The higher the DA of chitin, the lower the solubility in common solvents (Kurita 2001). Chitin is generally crystalline in nature, and the degree of crystallinity is a function of the DD (Rathke 1993). DD affects the chemical, physical, and biological properties of chitosan, such as adsorption, covalent linking, and encapsulation (Puvvada et al. 2012).

4.3.4 SOLUBILITY OF CHITIN

Chitin is highly hydrophobic and is insoluble in water and most organic solvents (Dutta et al. 2004). The semicrystalline structure of chitin with extensive intermolecular hydrogen bonding and cohesive energy density makes the solubility parameter of chitin to be very high, and thus, it will be insoluble in all the usual solvents (Kumar 2000; Rinaudo 2006). Both α- and β-forms of chitin are insoluble in all the common solvents. This insolubility is a major problem in view of the development of processing and applications of chitin. Chitin is infusible and sparingly soluble during transformation into different conformations (Figure 4.2).

Chitin is soluble in fluorinated solvents such as hexafluoroisopropanol and hexafluoroacetone (Capozza 1975), although the extent of solubility depends on the source of chitin (Rutherford and Austin 1978) and chloro alcohols in conjunction with aqueous solutions of mineral acids and dimethyl acetamide (DMAc) containing 5% lithium chloride (LiCl) (Rutherford and Austin 1978). The hydrolysis of chitin with concentrated acids under drastic conditions produces the relatively pure amino sugar, D-glucosamine. A 50% deacetylated chitin has been found to be soluble in water (Dutta et al. 2002). This water-soluble form of chitin is a useful starting material for its smooth modifications, through various reactions in solution phase.

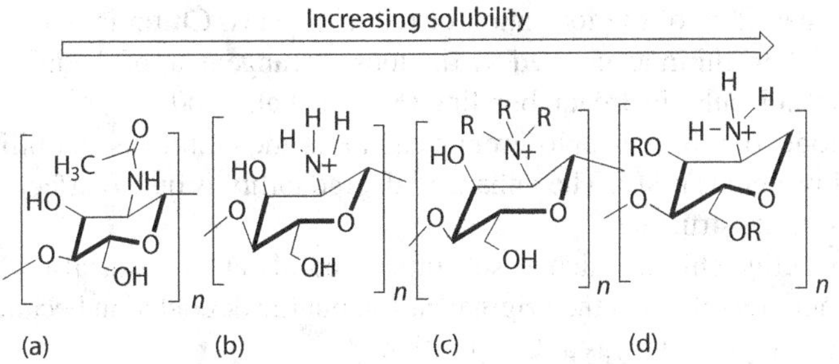

FIGURE 4.2   Solubility of chitin derivatives: (a) raw chitin (insoluble), (b) chitosan (acid soluble), (c) quaternized chitosan (soluble), and (d) substituted chitosan (soluble).

Highly benzoylated chitin is soluble in benzyl alcohol, dimethyl sulfoxide, formic acid, and dichloro acetic acid (Dutta et al. 2004). Methanol saturated with calcium chloride dihydrate, a solvent for nylons, has been recently reported to dissolve chitin, although anhydrous calcium chloride was apparently not suitable.

4.3.5   MOLECULAR WEIGHT AND DEGREE OF POLYMERIZATION OF CHITIN

The molecular weight of native chitin is usually larger than 1,000,000 Da (Li et al. 1992). The general methods used to determine the molecular weight of chitin are viscometry, light scattering, and gel permeation chromatography (GPC) (Hasegawa et al. 1993; Terbojevich et al. 1996). Chitin is usually present in a closely associated form with proteins and other substances, and hence, it is difficult to determine the molecular weight of native chitin. The main chitin chain can be depolymerized to some extent during isolation with acid and alkali. The degree of polymerization of chitin ranges between 2000 and 4000.

4.3.6   EFFECT OF TEMPERATURE AND TIME ON MOLECULAR WEIGHT

When the temperature and time are increased, the average molecular weight is reduced and the DD increases. The DD however increases only up to a particular extent, and it is not as elaborate as the decrease in average molecular weight. Lusena and Rose (1953) and Mima et al. (1983) carried out similar studies. They showed that higher temperatures increase the percentage of deacetylation and reduce molecular size, and that deacetylation proceeds rapidly to about 68% during the first hour of alkali treatment (in 50% NaOH), and with the reaction progressing, deacetylation reaches only 78% in 5 hours. Thus, alkali treatment beyond 2 hours does not deacetylate significantly, rather it only serves to degrade the molecular chain (Lusena and Rose 1953; Mima et al. 1983).

4.3.7   ENZYMATIC DEGRADATION

Chitin is generally biodegraded in nature by a number of microorganisms (Koga et al. 1999). The biodegradability of chitin and its derivatives is often conveniently evaluated in terms of susceptibility to lysozyme, and the degradation rate can be determined based on of the formation of reducing ends. Chitin is more susceptible to lysozyme than chitin as implied by the loose arrangement of the molecules with weaker intermolecular hydrogen bonding (Kurita et al. 2000).

The introduction of mercapto groups enhances the chitin susceptibility to lysozyme (Sashiwa et al. 1990). The enhanced degradability is due to effective destruction of crystalline structure.

Carboxymethyl chitin, which as substituent mainly at C-6, was also degraded by lysozyme more readily than the original chitin, but the degradation became slower if the carboxymethyl group was at C-3 position.

4.3.8 PROCESSABILITY

Chitin can easily be processed into gels, beads, powders, fibers, membranes, cotton, flakes, sponges, colloids, films, and spins.

4.4 DERIVATIVES OF CHITIN

Glycol chitin, a partially O-hydroxyethylated chitin, was the first derivative of practical importance (Kim et al. 1994; Hudson and Smith 1998).

The derivatives of chitin are classified into two main categories:

1. The *N*-acetyl groups are removed, and the exposed amino function then reacts with either acyl chlorides or anhydrides to give the group NHCOR.
2. The *N*-acetyl groups are removed, and the exposed amino functions are modified by reductive amination $NHCH_2COOH$.

Chemical modifications of chitin: As chitin is insoluble in most organic solvents, the solubilization of this rigid polysaccharide will be an essential step toward efficient modifications. Recent studies show that chitin actually becomes soluble in water or organic solvents with the destruction of its crystalline structure by proper structural modification.

4.4.1 ALKALI CHITIN

Chitin can be dissolved in sodium hydroxide to form alkali chitin. This product with about 50% deacetylation is soluble even in neutral water (Sannan et al. 1976; Dutta et al. 2002). Higher or lower deacetylation leads to formation of swollen gels. The DD should be 45%–55% for good water solubility.

4.4.2 CHITIN SPONGES

Chitin sponges prepared by freeze-drying methods exhibited many remarkable properties, including very low density, high porosity, good mechanical properties, and excellent oil absorption performance. The swelling property makes chitin-based sponges a versatile template for biomineralization in both calcification and silification reactions (Ehrlich 2010). The biomimetic potential of chitin-based composite biomaterials of poriferan origin is analyzed in detail in a recently published monograph entitled *Biomimetic Biomaterials: Structure and Applications* (Wysokowski et al. 2013).

4.4.3 CHITIN WHISKER

Chitin whisker, a kind of crystallite in nanoscale prepared by removing the amorphous phase of chitin, is an emerging nanofiller, which could enhance the mechanical and barrier properties of composites (Uddin et al. 2012; Rubentheren et al. 2015). Coating with chitin whiskers improves the physical properties of paper sheets that could be used as food packing materials (Li et al. 2015).

4.4.4 CARBOXYMETHYL CHITIN

The introduction of carboxymethyl group into chitin leads to the formation of anionic derivative. The carboxymethylation of chitin is conducted with alkali chitin and monochloroacetic acid. Uses of appropriate organic solvents facilitate the reaction (Zhou et al. 2006). Carboxymethylation is supposed to proceed preferentially at C-6 position. Carboxymethyl chitin is used as a drug carrier and biomaterial.

4.4.5 BIOLOGICAL ACTIVITY OF CHITIN IN AGRICULTURE

Chitin and its derivatives are biologically active during their interaction with plants and microorganisms. Four main approaches have been identified for chitin application in agriculture (see Tables 4.1 through 4.3):

1. Protection of plants from pests and diseases before and after harvest
2. Enhancement of antagonist microorganisms action and biological controls
3. Enhancement of the beneficial symbiotic plant–microorganism interactions
4. Regulation of plant growth and development

TABLE 4.1
Physical Form of Chitin Derivatives and Their Biomedical Application

Form of Material	Application
Solution	Baceteriostatic agent (Malette et al. 1983)
	Homeostatic agent (Allan et al. 1984)
	Cosmetics (Gross et al. 1980)
Whisker	Food packaging materials (Li et al. 2009)
Gel	Drug delivery vehicle (Jackson 1987)
	Spermicide (Smith 1984)
Powder	Surgical clove powder (Casey 1977)
	Enzyme immobilization (Lantero 1986)
Film/membrane	Dialysis membrane (Mima et al. 1983)
	Contact lens (Allan et al. 1984)
	Wound dressing (Widra 1986)
Sponge	Veterinary practices, filling agent for surgical tissue defects (Okamoto et al. 1993)
	Mucosal hemostatic agent (Itoi et al. 1985)
	Wound dressings (Kifune et al. 1987)
Miscellaneous pharmaceutical applications	Anticholesteremic materials (Nagyvary et al. 1979)

TABLE 4.2

Some Uses of Chitin and Its Derivatives in Agriculture

Use	Crop	Properties	Compound	Reference
Defensive enzyme stimulation	Rice	Inducer	Chitin	Hernández et al. (2007), Falcón et al. (2002), Hadwiger et al. (1994)
Mycorrhizal symbiosis stimulator	Tomato	Inducer of recognition mechanism	Chitin	Iglesias et al. (1994)
Nematocidal control	Tomato	Increase soil chitinolytic microbiotes	Chitin	Jin et al. (2005)
Biocontrol action enhancer	Peanut Apple	Stimulator substrate for hydrolase enzyme	Chitin	Backman et al. (1994)

TABLE 4.3

Application of Chitin and Its Derivatives

Specific Properties	Main Applications
Bioactivity	Prevention against microbial growth, antimicrobial additive to fibers and textile products, food packaging material, which act as an inhibitor of microbial contamination, stimulation of immunological system, anticholesterolemic agent, lowering of body overweight, wound healing, blood anticoagulant
Biodegradability	Carbon source for single-cell protein production, biodegradable radar countermeasure chaffs, biodegradable packaging materials, controlled release of drugs, agrochemicals, drug and nutrients, cosmetics and toiletries production
Reactivity of deacetylated amino groups	Enzyme immobilization, media for affinity chromatography and gel filtration, moisture retaining, antielectrostatic and hair-protecting products, formation of polyelectrolytes
Chelation ability	Reduction of surface water and wastewater pollutions by chelating heavy metal ions and radionuclides, inactivation of metalloenzymes influenced on undesirable changes of food
Adsorption capacity	Removal of phenols from wastewater, efficient elesctrostatic painting, recovery or separation of protein and other by-products, clarification of juices and beverages

4.5 CHITOSAN

Chitin is the raw material for all commercial productions of chitosan and glucosamine, with an estimated annual production of 2000 and 4000 tons, respectively. The difference between chitin and chitosan lies in the DD. The deacetylation process of chitin in the alkaline medium does generally not result in complete conversion

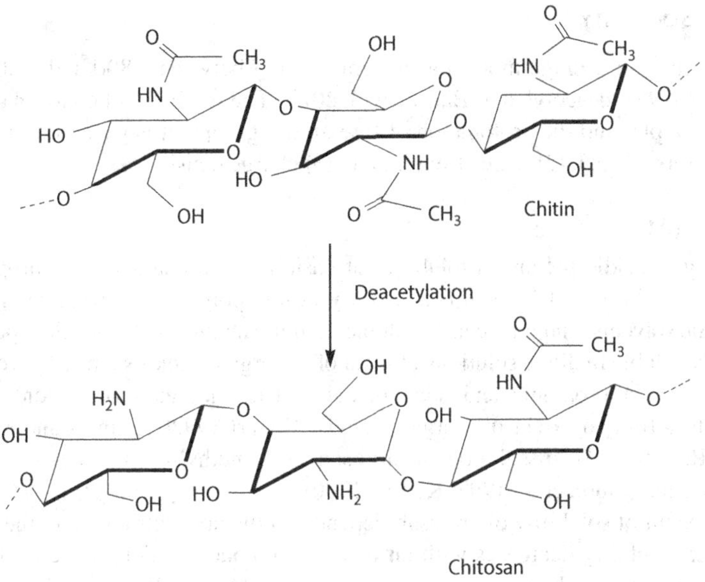

FIGURE 4.3 Preparation of chitosan.

into chitosan even in harsh treatments. The DD generally ranges from 70% to 95% depending on the method used (Figure 4.3).

Chitosan is a linear polysaccharide composed of randomly distributed β-(1–4)-linked D-glucosamine (deacetylated unit) and N-acetyl-D-glucosamine (acetylated unit) (Islam et al. 2013). It is a nontoxic polysaccharide, biocompatible, and biodegradable (Shigemasa et al. 1994), which forms films, and has antifungal (Hernández et al. 2007) and antibacterial (Gil et al. 2004) properties.

Chitin can be converted into chitosan by enzymatic preparations (Kafetzopoulos et al. 1993; Aiba 1994; Ilyina et al. 1999; Tokuyasu et al. 2000) or chemical process (Kurita et al. 1977; No and Meyers 1995). Chemical methods are used extensively for commercial purposes of chitosan preparation because of their low cost and suitability to mass production (No and Meyers 1995).

4.5.1 CHEMICAL REACTIVITY

Chitosan has three reactive groups: the primary (C-6) and secondary (C-3) hydroxyl groups on each repeat unit, and the amino (C-2) group on each deacetylated unit. These reactive groups are readily subject to chemical modifications to alter the mechanical and physical properties of chitosan. The typical reactions involving the hydroxyl groups are etherification and esterification. Selective O-substitution can be achieved by protecting the amino groups during the reaction (Badawy et al. 2004).

4.5.2 Solubility

Chitosan has an average molecular weight ranging between 3,800 and 20,000 Da, and is 66%–95% deacetylated (Bansal et al. 2011). The solubility of chitosan depends on the DD, pH, and the protonation of free amino groups. It is governed mainly by three factors: (1) pH, (2) ionic strength, and (3) charge density.

4.5.2.1 pH

Solubility at acidic pH and insolubility at basic pH is a characteristic property of commercial chitosan. Chitosan is a semicrystalline polymer and insoluble in water or organic solvents, and it is readily soluble in dilute acidic solutions below pH 6.0. It is readily soluble in dilute solutions of most of the organic acids such as hydrochloric acid, lactic acid, propionic acid, succinic acid, citric acid, and tartaric acid, but it is soluble to a limited extent in inorganic acids (Robert 1992b; Francis and Matthew 2000). Recently, the dissolution of chitosan in N-methylmorpholine-N-oxide has been reported (Dutta et al. 1997; Kumar 2000).

The extent of solubility of chitosan depends on the concentration and the type of acid. The solubility decreases with an increase in concentration of the acid. Nitric acid could dissolve chitosan but after dissolution (Muzzarelli 1973). Sulfuric acid does not dissolve chitosan because it would react with chitosan to form chitosan sulfate, which is a white crystalline solid (Muzzarelli 1973).

The solubility of chitosan in the acidic medium is due to the presence of primary amino groups with a pK_a value of 6.3. The presence of the amino groups indicates that the pH substantially alters the charged state and properties of chitosan (Yi et al. 2005).

Generally, chitosan solubility decreases with an increase in pH. Above pH 7, chitosan is insoluble in water, alkali, or aqueous solutions due to its stable and rigid crystalline structure. At higher pH, precipitation or gelation tends to occur, and the chitosan solution forms a poly-ion complex with an anionic hydrocolloid resulting in the gel formation (Kurita 1998).

4.5.2.2 Ionic Strength

The ionic strength of solvent also affects the solubility of chitosan (salting out effect). For example, the presence of copper and multivalent negative ions such as molybdate interacts with chitosan and limits its solubility in water.

4.5.2.3 Charge Density

The charge density of chitosan also referred to as the degree of protonation of amino groups determines the solubility of chitosan (Figure 4.4).

At low pH, the amines present in chitosan get protonated and become positively charged, which makes chitosan a water-soluble cationic polyelectrolyte. However, as the pH increases above 6, the amines present in chitosan become deprotonated and the polymer loses its charge and becomes insoluble. The soluble–insoluble transition occurs at its pK_a value changes around pH between 6 and 6.5.

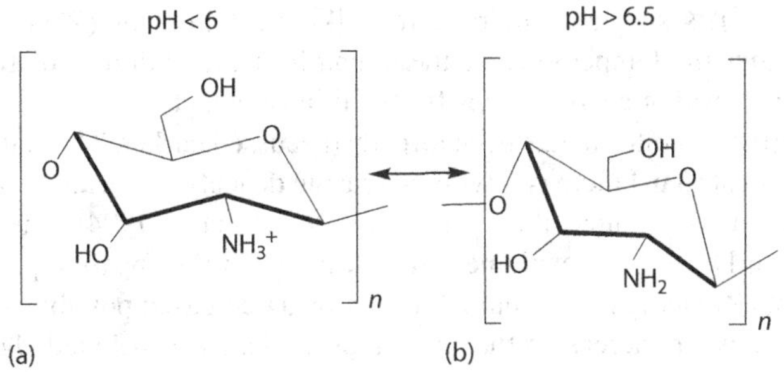

FIGURE 4.4 Charge density. (a) *Soluble*: electrostatic interactions with negatively charged molecules such as anionic glycosaminoglycans, proteoglycans, phospholoipids, and negatively charged liposomes. (b) *Insoluble*: hydrophobic interactions with, for example, fatty acids cholesterol and noncharged liposomes.

Chitosan is only soluble in aqueous solutions of some acids and some selective *N*-alkylidinations (Hirano 1997; Muzzarelli et al. 1997) and *N*-acylations (Li et al. 1997).

4.5.3 MOLECULAR WEIGHT AND VISCOSITY

The functional properties of chitosan are mainly dependent on its molecular weight or viscosity. Earlier studies demonstrated suggest that chitosan with high molecular weight (highly viscous) are more effective as food preservatives than those with low molecular weight. Chitosan is soluble in aqueous acid solutions, and the molecular weight of chitosan is estimated by either GPC or viscometry (Lee 1974; Shimojoh et al. 1998). Chitosan can be converted into chitin by N-acetylation under mild conditions, and the molecular weight can be measured by GPC in DMAc/LiCl (Hasegawa et al. 1993).

Chitosan is a pseudoplastic material and has an excellent viscosity enhancing the agent in the acidic environment. The viscosity of chitosan mainly depends on the concentration and temperature. An increase in concentration generally increases the viscosity of chitosan, and a decrease in temperature generally increases the viscosity of chitosan. Chitosan is generally hydrophilic in nature and form gels at the acidic medium. This type of gels was used in slow release of drug delivery system. The viscosity of the pharmaceutical chitosan is a very important aspect in handling a polymer for the drug delivery (Puvvada et al. 2012).

The DD also plays a significant role in affecting the molecular weight of chitosan. A lower DD leads to a higher molecular weight.

4.5.4 DEACETYLATION

The process of deacetylation involves the removal of acetyl groups from the molecular chain of chitin, leaving behind a complete amino group ($-NH_2$). Chitosan versatility depends mainly on this high degree of chemically reactive amino groups. To increase the amino group content of chitosan and higher deacetylation, chitosan (e.g., DD >90%) is subjected to repeated alkaline treatment (Wan et al. 2003). Increasing either the temperature or the strength of the alkaline solution can also enhance the removal of acetyl groups from chitin (Khan et al. 2001).

The solubility of chitosan has been already discussed earlier. The water solubility of chitosan at neutral pH increases with increasing deacetylation, and a chitosan with DA 0.6 is fully water soluble at all pH values (Vårum et al. 1994). The dependence of solubility on DA may be explained by a decrease in the apparent pK_a value with deacetylation, (Rinaudo and Domard 1989) or by a decreased possibility of aligning polymer chains when increasing the amount of randomly distributed GlcNAc units.

4.5.5 CHELATION PROPERTY OF CHITOSAN

Chitosan possess an excellent chelation property due to the presence of a large number of amino groups (Nomanbhay and Palanisamy 2005), and this biopolymer finds its application in water treatment. The polycationic nature of chitosan makes it to act as a good flocculating agent and act as a chelating agent and heavy metal trapper. It has been found that chitosan and its derivatives can remove heavy metals, dye ions, and oils from water (Ge and Huang 2010).

In heavy metal trapping, the nitrogen in the amino group acts as an electron donor, and it is responsible for selective chelation with metal ions (Siraj et al. 2012). Ogawa and Oka (1993) confirmed that the presence of amino group in chitosan is responsible for effective binding of metal ions. Hence, the content of higher free amino groups in chitosan should give higher metal ion adsorption rates.

4.5.6 ANTIMICROBIAL ACTIVITY

Friedman and Juneja (2010) suggest that low-molecular-weight chitosan at a pH below 6.0 presents optimal conditions for achieving desirable antimicrobial and antioxidative–preservative effects in liquid and solid foods. Kardas et al. (2012) described in his review that the chitosan and its derivatives offer a wide range of unique applications, including preservation of foods from microbial deterioration and formation of biodegradable films.

Chitosan was shown to have several advantages over other disinfectants, as it possesses a higher antimicrobial activity, a broader spectrum of activity, a higher kill rate, and a lower toxicity toward mammalian cells (Synowiecki and Al-khatteb 2003). Chitosans are more effective for gram-negative bacteria than for gram-positive bacteria (Muzzarelli et al. 1990; Rhoades and Roller 2000; Jeon et al. 2001). Younes et al. (2014) have clearly shown in their study that the chitosan with lower DA, lower molecular weight, and lower pH gives the larger efficiency of antimicrobial activity.

4.6   CHEMICAL MODIFICATION OF CHITOSAN

In order to improve or impart new properties to chitosan, chemical modification of chitosan is necessary. Chitosan has reactive amino, primary hydroxyl, and secondary hydroxyl groups, which can be used for chemical modifications under mild reaction conditions to alter its properties.

Various studies were conducted to make water-soluble derivatives of chitosan by chemical modification techniques, such as polyethylene glycol (PEG)-grafting (Ouchi et al. 1998; Sugimoto et al. 1998; Gorochovceva and Makuska 2004), sulfonation (Francis and Matthew 2000), partial N-acetylation (Kubota et al. 2000), N-acetylation (Kumar 2000; Francis and Matthew 2000), chitosan carrying phosphonic and alkyl groups (Ramos et al. 2003), hydroxypropyl chitosan (Xie et al. 2002), branching with oligosaccharides (Tommeraas et al. 2002), chitosan-saccharide derivatives (Yang and Chou 2002; Chung et al. 2005), O-succinyl-chitosan (Zhang et al. 2003), quaternization (Snyman et al. 2002), and carboxymethylation chitosan (Chen and Park 2003).

4.6.1 N-ALKYL CHITOSANS

N-alkyl chitosan can be synthesized through reductive amination procedure. The primary amino groups of chitosan undergo Schiff reaction with aldehyde and ketones to yield the corresponding aldimines and ketimines, which are reduced with reducing agents such as sodium borohydride ($NaBH_4$) (Ramos et al. 2003; Rabea et al. 2005) or sodium cyanoborohydride ($NaBH_3CN$) (Desbrières et al. 1996; Bobu et al. 2011), and potassium borohydride (KBH4) (Zhang et al. 2003; Liu et al. 2010) to form N-alkyl chitosans (Figure 4.5).

Chitosan modification into N-alkyl chitosan will give chitosan derivative, which is amphiphilic, because it has both hydrophilic and hydrophobic chains. The hydrophobic chain of N-alkyl chitosan will decrease chitosan water absorption capacity (Nicu et al. 2013), so it can be used as a waterproof coating in food packaging paper (Bobu et al. 2011).

N-alkyl chitosan with high degree of substitution (DS) is generally best suited for paper coating. It was supported by many researchers. Nikmawahda Sugita et al. (2015) prepared N-alkyl chitosan using aldehydes octanal, decanal, and dodecanal with alkyl DS 0.0374, 0.0351, and 0.0335, respectively. N-Octylchitosan having the highest DS value is the best to be used as a paper coating among them because it has the lowest water absorption capacity.

Mobarak and Abdullah (2010) reported N-dodecyl chitosan synthesis with a DS value of 0.25. Onesippe and Lagerge (2008a) synthesized N-dodecyl chitosan with DS 0.068 from chitosan having DD 75%.

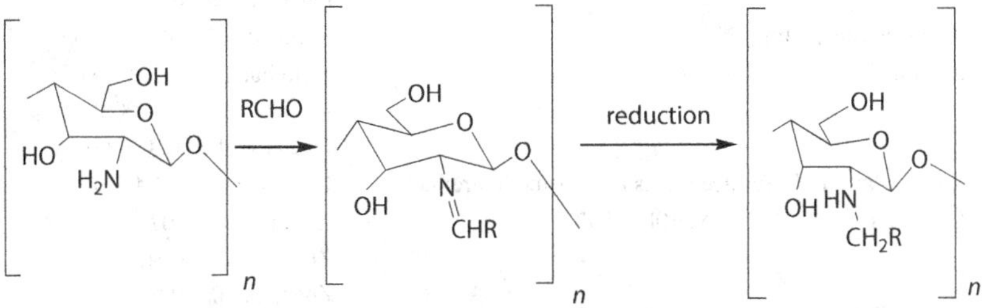

FIGURE 4.5 N-alkyl chitosan.

Liu et al. (2010) synthesized N-octyl-O-methoxypolyethyleneglycol from methoxypolyethylene glycol and chitosan having DD 95%, and the DS of obtained N-octylchitosan is 0.543.

N-Succinyl-N-octyl chitosan (SOCS), which can form micelles in aqueous media, was prepared by modifying the amino group with hydrophobic long-chain alkyl functionality and hydrophilic succinyl moiety. Doxorubicin (antitumor drug) was successfully loaded into SOCS micelles, and a sustained release of drug was observed.

Rinaudo and Domard (1989) prepared the N-alkyl chitosan derivatives and found the optimum alkyl chain length of C12 and grafting of 55 (Table 4.4).

4.6.2   QUATERNIZATION OF PRIMARY AMINE IN CHITOSAN

Generally, quaternization of amino group in chitosan increases the solubility of chitosan in water over a wide range of pHs (Verheul and Amidi 2008). In addition, the cationic character can be controlled and kept pH independent (Lee and Nah 2001). Typically, the reaction of chitosan with methyl iodide under basic condition is the most straightforward route for quaternizing chitosan (Sieval and Thanou 1998).

Chitosan can be modified into N,N,N-trimethyl chitosan chloride (TMC), which is a quaternary derivative of chitosan and has a superior aqueous solubility, intestinal permeability, and higher absorption over a wide range of pHs (Varkouhi and Verheul 2010). Among all the quaternized chitosans described in the literature, TMC is the most widely applied chitosan for gene therapy applications (Sieval and Thanou 1998; Thanou and Kotze 2000; Kean and Roth 2005). Depending on the degree of quaternization, the mucoadhesive property of chitosan is improved, and TMC is best used for gene delivery (Mourya and Inamdar 2008). TMC decreases the transepithelial electrical resistance, and therefore influences its drug absorption-enhancing properties.

TABLE 4.4
Application of N-Alkyl Chitosans

Application	Reference
Tissue engineering (scaffolds)	Cooney et al. (2009)
Sensor and fuel-cell applications (membrane)	Klotzbach et al. (2006)
	Klotzbach et al. (2008)
Model study of interaction with biological membranes	Lee et al. (2005)
	Lee et al. (2006)
Antibacterial coating	Maingam (2006)
DNA delivery	Ngimhuang et al. (2004)
	Rojanarata et al. (2008)
	Opanasopit et al. (2009)
Encapsulation of neutraceuticals and cosmetic products	Onesippe et al. (2008b)
Drug delivery (DOX, PTX, 10H CPT)	Xiang et al. (2007)
	Zhang et al. (2004)
	Zhang et al. (2008)
Membrane coating	de Britto and De Assis (2007)

Verheul and coworkers developed a synthetic route for the preparation of thiol-bearing TMC, which further enhances the delivery property of TMC (Varkouhi and Verheul 2010; Verheul and Van der wal 2010). The presence of thiol increased the mucoadhesion of chitosan derivatives by forming a disulfide bond with mucin proteins of the cell membrane (Langoth and Kahlbacher 2006; Yin and Ding 2009).

Chitosan can be modified into an ester form such as chitosan glucomate, chitosan succinate, and chitosan phthalate. These esteric forms have a different solubility profile. These esteric forms are insoluble in acidic conditions and provide a sustained release in basic conditions. Chitosan ester-based matrices have been used successfully in many formulations such as in colon-specific oral delivery of sodium diclofenac (Sinha and Kumria 2001).

4.6.3 GRAFTING OF CHITOSAN

Grafting of chitosan with succinic acid increases the solubility of chitosan in water. The grafting of carboxylic acids onto chitosan chains improved the transfection efficiency compared to pure chitosan but led to the formation of a weaker complex with DNA. To improve the transfection efficiency of chitosan, the grafting of cationic polymer chains onto chitosan was also investigated (Jiang and Kim 2007, 2009; Li and Guo 2010). Jere and Jiang (2009) successfully grafted low-molecular-weight poly(ethylene imine) (PEI) chains onto chitosan with the formation of the corresponding chitosan-*g*-PEI copolymer. Grafting of a carboxylic acid-bearing imidazole onto chitosan by amide formation, mediated by 1-ethyl-3-(3-dimethylaminopropyl) carbodiimide, was simple and reproducible, and improved the solubility and the buffering capacity of the chitosan derivatives (Ghosn and Kasturi 2008).

4.6.4 CHITOSAN OLIGOSACCHARIDE

Due to the poor solubility nature of chitosan, it is difficult to use in food and biomedical applications (Lodhi et al. 2014). Chitosan oligosaccharide (COS; D-glucosamine oligomer) is readily soluble in water because of its shorter chain length (Jeon et al. 2000). The low viscosity and greater solubility of COS at neutral pH have attracted the interest of many researchers to utilize chitosan in its oligosaccharide form (Table 4.5).

TABLE 4.5

Anticancer Derivatives of Chitosan Oligosaccharide

Chitosan Oligosaccharide Derivative	Application	Reference
Stearic acid-*g*-chitosan oligosaccharide	Anticancer agents	Huang et al. (2012)
Weight polyethyleneimine-conjugated stearic acid-*g*-chitosan oligosaccharide	Gene delivery and therapy	Hu et al. (2013)
Chitosan oligosaccharide-arachidic acid (CSOAA)	Doxorubicin delivery	Termsarasab et al. (2013)
Ferrocene-modified chitosan oligosaccharide nanoparticles	5-Fluorouracil delivery	Xu et al. (2014)

4.6.5 Carboxymethyl Chitosan

N-carboxymethyl chitosan was obtained in a water-soluble form by a proper selection of the reactant ratios, for example using equimolecular quantities of glyoxylic acid and amino groups (Muzzarelli 1988).

Chitosan is not suitable to bind directly onto Fe_3O_4 nanoparticles as it readily undergoes physisorption and aggregation. To overcome this problem, the derivative of chitosan is used with some physical and chemical modifications, which alters the magnetic property. Chang and Chen (2005) and Zhou et al. (2006) prepared carboxymethyl chitosan-Fe_3O_4 particles via carbodiimide activation. The final polymer magnetic microspheres had a high magnetic content and showed unique pH-dependent behaviors on the size and zeta potential.

Liang Guo et al. (2010) prepared Fe_3O_4/chitosan–polyacrylic acid (PAA) magnetic microspheres with high stability of magnetization. As this magnetic microsphere is solely made up of hydrophilic polymers, chitosan, and PAA that are nontoxic and biodegradable, it is used in bioapplications.

N-carboxymethyl chitosan is a chelating agent which is much more powerful than the parent chitosan for a number of metal ions with the notable exception of calcium. N-carboxymethyl chitosan and N-carboxyethyl chitosan are more effective bacteriostatic agents (Muzzarelli 1988).

4.6.6 Chitosan in Drug Delivery

Drug delivery system generally requires high molecular weight and high DD. Chitosan can be formulated as nanoparticles, microspheres (Berthold et al. 1996), and membrane sponge for drug delivery system (Puvvada et al. 2012).

4.6.7 Chitosan with Cross-Linking Agents

The solubility of chitosan is decreased due to the cross-linking with glutaraldehyde. Covalent interaction results in this cross-linking, which generally decreases the solubility behavior. Swelling property is also decreased with an increase in the concentration of cross-linking agent.

Allan et al. (1984) prepared chitosan-based vaginal tablets containing metronidazole by directly compressing the natural cationic polymer chitosan, loosely cross-linked with glutaraldehyde (Table 4.6).

4.7 CONCLUSION

The recourse to naturally occurring products with interesting antimicrobial and eliciting properties such as chitosan has been getting more attention in recent years. Chitin and chitosan were used extensively in all fields by modifying their physical and chemical properties because the source of the marine biopolymer is more and it should be eco-friendly. The modified form of chitin and chitosan was discussed with their applications.

TABLE 4.6

Applications of Chitosan by Improving Its Physicochemical Properties

Purpose	Reaction	Product
Reduces molecular weight (low viscosity, better solubility)	Depolymerization	Low-molecular-weight chitosan Chitosan oligomers
Improves cationic properties	Deacetylation Quaternization Addition of cationic moieties	Chitosan with high DD Quaternized chitosan Highly cationic derivatives
Improves chitosan water solubility	Alkylation, acylation Pegylation Hydroxyalkylation Carboxyalkylation	N-alkyl, acyl-chitosan PEG-chitosan Hydroxyalkyl-chitosan Carboxyalkyl chitosan
Amphoteric polyelectrolytes	Carboxyalkylation Phosphorylation Sulfatation	Carboxyalkyl chitosan Phosphonic-chitosan Sulfonic-chitosan
Cell targeting	Alkylation, cross-linking	Sugar modified chitosan
Photosensible derivatives	Azidation	Azidated-chitosan
Amphiphilic derivatives	Introduction of hydrophobic branches (alkylation, acylation, grafting, cross-linking)	N-alkyl chitosan Acyl-chitosan Graft derivatives Crown-ether derivatives Cyclodextrin derivatives
Miscellaneous	Several reactions (thiolation, Michael additon)	Thiol chitosan Thiourea-chitosan Chitosan-dentrimers

REFERENCES

Aiba, S.I. 1994. Preparation of N-acetylchitooligosaccharides by hydrolysis of chitosan with chitinase followed by N-acetylation. *Carbohydrate Research* 265: 323–328.

Allan, G.G., L.C. Altman, R.E. Bensinger, D.K. Ghosh, Y. Hirabayashi, A.N. Neogi, and S. Neogi. 1984. Biomedical applications of chitin and chitosan. In *Chitin, Chitosan and Related Enzymes*, J.P. Zikakis (ed.). Orlando, FL: Academic Press, pp. 119–134.

Backman, P.A., P.M. Brannen, and W.F. Mahaffee. 1994. Plant response and disease control following seed inoculation with *Bacillus subtilis*. *Proceedings of the Third International Workshop on Plant Growth-Promoting Rhizobacteria*, pp. 3–8.

Badawy, M.E.I., E.I. Rabea, and T.M. Rogge. 2004. Synthesis and fungicidal activity of new N, O-acyl chitosan derivatives. *Biomacromolecules* 5: 2.

Bansal, V., P.K. Sharma, N. Sharma, O.P. Pal, and R. Malviya. 2011. Applications of chitosan and chitosan derivatives in drug delivery. *Advances in Biological Research* 5(1): 28–37.

Berthold, A., K. Cremer, and J. Kreuter. 1996. Preparation and characterization of chitosan microspheres as drug carrier for prednisolone sodium phosphate as model for anti-inflammatory drugs. *Journal of Control Release* 39: 17–25.

Bobu, E., R. Nicu, M. Lupei, F.L. Ciolacu, and J. Desbrières. 2011. Synthesis and characterization of N-alkyl chitosan for papermaking applications. *Cellulose Chemistry Technology* 45(9–10): 619–625.

Capozza, R.C. 1975. German Patent no. 2,505,305.

Casey, D.J. 1977. Chitin derived surgical glove powder. U.S. Patent 4,064,564.

Cauchie, H.M. 2002. Chitin production by arthropods in the hydrosphere. *Hydrobiologia* 470: 63–96.

Chang, Y.C. and D.H. Chen. 2005. Adsorption kinetics and thermodynamics of acid dyes on a carboxymethylated chitosan-conjugated magnetic nanoadsorbent. *Macromolecule Bioscience* 5: 254–261.

Cheba, B.A. 2011. Chitin and chitosan. *Global Journal of Biotechnology & Biochemistry* 6(3): 149–153.

Chen, X. and H. Park. 2003. Chemical characteristics of O-carboxymethylchitosans related to preparation conditions. *Carbohydrate Polymers* 53: 355–359.

Chung, H.J., J.W. Bae, H.D. Park, J.W. Lee, and K.D. Park. 2005. Thermosensitive chitosans as novel injectable biomaterials. *Macromolecular Symposia* 224(1): 275–286.

Cooney, M.J., J. Petermann, C. Lau, and S.D. Minteer. 2009. Characterization and evaluation of hydrophobically modified chitosan scaffolds: Towards design of enzyme immobilized flow-through electrodes. *Carbohydrate Polymers* 75: 428–435.

de Britto, D. and O.B.G. De Assis. 2007. Synthesis and mechanical properties of quaternary salts of chitosan-based films for food application. *International Journal of Biological Macromolecules* 41: 198–203.

Desbrières, J., C. Martinez, and M. Rinaudo. 1996. Hydrophobic derivatives of chitosan: Characterization and rheological behavior. *International Journal of Biological Macromolecules* 19: 21–22.

Domard, A. 1996. Some physicochemical and structural basis for applicability of chitin and chitosan in chitin and chitosan. In *The Proceeding of the Second Asia Pacific Symposium*, W.F. Stevens, M.S. Rao, S. Chandrkrachang (eds.). Bangkok, Thailand: Asian Institute of Technology, pp. 1–12.

Dutta, P.K., M.N. Ravikumar, and J. Dutta. 2002. Chitin and Chitosan for versatile applications. *Journal of Macromolecular Science* C42: 307–354.

Dutta, P.K., J. Dutta, and V.S. Tripathi. 2004. Chitin and chitosan: Chemistry, properties and applications. *Journal of Scientific and Industrial research* 63: 20–31.

Dutta, P.K., P. Vishwanathan, L. Mimrot, and M.N.V. Ravikumar. 1997. Use of chitosan-amine-oxide gel as drug carriers. *Journal of Polymer Materials* 14: 531.

Ehrlich, H. 2010. Chitin and collagen as universal and alternative templates in biomineralization. *International Geology Review* 52: 661–699.

Ehrlich, H., M. Ilan, M. Maldonado, G. Muricy, G. Bavestrello, Z. Kljajic, J.L. Carballo, and et al. 2010. Three-dimensional chitin-based scaffolds from Verongida sponges (Demospongiae: Porifera), Part I-Isolation and identification of chitin. *International Journal of Biological Macromolecules* 47(2): 132–140.

Falcón, A.B., M.A. Ramírez, R. Márquez, and M. Hernández. 2002. Chitosan and its hydrolysateat tobacco-phytophthoraparasitica interaction. *Cultivos Tropicales* 23(1): 61.

Francis, S.J.K. and H.W.T. Matthew. 2000. Application of chitosan based polysaccharide biomaterials in cartilage tissue engineering: A review. *Biomaterials* 21: 2589–2598.

Friedman, M. and V.K. Juneja. 2010. Review of antimicrobial and antioxidative activities of chitosans in food. *Journal of Food Protection* 73: 1737–1761.

Gamayurova, V.S., M.N. Kotlyar, N.V. Shabrukova, and F.G. Khalitov. 1998. Thematic course: Natural polysaccharides. Part I. synthesis of soluble derivatives of chitin-glucan complex. *Chemistry and Computational Simulation Communications* 1: 73.

Guo, L., G. Liu, R.-Y. Hong., H.-Z. Li. 2010. Preparation and characterization of chitosan poly(acrylic acid) magnetic microspheres. *Marine Drugs* 8: 2212–2222.

Ge, H. and S. Huang. 2010. Microwave preparation and adsorption properties of EDTA-modified cross-linked chitosan. *Journal of Applied Polymer Science* 115(1): 514–519.

Ghosn, B. and S.P. Kasturi. 2008. Enhancing polysaccharide-mediated delivery of nucleic acids through functionalization with secondary and tertiary amines. *Current Topics in Medicinal Chemistry* 8: 331–340.

Gil, G., S. Del Monaco, P. Cerruti, and M. Galvagano. 2004. Selective antimicrobial activity of chitosan on beer spoilage bacteria and brewing yeast. *Biotechnology Letters* 26: 569–574.

Gorochovceva, N. and R. Makuska. 2004. Synthesis and study of water-soluble chitosan-O-poly (ethylene glycol) graft copolymers. *European Polymer Journal* 40(4): 685–691.

Gross, P., E. Konrad, and H. Mager. 1980. Hair shampoo and conditioning lotion. U.S. Patent 4,202,881.

Hadwiger, L.A., T. Ogawa, and H. Kuyama. 1994. Chitosan polymer sizes effective in inducing phytoalexin accumulation and fungal suppression are verified with synthesized oligomers. *Molecular Plant Microbe Interactions* 7(4): 531–533.

Hajji, S., I. Younes, O. Ghorbel-Bellaaj, R. Hajji, M. Rinaudo, M. Nasri, and K. Jellouli. 2014. Structural differences between chitin and chitosan extracted from three marine sources. *International Journal of Biological Macromolecules* 65: 298–306.

Hasegawa, M., A. Isogai, and F. Onabe. 1993. Preparation of low-molecular-weight chitosan using phosphoric acid. *Carbohydrate Polymers* 20: 279–283.

Hernández, R.M., A.N. Velázquez, and S. Bautista. 2007. Induction of defense response of Oryza sativa L. against Pyriculariagrisea (Cooke) Sacc by treating seeds with chitosan and hydrolyzed chitosan. *Pesticide Biochemistry and Physiology* 89: 206–15.

Hirano, S. 1997. *N*-acyl, *N*-arylidene- and *N*-alkylidenechitosans, and their hydrogels. In *Chitin Handbook*, R.A.A. Muzzarelli, M.G. Peter (eds.). Italy: European Kinetic Society, pp. 71–76.

Hu, F.Q., W.W. Chen, M.D. Zhao, H. Yuan, and Y.Z. Du. 2013. Effective antitumor gene therapy delivered by polyethylenimine-conjugated stearic acid-g-chitosan oligosaccharide micelles. *Gene Therapy* 120: 597–606.

Huang, X., X. Huang, X.H. Jiang, F.Q. Hu, Y.Z. Du, Q.F. Zhu, and C.S. Jin. 2012. In vitro antitumour activity of stearic acid-g-chitosan oligosaccharide polymeric micelles loading podophyllotoxin. *Journal of Microencapsulation* 29: 1–8.

Hudson, S.M., and C. Smith. 1998. Polysaccharide: Chitin and chitosan: Chemistry and technology of their use as structural materials. In *Biopolymers From Renewable Resources*, D.L. Kalpan (ed.). New York: Springer-Verlag, pp. 96–118.

Iglesias, R., A. Gutiérrez, and F. Fernández. 1994. The influence of chitin from lobster exoskeleton on seedling growth and mycorrhizal infection in tomato crop (*Licopersicumesculentum Mill.*). *Cultivos Tropicales* 15(2): 48–49.

Ilyina, A.V., N.Y. Tatarinova, and V.P. Varlamov. 1999. The preparation of low-molecular-weight chitosan using chitinolytic complex from *Streptomyces kurssanovii*. *Process Biochemistry* 34: 875–878.

Islam, S., L. Arnold, and R. Padhye. 2013. Application of chitosan on wool-viscose nonwoven for wound dressing. *Journal of Biobased Materials and Bioenergy* 7(4): 439–443.

Itoi, H., N. Komiyama, H. Sano, and H. Mandai. 1985. Pharmaceutical Bandages, Japanese Patent Kokai 60-142927.

Jackson, D.S. 1987. Chitosan-Glycerol-water gel. U.S. patent 4,659,700.

Jang, M.K., B.G. Kong, Y.I. Jeong, C.H. Lee, and J.W. Nah. 2004. Physicochemical characterization of α-chitin, β-chitin, and γ-chitin separated from natural resources. *Journal of Polymer Science Part A: Polymer Chemistry* 42: 3423–3432.

Jeon, Y.J., P.J. Park, and S.K. Kim. 2001. Antimicrobial effect of chitooligosaccharides produced by bioreactor. *Carbohydrate Polymers* 44: 71–76.

Jeon, Y.J., F. Shahidi, and S.K. Kim. 2000. Preparation of chitin and chitosan oligomers and their applications in physiological functional foods. *Food Reviews International* 16: 159–176.

Jere, D. and H.L. Jiang. 2009. Chitosan-graft-polyethylenimine for Akt1 siRNA delivery to lung cancer cells. *International Journal of Pharmaceutics* 378: 194–200.

Jiang, H.L. and Y.K. Kim. 2007. Chitosan-graft-polyethylenimine as a gene carrier. *Journal of Controlled Release* 117: 273–280.

Jiang, H.L. and Y.K. Kim. 2009. Mannosylated chitosan-graft-polyethylenimine as a gene carrier for Raw 264.7 cell targeting. *International Journal of Pharmaceutics* 375: 133–139.

Jin, R.D., J. Suh, R.D. Park, Y.W. Kim, H.B. Krishnan, and K. Kil Yong. 2005. Effect of chitin compost and broth on biological control of Meloidogyne incognita on tomato (*Lycopersiconesculentum Mill.*). *Nematology* 7(1): 125–132.

Kafetzopoulos, D., A. Martinou, and V. Bouriotis. 1993. Bioconversion of chitin to chitosan: Purification and characterization of chitin deacetylase from Mucorrouxii. *Proceedings of the National Academy of Sciences* 90: 2564–2568.

Kardas, I., M.H. Struszczyk, M. Kucharska,. L.A.M. Van den Broek, J.E.G. Van Dam, and D. Ciechańska. 2012. Chitin and chitosan as functional biopolymers for industrial applications. In *The European Polysaccharide Network of Excellence (EPNOE). Research Initiatives and Results*, P. Narvard (ed.). Wien, Austria: Springer-Verlag, pp. 329–374.

Kean, T. and S. Roth. 2005. Trimethylatedchitosans as non-viral gene delivery vectors: Cytotoxicity and transfection efficiency. *Journal of Controlled Release* 103: 643–653.

Khan, T.A., K.K. Peh, and H.S. Ch'ng. 2001. Reporting degree of deacetylation values of chitosan: Influence of analytical methods. *Journal of Pharmacy and Pharmaceutical Sciences* 5(3): 205–212.

Kifune, K., Y. Yamaguchi, and H. Tanae. 1987. Wound Dressing, U.S. Patent 4,651,725.

Kim, S.J., S.S. Kim, and Y.M. Lee. 1994. Synthesis and characterization of ether-type chitin derivatives. *Macromolecular Chemistry and Physics* 195(5): 1687–1693.

Klotzbach, T., M. Watt, Y. Ansari, and S.D. Minteer. 2006. Effects of hydrophobic modification of chitosan and nafion on transport properties, ion-exchange capacities, and enzyme immobilization. *Journal of Membrane Science* 282: 276–283.

Klotzbach, T.L., M. Watt, Y. Ansari, and S.D. Minteer. 2008. Improving the micro environment for enzyme immobilization at electrodes by hydrophobically modifying chitosan and Nafion polymers. *Journal of Membrane Science* 311: 81–88.

Knorr, D. 1984. Use of chitinous polymers in food. *Food Technology* 38(1): 85–97.

Koga, D., R.H. Chen, and H.C. Chen (eds.). 1999. *Advances in Chitin Science*, vol. 3. Taipei, Taiwan: Rita Advertising, p. 16.

Kubota, N., N. Tastumoto, T. Sano, and K. Toya. 2000. A simple preparation of half Nacetylated chitosan highly soluble in water and aqueous organic solvents. *Carbohydrate Research* 324(4): 268–274.

Kuhlmann, K., A. Czupala, J. Haunhorst, A. Weiss, T. Prasch, and U. Schorken. 1999. Preparation and Characterization of Chitosan from Mucorales. *In Advances in Chitin Science*, Vol 4, M.G. Peter, A. Domard, R.A.A. Muzzarelli (eds.). European Chitin Society, pp. 7–15.

Kumar, M.N.V.R. 2000. A review of chitin and chitosan applications. *Reactive and Functional Polymers* 46: 1–27.

Kurita, K. 1998. Polymer degradation and stability. *Macromolecular Chemistry* 59(1): 117–120.

Kurita, K. 2001. Controlled functionalization of polysaccharide chitin. *Progress in Polymer Science* 26: 1921–1971.

Kurita, K., S. Ishii, K. Tomita, S.I. Nishimura, and K. Shimoda. 1994. Reactivity characteristics of squid β-chitin ascompared with those of shrimp chitin: High potentials of squid chitin as a starting material for facile chemical modifications. *Journal of Polymer Science Part A: Polymer Chemistry* 32: 1027–1032.

Kurita, K., Y. Kaji, T. Mori, and Y. Nishiyama. 2000. Enzymatic degradation of β-chitin: Susceptibility and the influence of deacetylation. *Carbohydrate Polymers* 42: 19–21.

Kurita, K., T. Sannan, and Y. Iwakura. 1977. Studies on chitin, 4: Evidence for formation of block and random copolymers of N-acetyl-D-glucosamine and D-glucosamine by hetero- and homogeneous hydrolyses. *Macromolecular Chemistry* 178: 3197–3202.

Langoth, N. and H. Kahlbacher. 2006. Thiolated chitosans: Design and in vivo evaluation of a mucoadhesive buccal peptide drug delivery system. *Pharmaceutical Research* 23: 573–579.

Lantero, O.J. 1986. Immobilization of Biocatalysts. Canadian Patent 1,210,717.

Lee, V. 1974. *Solution and Shear Properties of Chitin and Chitosan.* Ann Arbor, MI: University Microfilms.

Lee, J.H., J.P. Gustin, T. Chen, G.F. Payne, and S.R. Raghavan. 2005. Vesicle biopolymer gels: Networks of surfactant vesicles connected by associating biopolymers. *Langmuir* 21: 26–33.

Lee, M., Y.W. Cho, J.H. Park, H. Chung, S.Y. Jeong, and K. Choi. 2006. Size control of self-assembled nano particles by an emulsion/solvent evaporation method. *Colloid and Polymer Science* 284: 506–512.

Lee, M. and J.W. Nah. 2001. Water-soluble and low molecular weight chitosan-based plasmid DNA delivery. *Pharmaceutical Research* 18: 427–431.

Li, Q., E.T. Dunn, E.W. Grandmaison, and M.F.A. Goosen. 1992. Applications and properties of chitosan. *Journal of Bioactive and Compatible Polymers* 7: 370–397.

Li, Q., E.T. Dunn, E.W. Grandmaison, and M.F.A. Goosen. 1997. Applications and properties of chitosan. In *Applications of Chitin and Chitosan*, M.F.A. Goosen (ed.). Lancaster, England: Technomic Publishing Company, pp. 3–29.

Li, Q., J. Zhou, and L. Zhang. 2009. Structure and properties of the nanocomposite films of chitosan reinforced with cellulose whisker. *Journal of Polymer Science, Part B* 47(11): 1069–1077.

Li, Z., R. Yang, M. Zhang, and B. Wang. 2015. Structure and properties of chitin whisker reinforced for food packaging application. *BioResources* 10(2): 2995–3004.

Li, Z.T. and J. Guo. 2010. Chitosan-graft-polyethylenimine with improved properties as a potential gene vector. *Carbohydrate Polymers* 80: 254–259.

Liu, G., J. Gan, A. Chen, Q. Liu, and X. Zhao. 2010. Synthesis and characterization of an amphiphilic chitosan bearing octyl and methoxy polyethylene. *Journal of Natural Science* 2(7): 707–712.

Lodhi, G., Y.S. Kim, J.W. Hwang, S.K. Kim, Y.J. Jeon, J.Y. Je, C.B. Ahn, S.H. Moon, and P.J. Park. 2014. Chitooligosaccharide and its derivatives: Preparation and biological applications. *Biomed Research International* 654913: 1–13.

Lusena, C.V. and R.C. Rose. 1953. Preparation and viscosity of chitosan. *Journal of Fish Research* 10: 521–522.

Maingam, K. 2006. Comblikepoly(ethyleneoxide)/hydrophobic C6 branched chitosan surfactant polymers as anti-infection surface modifying agents. *Colloids and Surfaces B: Biointerfaces B* 49: 117–125.

Malette, W.G., H.J. Quigley, R.D. Gaines, N.D. Johnson, and W.G. Rainer. 1983. Chitosan: A new hemostatic. *The Annals of Thoracic Surgery* 36(1): 55–58.

Mima, S., M. Miya, R. Iwamoto, and S. Yoshikana. 1983. Highly Deacetylated chitosan and its properties. *Journal of Applied Polymer Science* 28: 1909–1917.

Mobarak, N.N. and M.P. Abdullah. 2010. Synthesis and characterization of several lauryl chitosan derivatives. *Malaysian Journal of Analytical Sciences* 14(2): 82–99.

Mourya, V.K. and N.N. Inamdar. 2008. Chitosan-modifications and applications: Opportunities galore. *Reactive and Functional Polymers* 68: 1013–1051.

Muzzarelli, R., R. Tarsi, O. Filippini, E. Giovanetti, G. Biagini, and P.E. Varaldo. 1990. Antimicrobial properties of N-carboxybutyl chitosan. *Antimicrobial Agents and Chemotherapy* 34(10): 2019–2023.

Muzzarelli, R.A.A. 1973. *Natural Chelating Polymers; Alginic Acid, Chitin and Chitosan* Oxford, New York: Pergamon Press.

Muzzarelli, R.A.A. 1977. *Chitin*. Kidlington, Oxford: Pergamon Press.

Muzzarelli, R.A.A. 1988. Carboxymethylated chitins and chitosans. *Carbohydrate Polymers* 8: 1–21.

Muzzarelli, R.A.A., C. Muzzarelli, and M. Terbojevich. 1997. Chitin chemistry, upgrading a renewable resource. *Carbohydrates in Europe* 19: 10–17.

Nagyvary, J.J., J.D. Falk, M.L. Hill, M.L. Schmidt, A.K. Wilkins, and E.L. Bradbury. 1979. The hypolipidemic activity of chitosan and other polysaccharides in rats. *Nutrition Reports International* 20: 677–684.

Ngimhuang, J., J.I. Furukawa, T. Satoh, T. Furuike, and N. Sakairi. 2004. Synthesis of a novel polymeric surfactant by reductive *N*-alkylation of chitosan with 3-O-dodecyl-D-glucose. *Polymer* 45: 837–841.

Nicu, R., M. Lupei, T. Balan, and E. Bobu. 2013. Alkyl–chitosan as paper coating material to improve water barrier properties. *Cellulose Chemistry and Technology* 47(7–8): 623–630.

Nikmawahda, H.T., P. Sugita, and B. Arifin. 2015. Synthesis and characterization of N-alkylchitosan as well as its potency as a paper coating material. *Advances in Applied Science Research* 6(2): 141–149.

No, H.K. and S.P. Meyers. 1995. Preparation and characterization of chitin and chitosan-A review. *Journal of Aquatic Food Product Technology* 2: 27–52.

Noishiki, Y., H. Takami, Y. Nishiyama, M. Wada, S. Okada, and S. Kuga. 2003. Alkali-induced conversion of β-chitin to α-chitin. *Biomacromolecules* 4: 896–899.

Nomanbhay, S.M. and K. Palanisamy. 2005. Removal of heavy metal from industrial waste-water using chitosan coated oil palm shell charcoal. *Electronic Journal of Biotechnology* 8(1): 43–53.

Ogawa, W. and N. Oka. 1993. X-ray study of chitosan-transition metal complexes. *Chemistry of Materials* 5(5): 726–728.

Okamoto, Y., S. Minami, A. Matsuhashi, H. Sashiwa, H. Saimoto, Y. Shigemasa, T. Tanigawa, Y. Tanaka, and S. Tokura. 1993. Application of polymeric *N*-acetyl-D-glucosamine (chitin) to veterinary practice. *The Journal of Veterinary Medical Science* 55(5): 743–774.

Onesippe, C. and S. Lagerge. 2008a. Study of the complex formation between sodium dodecyl sulfate and hydrophobically modified chitosan. *Carbohydrate Polymers* 74: 648–658.

Onésippe, C. and S. Lagerge. 2008b. Studies of the association of chitosan and alkylated chitosan with oppositely charged sodium dodecyl sulfate. *Colloid Surfaces A* 330: 201–206.

Opanasopit, P., M. Petchsangsai, T. Rojanarata, T. Ngawhirunpat, W. Sajomsang, and U. Ruktanonchai. 2009. Methylated *N*-(4-*N*,*N*-dimethylaminobenzyl) chitosan as effective gene carriers: Effect of degree of substitution. *Carbohydrate Polymers* 75: 143–149.

Ouchi, T., H. Nishizawa, and Y. Ohya. 1998. Aggregation phenomenon of PEG-grafted chitosan in aqueus solution. *Polymer* 39(21): 5171–5175.

Percot, A., C. Viton, and A. Domard. 2003. Optimization of chitin extraction from shrimp shells. *Biomacromolecules* 4: 1218.

Pillai, C.K.S., W. Paul, and C.P. Sharma. 2009. Chitin and chitosan polymers: Chemistry, solubility and fiber formation. *Progress in Polymer Science* 34(7): 641–678.

Puvvada, Y.S., S. Vankayalapati, and S. Sukhavasi. 2012. Extraction of chitin from chitosan from exoskeleton of shrimp for application in the pharmaceutical industry. *International Current Pharmaceutical Journal* 1(9): 258–263.

Rabea, E.I., M.E.I. Badawy, T.M. Rogge, C.V. Stevens, G. Smagghe, M. Hofte, and W. Steurbaut. 2005. Insecticidal and fungicidal activity of new synthesized chitosan derivatives. *Pest Management Science* 61(10): 951–960.

Ramos, V.M., N.M. Rodriguez, M.S. Rodriguez, A. Heras, and E. Agullo. 2003. Modified chitosan carrying phosphonic and alkyl groups. *Carbohydrate Polymers* 51: 425–429.

Rathke, T. 1993. Determination of the degree of N-deacteylation in chitin and chitosan as well as their monomer sugar ratios by near infrared spectroscopy. *Journal of Polymer Science Part A: Polymer Chemistry* 31: 749–753.

Rhoades, J. and S. Roller. 2000. Antimicrobial actions of degraded and native chitosan against spoilage organisms in laboratory media and foods. *Applied and Environmental Microbiology* 66: 80–86.

Rinaudo, M. 2006. Chitin and chitosan: Properties and applications. *Progress in Polymer Science* 31(7): 603–632.

Rinaudo, M. and A. Domard. 1989. Solution properties of chitosans. In *Chitin and Chitosan*, G. Skjak-Braek, T. Anthonsen, P. Sandford (eds.). London, UK: Elsevier, pp. 71–86.

Roberts, G.A.F. 1992a. *Chitin Chemistry*, 1st edition. London, UK: MacMillan.

Roberts, G.A.F. 1992b. Solubility and solution behavior of chitin and chitosan. In *Chitin Chemistry*, G.A.F. Roberts (ed.). Basingstoke, UK: MacMillan, pp. 274–329.

Rojanarata, T., M. Petchsangsai, P. Opanasopit, T. Ngawhirunpat, U. Ruktanonchai, W. Sajomsang, and S. Tantayanon. 2008. Methylated N-(4-N,N-dimethylaminobenzyl) chitosan for novel effective gene carriers. *European Journal of Pharmaceutics and Biopharmaceutics* 70: 207–214.

Rubentheren, V., T.A. Ward, C.Y. Chee, and C.K. Tang. 2015. Processing and analysis of chitosan nanocomposites reinforced with chitin whiskers and tannic acid as a crosslinker. *Carbohydrate Polymer* 115: 379–387.

Rudall, K.M. and W. Kenchington. 1973. The chitin system. *Biological Reviews* 49: 597–636.

Rutherford, F. and P.R. Austin. 1978. In *Proceedings of First International Conference on Chitin and Chitosan*, R.A.A. Muzzarelli, E.R. Pariser (eds.). Cambridge, MA: MIT Press, pp. 182–192.

Sannan, T., K. Kurita, and Y. Iwakura. 1976. Studies on chitin, effect of deacetylation on solubility. *Die Makromolekulare Chemie* 177: 3589–3600.

Sashiwa, H., H. Saimoto, Y. Shigemasa, R. Ogawa, and S. Tokura. 1990. Lysozyme susceptibility of partially deacetylated chitin. *International Journal of Biological Macromolecules* 12: 295.

Shigemasa, Y., K. Saito, H. Sashiwa, and H. Saimoto. 1994. Enzymatic degradation of chitins and partially deacetylated chitins. *International Journal of Biological Macromolecules* 16: 43–49.

Shimojoh, M., M. Fukushima, and K. Kurita. 1998. Low-molecular-weight chitosans derived from beta-chitin: Preparation, molecular characteristics and aggregation activity. *Carbohydrate Polymers* 35: 223–231.

Sieval, A.B. and M. Thanou. 1998. Preparation and NMR characterization of highly substituted N-trimethyl chitosan chloride. *Carbohydrate Polymers* 36: 157–165.

Sinha, V.R. and R. Kumria. 2001. Polysaccharides in colon-specific drug delivery. *International Journal of Pharmaceutics* 224(1–2): 19–38.

Siraj, S., M.D.M. Islam, P.C. Das, S.M.D. Masum, I.A. Jahan, M.D. Ahsan, and M.D. Shajahan. 2012. Removal of chromium from tannery effluent using chitosan-charcoal composite. *Journal of Bangladesh Chemical Society* 25(1): 53–61.

Smith, R.L. 1984. Chitosan as a Contraceptive, U.S. Patent 4,474,769.

Snyman, D., J.H. Hamman, J.S. Kotze, J.E. Rollings, and A.F. Kotze. 2002. The relationship between the absolute molecular weight and the degree of quaternization of N-trimethyl chitosan chloride. *Carbohydrate Polymers* 50(2): 145–150.

Struszczyk, M.H., R. Halweg, and M.G. Peter. 1999. Comparative analysis of chitosans from insects and Crustacea. In *Advances in Chitin Science*, Vol 4, M.G. Peter, A. Domard, R.A.A. Muzzarelli (eds.). European Chitin Society, pp. 40–49.

Sugimoto, M., M. Morimoto, and H. Sashiwa. 1998. Preparation and characterization of water-soluble chitin and chitosan derivatives. *Carbohydrate Polymers* 36(1): 49–59.

Synowiecki, J. and N.A.A. Al-khatteb. 2003. Production, properties and some new applications of chitin and its derivatives. *Critical Reviews in Food Science and Nutrition* 43:144–171.

Tanner, S.F., H. Chanzy, M. Vincendon, J.C. Roux, and F. Gaill. 1990. High resolution solid-state carbon-13 nuclear magnetic resonance study of chitin. *Macromolecules* 23: 3576–3583.

Terbojevich, M., A. Cosani, and R.A.A. Muzzarelli. 1996. Molecular parameters of chitosans depolymerized with the aid of papain. *Carbohydrate Polymers* 29: 63.

Termsarasab, U., H.J. Cho, D.H. Kim, S. Chong, S.J. Chung, C.K. Shim, H.T. Moon, and D.D. Kim. 2013. Chitosan oligosaccharide-arachidic acid-based nanoparticles for anticancer drug delivery. *International Journal of Pharmaceutics* 441: 373–380.

Thanou, M.M. and A.F. Kotze. 2000. Effect of degree of quaternization of N-trimethyl chitosan chloride for enhanced transport of hydrophilic compounds across intestinal Caco-2 cell monolayers. *Journal of Controlled Release* 64: 15–25.

Tokuyasu, K., M. Mitsutomi, I. Yamaguchi, K. Hayashi, and Y. Mori. 2000. Recognition of chitooligosaccharides and their *N*-acetyl groups by putative subsites of chitin deacetylase from a deuteromycete, Colletotrichumlindemuthianum. *Biochemistry* 39: 8837–8843.

Tolaimate, A., J. Desbrieres, M. Rhazi, and A. Alagui. 2003. Contribution to the preparation of chitins and chitosans with controlled physico-chemical properties. *Polymer* 44: 7939–7952.

Tommeraas, K., M. Koping-Hoggard, K.M. Varum, B.E. Christensen, P. Artursson, and O. Smidsrod. 2002. Preparation and characterisation of chitosans with oligosaccharide branches. *Carbohydrate Research* 337(24): 2455–2462.

Uddin, A.J., J. Araki, M. Fujie, S. Sembo, and Y. Gotoh. 2012. Interfacial interaction and mechanical properties of chitin whisker–poly(vinyl alcohol) gel-spun nanocomposite fibers. *Polymer International* 61(6): 1010–1015.

Varkouhi, A.K. and R.J. Verheul. 2010. Gene silencing activity of Si RNA polyplexes based on thiolated N, N, N-trimethylated chitosan. *Bioconjugate Chemistry* 21: 2339–2346.

Vårum, K.M., M.H. Ottoy, and O. Smidsrod. 1994. Water-solubility of partially N-acetylated chitosans as the function of pH. Effect of chemical composition and depolymerization. *Carbohydrate Polymers* 25 (2): 65–70.

Verheul, R.J. and M. Amidi. 2008. Synthesis, characterization and in vitro biological properties of O-methyl free *N,N,N*-trimethylated chitosan. *Biomaterials* 29: 642–3649.

Verheul, R.J. and S. Van der Wal. 2010. Tailorable thiolated trimethylchitosans for covalently stabilized nanoparticles. *Biomacromolecules* 11: 1965–1971.

Wan, Y., K.A.M. Creber, V.B. Peppley, and T. Bui. 2003. Ionic conductivity of chitosan membranes. *Polymer* 44: 1057–1065.

Widra, A. 1986. Hydrophilic Biopolymeric copolyelectrolyte, and Biodegradable Wound Dressing Comprising Same. U.S. Patent 4,570,629.

Wysokowski, M., V.V. Bazhenov, M.V. Tsurka, R. Galli, A.L. Stelling, H. Stöcker, S. Kaiser, E. Niederschlag, G. Gärtner, and T. Behm. 2013. Isolation and identification of chitin in three-dimensional skeleton of *Aplysina fistularis* marine sponge. *International Journal of Biological Macromolecules* 62: 94–100.

Xiang, Y.X., L. Ling, Z. Jianping, L. Shiyue, Y. Jie, Y. Xiaojin, and R. Jinsheng. 2007. Preparation and characterization of N-succinyl-N-octyl chitosan micelles as doxorubicin carriers for effective anti-tumor activity. *Colloids and Surfaces B* 55: 222–228.

Xie, W.M., P.X. Xu, W. Wang, and Q. Lu. 2002. Preparation and antibacterial activity of water-soluble chitosan derivatives. *Carbohydrate Polymers* 50(1): 35–40.

Xu, Y., L. Wang, Y.K. Li, and C.Q. Wang. 2014. Oxidation and pH responsive nanoparticles based on ferrocene-modified chitosan oligosaccharide for 5-fluorouracil delivery. *Carbohydrate Polymers* 114: 27–35.

Yang, T.C. and C.C. Chou. 2002. Preparation, water solubility and rheological property of the N-alkylated mono or disaccharide chitosan derivatives. *Food Research International* 35: 707–713.

Yi, H., L.Q. Wu, W.E. Bentley, R. Ghodssi, G.W. Rubloff, and J.N. Culver. 2005. Biofabrication with chitosan. *Biomacromolecules* 6: 2881–94.

Yin, L.C. and J.Y. Ding. 2009. Drug permeability and mucoadhesion properties of thiolatedtri-methyl chitosan nanoparticles in oral insulin delivery. *Biomaterials* 30: 5691–5700.

Younes, I., S. Sellimi, M. Rinaudo, K. Jellouli, and M. Nasri. 2014. Influence of acetylation degree and molecular weight of homogeneous chitosans on antibacterial and antifungal activities. *International Journal of Food Microbiology* 185: 57–63.

Zhang, C., Q. Ping, H. Zhang, and J. Shen. 2003. Preparation of N-alkyl-O-sulfate chitosan derivatives and micellar solubilization of taxol. *Carbohydrate Polymers* 54: 137–141.

Zhang, C., P. Qineng, and H. Zhang. 2004. Self-assembly and characterization of paclitaxel-loaded N-octyl-O-sulfate chitosan micellar system. *Colloids and Surfaces B: Biointerfaces* 39: 69–75.

Zhang, C., G. Qu, Y. Sun, X. Wu, Z. Yao, and Q. Guo. 2008. Pharmacokinetics, bio distribution, efficacy and safety of N-octyl-O-sulfate chitosan micelles loaded with paclitaxel. *Biomaterial* 29: 1233–1241.

Zhang, H., R. Li, and W. Liu. 2011. Effects of chitin and its derivative chitosan on postharvest decay of fruits: A review. *International Journal of Molecular Sciences* 12(2): 917–934.

Zhou, L.M., Y.P. Wang, Z.R. Liu, and Q.W. Huang. 2006. Carboxymethyl chitosan-Fe_3O_4 nanoparticles: Preparation and adsorption behavior toward Zn^{2+} ions. *Carboxymethyl Chitosan-Fe_3O_4 Nanoparticles: Preparation and Adsorption Behavior Toward Zn^{2+} ions* 22: 1342–1346.

5 Chemical Modification of Chitin and Chitosan for Their Potential Applications

Mohamed E.I. Badawy and Entsar I. Rabea

CONTENTS

5.1   INTRODUCTION

Evolution and development of absorbable/biodegradable polysaccharides was associated mostly with chitin and chitosan biopolymers. Chitin is a naturally abundant polysaccharide and the supporting material of crustaceans, insects, and fungi (Austin et al. 1981). It consists of β-(1–4)-2-acetamido-2-deoxy-β-D-glucose (GlcNAc) units through a β-(1→4) linkage. However, chitosan is composed of >70%

of β-(1-4)-2-deoxyβ-D-glucopyranose (GlcN) and <30% of GlcNA units linked by β-1,4-glucosidic bonds and obtained through deacetylation (DA) process of purified chitin using hot alkali (Sandford 1989; No and Meyer 1995; Sandford 2003; Tharanathan and Kittur 2003; Dutta et al. 2004; Pillai et al. 2009). A sharp classification with respect to the degree of N-DA has not been defined between chitin and chitosan (Muzzarelli 1973; Muzzarelli et al. 1997; Zikakis et al. 1982; Zikakis 2012). Chitin and chitosan are of commercial interest because of their high content of nitrogen (~6.0%–7.0%) compared to the cellulose (1.25%). This makes both of them useful chelating agents (Muzzarelli and Tubertini 1969; Muzzarelli 1973; Hall and Yalpani 1980a; Varma et al. 2004; Kyzas and Bikiaris 2015).

5.2 CHEMICAL REACTIVITY OF CHITIN AND CHITOSAN

Chitin and chitosan are interesting biopolymers because of the presence of the reactive function groups, which could be suitably modified to impart the desired properties and distinctive physicochemical and biological properties (Muzzarelli 1977; Hudson and Smith 1998; Kurita et al. 2002; Tharanathan and Kittur 2003; Rinaudo 2006; Campana-Filho et al. 2007). The free NH_2 group at the C-2 position is the important point of difference between chitin and chitosan. Chitin and chitosan have two reactive hydroxyl groups, which could be chemically modified to enhance their properties (Dumitriu 1996). The possible reaction sites for chitin and chitosan are shown in Figure 5.1. Several research groups have studied the various aspects of chemical modification of both polymers (Kurita 1986; Kurita et al. 2002; Chen and Park 2003; Dutta et al. 2004; Kumar et al. 2004; Jayakumar et al. 2005; Prashanth and Tharanathan 2007; d'Ayala et al. 2008; Jayakumar et al. 2008b; Mourya and Inamdar 2008; Prabaharan 2008; Pillai et al. 2009). The amino group of chitosan chain gives rise to chemical reactions such as acetylation, quaternization, Schiff's bases, reductive amination, acylation, phosphorylation, and chelation of metals to produce many products that have promising properties such as antimicrobial, antiviral, nontoxic, nonallergenic, total biocompatibility, and biodegradability. The hydroxyl functional groups of both chitin and chitosan also give various reactions such as O-acetylation, H-bonding with polar atoms,

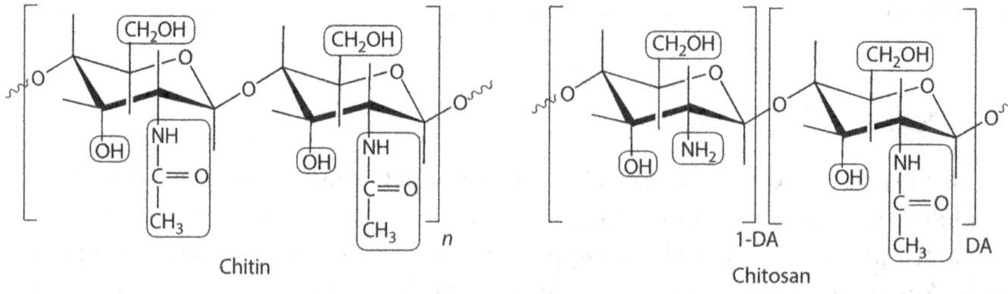

FIGURE 5.1 Chemical structures and illustrations of the possible reaction sites in the chitin (GlcNAc units) and chitosan (GlcN and remaining of GlcNAc units).

etherification, esterification, cross-linking, and graft copolymerization. Due to the rigid crystanility and insolubility of chitin (Muzzarelli 1977; Muzzarelli et al. 1986a; Rinaudo 2006), most research studies have been focused on the chemical modification of chitosan with regard to preparing compounds having well-defined structures and advanced properties and functions.

Compared to the present synthetic polymers, chitin and chitosan have biocompatibility, biodegradability, and low mammalian toxicity properties that make such polymers useful in different applications in the environment. However, these polymers also exhibit a limitation in their solubility, reactivity, and processability (Ilium 1998). Therefore, much attention has been paid to modification of the chemical structure of chitin and chitosan which are potential polysaccharides resources (Nishimura et al. 1991; Alves and Mano 2008; Venditti et al. 2015). Although several works have been reported to obtain the functional derivatives of chitosan by chemical modification, very few attained solubility in general organic solvents (Toffey et al. 1996; Knaul and Creber 1997; Sashiwa et al. 2002b) and some binary solvent systems (Sakamoto et al. 1994; Tseng et al. 1995a). Several works modified chitosan structure by chemical or enzymatic methods to obtain high biologically active compounds and improve solubility in general organic solvents and aqueous solutions at a wide range of the pH (Muzzarelli 1983; Kurita 1986; Loubaki et al. 1991; Lillo and Matsuhiro 1997; Muzzarelli 1988; Amiji 1997; Kurita et al. 2002; Changhong et al. 2003; Chen and Park 2003; Amaral et al. 2005; Alves and Mano 2008; Badawy 2008; Badawy and Rabea 2012; de Oliveira Pedro et al. 2013; Badawy and Rabea 2014). This chapter is an attempt to discuss the major importance of chemical modifications of chitin and chitosan with their applications in different areas.

5.3 CHITIN DERIVATIVES OF MAJOR IMPORTANCE

Structure modification of a chitin molecule is generally difficult, because it is a highly crystalline polymer with a strongly hydrogen-bonded network composition. Generally, the reactivity of chitin, under heterogeneous conditions, can be increased with decreasing the degree of crystallinity, and the reaction in the amorphous region would proceed more efficiently than that in the crystalline form. Therefore, for the products obtained under heterogeneous conditions, it would be difficult to control the degree of substitution (DS), solubility, and other properties. Under alkaline conditions, some N-DA of chitin can be occurred with formation of free amino groups (Shigemasa et al. 1999). The most important derivative of chitin is the chitosan that obtained by DA of chitin under alkaline conditions or by enzymatic hydrolysis in the presence of a chitin deacetylase (Rinaudo 2006). Hydrolysis of acetamide groups of chitin to form chitosan as a DA process is carried out by two main procedures: the Broussignac process (Broussignac 1968), in which chitin is treated with a mixture of solid potassium hydroxide (50%, w/w) in 96% ethanol and monoethylene glycol (1:1), and the Kurita process (Kurita et al. 1993a), in which chitin is treated with hot aqueous sodium hydroxide solution (50%, w/v). The latter method is preferred for industrial purposes. The concentration of alkali and the temperature of

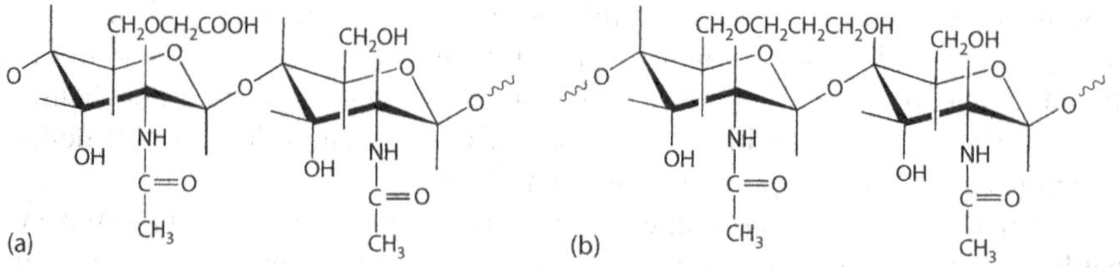

FIGURE 5.2 Chemical structures of CM-chitin (a) and HPC (b).

reaction are the important parameters affecting the DA and the degradation of the polysaccharide chain.

A number of water-soluble chitin derivatives have been prepared such as carboxymethyl chitin (CM-chitin), hydroxypropyl chitin (HPC), and dihydroxypropyl chitin. These products were prepared through alkali chitin suspension under heterogeneous conditions (Tokura et al. 1983; Muzzarelli 1988; Kurita et al. 1989a). CM-chitin derivatives (Figure 5.2a) are good candidates in tissue engineering and other biomedical applications, for metal ions adsorption, and as antimicrobial agents (Tokura et al. 1990; Jayakumar et al. 2010; Narayanan et al. 2014; Azuma et al. 2015). The carboxymethylation of chitin is prepared similarly to that of cellulose, in which chitin is treated with monochloroacetic acid in the presence of strong alkaline media. The reaction takes place preferentially at C-6 hydroxyl groups; however, sometimes >50% of acetamido groups are certainly hydrolyzed under the strongly basic conditions. In a modified method by Trujillo (1968), dimethyl sulfoxide (DMSO) is used to swell chitin, and the slurry formed is stirred for 1 h with 65% NaOH to produce CM-chitin (Trujillo 1968).

The method of cellulose derivatization is also used to prepare HPC (Figure 5.2b), a water-soluble derivative (Park and Park 2001; Chow and Khor 2002; Liu et al. 2003; Li et al. 2015). HPC was obtained from chitin powder dispersed in water with propylene oxide (PO) or by the reaction of chitin with PO under homogeneous conditions using a LiCl/dimethylacetamide (DMAc) solvent system (Park and Park 2001). Partially N-deacetylated chitin (DAC) derivatives were synthesized through ring-opening mechanisms with cyclic acid anhydrides in LiCl/DMAc and in aqueous MeOH as a solvent system (Sashiwa and Shigemasa 1999; Shigemasa et al. 1999). Reaction of partially DAC with aromatic cyclic acid anhydrides such as succinic, maleic, glutaric, phthalic, trimellitic, and pyromellitic was also carried out under homogeneous conditions in organic aprotic solvents with highly swollen precipitate of water-soluble chitin (50% DA). In this reaction, the cyclic acid anhydrides were supposed to react rapidly and primarily with the free amino groups in the water-soluble chitin, but to a much lower extent with the hydroxyl group leading to the formation of ester linkage (Figure 5.3). The resulting amic acid-chitins were converted into the corresponding imide-chitins by heating. In addition, this treatment can also remove the acid anhydrides reacted at the hydroxyl group producing N-substituted derivatives with high solubility in aqueous alkaline solutions and in organic solvents (Kurita et al. 1982; Shigemasa et al. 1999). In addition,

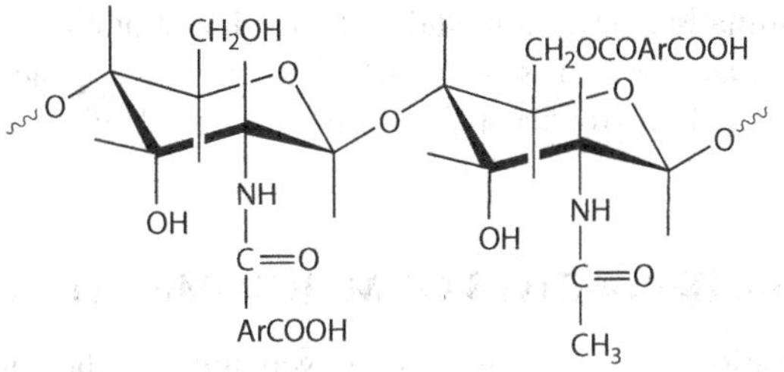

FIGURE 5.3 Chemical structures of N,O-(aryl) chitin produced from the reaction of partially DAC with aromatic cyclic acid anhydrides.

N-alkylation of DAC derivatives was prepared in aqueous methanol with different aldehydes, monosaccharides, and disaccharides, and the water solubility at various pHs was evaluated (Sashiwa and Shigemasa 1999).

N- and O-sulfated chitins, as water-soluble derivatives, were prepared under heterogeneous conditions, and various reagents have been used, including concentrated sulfuric acid, oleum, sulfur trioxide/pyridine, sulfur trioxide/sulfur dioxide, and chlorosulfonic acid, but the last one is most commonly used (Muzzarelli 1977; Muzzarelli et al. 1986a; Nishimura et al. 1986; Tokura et al. 1994). The reaction of chitin with phosphorous pentoxide formed water-soluble phosphorylated chitin (P-chitin) with high DS. P-chitin was prepared by heating chitin with orthophosphoric acid and urea in dimethylformamide (DMF) (Sakaguchi and Nakajima 1982; Nishi et al. 1984; Nishi 1986; Nishi et al. 1986; Nishi et al. 1987; Jayakumar et al. 2006; Jayakumar et al. 2008b; Jayakumar et al. 2009) (Scheme 3.20). P-chitin and deacetylated chitin (DA-chitin) derivatives were prepared with sufficiently high DS under homogeneous conditions by the reaction of chitin or DA-chitins with phosphorus pentoxide in methanesulfonic acid (Nishi et al. 1984; Nishi et al. 1986; Andrew et al. 1998). The phosphorylation reactions of chitin in phosphorous pentoxide-methane sulfonic acid were found to be very proficient, and the products possessed good solubility in many kinds of solvents (Somorin et al. 1979; Kaifu et al. 1981; Nishi et al. 1986; Nishi et al. 1987; Jayakumar et al. 2008b). P-chitin was also synthesized by mixing chitin with sodium pyrophosphate (Yalpani 1992).

Organosoluble chitin derivatives were also prepared and used as precursors for regioselective modifications such as introduction of various sugar groups resulting in nonnatural branched chitin products (Kurita 1998). Several scientists reported that the reactivity of β-chitin was higher than that of α-chitin. The resulting chitin derivatives were evaluated in their solubility, lysozyme susceptibility, and antimicrobial activity. Fluorination of chitin was achieved by facile homogenation reaction of chitin with diethyl amino sulfur trifluoride ($C_4H_{10}NSF_3$) with DS of 50%–98% according to the reaction time. The reaction of chitin with pentafluorobenzoyl chloride, trifluoromethylbenzoyl chloride, and pentafluoropropionic anhydride produced fluoro-chitin derivatives with DS of 5%, 10%, and 40%, respectively (Chow and Khor 2002). Other chitin derivatives have been prepared and characterized in the literature such as (diethylamino) ethyl chitin (Kurita et al. 1990), mercapto chitin (Kurita et al. 1993b; Kurita et al. 1997b), and chitin carbamates (Vincendon 1993). Moreover, chlorination, bromination, acylation, and carbamoylation of chitin were also studied in the LiCl/DMAc as a solvent system, which gave a homogeneous reaction mixture (McCormick and Lichatowich 1979; Terbojevich et al. 1988; Tseng et al. 1995b; Tseng et al. 1997).

5.4 CHITOSAN DERIVATIVES OF MAJOR IMPORTANCE

Chemical modification of chitosan is progressively more studied as it has the potential of providing new applications in different fields such as biotechnology, pharmaceutics, cosmetics, and agriculture. However, its low solubility at pH >6.5 is the major limiting factor in its utilization, that is, its application in biology, because many enzyme assays are performed in neutral media. Therefore, the preparation of water-soluble chitosans could enhance their biological and physiological potential (Rabea et al. 2003; Alves and Mano 2008; Mourya and Inamdar 2008).

As previously discussed in Section 5.2, the structure of chitosan is useful to the synthetic organic chemist interested in site-specific modifications. Modification does not change the original structure of chitosan but brings new compound or improved properties. From the synthetic point, all of the chemical modifications have been performed on the primary amino group (at C-2) or the two hydroxyl groups (at C-3 and C-6) of the chitosan molecule such as N-reductive amination, quaternization, hydroxyalkylation, N,O-carboxymethylation, N,O-acylation, phosphorylation, N,O-phthaloylation, N,O-succinylation, chitosan-amino acid and chitosan-peptide conjugates, and graft copolymerization (Kast and Bernkop-Schnürch 2001; Sashiwa et al. 2002c; Chen and Park 2003; Le Tien et al. 2003; Park et al. 2003; Sashiwa et al. 2003; Zhang et al. 2003a; Badawy et al. 2004; Dutta et al. 2004; Gorochovceva and Makuška 2004; Kumar et al. 2004; Ge and Luo 2005; Jayakumar et al. 2005; Rabea et al. 2006; Alves and Mano 2008; Badawy 2008; Kim et al. 2008; Mourya and Inamdar 2008; Badawy and Rabea 2014). The advantage of chitosan over other polysaccharides is that its chemical structure allows specific modifications without too many difficulties at C-2 position. Specific groups can be introduced to design polymers for selected applications. However, chitosan is still less accessible to potential reactants probably because of the characteristic crystalline structures with strong intermolecular forces. The chemical reactions of chitosan are usually accompanied by some difficulties arising from limited solubility, poor reactivity, and the multifunctionalities. The following are the most important common chemical modifications of chitosan that currently have prominent places in advanced research in different application areas.

5.4.1 SCHIFF BASES AND THEIR REDUCTIVE AMINATION PRODUCTS

The amino group attached at C-2 in the GlcN residue of chitosan is more reactive toward electrophiles than toward hydroxyl groups at C-3 and C-6. As a result, chitosan can be modified under mild conditions, often resulting in regioselectivity for the C-2 amino group. The Schiff base reaction between amino groups in

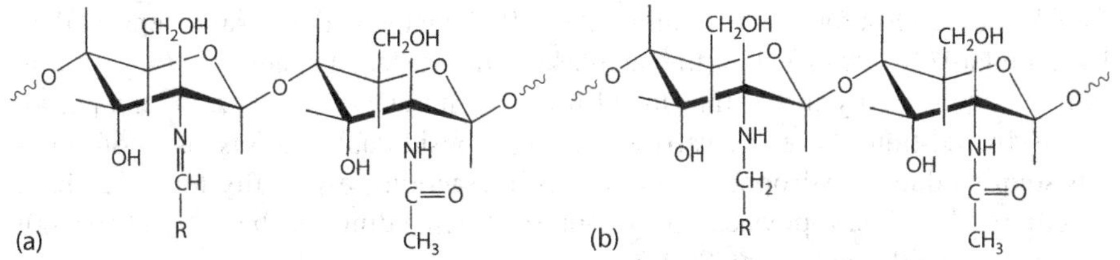

FIGURE 5.4 Chemical structures of Schiff base of chitosan (a) and *N*-alkyl or *N*-aryl chitosan (b). R = alkyl or phenyl substituent.

chitosan and aldehydes or ketones gives the corresponding aldimines and ketimines (Figure 5.4a), which are converted into *N*-alkyl or *N*-aryl derivatives (Figure 5.4b), upon reduction with borohydride (Kim et al. 1997; Jia and Xu 2001; Badawy and Rabea 2013; Badawy and Rabea 2014; Kenawy et al. 2015). These reactions are facile, and the DS is generally high. Intramolecular hydrogen bonds in these products are apparently weakened by the presence of the bulky substituents, and thus, these products are less susceptible to hydrolysis and hydrophobic associating water-soluble polymers (Toffey et al. 1996). However, these derivatives are soluble in aqueous diluted acids.

The imine linkage formed by Schiff reaction is rapidly hydrolyzed under acidic conditions to regenerate the free amino group; however; it is fairly stable in neutral and alkaline media. Therefore, aldehydes can be used for protecting the amino groups of chitosan to allow hydroxyl groups to be modified. Based on this approach, the full acylation of chitosan was attained, which was difficult by direct reaction. For example, fully acetylated chitin was prepared by a series of reactions involving the protection of the amino groups with an aldehyde, O-acetylation with acetic anhydride, deprotection, and N-acetylation (Moore and Roberts 1982).

Using the reductive amination reaction, many chitosan-based amphiphilic products having more hydrophobic substituents were prepared with different chain lengths (from C3 to C14) and controlled DS (usually <10% to maintain water solubility under acidic conditions) (Desbrieres et al. 1996; Muzzarelli et al. 2000; Rabea et al. 2006). The resulting derivatives were soluble in dilute acetic acid and had film-forming properties. The derivatives having side chains higher than C_8 showed an affinity to soluble in organic solvents. *N*-alkyl chitosan derivatives with good solubility under acidic conditions, including *N*-propyl, *N*-butyl, *N*-hexyl, *N*-heptyl, *N*-octyl, *N*-decanyl, and *N*-lauryl, were synthesized and reported elsewhere (Muzzarelli 1983; Desbrieres et al. 1996; Kim et al. 1997; Sashiwa and Shigemasa 1999; Dong et al. 2001; Desbrieres 2004; Badawy 2010; Sahariah et al. 2015). These derivatives have a number of very interesting properties and are industrially important as they show unusual and interesting rheological properties, which are thought to arise from the intermolecular association of adjacent hydrophobic substituents. They exhibit surface activity and they were compared with the corresponding low-molecular-weight (MW) surfactants (Desbrieres et al. 1996;

Babak et al. 2000); for the same amount of alkyl chains with the same length, they have a relatively low effect on the decrease of the surface tension, but they greatly improve the stability of the interfacial film (Vikhoreva et al. 1997; Olteanu et al. 2003). In addition, these derivatives increase considerably the viscosity of aqueous solution due to hydrophobic interchain interactions; especially for C-12 chain length and low DS, a physical gel is obtained depending on the pH and the salt concentration (Rinaudo et al. 2005).

N-aryl derivatives of chitosan with different electron-donating and electron-withdrawing substituents had been synthesized by the reaction of chitosan with aromatic aldehydes. These *N*-aryl chitosan derivatives were prepared from the corresponding Schiff base intermediates, followed by reduction with sodium cyanoborohydride (Rabea et al. 2005; Guo et al. 2007a; Badawy 2008; Sajomsang et al. 2009a; Badawy and Rabea 2013; Badawy and Rabea 2014). Under the reaction conditions employed, the aromatic aldehydes with electron-donating substituents were shown to be less reactive than aldehydes with electron-withdrawing substituents, largely due to the resonance effects. These derivatives showed a high antimicrobial activity against plant pathogenic bacteria and fungi. *N*-arylidene-chitosan phenylcarbamate derivatives (Figure 5.5) prepared by treating chitosan with aromatic aldehydes and then with phenyl isocyanate were used as chiral stationary phases for optical resolutions using high-performance liquid chromatography. Among some derivatives, the one carrying naphthylidene groups exhibited a particularly high-resolution performance (Ohga et al. 1991). In addition, heterocyclic aldehydes, including furan-2-carbaldehyde, 5-methylfuran-2-carbaldehyde, 3-pyridine carboxyaldehyde, benzo[*d*][1,3]dioxole-5-carbaldehyde, and 4-oxo-4*H*-chromene-3-carbaldehyde, were reacted with chitosan by one equivalent at room temperature and then reduction by 10% (w/v) sodium borohydride solution to produce *N*-(heterocyclic) chitosan derivatives (Figure 5.6) with DS ranged from 0.30 to 0.43 (Badawy 2008). *N*-(4-Pyridylmethyl) chitosan (Figure 5.6d) was also prepared, with different DS values, by reacting chitosan with 4-pyridinecarboxaldehyde in acidic media through the Schiff base intermediate according to Rodrigues method (Rodrigues et al. 1998) and then reduction by sodium borohydride or sodium cyanoborohydride (Baba and Hirakawa 1992; Sajomsang et al. 2008a; Sajomsang et al. 2008b).

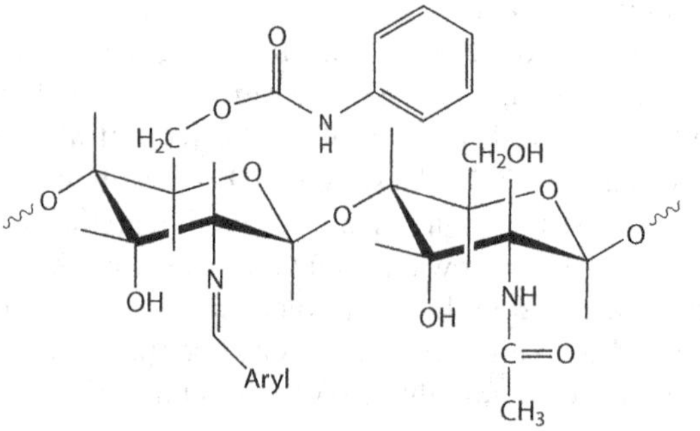

FIGURE 5.5   Chemical structures of *N*-arylidene-chitosan phenylcarbamate derivatives.

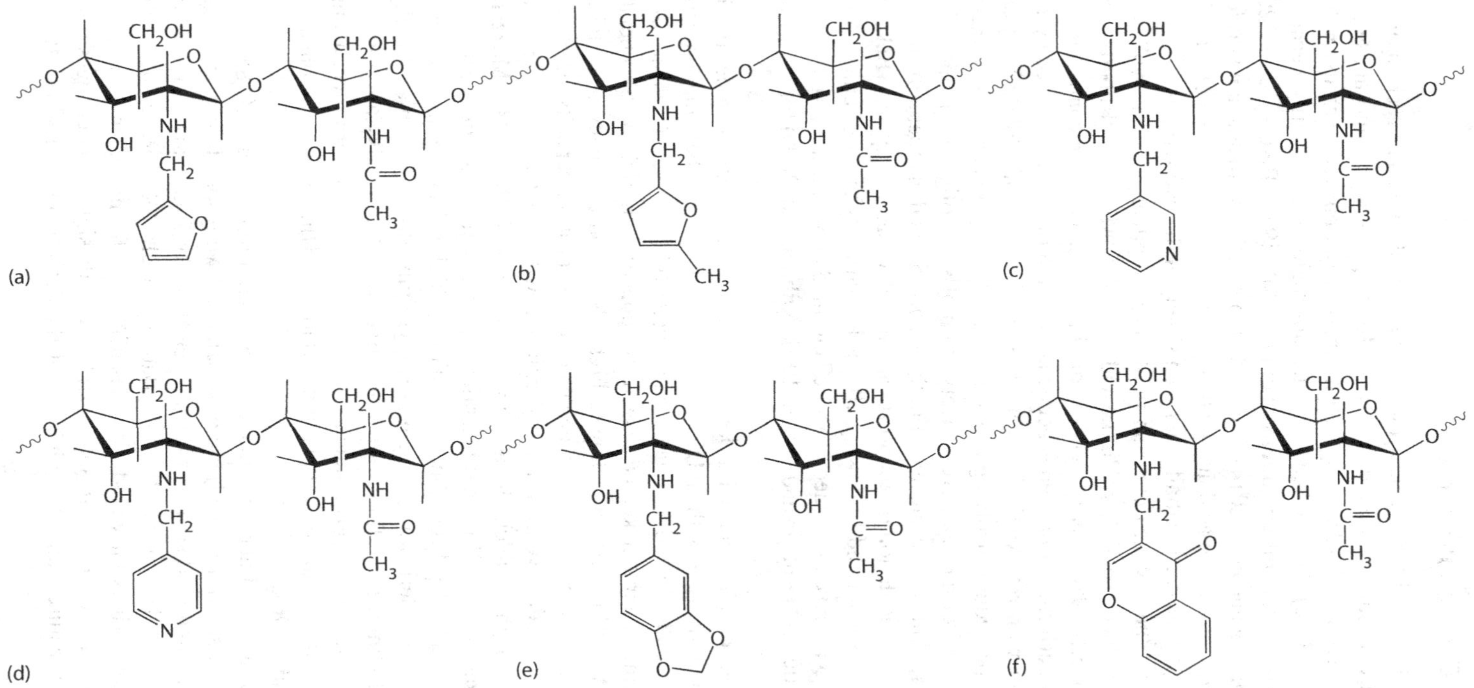

FIGURE 5.6 Chemical structures of N-(heterocyclic) chitosan derivatives N-(furan-2-ylmethyl) chitosan (a), N-((5-methylfuran-2-yl)methyl) chitosan, (b) N-(pyridin-3-ylmethyl) chitosan, (c) N-(pyridin-4-ylmethyl) chitosan (d), N-(benzo[d][1,3]dioxol-5-ylmethyl) chitosan (e), and N-(methyl-4H-chromen-4-one) chitosan (f).

5.4.2 Acyl Chitosan Products

Acylation of chitosan is the typical method that involves reacting chitosan with either an acid chloride or an acid anhydride forming N-(acyl) chitosan, O-(acyl) chitosan, N,O-(acyl), N-(hydroxyacyl) chitosan, or N-(carboxyacyl) chitosan derivatives (Figure 5.7a–e), but the reactions are not regioselective partly because of the heterogeneous reaction conditions (Hirano et al. 1976; Badawy et al. 2004; Ma et al. 2009; Shibano et al. 2014). The acylation reaction with acid anhydrides in a mixture of aqueous acetic acid and methanol was shown to proceed efficiently at the free amino groups preferentially and then slowly at the hydroxyl groups. Under these conditions, the acylated chitosan products precipitate or form swollen gels because of the reduced solubility (Hirano and Ohe 1975; Moore and Roberts 1980a; Moore and Roberts 1980b). N-acetylation of chitosan can also be controlled when the reaction is performed in aqueous acetic acid media or in a mixture of pyridine and chloroform with reflux (Kurita et al. 1989b; Kubota et al. 2000; Zong et al. 2000). A mild procedure involving acetic anhydride in aqueous methanol (neutral or basic) was used for the selective N-acetylation of some oligosaccharides of chitosan. However, chitosan was insoluble in these solvents and in other solvents commonly used for the acylation of amino sugars and glycosaminoglycans (Baker and Schaub 1954; Roseman and Ludowieg 1954). Partial acetylation of chitosan (DA <50%) was also achieved in aqueous acetic acid/methanol mixture (Aiba 1989) or in aqueous acetic acid (Kubota and Eguchi 1997; Kubota et al. 2000) forming water-soluble derivatives.

The reaction of chitosan with ketones such as 2,4-pentanedione resulted in N-acylvinyl derivative with a DS of 1.0. It had strong chelating properties toward heavy metals, including Cu(II) and Co(II) (Gómez-Guillén et al. 1992). 2-Formylpyridine is another ketone reagent for constructing a favorable chelating site on chitosan, and the product showed high adsorption efficiency of metal cations (Tong et al. 1991). In order to enhance the adsorption capacity of chitosan for metal cations, reductive alkylation of chitosan with salicylaldehyde (Hall and Yalpani 1980a) or phthalaldehydic acid (Muzzarelli and Tanfani 1982; Muzzarelli et al. 1982b) was examined, and a substantial improvement in chelation was accomplished. Efforts have also been done for achieving high selectivity in metal cation adsorption, and some derivatives such as N-(2-pyridylmethyl), N-(2-thienylmethyl), and N-(3-(methylthio) propyl) chitosans prepared by reductive alkylation with the corresponding aldehydes showed much improved selectivity toward precious metals, including gold, palladium, and platinum (Baba and Hirakawa 1992; Baba et al. 1994; Baba et al. 1996).

N-Saturated fatty acyl derivatives of chitosan were prepared in 75%–85% yields by N-acylation of sodium N-(acyl) chitosan salts and were soluble in water and in aqueous alkaline and acid solutions (Hirano et al. 1976; Zhang and Hirano 1995; Hirano et al. 2002; Hirano et al. 2003; Badawy et al. 2004; Rodrigues 2005). N-acylation with various fatty acid chlorides (C6–C16) formed hydrophobic products with an increase of the chain substituent and made significant changes in chitosan structural features, and the solubility of the derivatives varies with the acyl

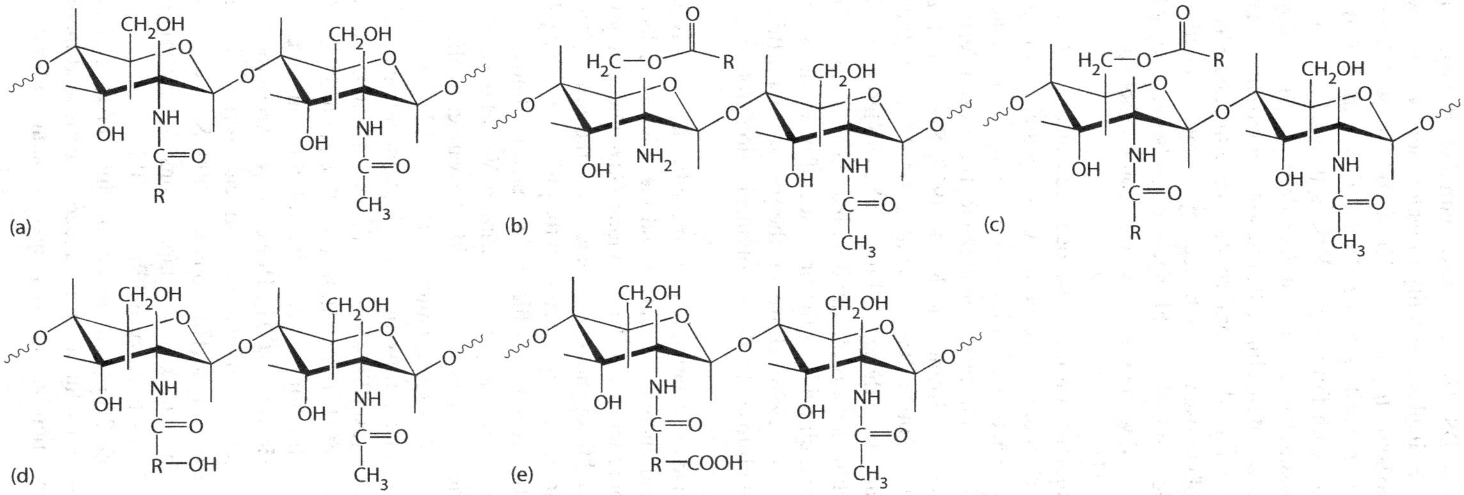

FIGURE 5.7 Chemical structures of *N*-(acyl) chitosan derivatives (a), *N*-(carboxyacyl) chitosan derivatives (b), *N*-(hydroxyacyl) chitosan derivatives (c), *O*-(acyl) chitosan derivatives (d), and *N,O*-(acyl) chitosan derivatives (e). R = alkyl or phenyl substituent.

chain length and also the DS. The derivatives with a short chain length (up to C8) and low to moderate DS display solubility in water; however, one with higher DS exhibits very little or no solubility in water. The derivatives with longer chain length are not soluble in water, regardless of the DS. Le Tein et al. (2003) added that the N-acylation of chitosan with fatty acyl chlorides (C8–C16) produced hydrophobic products for use as suitable carriers for drug delivery. Anacardoylated chitosan exhibited sustained release of insulin in the intestinal environment, and the released insulin was stable and retained its conformation (Shelma and Sharma 2010). The bioadhesive property of chitosan was enhanced by N-acylation with fatty acid chlorides. Chitosan modified with oleoyl chloride showed better mucoadhesion properties than chitosan modified with lower fatty acid groups (Shelma and Sharma 2010; Shelma and Sharma 2011).

In addition, acyl substitution could be occurred at both O- and N-positions with an excess of acid chloride as a reactant. N,O-Acylated chitosans (Figure 5.7c) were prepared via the reaction of chitosan dissolving in methane sulfonic acid with different acyl chlorides forming the N,O-(acyl) chitosan derivatives with the majority of O-substitution (Hirano and Koide 1978; Sashiwa et al. 2000c; Seo et al. 2001; Sashiwa et al. 2002a; Badawy et al. 2004; Ma et al. 2009). Under suitable conditions comparable to those used for the benzoylation of chitin (Somorin et al. 1979), benzoyl chitosan was obtained with a DS of up to 2.5 by the reaction of chitosan with benzoyl chloride in the presence of methane sulfonic acid (Inui et al. 1998; Uragami et al. 1998). However, the problem with this method is the decrease in the MW of chitosan by the depolymerization process occurred during the reaction.

Although the selective O-acylation in methane sulfonic acid was performed (Seo et al. 2001), the detailed chemical structure and the shielding effect on the amino group by methanesulfonic acid are still not obvious. O,O-(Didecanoyl) chitosan preparation was also achieved throughout the protection of the amino group by phthaloyl moiety as an intermediate, then deprotection of the phthaloyl group (Nishimura et al. 1990). Whole N-acylation has been achieved by reacting chitosan with cyclic acid anhydrides in aqueous solution at pH 4–8 forming N-(carboxyacyl) chitosans that were productively changed into the related imido derivatives by thermal dehydration (Satoh et al. 2003). N-(Carboxyacyl) chitosans (Figure 5.7e) were also prepared by reactions with intramolecular carboxylic anhydrides, including maleic, glutaric and phthalic (Hirano and Moriyasu 1981; Satoh et al. 2003; Hirano and Moriyasu 2004), and succinic (Yamaguchi et al. 1981; Satoh et al. 2003) anhydrides. As interrelated derivatives, other cyclic phthalimido derivatives of chitosan were reported (Kurita et al. 1982; Hirano and Moriyasu 2004). However, N-(carboxyacyl) chitosans filaments were obtained by reaction of chitosan with carboxylic anhydrides in methanol at room temperature overnight (Hirano et al. 2000; Sashiwa et al. 2000c). The products could be used in many kinds of applications as their solubility in a wide pH range (Hirano et al. 2002). Badawy and Rabea (2012) synthesized N-carboxyacyl chitosans with DS of 0.09–0.86 by treatment of chitosan with glutaric anhydride at different molar ratios in a solution of 2% aqueous acetic acid-methanol (1:1, v/v) and evaluated their antimicrobial activity against plant pathogens. As a result,

N-(4-carboxybutyroyl) chitosan derivatives (DS = 0.09, 0.26, 0.45, 0.52, and 0.86) were isolated with 80%–93% yields.

5.4.3 PHTHALOYL CHITOSAN PRODUCTS

Phthaloylation of chitosan can be a practical way for solubilization in organic solvents because the phthaloyl group is bulky and eliminates hydrogen from the amino group to prevent hydrogen bonding. In addition, this reaction is used for protection of the amino groups to facilitate some reactions that take place on the hydroxyl groups at C-3 and C-6. Therefore, the *N*-phthaloyl group can be indispensable for both protection and solubilization. The reaction was carried out by treating a chitosan suspension in DMF with excess phthalic anhydride (three equivalents of phthalic anhydride to chitosan) at 120°C–130°C, and the resulting products, *N*-(phthaloyl) chitosan or *N*-,*O*-(phthaloyl) chitosan (Figure 5.8), showed high solubility in organic solvents such as DMSO (Kurita et al. 1982; Nishimura et al. 1990). In this reaction, partial O-phthaloylation also occurred; however, the DS was higher than 1.0. Although the phthalimide group was sensitive to alkali, an ester exchange reaction with sodium in methanol removed the *O*-acetyl groups to give *N*-(phthaloyl) chitosan with a DS of 1.0 (Kurita et al. 2000). When fully deacetylated chitosan was phthaloylated, the product showed higher solubility in aprotic polar organic solvents such as pyridine, DMSO, DMAc, and DMF (Nishimura et al. 1990).

Microwave heating was used as an alternative technique in production of phthaloyl chitosan (Liu et al. 2004). In this method, chitosan reacted with phthalic anhydride in DMF; the mixture was irradiated in a microwave oven at pointed power for a predetermined time under a nitrogen atmosphere. The reaction product was precipitated in ice water, washed completely with ethanol, and dried under vacuum at 40°C.

Phthaloyl chitosan, either N,O-phthaloylated or N-phthaloylated chitosan, can be used as a key intermediate for many modification reactions that take place regioselectively in

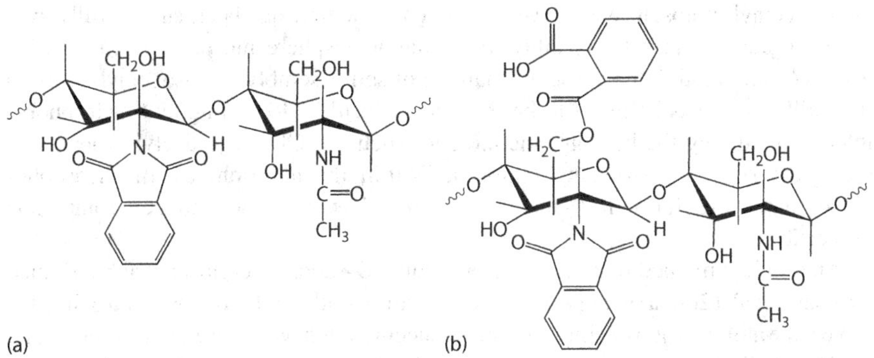

(a)   (b)

FIGURE 5.8 Chemical structures of *N*-(phthaloyl) chitosan (a) and *N*,*O*-(phthaloyl) chitosan (b) derivatives.

homogeneous solutions in organic solvents (Nishimura et al. 1991; Kurita et al. 1998). Triphenylmethylation, for example, takes place quantitatively at C-6 hydroxyl groups in pyridine. Even if *N*-(phthaloyl) chitosan having some *O*-phthaloyl groups is used as a starting material, the *O*-phthaloyl groups are replaced completely by triphenylmethyl groups. The product is a precursor for regioselective substitution at C-3. Subsequent acetylating at C-3 and detriphenylmethylation affords a derivative with a free hydroxyl group at C-6, which allows regioselective substitution at C-6. All of these transformations proceed smoothly in solution and are quantitative in terms of the DS. Another important kind of possible modification reactions of phthaloylated chitosan is a glycosylation to introduce sugar branches at C-6. This reaction is very important in view of the biological activity (Kurita et al. 1997a; Kurita et al. 2003; Yang et al. 2004; Ješelnik and Žagar 2014; Sugita et al. 2014). Therefore, phthaloylated chitosan is thus a suitable precursor for a wide range of site-specific modification reactions to prepare well-defined molecular environments on chitosan and is the first example that has enabled perfect discrimination of the three kinds of functional groups in chemical reactions.

5.4.4 Succinyl Chitosan Products

N-succinyl-chitosan (Figure 5.9a) was obtained by introduction of succinyl groups into chitosan N-terminal of the glucosamine units. However, succinyl moiety was introduced into O-terminal (Figure 5.9b) of the glucosamine units after protection of the free amino groups and then removal of the protecting moiety. The degree of succinylation chitosan could be easily modified by changing reaction conditions using succinic anhydride (Yamaguchi et al. 1981; Onishi et al. 2001; Kato et al. 2002; Zhang et al. 2003b; Kato et al. 2004; Aiping et al. 2006; Li et al. 2007; Woraphatphadung et al. 2015).

N-succinyl-chitosan/alginate hydrogel beads were prepared by dropping a mixture of succinyl chitosan and alginate into a Ca^{2+} solution (Li et al. 2007; Dai et al. 2008). The preparation method was adapted by different factors to control the swelling performance of the nifedipine drug, and the release cinitics of the nifedipine was tested in simulated gastric and intestinal fluid.

N-succinyl-chitosan, with a well-designed structure, has been successfully synthesized, and it can self-assembly to regular nanosphere morphology in distilled water (Aiping et al. 2006). The mechanism of self-assembly of *N*-succinyl-chitosan in distilled water is believed to be the intermolecular H-bonding and hydrophobic interaction among the hydrophobic moieties such as $-CH_2CH-$, acetyl groups, and glucosidic rings in *N*-succinyl-chitosan. Within the nanospheres, the hydrophobic domains are formed. *N*-succinyl-chitosan has nontoxic and cell-compatible properties.

An efficient method to prepare water-soluble *O*-succinyl-chitosan was performed by Zhang et al. (2003a) using a three-step reaction. Phthaloyl group was introduced to protect the amino group of chitosan, and *O*-succinylation was then achieved and finally the *N*-phthalimido group was removed by using hydrazine monohydrate (Zhang et al. 2003b). Woraphatphadung and coauthors synthesized a pH-responsive *N*-naphthyl-*N,O*-succinyl chitosan and evaluated the influence of drug (meloxicam)-loaded micelle methods on the loading efficiency, particle size, and micelle stability. This

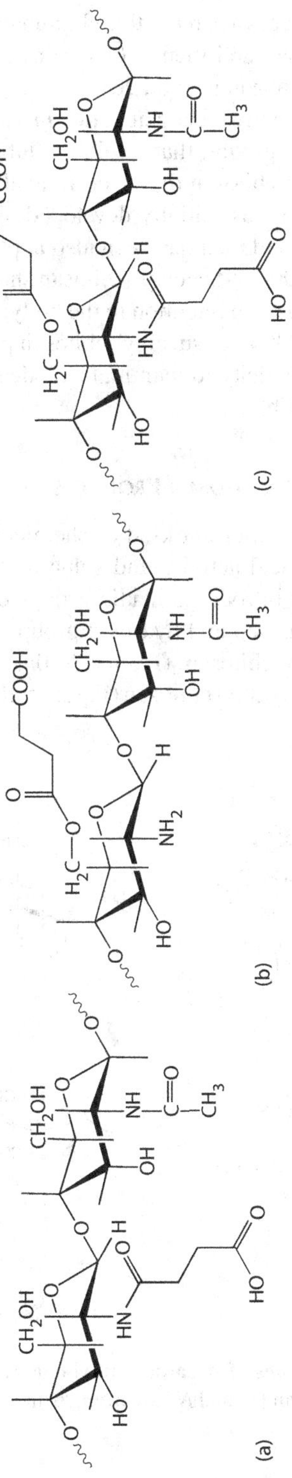

FIGURE 5.9 Chemical structures of *N*-(succinyl) chitosan (a), *O*-(succinyl) chitosan (b), and *N,O*-(succinyl) chitosan (c) derivatives.

product was synthesized by successive reductive N-amination with 2-naphthaldehyde to produce *N*-naphthyl chitosan and then N,O-succinylation was conducted using succinic anhydride (Woraphatphadung et al. 2015).

Succinyl chitosan has distinctive characteristics *in vitro* and *in vivo* due to the presence of several carboxyl groups that exhibit solubility in different aqueous media compared to the native chitosan dissolved in acidic water only (Yamaguchi et al. 1981). Succinyl chitosan was initially developed as a wound dressing material (Kuroyanagi et al. 1994), and then has been also applied as a cosmetic material (Izume 1998; Tajima et al. 2000). *N*-Succinyl-chitosan showed biocompatibility, low toxicity to mammals, and long-term retention in the body; therefore, it has been used as a drug carrier (Kato et al. 2004). *O*-succinyl-chitosan possesses many advantages such as water solubility, low toxicity to mammals, biodegradability, and antimicrobial activity (Zhang et al. 2003b).

5.4.5 CARBOXYALKYL (ARYL) CHITOSAN PRODUCTS

Carboxyalkylation is another important kind of chemical modification of chitosan that could enhance its biological activity and solubility in aqueous solution. The process of carboxyalkylation introduces acidic groups on the polymer backbone. In this reaction, both amino group and hydroxyl group could be carboxyalkylated and produce *N*-carboxyalkyl chitosan (Figure 5.10a), *O*-carboxyalkyl chitosan (Figure 5.10b), and *N,O*-carboxyalkyl chitosan (Figure 5.10c) derivatives (Muzzarelli

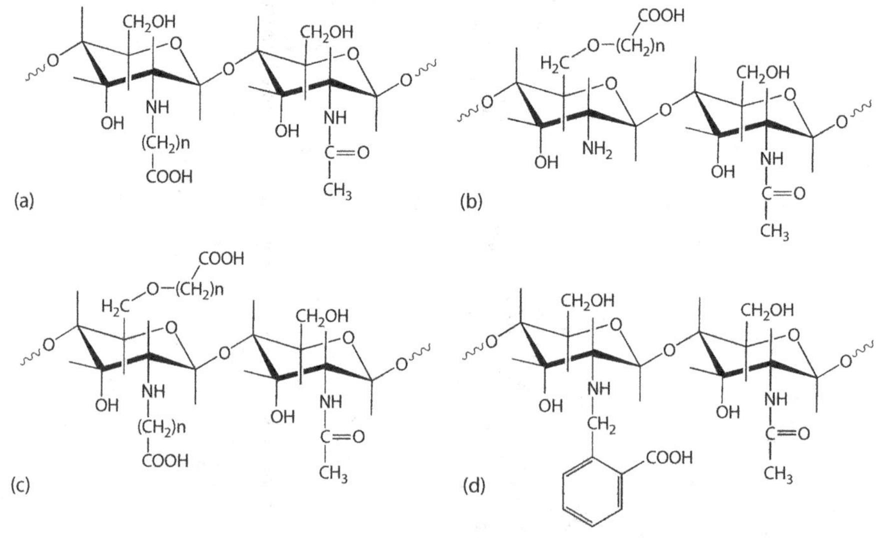

FIGURE 5.10 Chemical structures of *N*-carboxyalkyl chitosan (a), *O*-carboxyalkyl chitosan (b), *N,O*-carboxyalkyl chitosan (c), and *N*-(2-carboxybenzyl) chitosan (d) derivatives.

et al. 1982a; Kim and Choi 1998; Badawy et al. 2004; Mourya et al. 2010). The introduction of carboxyalkyl groups into chitosan leads to the formation of anionic derivatives. By varying the DS of the carboxyl-bearing group, we can obtain various charge densities on the molecular chain, which provide a convenient way to control pH-dependent behavior. As in the preparation of carboxymethyl cellulose and CM-chitin, the carboxymethyl chitosan (CM-chitosan) has been synthesized in different ways as direct alkylation, Michael addition, and reductive alkylation, and characterized by infrared (IR) and nuclear magnetic resonance (NMR) spectroscopy, titrimetry, viscometry, gel permeation chromatography (GPC), X-ray diffraction, and capillary zone electrophoresis (Trujillo 1968; Muzzarelli and Tanfani 1982; Kittur et al. 2002). The carboxymethyl group can be linked to the O- or N-position of chitosan chain. Compared with other water-soluble carboxyalkyl chitosan derivatives, CM-chitosan has been widely studied because of its ease of synthesis, ampholytic character, and possibilities of abundant of applications. It has properties such as metal ion chelation, sorption, moisture retention, antioxidant, and antimicrobial. CM-chitosan is also currently used in controlled release of pharmaceutical drugs, DNA delivery. In addition, it can be further modified with alkylation, acylation, and grafting.

The carboxymethyl groups are introduced in both the hydroxyl and amino groups to give N,O-carboxymethylated chitosans (CM-chitosans) (Carolan et al. 1991; Rinaudo et al. 1992; Chen et al. 2004a; Chen et al. 2004b; Ge and Luo 2005; Lin et al. 2005). The water solubility of CM-chitosans mainly depends on the modifying conditions and the degree of carboxymethylation where the CM-chitosans prepared at a temperature range of 0°C–20°C were highly soluble in water; however, those prepared at a temperature between 20°C and 60°C were insoluble. Generally, the limit solubility at different values of the pH was varied with the carboxymethylation degree. The increase in the temperature increased the carboxymethylation degree and thus decreased the solubility at lower pH; however, the increase of the solvent ratio (water/isopropanol) in the reaction medium decreased the degree of the carboxymethylation, which significantly increased the insolubility at higher pH values (Qian et al. 1996; Liu et al. 2001; Chen and Park 2003; Chen et al. 2004b).

In contrast to the CM-chitosans prepared by the conventional carboxymethylation with chloroacetic acid, N-CM-chitosan prepared by reductive alkylation is a well-defined derivative, because the reaction is regioselective at the amino group. Reductive alkylation is thus indispensable for introducing carboxymethyl groups into chitosan. First, chitosan reacts readily with glyoxylic acid in aqueous acidic solution to form a Schiff base that is converted into N-(carboxymethyl) chitosan on reduction (Muzzarelli and Tanfani 1982; Muzzarelli et al. 1982a). N,N-Dicarboxymethylation appears to take place under appropriate conditions (Muzzarelli et al. 1994a). The derivative is water soluble, and the flow behavior is examined (Delben et al. 1990). In a similar manner, several other N-carboxyalkylated chitosans have been prepared from carboxylic acids having an aldehyde or ketone group, including pyruvic acid, β-hydroxypyruvic acid,

2-ketoglutaric acid, dehydroascorbic acid (Muzzarelli et al. 1986b), and 2-oxopro-pionic acid (Shigemasa et al. 1995).

The other synthetic route that is selective in the formation of N-carboxyalkylation uses carboxyaldehydes in a reductive amination sequence (Muzzarelli et al. 1982a). The carboxyl-bearing aromatic substitution can be done with aromatic aldehydes. N-(2-Carboxybenzyl) chitosan (Figure 5.10d) was prepared by reductive amination sequence with 2-carboxy benzaldehyde and cross-linked with glutaraldehyde to develop pH-sensitive hydrogel for colon-specific drug delivery of 5-fluorouracil (Kumar et al. 2004; Lin et al. 2007). α-Keto acids such as pyruvic acid, β-hydroxypyruvic acid, phenylpyruvic acid, hydroxyphenylpyruvic acid, α-ketoglutaric acid, and levulinic acid are some of the other carboxyaldehydes being employed for carboxyalkylation of chitosan.

5.4.6 HYDROXYALKYL CHITOSAN PRODUCTS

Hydroxyalkyl chitosans are usually prepared by the reaction of chitosan with epoxides (ethylene oxide, PO, butylene oxide) and glycidol. Depending on the reaction conditions, such as the pH, the solvent system, and the temperature, the reaction may take place at the amino or hydroxy groups forming N-(hydroxyalkyl) chitosan (Figure 5.11a) or O-(hydroxyalkyl) chitosan (Figure 5.11b) or a mixture of both types (Figure 5.11c). Under neutral and acidic conditions, N-alkylation has been occurred, whereas under alkaline conditions, the strong nucleophilic oxygen ions will react more rapidly forming the O-alkylation. Under these conditions, the DS is higher than 2, which indicates poly(alkylenoxide) chain formation (Lang et al. 1988; Lang et al. 1990a; Swain et al. 2015). Therefore, the ratio of O/N-substitution (hydroxypropylation of chitosan by PO) is determined by the choice of catalyst (NaOH or HCl) and the reaction temperature (Maresh et al. 1989). Hydroxyalkylations with 2-chloroethanol and 3-chloropropane-1,2-diol are also reported (Tokura et al. 1994).

N-Hydroxypropyl chitosan as an antimicrobial agent and as a temperature-sensitive injectable carrier for cells is prepared without addition of catalyst, whereas acid catalysis leads to mainly N- but some O-alkylation product. In the presence of a basic catalyst, O-alkylation is preferred with a tendency to yield oligomers at a temperature higher than 40°C (Maresh et al. 1989; Peng et al. 2005; Dang et al. 2006). The substitution of 2,3-dihydroxypropyl groups to chitosan can be occurred on both the reactive hydroxyl group and the amino group of chitosan. However, N-substitution was reported to be more preferred than O-substitution except in the preparation of hydroxyalkyl chitosans via alkali chitosan (Lang et al. 1997). O-Hydroxyethyl chitosan (glycol chitosan) was also synthesized by the reaction of chitosan with 2-chloroethanol in the alkaline medium (Ronghua et al. 2003; Xie et al. 2007). In addition, this product was developed as a self-assembled nanoparticle for carrier of paclitaxel and doxorubicin and as a stabilizer for protein encapsulated into a poly(lactide-co-glycolide) microparticle (Kim et al. 2006; Park et al. 2006; Lee et al. 2007).

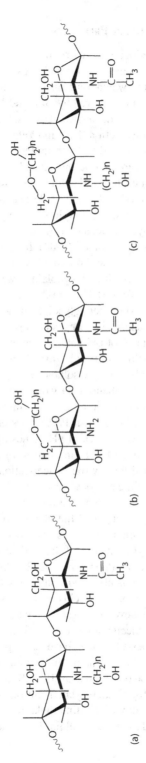

FIGURE 5.11 Chemical structures of *N*-hydroxyalkyl chitosan (a), *O*-hydroxyalkyl chitosan (b), and *N,O*-hydroxyalkyl chitosan (c) derivatives.

5.4.7 SUGAR-MODIFIED CHITOSAN PRODUCTS

Carbohydrates containing a reducing end group such as D-glucose, D-galactose, lactose, maltose, melibiose, maltotoriose, and cellobiose were reacted in the open-chain form with chitosan forming water-soluble sugar-modified chitosan derivatives (Figure 5.12). The reaction was first prepared by Hall and Yalpani who reported that the unmodified sugars or sugar-aldehyde derivatives were linked to the C-2 position of chitosan by reductive N-alkylation reaction (Hall and Yalpani 1980b; Yalpani and Hall 1984; Holme and Hall 1991a; Holme and Hall 1991b; Park et al. 2003). Carbohydrates that contain an aldehyde group can also be introduced without ring opening at the C-6 position of chitosan (Holme and Hall 1992). Sashiwa and Shigemasa (1999) prepared different kinds of N-alkylated chitosan derivatives using triose (glyceraldehyde), pentose (D-ribose, D-arabinose, D-xylose, 2-deoxy-D-ribose), and hexose (2-deoxy-D-glucose, 3-O-methyl-D-glucose, D-mannose, L-fucose, L-rhamnose) according to the method of Yalpani and Hall (1984). In case of using glycolaldehyde (dimer), only water-insoluble material was obtained, which would be caused by the cross-linking formation between substituted glycolaldehyde dimers. Although the DS value of these derivatives varied from 0.37 to 1.02 under the same conditions, they were soluble in dilute acidic solution except glycolaldehyde. The chitosan derivatives with D-arabinose, 2-deoxy-D-glucose, lactose, cellobiose, and maltose rapidly dissolved in water and at a wide range of pH values. The N-alkylated derivatives with DL-glyceraldehyde, D-ribose, D-glucose, D-galactose, D-mannose, and L-fucose were insoluble in distilled water directly but were soluble at all pH regions after dissolving them in dilute HCl solution. These phenomena would be explained by the fact that the hydration in the acidic medium would be an important process to dissolve these derivatives in water (Sashiwa and Shigemasa 1999). Park et al. (2003) enhanced the water solubility of chitosan in a wide range of pH values by attaching a hydrophilic sugar moiety, gluconic acid, through the formation of an amide bond. This sugar-bearing chitosan was further modified by the N-acetylation in an alcoholic aqueous solution. Thereafter, the effects of the gluconyl group and the DA on the water solubility at different pH values and on the biodegradability of chitosan were investigated.

Sialic acid, the most established sugar of the glycolipids and glycoproteins present in the surface of the mammalian cells, was also incorporated into chitosan by reductive alkylation with a formyl derivative of the acid, and the products were characterized by interaction with lectins (Sashiwa et al. 2000b). Sialic acid dendrimers provided another form of chitosan/sialic acid conjugates that might be interesting because of a high local concentration of the clustering sugar moieties (Sashiwa et al. 2001a; Sashiwa et al. 2002d). However, chitosan–sialic acid product was insoluble in water; therefore, consecutive N-succinylation was performed to obtain water-soluble derivatives. Many different types of spacer have been prepared on sialic acid or α-galactosyl-bound chitosans and tested as potent inhibitors of influenza viruses or blocking agents for acute rejection (Gamian et al. 1991; Sashiwa et al. 2000a; Sashiwa et al. 2000b; Sashiwa et al. 2001b). Galactosylated chitosan obtained by reacting lactobionic acid and chitosan with 1-ethyl-3-(3-dimethylaminopropyl)-carbodiimide and N-hydroxysuccinimide was used as an extracellular matrix for hepatocyte attachment (Park et al. 2003).

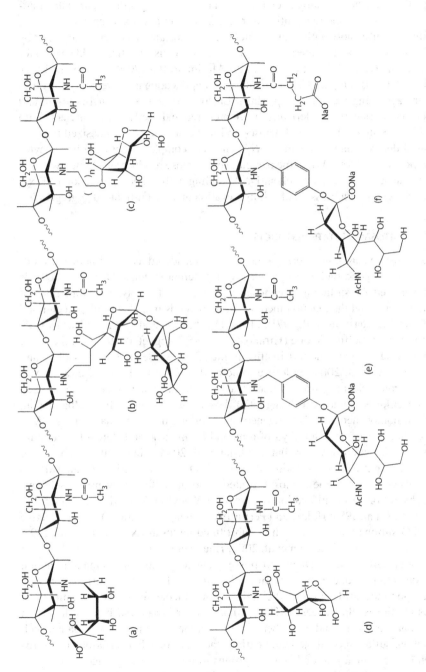

FIGURE 5.12 Chemical structures of sugar-modified chitosan products: pentose-chitosan (a), di saccharides-chitosan (chitosan-lactose) (b), polysac-charides-chitosan (c), gluconic acid-chitosan (d), sialic acid-chitosan (e), and sialic acid-succinyl-chitosan (f) derivatives.

The sugar-bound chitosans had been first investigated mainly in rheological studies, and then they have usually been used to introduce cell-specific sugars into chitosan after discovering the recognition of bacterial and viral cells using sugars. These derivatives such as those with D- and L-fucose are important as they are recognized by the corresponding specific interactions with lectin and cells, and thus could be used for drug targeting (Li et al. 1999; Li et al. 2000; Morimoto et al. 2001; Yang et al. 2002). Donati et al. (2005) prepared lactose-chitosan for application in the repair of the articular cartilage using the similar approach. Lactosaminated N-succinyl-chitosan and its fluorescein thiocarbanyl derivative were prepared and used as drug carriers (Kato et al. 2001a; Kato et al. 2001b). Lactose-modified chitosan was synthesized to make a plasmid deoxyribonucleic acid (pDNA)/chitosan complex specific to hepatocytes (Hashimoto et al. 2006). When the percentage of lactose residues substituted was 8%, lactose-chitosan showed an excellent DNA-binding ability, good protection of DNA from nuclease, and suppression of self-aggregation and serum-induced aggregation.

5.4.8 CHITOSAN SULFATE PRODUCTS

Chitosan sulfates are amphoteric in nature and considered as very important products possessing good biological properties in different systems. Different methods have been used for sulfation of chitosan molecules that involved combinations of sulfating agents and the reaction media. These methods include use of concentrated sulfuric acid (Nagasawa et al. 1971), oleum (Vikhoreva et al. 2005), sulfur trioxide or sulfur trioxide/sulfur dioxide (Hirano et al. 1985; Naggi et al. 1986), a mixture of sulfur trioxide and pyridine or trimethylamine (Gamzazade et al. 1997; Holme and Perlin 1997; Je et al. 2005), chlorosulfonic acid-sulfuric acid (Naggi et al. 1986), 2-sulfobenzoic acid anhydride (Chen et al. 1998), and the most commonly used reagent is chlorosulfonic acid (Naggi et al. 1986; Hagiwara et al. 1999; Zhang et al. 2003a) in homogeneous or heterogeneous conditions in the media such as DMF, DMF-dichloroacetic acid, tetrahydrofuran, and formic acid at different temperature ranges or under microwave irradiation (Xing et al. 2004; Xing et al. 2005b). Using all these reagents, N,O-disubstituted and N,O,O-trisubstituted chitosan sulfates are obtained instead of the monosubstituted chitosan sulfate. However, a selective monosubstitution of O-sulfonation occurs with N-acyl or N-alkyl chitosan derivatives (Hirano et al. 1985; Holme and Perlin 1997; Zhang et al. 2003a), and a selective N- or N,O-sulfonation occurs with O-substituted chitosan (Nishimura et al. 1998; Hagiwara et al. 1999; Vongchan et al. 2002; Huang et al. 2004).

Chitosan sulfates have shown to possess anticoagulant and hemagglutination inhibition activities due to the structural similarity to heparin. Heparin is a highly sulfated polysaccharide used medicinally as an anticoagulant in the treatment of various cardiovascular diseases. The similarity of chitosan and heparin has been pointed out previously, and a number of modifications have been investigated, such as sulfation, sulfation combined with carboxylation, or depolymerization, and introduction of the sulfoamino or N-formyl groups to give chitosan products having an anticoagulant activity (Muzzarelli et al. 1984; Muzzarelli et al. 1986b; Hirano 1999; Drozd et al. 2001; Jayakumar et al. 2007; Cao et al. 2014). Moreover, other research studies relate to the anticoagulant activity of such products as chitosan-dextran sulfate and chitosan-(carboxymethyl) dextran complexes and dextrans containing carboxymethyl, sulfate, benzyl sulfate, and α-amino acid groups. Other biological activities demonstrated by chitosan sulfates include antisclerotic, antiviral, anti-HIV, antibacterial, antioxidant, and enzyme inhibition activities (Hirano et al. 1985; Nishimura et al. 1998; Vongchan et al. 2002; Huang et al. 2004; Xing et al. 2005b; Jayakumar et al. 2007; Zhang et al. 2008a; Zhang et al. 2008b; Qu et al. 2009).

5.4.9 PHOSPHORYLATED CHITOSAN PRODUCTS

The production of anionic carbohydrate polymers containing heteroatoms such as phosphorus is very useful as anticoagulants, metal-chelating agents, and fire-retardant materials. Therefore, several techniques are used in the incorporation of phosphorous moiety into chitosan due to the interesting biological and metal chelating properties of the products (Nishi 1986; Nishi et al. 1986; Wang et al. 2001; Amaral et al. 2005; Jayakumar et al. 2008a; Jayakumar et al. 2008b; Wang and Liu 2014; Dadhich et al. 2015). Phosphorylated chitosan (P-chitosan) was prepared by reacting chitosan with orthophosphoric acid and urea in DMF by heating (Sakaguchi and Nakajima 1982; Wan et al. 2003; Jayakumar et al. 2006). P-chitosan was also prepared by the reaction of chitosan with phosphorous pentoxide in methane sulfonic acid (Nishi et al. 1984; Nishi et al. 1986) or mixing chitosan with sodium pyrophosphate (Yalpani 1992). The phosphorylation reactions in the presence of phosphorous pentoxide–methane sulfonic acid were found to be very efficient reactions and give high DS of the products with an increasing amount of phosphorous pentoxide. However, P-chitosans with high DS were insoluble in water, whereas those with low DS were highly soluble. The low solubility of high-DS P-chitosan may lead to the formation of intermolecular salt linkage between the amino and phosphate groups that form poly-ion complex. Nishi et al. (1987) synthesized P-chitosan by the cross-linking reaction of chitosan with adipoyl chloride and phosphorous pentoxide in methane sulfonic acid and used the product as an adsorbent of metal ions in water. Grafting mono(2-methacryloyl oxyethyl) acid phosphate onto chitosan produced P-chitosan with improved antimicrobial activities of the product (Jung et al. 1999). Lee et al. (2000) added that the chitosan tripolyphosphate was prepared using an ionotropic cross-linking technique in one step without using other hazardous cross-linking reagents such as glutaraldehyde and ethylene glycol diglycidyl ether.

The incorporation of methylene phosphonic groups into chitosan chain significantly increased its solubility in neutral solutions without declining its filmogenic properties (Heras et al. 2001). The reaction of phosphonic acid with chitosan according to the Moedritzer and Irani (1966) method was replaced by a mixture of phosphoric acid and formaldehyde forming a water-soluble N-methylene phosphonic chitosan (NMPC, Figure 5.13a and b). NMPC was also prepared from chitosan with different DAs and time intervals (Ramos et al. 2003a; Ramos et al. 2003b). A significant decrease in the viscosity and MW of the NMPC product was observed and was dependent on the reaction time, and the crystallinity of the product was considerably decreased.

Wang et al. (2011) prepared water-soluble phosphonium chitosan derivatives (WSPCSs) with two different DS values (3.6% and 4.2%) of quaternary phosphonium in a homogeneous system at 25°C. The WSPCSs showed low crystallinity, good

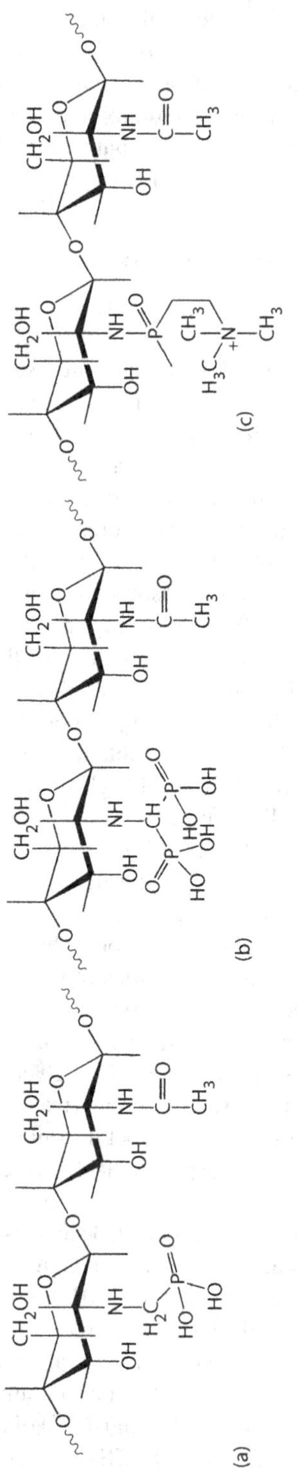

FIGURE 5.13 Chemical structures of phosphorylated chitosan products: *N*-methylenephosphonic chitosan (a), *N,N*-(di-methylenephosphonic) chitosan (b), and phosphorylcholine chitosan (c).

solubility in water, satisfying affinity in DMSO, pyridine, $CHCl_3$, and low toxicity to L929 cell lines. Lebouc et al. (2005) studied the phosphonomethylation reaction on chitosan by NMR spectroscopy. The experimental conditions for the phosphono-methylation of chitosan amino functions have been evaluated to conclude that this reaction was possible if it was carried out with a large excess of phosphorous acid and formaldehyde added simultaneously and heated for at least 6 hours (better yield was obtained within 24 hours) at 70°C. The peak at 7.0 ppm in ^{31}P-NMR spectrum has unequivocally confirmed the introduction of the α-aminomethylphosphonic acid function to chitosan and the doublet at 54.20 ppm associated with a large scalar coupling in ^{13}C-NMR. However, ^{13}C- and ^{1}H-NMR analyses revealed the presence of a side reaction, which occurs according to a mechanism based on the Leuckart–Wallart reaction, leading to the N-(methyl) and N,N-(dimethyl) chitosan. Reaction of chitosan with 2-chloro-1,3,2-dioxaphospholane under homogeneous or heterogeneous conditions produced phosphorylcholine chitosan (Figure 5.13c), which showed good anti-blood coagulation properties (Meng et al. 2007).

5.4.10 THIOLATED CHITOSAN PRODUCTS

The thiol group is a chemical analoge of the hydroxyl group and, thus, indicates the great potential of enhancing the properties of chitosan molecule. Thiolated chitosans are prepared by coupling the reagents containing thiol groups to the primary amino groups of chitosan via amide or amidine bond formation. The carboxylic acid group present in some reagents containing thiol groups such as cysteine and thioglycolic acid reacts with the amino group of chitosan forming a water-soluble carbodiimide product (Bernkop-Schnürch et al. 1999b; Kast and Bernkop-Schnürch 2001; Bernkop-Schnürch et al. 2001; Bernkop-Schnürch et al. 2003; Bernkop-Schnürch et al. 2004). The disulfide bonds can be formed by oxidation with air condition through the reaction; therefore, this undesirable product can be avoided by performing the reaction at a low pH of 5 which the thiolate anions concentration is little. Otherwise, the coupling reaction between the thiol group and the amino group of chitosan can be performed in the inert environment. For the formation of amidine bonds, 2-iminothiolane is usually used as a coupling reagent, which is a straightforward one-step coupling reaction (Andreas et al. 2003). Moreover, the thiol group of the reagent in this kind of the reaction is protected from the oxidation process. It was reported that a degree of modification of 25–250 mmol thiol groups per 1 g of chitosan showed the highest enhancement in the mucoadhesive and permeation properties. Finally, the concentration thiol groups immobilized into reduced and oxidized forms of thiolated chitosans can be determined using Ellman's reagent (5,5'-dithiobis-(2-nitrobenzoic acid) or DTNB) (Bernkop-Schnürch et al. 2003) with or without prior quantitative reduction of disulfide bonds by borohydride reagent (Leitner et al. 2003).

At present, four types of thiolated chitosans have been generated: chitosan–cysteine, chitosan–thioglycolic acid, chitosan–4-thiobutylamidine, and chitosan–thioethylamidine conjugates (Figure 5.14) (Bernkop-Schnürch et al. 1999a; Andreas et al. 2003; Bernkop-Schnürch et al. 2004; Kafedjiiski et al. 2005; Sreenivas and Pai 2008; Werle and Bernkop-Schnürch 2008; Sarti and Bernkop-Schnürch 2011; Han et al. 2012). Among them, the chitosan–thioglycolic conjugate has exhibited

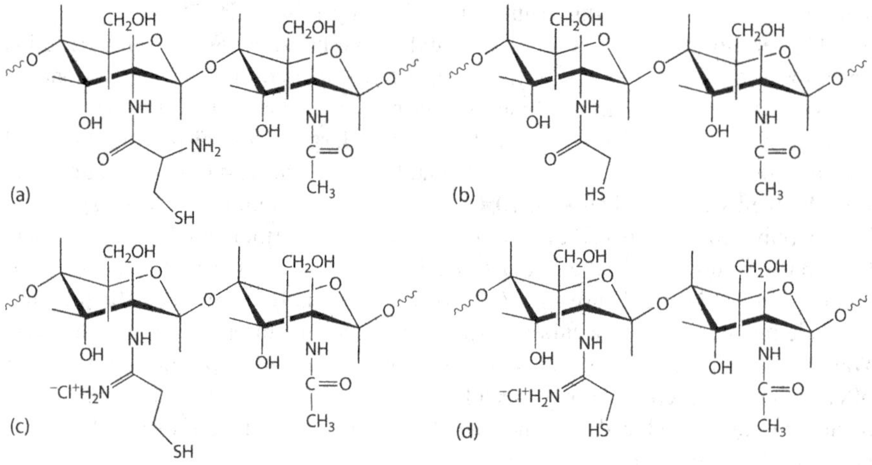

FIGURE 5.14 Chemical structures of thiolated chitosan products: chitosan-cysteine (a), chitosan-thioglycolic acid (b), chitosan-4-thiobutylamidine (c), and chitosan-thioethylamidine (d).

promising properties for tissue engineering because of its high solubility in water, well-situated biodegradation, and *in situ* gelling at physiological pH values (Hornof et al. 2003). However, all thiolated chitosans have numerous beneficial properties especially in a significant improvement of the mucoadhesive and permeation characters (Bernkop-Schnürch et al. 1999a; Kast and Bernkop-Schnürch 2001; Andreas et al. 2003; Bernkop-Schnürch et al. 2003; Roldo et al. 2004; Bravo-Osuna et al. 2007). Their strong cohesive properties make them extremely appropriate agents in the controlling of drug release doses (Kast and Bernkop-Schnürch 2002; Bernkop-Schnürch et al. 2003). The improvement of mucoadhesion properties of thiolated chitosans may be referring to the formation of covalent bonds between chitosan molecule and the mucus layer. Thiolated chitosans have been also used as scaffold materials in tissue engineering and as coating materials for stents (Bernkop-Schnürch et al. 2004).

5.4.11 QUATERNARY AMMONIUM CHITOSAN PRODUCTS

Quaternary ammonium chitosan products are the most promising derivatives of a chitosan molecule due to their multifunction along with favorable solubility at neutral and a wide range of the pH (Spinelli et al. 2004; Belalia et al. 2008; Mourya and Inamdar 2008; Tan et al. 2013; Badawy and Rabea 2014; Feng et al. 2015). These derivatives can be obtained in two different ways: by quaternization of the amino groups of chitosan with a suitable alkylating agent or by addition of a substituent containing a quaternary ammonium group (Spinelli et al. 2004). *N,N,N*-Trimethyl chitosan (TMC; Figure 5.15a), the simplest form of quaternized chitosan, is generally prepared by treating chitosan with formaldehyde to form a Schiff base, followed by reduction of the product to yield the corresponding *N*-alkyl chitosan. Then excess of methylation process with methyl iodide is carried out, generating the quaternary salt,

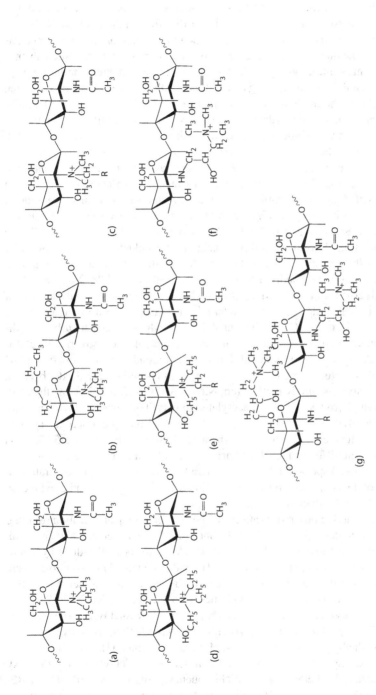

FIGURE 5.15 Chemical structures of TMC (a), TMCMC (b), *N,N,N*-dimethylalkyl chitosans (c), *N,N,N* triethylammonium chitosan (d), *N,N*-(diethyl),*N*-(aryl) chitosans (e), *N*-(2-hydroxyl) propyl-3-trimethylammonium chitosan (f), and N-substituted CMC-Quat-188 derivatives (g). R = alkyl or phenyl substituent.

or reaction of chitosan with excess of methyl iodide under strong alkaline conditions using N-methyl-2-pyrrolidone (NMP) as a solvent and sodium iodide as a catalyst (Domard et al. 1986). The authors established that the combination of NMP and NaOH was preferred for the quaternization much better than organic bases such as triethylamine. The quaternization mechanism is based on the nucleophilic substitution of the primary amino group at the C-2 position with iodomethane in the presence of sodium iodide solution. Dung et al. (1994) synthesized the TMC in a one-step reaction similar to the method used by Domard et al. (1986), but it was different in the concentration of sodium hydroxide and the reaction time. Other attempts such as treating chitosan with dimethylsulfate were achieved (de Britto and Assis 2007); however, almost all the reactions are carried out under strong basic conditions with high temperature, resulting in undesirable O-methylation that cannot be controlled and decrease the solubility of TMC in aqueous medium. To avoid O-methylation reaction, trimethylation was employed by reacting chitosan with methyl iodide at lower temperature by using DMF/H_2O mixture as a solvent instead of NMP and without catalyst (Rúnarsson et al. 2007). TMC was performed by Eschweiler–Clarke reaction by treating chitosan with formic acid and formaldehyde first, followed by methylation with excessive methyl iodide in NMP at 40°C in the absence of a mixture of sodium iodide and sodium hydroxide (Verheul et al. 2008; Xu et al. 2010; Patrulea et al. 2015). In this reaction, O-methylation did not occur, and the MW of O-methyl free TMC chloride salt considerably increased, with an increase of the degree of quaternization (DQ) (Verheul et al. 2008). TMC was further carboxymethylated by monochloroacetic acid to obtain N,N,N-trimethyl-O-carboxymethyl chitosan (TMCMC; Figure 5.15b) (Xu et al. 2010). It was found that the O-methyl TMC showed a high structural heterogeneity compared to O-methyl free TMC, because that presents in its structure N-methylated, N,N-dimethylated, N,N,N-trimethylated, and O-methylated groups and at rest acetylated moiety. This structural dissimilarity alters considerably the physicochemical properties and biological activity of such compounds (Verheul et al. 2008). N-Triethylated chitosan (TEC; Figure 5.15d) was prepared based on different DQs for pharmacological and pharmaceutical applications. Chitosan was dispersed in NMP and stirred for 4 hours at room temperature in the presence of aqueous sodium hydroxide solution, sodium iodide, and ethyl iodide (Sieval et al. 1998; Avadi et al. 2003).

The alkyl and aryl chitosan derivatives can be subjected to quaternization resulting in water-soluble products (Figure 5.15c) (Jia and Xu 2001; Avadi et al. 2004; Guo et al. 2007b; Badawy 2010; Badawy and Rabea 2014). TMC, N-propyl-N,N-dimethyl chitosan, and N-furfuryl-N,N-dimethyl chitosan and of N-diethylmethylamino chitosan were synthesized via Schiff base reaction first followed by reduction, and then the N-alkyl or aryl chitosan products were reacted with methyl iodide (Jia and Xu 2001). TEC and N,N-(diethyl), N-(aryl) chitosans (Figure 5.15e) include N,N-(diethyl), N-(benzyl) chitosan, N,N-(diethyl), N-(p-methylbenzyl) chitosan, N,N-(diethyl), N-(p-cyanobenzyl) chitosan, N,N-(diethyl), N-(p-fluorobenzyl) chitosan, N,N-(diethyl), N-(p-nitrobenzyl) chitosan, N,N-(diethyl), N-(o-fluorobenzyl) chitosan, N,N-(diethyl), N-(o,p-diethoxy benzyl) chitosan, N,N-(diethyl), N-(o,p-dichlorobenzyl) chitosan, N,N-(diethyl), N-(2-chloro,6-fluorobenzyl) chitosan, N,N-(diethyl), N-(cinnamyl) chitosan, N,N-(diethyl), N-(cuminyl) chitosan, and N,N-(diethyl), N-(p-dimethylaminobenzyl) chitosan, which were prepared via reductive amination reaction of chitosan with aromatic aldehydes and then quaternized by nucleophilic substitution of product amine protons with ethyl groups of ethyl iodide leading to water-soluble chitosan compounds (Badawy and Rabea 2014). Finally, the counterion I⁻ was exchanged in the presence of sodium chloride in a methanol/water medium with Cl⁻ to obtain N,N,N-(diethylaryl) chitosan chloride having higher solubility than the iodide counterpart.

Glycidyltrimethylammonium chloride (GTMAC) has been widely used as a quarternizing agent of chitosan resulting in N-(2-hydroxy)propyl-3-trimethylammonium chitosan chloride (HTCC; Figure 5.15f) because it has a quaternary ammonium group itself (Loubaki et al. 1991; Xu et al. 2003; Lim and Hudson 2004; Sun et al. 2006a; Peng et al. 2010; Tan et al. 2013; Rwei et al. 2014; Feng et al. 2015; Yang et al. 2015). The reaction between the amino group of chitosan and GTMAC increased the chains of the chitosan derivative obtained (Peng et al. 2010). In this case, the complete N-monoalkylation can be performed in water at 60°C for 15 hours (Sajomsang et al. 2010). Under the basic conditions, Daly and Manuszak-Guerrini (2001) prepared HTCC from (3-chloro-2-hydroxypropyl)trimethylammonium chloride (Quat-188 salt). The presence of the hydroxyl groups in the O,N-(2-hydroxy)propyl-3-trimethylammonium chains enhanced the polarity of the product compared to TMC, which increased the biological activity. N-Substituted CM-chitosan derivatives having a variety of N-aryl substituents bearing either electron-donating or electron-withdrawing groups were also quaternized by Quat-188 salt with iodine as a catalyst in a heterogeneous condition of alkaline media producing N-substituted CM-chitosan-Quat-188 derivatives (Figure 5.15g) (Sajomsang et al. 2009b; Mohamed et al. 2013). Quat-188 readily formed the consequent epoxide which reacted with the primary amino groups of CM-chitosan via nucleophilic substitution, and then the quaternary groups were linked to chitosan chains (Peng et al. 2010; Sajomsang et al. 2010). Keeping the DQ on the CM-chitosan backbone constant, the antimicrobial activity of N-quaternized CM-chitosan derivatives was affected not only by the nature of the microorganisms but also by the nature, position, and number of the substituent groups on the phenyl ring.

The DQ is usually determined by different techniques including pH-metric titration, IR, ¹H-NMR spectroscopy, potentiometry, and conductimetry (Domard et al. 1986; Sieval et al. 1998; Thanou et al. 2000; Avadi et al. 2003; Curti et al. 2003; de Britto and Assis 2007). The DQ calculated by H-NMR spectroscopy based on the integral area of one hydrogen from the methyl protons in the range of δ 1.30–1.50 ppm and the integral area of one hydrogen from the protons of H-1, 2, 3, 4, 5, and 6 of GlcN unit in the range of δ 3.15–4.20 ppm in ¹H-NMR spectra of the quaternary ammonium chitosan compounds (Sajomsang et al. 2010; Badawy and Rabea 2014). N-(Alkyl) chitosan derivatives were also quaternized using methyl iodide to produce water-soluble cationic polyelectrolytes (Kim et al. 1997; Kim and Choi 2002). The degree of trimethylation for TMC was calculated using the combined integral methods of peak areas in NMR spectra according to the following equation:

$$N,N,N\text{-Trimethylation}(\%) = \frac{\left[N(CH_3)3 \right]}{\left[H2,\ H3,\ H4,\ H5,\ H6,\ H6' \right] \times 6/9} \times 100$$

where $[N(CH_3)_3]$ is the integral of the N,N,N-trimethyl singlet peak ($\delta = 3.1$ ppm) (Rúnarsson et al. 2007).

As the reaction is performed in a heterogeneous medium, the monomethylated, dimethylated, and trimethylated products are formed indiscriminately. This complex of the products leads to misinterpretation of spectra obtained from ^{1}H-NMR spectroscopy, whereas the solid-state ^{13}C-NMR technique can be successively used as an alternative technique to determine the DQ of the TMC (de Britto and Assis 2007; de Britto et al. 2008). The potentiometric method for determination of DQ depends on the titration of the chloride ion present in quaternary ammonium chitosan chloride with aqueous silver nitrate solution, using a calomel electrode as the reference and a silver electrode for the measurement (Domard et al. 1986; Curti et al. 2003). DQ is calculated as follows:

$$DQ = \frac{CV/1000}{\left(CV/1000\right)+\left(W-\left(CVM_2/1000\right)\right)/M_1}$$

where:
    C (mol/L) is the concentration of $AgNO_3$ solution
    V (mL) is the volume of $AgNO_3$ solution
    W (g) is the weight of quaternary chitosan
    M_1 (mol/g) is the molar mass of glucosamine
    M_2 (mol/g) is the molar mass of quaternary chitosan

Quaternary ammonium chitosans have positive charges as a result of the protonation of the amino groups of chitosan under acidic conditions, which are the driving force for chitosan solubilization especially at physiological pH conditions. Due to the unique properties of chitosan quaternary ammonium products, they are extensively used in different areas such as cosmetics (Lang and Wendel 1990; Lang et al. 1990b; Jimtaisong and Saewan 2014), wastewater treatment (Bhatnagar and Sillanpää 2009; Lin et al. 2014; Farah et al. 2015), and pharmaceutical and drug delivery carriers (Uchegbu et al. 2001; Thanou et al. 2002; Mourya and Inamdar 2009; Li et al. 2014; Dai et al. 2015). In addition, this kind of products showed high activities against microorganisms as a result of the presence of permanent positive charge that can interact with anionic compounds and macromolecular structures of the microbial cells of bacteria and fungi (Kim et al. 1997; Jia and Xu 2001; Rúnarsson et al. 2007; Sajomsang et al. 2010; Li et al. 2011; Muñoz-Bonilla and Fernández-García 2012; Sajomsang et al. 2012; Carmona-Ribeiro and de Melo Carrasco 2013; Martins et al. 2014; Khalil et al. 2015). Some authors reported that the antibacterial activity of quaternary ammonium chitosans is stronger than that of unmodified chitosan, and the antibacterial property depends on the DQ and the pH of the assays. Jia and Xu (2001) reported that the N-propyl-N,N-dimethyl chitosan has the bactericidal activity against *Escherichia coli* 20 times higher than that of chitosan with 96% DA. Other authors reported that the antimicrobial activity of TMC is approximately 500 times higher than that of chitosan (Xie et al. 2002; Xu et al. 2010; Tan et al. 2013). Another work showed that the quaternization of heterocyclic chitosan derivatives significantly enhanced the antimicrobial activity against *Mycobacterium smegmatis* (MTCC 943) and *Pseudomonas aeroginosa* (MTCC 4676) at 500 mg/L, whereas chitosan was not effective at the same concentration (Chethan et al. 2013). *N*-[(2-Hydroxy-3-trimethylammonium)propyl chitosan and TMC, having the same MW, were synthesized and found to have good antibacterial activities against *E. coli* and *Staphylococcus aureus* at pH 7.1 (Huang et al. 2013). Xu et al. (2011) added that *N,N,N*-trimethyl-*O*-(2-hydroxy-3-trimethylammonium propyl) chitosans with different degrees of O-substitution showed a high antibacterial activity compared with TMC, and the activity was increased with an increase in the DS value.

   N,N,N-Dimethylalkyl chitosans (Figure 5.15c) significantly improved the antifungal activity against *Botrytis cinerea*, *Fusarium oxysporum*, and *Pythium debaryanum* (Badawy 2010). *N,N,N*-Dimethylpentyl chitosan and *N,N,N*-dimethyloctyl chitosan were the highest in mycelial growth inhibition of *B. cinerea* (EC_{50} = 908 and 383 mg/L, respectively), *F. oxysporum* (EC_{50} = 871 and 812 mg/L, respectively), and *P. debaryanum* (EC_{50} = 624 and 440 mg/L, respectively). Furthermore, spore germination of *B. cinerea* and *F. oxysporum* was greatly affected at the concentrations ranged from 50 to 1000 mg/L, and the activity was increased with an increase in the alkyl substituent chain. Another series of *N*-(aryl) and quaternary *N*-(aryl) chitosan derivatives were prepared and evaluated by *in vitro* and *in vivo* assays against *B. cinerea* (Badawy and Rabea 2014). All quaternized chitosans were more active (*in vitro*) than *N*-(aryl) chitosan derivatives and *N,N,N*-(diethylcinnamyl) chitosan was the most potent (EC_{50} = 1147 mg/L) against mycelia; however, *N,N,N*-(diethyl-*p*-dimethylaminobenzyl) chitosan was the most active (EC_{50} = 334 mg/L) against the spores. In the *in vivo* experiment, by application of compounds on tomato plants prior to inoculation with fungal spores, no disease incidence (0.0%) was observed with both compounds at 1000 mg/L. In this experiment, spray liquid chitosans improved total phenolic content and guaiacol peroxidase in tomato leaves compared with the control. In another study, these derivatives exhibited high activity against the mycelial growth of *B. cinerea*, *Botryodiplodia theobromae*, *F. oxysporum*, and *Phytophthora infestans* and inhibited, *in vivo*, exocellular enzymes, including polygalacturonase, pectinlyase, polyphenol oxidase, and cellulase at 1000 mg/L. The results demonstrated that the grafting of aryl moiety onto chitosan molecule followed by quaternization of the derivatives successfully inhibited microbial growth. Guo et al. (2007a) added that the quaternized phenyl and hydroxyphenyl chitosan derivatives had better antifungal activity against *B. cinerea* than chitosan, chitosan-Schiff bases, and N-substituted chitosan derivatives, and the inhibitory indices of quaternary phenyl chitosan or quaternary hydroxyphenyl chitosan were 81.2% and 58.6% at 1000 mg/L, respectively (Guo et al. 2007a). The same research group (Guo et al. 2007b) in another study found that four quaternized chitosans *N*-(2-hydroxyl-phenyl)-*N,N*-dimethyl chitosan, *N*-(5-chloro-2-hydroxyl-phenyl)-*N,N*-dimethyl chitosan, *N*-(2-hydroxyl-5-nitro-phenyl)-*N,N*-dimethyl chitosan, and *N*-(5-bromic-2-hydroxyl-phenyl)-*N,N*-dimethyl chitosan showed higher antifungal activity against *B. cinerea* and *Colletotrichum lagenarium* than chitosan, and the inhibitory indices, at 1000 mg/L, were 58.6%, 86.7%, 68.8%, and 66.6%, respectively, for *B. cinerea*, and 55.8%, 72.6%, 63.6%, and 79.5% for *C. lagenarium*, respectively.

The antifungal activity of chitosan can be improved by increasing the DS of alkyltrimethyl ammonium groups on the polymer chain. This fact was confirmed by de Oliveira Pedro et al. (2013), who reported that the inhibition indices of propyl and pentyl(trimethylammonium) chitosans increased with an increase in the DS, and both derivatives exhibited the inhibition values 3 and 6 times, respectively, higher than those obtained with chitosan against *A. flavus*. Sajomsang and coauthors studied the antimicrobial activity of TMC, *N*-(4-*N,N,N*-trimethylcinnamyl) chitosan (TMCMCHT) and *N*-(4-pyridylmethyl) chitosan (PyMCHT) derivatives containing *N,N,N*-trimethylammonium moieties. These compounds possessed a high positive charge density and a strong bactericidal activity at neutral pH, and TMCMCHT exhibited the higher effect than TMC, whereas PyMCHT reduced the activity against *E. coli* (ATCC 25922) and *S. aureus* (ATCC 6538) at the same DQ level (Sajomsang et al. 2009a; Sajomsang et al. 2009b; Sajomsang 2010; Sajomsang et al. 2010). Recently, quaternary *N*-alkyl and *N,N*-dialkyl chitosan derivatives have been synthesized and studied for the antibacterial activity against Gram-positive *S. aureus* and *Enterococcus faecalis*, and Gram-negative *E. coli* and *P. aeruginosa* (Sahariah et al. 2015). It was found that the activity was positively correlated with the alkyl chain length, and the most active chitosan derivatives were found to be more selective for killing bacteria than the quaternary ammonium disinfectants cetylpyridiniumchloride and benzalkoniumchloride.

5.4.12 CHITOSAN OLIGOMERS

Chitosan has several drawbacks to be utilized in biological applications, including poor solubility under physiological conditions. Therefore, high-MW chitosan molecule can be subjected to the depolymerization process producing low-MW chitosan, oligosaccharide (chitooligomers), and monomers that have low viscosity and greater solubility in neutral media and can be applied in many applications in different areas (Prashanth and Sugano et al. 1988; Inui et al. 1995; Tharanathan 2007). Different methods including chemical (oxidative–reductive, free radical depolymerization, acid and alkaline hydrolysis), ultrasonic degradation, and enzyme-catalyzed hydrolysis have been studied for the preparation of chitosan oligomers (Domard and Cartier 1989; Aiba 1994a; Jeon and Kim 2000; Vårum et al. 2001; Roy et al. 2003; Il'Ina and Varlamov 2004; Kim and Rajapakse 2005; Ramírez-Coutiño et al. 2006). However, chemical hydrolysis is widely used in the industrial-scale production. Depolymerization occurs via cleavage of the glycosidic bonds. The depolymerization by chemical methods are limited to acidic hydrolysis with traditional heating methods and have some disadvantages such as high cost, low yield, not specific; residual acidity, and higher risk associated with the environmental pollution, and the hydrolysis goes randomly generating a large amount of monomers, such as D-glucosamine, as the reaction time increases (Kim and Rajapakse 2005; Uryash et al. 2007). Studies recommended nitrous acid, hydrochloric acid, phosphoric acid, and hydrogen peroxide for chitosan depolymerization (Allan and Peyron 1995b; Chang et al. 2001; Vårum et al. 2001; Jia and Shen 2002; Kato et al. 2002; Tian et al. 2003; Tian et al. 2004). The reaction of nitrous acid (HONO) with chitosan molecule is particularly advantageous because it is selective, rapid, and easily controlled, and the reaction products are well established stoichiometry (Tømmeraas et al. 2001; Vårum et al. 2001; Mao et al. 2004; Galed et al. 2005). Nitrosating agents originating from HONO selectively attack the glucosamine but not the N-acetylglucosamine moieties, and subsequently cleave the anhydroglyco-sidic linkages of the polymer chain (Defaye et al. 1994). One mole of HONO is consumed per mole of amine group reacted, and a 2,5-anhydro-D-mannose unit is formed at the reducing end of the cleaved polymer (Sashiwa et al. 1993 and Tommeraas et al. 2001). Janes and Alonso (2003) reported that $NaNO_2$ showed the best performance. Depolymerization in concentrated nitrous acid produced chito-san oligomers with a DP of 9–18, but it was difficult to obtain oligomers with a DP below 10, and the final products contained 2,5-anhydromannose residues by deami-nation (Peniston and Johnson 1980; Allan and Peyron 1995a; Allan and Peyron 1995b; Furusaki et al. 1996).

Hydrogen peroxide can also be conveniently used to depolymerize chitosan by means of generation of hydroxyl radicals (Tian et al. 2003; Tian et al. 2004). Use of a hot phosphoric acid has also been reported for preparing chitosan oligomers (Jia and Shen 2002). The yields were reported as 10%–20% for products with a DP of 6–8, and neutralization and desalting steps were recommended. In addition, two types of chitosan oligomers with DPs of 7.3 and 16.8 were also prepared by homogeneous hydrolysis of chitosan in 85% phosphoric acid at room temperature, but long reaction times of more than 4 weeks were required (Hasegawa et al. 1993).

The depolymerization can also be achieved using microwave technology assisted by the addition of salts under homogeneous reaction conditions, which produces low-MW chitosan in a shorter time (Ren et al. 2005; Xing et al. 2005a; Omari et al. 2012). The enzymatic processes for chitosan oligomer production are now preferred over chemical methods and generally carried out in batch reactors (Aiba 1994b; Muzzarelli et al. 1995; Kim et al. 1998; Kuroiwa et al. 2002; Tharanathan 2004; Cabrera and Van Cutsem 2005; Kim and Rajapakse 2005; Yao et al. 2014; Kumar and; Mawad et al. 2015). Chitinolytic enzymes such as chitinase, chitosanase, papin, and lysozyme are widely distributed in a variety of organisms ranging from bacte-ria to animals. Enzymatic hydrolysis for chitooligosaccharides (COS) production is preferable because these methods obtain greater yields of oligomers with a higher DP (Uchida et al. 1989; Muzzarelli et al. 1994b; Jeon and Kim 2000; Chen et al. 2003; Kim and Mendis 2006). According to the cleavage sites, chitinases can be classi-fied into two main categories: endo-chitinases and exo-chitinases. Endo-chitinases (EC 3.2.1.14) generally cleave the linkage of GlcNAc–GlcNAc, GlcN–GlcNAc, and GlcNAc–GlcN in chitin to release soluble chitin oligomers with variable DPs (Hayes et al. 2008). Exo-chitinases can be divided into two subcategories: N,N'-diacetylchitobiohydrolase (chitobiase, EC 3.2.1.29) and β-N-acetylglucosaminidase (GlcNAc-ase, EC 3.2.1.30). Chitobiases catalyze the progressive release of chitobiose from either the nonreducing end or the reducing end of chitin. GlcNAc-ases progres-sively break down chitin polymers or oligomers from the nonreducing or reducing end of the molecule, releasing β-D-GlcNAc or α-D-GlcNAc, respectively (Kim 2010; Zhao et al. 2010; Zhao et al. 2011). Chitosanase from *Bacillus* sp. has previously been used to hydrolyze deacetylated chitosan in batch fermenters (Izume and Ohtakara 1987; Jeon and Kim 2000). Even though microbial chitosanases are excellent for

COS production, they are considered too expensive for industrial-scale production (Kim and Rajapakse 2005). Thus, other sources are generally considered to produce COS at low cost (Zhang et al. 2006).

5.4.13 CHITOSAN–METAL COMPLEXES

Chitosan has amino groups that are known to have coordination behavior and easily forms complexes with transition metals such as cadmium, zinc, or cupric ions giving chitosan–metal complexes (Ogawa et al. 1993; Varma et al. 2004; Chauhan 2015). For large-scale use of chitosan, most research studies are concerned with metal-chelating agents for the recovery or removal of metallic impurities from wastewaters (Muzzarelli 1973; Bassi et al. 2000; Guibal 2004; Varma et al. 2004; Verbych et al. 2005). Binding of chitosan with alkaline earth metals is extensively studied and investigated (Deans and Dixon 1992; Peniche-Covas et al. 1992; Oshita et al. 2001; Crini et al. 2014; Galhoum et al. 2015). Chitosan has chelating capacities of >1 mmol/g for toxic heavy metals, with the exception of chromium and mercury that the maximum adsorption capacities are shown to be 558 and 1123 mg/g of chitosan, respectively (Bailey et al. 1999; Varma et al. 2004).

The metal–complex formation mainly depends on the amino groups that contain nitrogen as an electron donor, and the hydroxyl groups can participate in the linkage between chitosan and metal ions. The combination mechanism of both reactive groups with metal ions depends on the ion type and the pH of the solution (Domard 1987; Ogawa et al. 1993; Wang et al. 2004). Another proposed mechanism was also described based on the Lewis acid–base theory that proved the metal ions acting as the acid which are accept of a pair of electrons donated by chitosan that acting as the base. Based on this information, the proposed structure of a chitosan–metal complex is shown in Figure 5.16 (Wang et al. 2004). The metal ion like a bridge connected one or more chains of chitosan by interacting with hydroxyl and amino groups. The product of chitosan binding with metal, through nitrogen, oxygen, or both of them, has some potential donor atoms free that enhance the biological activity of the complex (Wang et al. 2005). However, the influence of the property of metal ions, molecular parameters, and environmental factors on the biological activity of chitosan–metal complexes was not clear up to date.

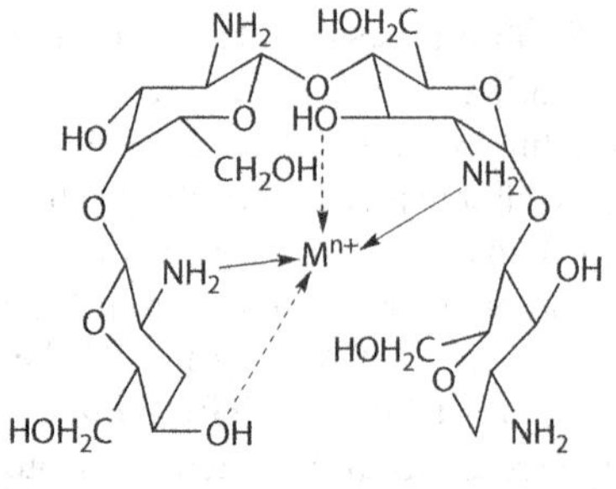

FIGURE 5.16   The reasonable structure of chitosan–metal complexes.

This chelation depends on the physical state of chitosan (powder, gel, fiber, film). Better chelation is obtained for greater DDA. Thus, chelation is related to the free amino group content as well as its distribution along chitosan molecule (Kurita et al. 1979). It is also related to the DP of oligochitosans; the complex starts to form a chelation when DP is 46 (Rhazi et al. 2002). In addition, the nature of the metal cation (valance, divalent, and trivalent cations) is very important in the mechanism of interaction (Rhazi et al. 2002; Vold et al. 2003). The chelation capacity was found to be increased from 0.02 mmol/g chitosan for divalent ions such as Co(II) and Ca(II) to 1.2 for Cu(II). However, in case of the trivalent ions, the chelating efficiency was ranged from 0.2 mmol/g chitosan for Pr(III) and Cr(III) to 1.47 for Eu(III) and Nd(III) (Rhazi et al. 2002). Moreover, the effect of the type of the anion was also studied (Mitani et al. 1991): for example, sulfate increases the fixation on swollen chitosan beads. In another study, chitosan powder was dispersed in silver nitrate solution or used to fill a column to adsorb mercuric ions from a chloride solution (Peniche-Covas et al. 1992; Peniche-Covas et al. 1988). It was shown that the conditions for using chitosan or chemical modification of chitosan also play a large role in the adsorption and kinetics of retention (Annachhatre et al. 1996; Hsien and Rorrer 1997; Wu et al. 2001; Ruiz et al. 2002; Zhou et al. 2009). There are several research articles and reviews on chitosan modification via protonation, cross-linking, carboxylation, and grafting techniques in efforts to improve complex formation with metal ions (Yalpani and Hall 1984; Hon and Tang 2000; Varma et al. 2004; Bhatnagar and Sillanpää 2009; Kyzas et al. 2009; Miretzky and Cirelli 2009; Boamah et al. 2015). Among these derivatizations, chitosans modified with a carboxylic group (carboxylate chitosan derivative) have multifunctional groups of carboxyl, amino, and hydroxyl are superior for removal of metal ions (Muzzarelli et al. 1982a; Hon and Tang 2000; Tang and Hon 2001; Sun and Wang 2006; Sun et al. 2006b; Boamah et al. 2015). N-CM-chitosan was highly documented product in chelation capacity of cobalt, copper, nickel, cadmium, and lead ions compared to chitosan alone (Muzzarelli et al. 1982a; Dobetti and Delben 1992; Wan Ngah and Liang 1999; Boamah et al. 2015).

Cross-linking of chitosan by di/polyfunctional reagents, such as glutaraldehyde, epichlorohydrin, ethylene glycol diglycidyl ether, iminodiacetic acid, and organic diisocyanates, is generally carried out to enable it to be used for metal complexation. The adsorption capacity depends on the extent of cross-linking and usually decreases with an increase in the extent of cross-linking (Baba et al. 1994; Tikhonov et al. 1996; Shim and Ryu 1998; Varma et al. 2004). High adsorbents for heavy metals such as Hg(II) and Cd(II) can be prepared by chitosan in cross-linking with organic diisocyanates such as hexamethylene diisocyanate and nitriloacetic acid resulting in superior adsorption efficiency (Tikhonov et al. 1996). Chitosan-glutaraldehyde (chitosan-GLA; Figure 5.17a), chitosan-glyoxal (Figure 5.17b), chitosan-epichlorohydrin (chitosan-ECH; Figure 5.17c), and chitosan-ethylene glycol diglycidyl ether (chitosan-EGDE; Figure 5.17d), respectively, were also extensively studied in removal of metal ions from environmental waste samples (Ngah et al. 2002; Webster et al. 2007; Chen et al. 2008; Miretzky and Cirelli 2009; Laus et al. 2010; Monier et al. 2010; Ngah et al. 2011; Sahin et al. 2011). Although cross-linking reduces the adsorption capacity, it enhances the

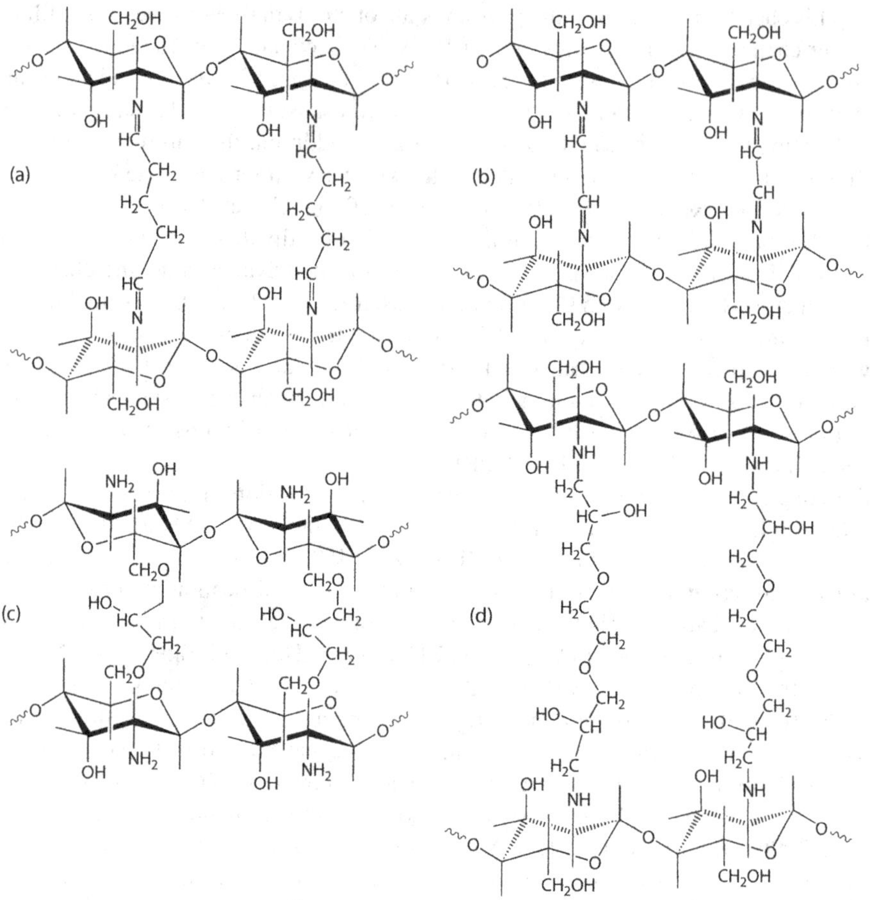

FIGURE 5.17 Chemical structures of chitosan-GLA (a), chitosan-glyoxal (b), chitosan-ECH (c), and chitosan-EGDE (d).

resistance of chitosan against acid, alkali, and chemicals (Inoue et al. 1993). The cross-linked chitosans are also very stable and maintain their strength even in acidic and basic solutions. It was reported that GLA, ECH, and EGDE prepared in the form of beads showed high adsorption efficiency for Cu(II). The uptakes of Cu(II) ions on the beads were 80.71 mg Cu(II)/g chitosan, on chitosan-GLA beads were 59.67 mg Cu(II)/g chitosan-GLA, on chitosan-ECH beads were 62.47 mg Cu(II)/g chitosan-ECH, and on chitosan-EGDE beads were 45.94 mg Cu(II)/g chitosan-EGDE (Ngah et al. 2002).

Recently, chitosan–metal complexes have been studied for removal and degradation of hazardous pesticides from wastewaters (Zhang et al. 2015). Three types of MW chitosans (high, medium, and low) were selected as ligands to synthesize chitosan- coordination complexes with Mg(II), Ca(II), Fe(III), and Zn(II), and were used for degradation of dichlorvos, omethoate, dimethoate, and chlorpyrifos as organophosphorous pesticides in a heterogeneous system. The chitosan–metal complexes especially with low MW showed high hydrolysis of these pesticides. It was found that the half-life of dichlorvos hydrolyzed by chitosan-Fe(III) was 52 hours, at pH 7.0°C and 20°C, whereas that of spontaneous dichlorvos hydrolysis was 105 hours. The degradation ratio of omethoate and dimethoate increased up to 38% and 52%, respectively, which were 34% and 48% higher than the control after 6 days at pH 7.0 and 20°C (Zhang et al. 2015).

5.5 CONCLUSION

Chitin and chitosan are the natural polymers available, and each of them has reactive functional groups that can be structurally modified by different techniques. Their unique physicochemical and biological characteristics make them worthy in regard to many applications in different areas. However, as their use is limited because they do not dissolve in neutral and basic aqueous media, their application as unmodified molecules is difficult. The chemical modification of chitin and chitosan provides derivatives that are soluble at a wide range of pH values. Moreover, the modification can be used to attach various functional groups and to control hydrophobic, cationic, and anionic properties. The derivatives obtained show improvement in their physicochemical properties along with the modification obtained by attachment of a particular substituent. Therefore, there is great opportunity to the research/development scientist to develop novel chitin and chitosan polymers by their structure modification.

REFERENCES

Aiba, S. 1989. Studies on chitosan: 2. Solution stability and reactivity of partially N-acetylated chitosan derivatives in aqueous media. *International Journal of Biological Macromolecules* 11: 249–252.

Aiba, S. 1994a. Preparation of N-acetylchitooligosaccharides by hydrolysis of chitosan with chitinase followed by N-acetylation. *Carbohydrate Research* 265: 323–328.

Aiba, S. 1994b. Preparation of N-acetylchitooligosaccharides from lysozymic hydrolysates of partially N-acetylated chitosans. *Carbohydrate Research* 261: 297–306.

Aiping, Z., C. Tian, Y. Lanhua, W. Hao, and L. Ping. 2006. Synthesis and characterization of N-succinyl-chitosan and its self-assembly of nanospheres. *Carbohydrate Polymers* 66: 274–279.

Allan, G.G. and M. Peyron. 1995a. Molecular weight manipulation of chitosan II: Prediction and control of extent of depolymerization by nitrous acid. *Carbohydrate Research* 277: 273–282.

Allan, G.G. and M. Peyron. 1995b. Molecular weight manipulation of chitosan. I: Kinetics of depolymerization by nitrous acid. *Carbohydrate Research* 277: 257–272.

Alves, N.M. and J.F. Mano. 2008. Chitosan derivatives obtained by chemical modifications for biomedical and environmental applications. *International Journal of Biological Macromolecules* 43: 401–414.

Amaral, I.F., P.L. Granja, and M.A. Barbosa. 2005. Chemical modification of chitosan by phosphorylation: An XPS, FT-IR and SEM study. *Journal of Biomaterials Science, Polymer Edition* 16: 1575–1593.

Amiji, M.M. 1997. Synthesis of anionic poly (ethylene glycol) derivative for chitosan surface modification in blood-contacting applications. *Carbohydrate Polymers* 32: 193–199.

Andreas, B., M. Hornof, and T. Zoidl. 2003. Thiolated polymers–thiomers: Modification of chitosan with 2-iminothiolane. *International Journal of Pharmaceutics* 260: 229–237.

Andrew, C.W., E. Khor, and G.W. Hastings. 1998. The influence of anionic chitin derivatives on calcium phosphate crystallization. *Biomaterials* 19: 1309–1316.

Annachhatre, A.P., N.N. Win, and S. Chandrkrachang. 1996. Adsorption of copper on chitosan. In *Chitin and Chitosan-Environmental Friendly and Versatile Biomaterials Proceedings of the Second Asia Pacific Symposium.* Bangkok, Thailand: Asian Institue of Technology, pp. 169–173.

Austin, P.R., C. Brine, J. Castle, and J. Zikakis. 1981. Chitin: New facets of research. *Science* 212: 749–753.

Avadi, M., M. Zohuriaan-Mehr, P. Younessi, M. Amini, M.R. Tehrani, and A. Shafiee. 2003. Optimized synthesis and characterization of N-triethyl chitosan. *Journal of bioactive and compatible polymers* 18: 469–479.

Avadi, M.R., G. Mahdavi, A.M. Sadeghi, M. Erfan, M. Amini, M.R. Tehrani, and A. Shafiee. 2004. Synthesis and characterization of N-diethyl methyl chitosan. *Iranian Polymer Journal* 13: 431–436.

Azuma, K., M. Nishihara, H. Shimizu, Y. Itoh, O. Takashima, T. Osaki, N. Itoh, T. Imagawa, Y. Murahata, and T. Tsuka. 2015. Biological adhesive based on carboxymethyl chitin derivatives and chitin nanofibers. *Biomaterials* 42: 20–29.

Baba, Y. and H. Hirakawa. 1992. Selective adsorption of Palladium (II), Platinum (IV), and Mercury (II) on a new chitosan derivative possessing pyridyl group. *Chemistry Letters* (10): 1905–1908.

Baba, Y., H. Hirakawa, and Y. Kawano. 1994. Selective adsorption of precious metals on sulfur-containing chitosan derivatives. *Chemistry Letters* (1): 117–120.

Baba, Y., Y. Kawano, and H. Hirakawa. 1996. Highly selective adsorption resins. I. preparation of chitosan derivatives containing 2-pyridylmethyl, 2-thienylmethyl, and 3-(methylthio) propyl groups and their selective adsorption of precious metals. *Bulletin of the Chemical Society of Japan* 69: 1255–1260.

Babak, V., E. Merkovich, J. Desbrieres, and M. Rinaudo. 2000. Formation of an ordered nanostructure in surfactant-polyelectrolyte complexes formed by interfacial diffusion. *Polymer Bulletin* 45: 77–81.

Badawy, M.E.I. 2008. Chemical modification of chitosan: Synthesis and biological activity of new heterocyclic chitosan derivatives. *Polymer International* 57: 254–261.

Badawy, M.E.I. 2010. Structure and antimicrobial activity relationship of quaternary N-alkyl chitosan derivatives against some plant pathogens. *Journal of Applied Polymer Science* 117: 960–969.

Badawy, M.E.I. and E.I. Rabea. 2012. Characterization and antimicrobial activity of water-soluble N-(4-carboxybutyroyl) chitosans against some plant pathogenic bacteria and fungi. *Carbohydrate Polymers* 87: 250–256.

Badawy, M.E.I. and E.I. Rabea. 2013. Synthesis and structure–activity relationship of N-(cinnamyl) chitosan analogs as antimicrobial agents. *International Journal of Biological Macromolecules* 57: 185–192.

Badawy, M.E.I. and E.I. Rabea. 2014. Synthesis and antifungal property of N-(aryl) and quaternary N-(aryl) chitosan derivatives against *Botrytis cinerea*. *Cellulose* 21: 3121–3137.

Badawy, M.E.I., E.I. Rabea, T.M. Rogge, C.V. Stevens, G. Smagghe, W. Steurbaut, and M. Höfte. 2004. Synthesis and fungicidal activity of new N,O-acyl chitosan derivatives. *Biomacromolecules* 5: 589–595.

Bailey, S.E., T.J. Olin, R.M. Bricka, and D.D. Adrian. 1999. A review of potentially low-cost sorbents for heavy metals. *Water Research* 33: 2469–2479.

Baker, B. and R.E. Schaub. 1954. Puromycin. Synthetic studies. III. Synthesis of 3-amino-D-ribose, an hydrolytic fragment. *The Journal of Organic Chemistry* 19: 646–660.

Bassi, R., S.O. Prasher, and B. Simpson. 2000. Removal of selected metal ions from aqueous solutions using chitosan flakes. *Separation Science and Technology* 35: 547–560.

Belalia, R., S. Grelier, M. Benaissa, and V. Coma. 2008. New bioactive biomaterials based on quaternized chitosan. *Journal of Agricultural and Food Chemistry* 56: 1582–1588.

Bernkop-Schnürch, A., U. Brandt, and A. Clausen. 1999a. Synthesis and in vitro evaluation of chitosan-cysteine conjugates. *Scientia Pharmaceutica* 67: 196–208.

Bernkop-Schnürch, A., A.E. Clausen, and M. Hnatyszyn. 2001. Thiolated polymers: Synthesis and in vitro evaluation of polymer–cysteamine conjugates. *International Journal of Pharmaceutics* 226: 185–194.

Bernkop-Schnürch, A., M. Hornof, and D. Guggi. 2004. Thiolated chitosans. *European Journal of Pharmaceutics and Biopharmaceutics* 57: 9–17.

Bernkop-Schnürch, A., M. Hornof, and T. Zoidl. 2003. Thiolated polymers-thiomers: Synthesis and in vitro evaluation of chitosan–2-iminothiolane conjugates. *International Journal of Pharmaceutics* 260: 229–237.

Bernkop-Schnürch, A., V. Schwarz, and S. Steininger. 1999b. Polymers with thiol groups: A new generation of mucoadhesive polymers. *Pharmaceutical Research* 16: 876–881.

Bhatnagar, A. and M. Sillanpää. 2009. Applications of chitin-and chitosan-derivatives for the detoxification of water and wastewater—a short review. *Advances in Colloid and Interface Science* 152: 26–38.

Boamah, P.O., Y. Huang, M. Hua, Q. Zhang, J. Wu, J. Onumah, L.K. Sam-Amoah, and P.O. Boamah. 2015. Sorption of heavy metal ions onto carboxylate chitosan derivatives—A mini-review. *Ecotoxicology and Environmental Safety* 116: 113–120.

Bravo-Osuna, I., C. Vauthier, A. Farabollini, G.F. Palmieri, and G. Ponchel. 2007. Mucoadhesion mechanism of chitosan and thiolated chitosan-poly (isobutyl cyanoacrylate) core-shell nanoparticles. *Biomaterials* 28: 2233–2243.

Broussignac, P. 1968. Chitosan: A natural polymer not well known by the industry. *Chimie et Industrie, Genie Chimique* 99: 1241–1247.

Cabrera, J.C. and P. Van Cutsem. 2005. Preparation of chitooligosaccharides with degree of polymerization higher than 6 by acid or enzymatic degradation of chitosan. *Biochemical Engineering Journal* 25: 165–172.

Campana-Filho, S.P., D. de Britto, E. Curti, F.R. Abreu, M.B. Cardoso, M.V. Battisti, P.C. Sim, R.C. Goy, R. Signini, and R.L. Lavall. 2007. Extraction, structures and properties of alpha- and beta-chitin. *Quimica Nova* 30: 644–650.

Cao, L., J. Wang, J. Hou, W. Xing, and C. Liu. 2014. Vascularization and bone regeneration in a critical sized defect using 2-N, 6-O-sulfated chitosan nanoparticles incorporating BMP-2. *Biomaterials* 35: 684–698.

Carmona-Ribeiro, A.M. and L.D. de Melo Carrasco. 2013. Cationic antimicrobial polymers and their assemblies. *International Journal of Molecular Sciences* 14: 9906–9946.

Carolan, C., H. Blair, S. Allen, and G. Mckay. 1991. N,O-Carboxymethyl chitosan, a water soluble derivative and potential green food preservative. *Chemical Engineering Research & Design* 69: 195–196.

Chang, K.L.B., M.C. Tai, and F.H. Cheng. 2001. Kinetics and products of the degradation of chitosan by hydrogen peroxide. *Journal of Agricultural and Food Chemistry* 49: 4845–4851.

Changhong, P., Y. Weijun, and T. Motang. 2003. Chemical modification of chitosan: Synthesis and characterization of chitosan-crown ethers. *Journal of Applied Polymer Science* 87: 2221–2225.

Chauhan, S. 2015. Modification of chitosan for sorption of metal ions. *Journal of Chemical & Pharmaceutical Research* 7(4): 49–55.

Chen, X.G. and H.J. Park. 2003. Chemical characteristics of O-carboxymethyl chitosans related to the preparation conditions. *Carbohydrate Polymers* 53: 355–359.

Chen, C.S., W.Y. Liau, and G.J. Tsai. 1998. Antibacterial effects of *N*-sulfonated and *N*-sulfobenzoyl chitosan and application to oyster preservation. *Journal of Food Protection* 61: 1124–1128.

Chen, A.H., S.C. Liu, C.Y. Chen, and C.Y. Chen. 2008. Comparative adsorption of Cu (II), Zn (II), and Pb (II) ions in aqueous solution on the crosslinked chitosan with epichlorohydrin. *Journal of Hazardous Materials* 154: 184–191.

Chen, L., Z. Tian, and Y. Du. 2004a. Synthesis and pH sensitivity of carboxymethyl chitosan-based polyampholyte hydrogels for protein carrier matrices. *Biomaterials* 25: 3725–3732.

Chen, S.C., Y.C. Wu, F.L. Mi, Y.H. Lin, L.C. Yu, and H.W. Sung. 2004b. A novel pH-sensitive hydrogel composed of N,O-carboxymethyl chitosan and alginate cross-linked by genipin for protein drug delivery. *Journal of Controlled Release* 96: 285–300.

Chen, S.H., Y.H. Yen, C.L. Wang, and S.L. Wang. 2003. Reversible immobilization of lysozyme via coupling to reversibly soluble polymer. *Enzyme and Microbial Technology* 33: 643–649.

Chethan P., B. Vishalakshi, L. Sathish, K. Ananda, and B. Poojary. 2013. Preparation of substituted quaternized arylfuran chitosan derivatives and their antimicrobial activity. *International Journal of Biological Macromolecules* 59: 158–164.

Chow, K.S. and E. Khor. 2002. New flourinated chitin derivatives: Synthesis, characterization and cytotoxicity assessment. *Carbohydrate Polymers* 47: 357–363.

Crini, G., N. Morin-Crini, N. Fatin-Rouge, S. Deon, and P. Fievet. 2014. Metal removal from aqueous media by polymer-assisted ultrafiltration with chitosan. *Arabian Journal of Chemistry*. doi:10.1016/j.arabjc.2014.05.020.

Curti, E., D. de Britto, and S.P. Campana Filho. 2003. Methylation of chitosan with iodomethane: Effect of reaction conditions on chemoselectivity and degree of substitution. *Macromolecular Bioscience* 3: 571–576.

Dadhich, P., B. Das, and S. Dhara. 2015. Microwave assisted rapid synthesis of N-methylene phosphonic chitosan via Mannich-type reaction. *Carbohydrate Polymers* 133: 345–352.

Dai, C., H. Kang, W. Yang, J. Sun, C. Liu, G. Cheng, G. Rong, X. Wang, X. Wang, and Z. Jin. 2015. O-2'-hydroxypropyltrimethyl ammonium chloride chitosan nanoparticles for the delivery of live Newcastle disease vaccine. *Carbohydrate Polymers* 130: 280–289.

Dai, Y.N., P. Li, J.P. Zhang, A.Q. Wang, and Q. Wei. 2008. A novel pH sensitive N-succinyl chitosan/alginate hydrogel bead for nifedipine delivery. *Biopharmaceutics & Drug Disposition* 29: 173–184.

Daly, W.H. and M.A. Manuszak-Guerrini. 2001. Biocidal chitosan derivatives for cosmetics and pharmaceuticals. US Patent 6,306,835, October 23, 2001.

Dang, J.M., D.D. Sun, Y. Shin-Ya, A.N. Sieber, J.P. Kostuik, and K.W. Leong. 2006. Temperature-responsive hydroxybutyl chitosan for the culture of mesenchymal stem cells and intervertebral disk cells. *Biomaterials* 27: 406–418.

d'Ayala, G.G., M. Malinconico, and P. Laurienzo. 2008. Marine derived polysaccharides for biomedical applications: Chemical modification approaches. *Molecules* 13: 2069–2106.

de Britto, D. and O.B. Assis. 2007. A novel method for obtaining a quaternary salt of chitosan. *Carbohydrate Polymers* 69: 305–310.

de Britto, D., L.A. Forato, and O.B. Assis. 2008. Determination of the average degree of quaternization of *N,N,N*-trimethylchitosan by solid state ^{13}C-NMR. *Carbohydrate Polymers* 74: 86–91.

Deans, J.R. and B.G. Dixon. 1992. Uptake of Pb^{2+} and Cu^{2+} by novel biopolymers. *Water Research* 26: 469–472.

Defaye, J., A. Gadelle, and C. Pedersen. 1994. A convenient access to β-(1 → 4)-linked 2-amino-2-deoxy-d-glucopyranosyl fluoride oligosaccharides and β-(1 → 4)-linked 2-amino-2-deoxy-d-glucopyranosyl oligosaccharides by fluorolysis and fluorohydrolysis of chitosan. *Carbohydrate Research* 261: 267–277.

Delben, F., R. Lapasin, and S. Pricl. 1990. Flow properties of N-(carboxymethyl) chitosan aqueous systems in the sol and gel domains. *International Journal of Biological Macromolecules* 12: 9–13.

de Oliveira Pedro, R., M. Takaki, T.C.C. Gorayeb, V.L.D. Bianchi, J.C. Thomeo, M.J. Tiera, and V.A. de Oliveira Tiera. 2013. Synthesis, characterization and antifungal activity of quaternary derivatives of chitosan on *Aspergillus flavus*. *Microbiological Research* 168: 50–55.

Desbrieres, J. 2004. Autoassociative natural polymer derivatives: The alkylchitosans. rheological behaviour and temperature stability. *Polymer* 45: 3285–3295.

Desbrieres, J., C. Martinez, and M. Rinaudo. 1996. Hydrophobic derivatives of chitosan: Characterization and rheological behaviour. *International Journal of Biological Macromolecules* 19: 21–28.

Dobetti, L. and F. Delben. 1992. Binding of metal cations by N-carboxymethyl chitosans in water. *Carbohydrate Polymers* 18: 273–282.

Domard, A. 1987. pH and cd measurements on a fully deacetylated chitosan: Application to Cu II—polymer interactions. *International Journal of Biological Macromolecules* 9: 98–104.

Domard, A. and N. Cartier. 1989. Glucosamine oligomers: 1. Preparation and characterization. *International Journal of Biological Macromolecules* 11: 297–302.

Domard, A., M. Rinaudo, and C. Terrassin. 1986. New method for the quaternization of chitosan. *International Journal of Biological Macromolecules* 8: 105–107.

Donati, I., S. Stredanska, G. Silvestrini, A. Vetere, P. Marcon, E. Marsich, P. Mozetic, A. Gamini, S. Paoletti, and F. Vittur. 2005. The aggregation of pig articular chondrocyte and synthesis of extracellular matrix by a lactose-modified chitosan. *Biomaterials* 26: 987–998.

Dong, Y., C. Xu, J. Wang, Y. Wu, Y. Ruan, and M. Wang. 2001. Influence of degree of N-butyrylation on critical concentration of N-butyrylated chitosan/dichloroacetic acid liquid crystalline solution. *Polymer Bulletin* 45: 495–500.

Drozd, N.N., A.I. Sher, V.A. Makarov, L.S. Galbraikh, G.A. Vikhoreva, and I.N. Gorbachiova. 2001. Comparison of antithrombin activity of the polysulphate chitosan derivatives in in vivo and in vitro system. *Thrombosis research* 102: 445–455.

Dumitriu, S. 1996. *Polysaccharides in Medicinal Applications*. Boca Raton, FL: CRC Press.

Dung, P.I., M. Milas, M. Rinaudo, and J. Desbrières. 1994. Water soluble derivatives obtained by controlled chemical modifications of chitosan. *Carbohydrate Polymers* 24: 209–214.

Dutta, P.K., J. Dutta, and V. Tripathi. 2004. Chitin and chitosan: Chemistry, properties and applications. *Journal of Scientific and Industrial Research* 63: 20–31.

Farah, S., O. Aviv, N. Laout, S. Ratner, N. Beyth, and A.J. Domb. 2015. Quaternary ammonium polyethylenimine nanoparticles for treating bacterial contaminated water. *Colloids and Surfaces B:Biointerfaces* 128: 614–619.

Feng, H., W. Xia, C. Shan, T. Zhou, W. Cai, and W. Zhang. 2015. Quaternized chitosan oligomers as novel elicitors inducing protection against B. cinerea in Arabidopsis. *International Journal of Biological Macromolecules* 72: 364–369.

Furusaki, E., Y. Ueno, N. Sakairi, N. Nishi, and S. Tokura. 1996. Facile preparation and inclusion ability of a chitosan derivative bearing carboxymethyl-β-cyclodextrin. *Carbohydrate Polymers* 29: 29–34.

Galed, G., B. Miralles, I. Paños, A. Santiago, and Á. Heras. 2005. N-Deacetylation and depolymerization reactions of chitin/chitosan: Influence of the source of chitin. *Carbohydrate Polymers* 62: 316–320.

Galhoum, A.A., M.G. Mahfouz, S.T. Abdel-Rehem, N.A. Gomaa, A.A. Atia, T. Vincent, and E. Guibal. 2015. Diethylenetriamine-functionalized chitosan magnetic nano-based particles for the sorption of rare earth metal ions [Nd (III), Dy (III) and Yb (III)]. *Cellulose* 22: 1–17.

Gamian, A., M. Chomik, C.A. Laferrière, and R. Roy. 1991. Inhibition of influenza A virus hemagglutinin and induction of interferon by synthetic sialylated glycoconjugates. *Canadian journal of microbiology* 37: 233–237.

Gamzazade, A., A. Sklyar, S. Nasibov, I. Sushkov, A. Shashkov, and Y. Knirel. 1997. Structural features of sulfated chitosans. *Carbohydrate Polymers* 34: 113–116.

Ge, H.C. and D.K. Luo. 2005. Preparation of carboxymethyl chitosan in aqueous solution under microwave irradiation. *Carbohydrate Research* 340: 1351–1356.

Gómez-Guillén, M., A. Gómez-Sánchez, and M.E. Martín-Zamora. 1992. A derivative of chitosan and 2, 4-pentanedione with strong chelating properties. *Carbohydrate Research* 233: 255–259.

Gorochovceva, N. and R. Makuška. 2004. Synthesis and study of water-soluble chitosan-O-poly (ethylene glycol) graft copolymers. *European Polymer Journal* 40: 685–691.

Guibal, E. 2004. Interactions of metal ions with chitosan-based sorbents: A review. *Separation and Purification Technology* 38: 43–74.

Guo, Z., R. Xing, S. Liu, Z. Zhong, X. Ji, L. Wang, and P. Li. 2007a. Antifungal properties of schiff bases of chitosan, N-substituted chitosan and quaternized chitosan. *Carbohydrate Research* 342: 1329–1332.

Guo, Z., R. Xing, S. Liu, Z. Zhong, X. Ji, L. Wang, and P. Li. 2007b. The influence of the cationic of quaternized chitosan on antifungal activity. *International Journal of Food Microbiology* 118: 214–217.

Hagiwara, K., Y. Kuribayashi, H. Iwai, I. Azuma, S. Tokura, K. Ikuta, and C. Ishihara. 1999. A sulfated chitin inhibits hemagglutination by theileria sergenti merozoites. *Carbohydrate Polymers* 39: 245–248.

Hall, L.D. and M. Yalpani. 1980a. Enhancement of the metal-chelating properties of chitin and chitosan. *Carbohydrate Research* 83: C5–C7.

Hall, L.D. and M. Yalpani. 1980b. Formation of branched-chain, soluble polysaccharides from chitosan. *Journal of the Chemical Society, Chemical Communications* 23: 1153–1154.

Han, B., Y. Wei, X. Jia, J. Xu, and G. Li. 2012. Correlation of the structure, properties, and antimicrobial activity of a soluble thiolated chitosan derivative. *Journal of Applied Polymer Science* 125: E143–E148.

Hasegawa, M., A. Isogai, and F. Onabe. 1993. Preparation of low-molecular-weight chitosan using phosphoric acid. *Carbohydrate Polymers* 20: 279–283.

Hashimoto, M., M. Morimoto, H. Saimoto, Y. Shigemasa, and T. Sato. 2006. Lactosylated chitosan for DNA delivery into hepatocytes: The effect of lactosylation on the physicochemical properties and intracellular trafficking of pDNA/chitosan complexes. *Bioconjugate chemistry* 17: 309–316.

Hayes, M., B. Carney, J. Slater, and W. Brück. 2008. Mining marine shellfish wastes for bioactive molecules: CHITIN and chitosan ndash; Part A: extraction methods. *Biotechnology Journal* 3: 871–877.

Heras, A., N. Rodriguez, V. Ramos, and E. Agullo. 2001. N-methylene phosphonic chitosan: A novel soluble derivative. *Carbohydrate Polymers* 44: 1–8.

Hirano, S. 1999. Chitin and chitosan as novel biotechnological materials. *Polymer International* 48: 732–734.

Hirano, S. and Y. Koide. 1978. Preparation of some novel N,O-acylchitosans. *Carbohydrate Research* 65: 166–168.

Hirano, S. and T. Moriyasu. 1981. N-(carboxyacyl) chitosans. *Carbohydrate Research* 92: 323–327.

Hirano, S. and T. Moriyasu. 2004. Some novel N-(carboxyacyl) chitosan filaments. *Carbohydrate Polymers* 55: 245–248.

Hirano, S. and Y. Ohe. 1975. A facile N-acylation of chitosan with carboylic anhydrides in acidic solutions. *Carbohydrate Research* 41: C1–C2.

Hirano, S., Y. Ohe, and H. Ono. 1976. Selective N-acylation of chitosan. *Carbohydrate Research* 47: 315–320.

Hirano, S., Y. Tanaka, M. Hasegawa, K. Tobetto, and A. Nishioka. 1985. Effect of sulfated derivatives of chitosan on some blood coagulant factors. *Carbohydrate Research* 137: 205–215.

Hirano, S., Y. Yamaguchi, and M. Kamiya. 2002. Novel N-saturated-fatty-acyl derivatives of chitosan soluble in water and in aqueous acid and alkaline solutions. *Carbohydrate Polymers* 48: 203–207.

Hirano, S., Y. Yamaguchi, and M. Kamiya. 2003. Water-Soluble N-(n-Fatty acyl) chitosans. *Macromolecular Bioscience* 3: 629–631.

Hirano, S., M. Zhang, B. Chung, and S. Kim. 2000. The N-acylation of chitosan fibre and the N-deacetylation of chitin fibre and chitin–cellulose blended fibre at a solid state. *Carbohydrate Polymers* 41: 175–179.

Holme, K.R. and L.D. Hall. 1991a. Chitosan derivatives bearing C_{10}-alkyl glycoside branches: A temperature-induced gelling polysaccharide. *Macromolecules* 24: 3828–3833.

Holme, K.R. and L.D. Hall. 1991b. Novel metal chelating chitosan derivative: Attachment of iminodiacetate moieties via a hydrophilic spacer group. *Canadian Journal of Chemistry* 69: 585–589.

Holme, K.R. and L.D. Hall. 1992. Preparation and characterization of N-[2-(glycosyloxy)-ethyl] chitosan derivatives. *Carbohydrate Research* 225: 291–306.

Holme, K.R. and A.S. Perlin. 1997. Chitosan N-sulfate. A water-soluble polyelectrolyte. *Carbohydrate Research* 302: 7–12.

Hon, D.N.S. and L.G. Tang. 2000. Chelation of chitosan derivatives with zinc ions. I. O,N-Carboxymethyl chitosan. *Journal of Applied Polymer Science* 77: 2246–2253.

Hornof, M.D., C.E. Kast, and A. Bernkop-Schnürch. 2003. In vitro evaluation of the viscoelastic properties of chitosan–thioglycolic acid conjugates. *European Journal of Pharmaceutics and Biopharmaceutics* 55: 185–190.

Hsien, T.Y. and G.L. Rorrer. 1997. Heterogeneous cross-linking of chitosan gel beads: Kinetics, modeling, and influence on cadmium ion adsorption capacity. *Industrial & Engineering Chemistry Research* 36: 3631–3638.

Huang, J., H. Jiang, M. Qiu, X. Geng, R. Yang, J. Li, and C. Zhang. 2013. Antibacterial activity evaluation of quaternary chitin against *Escherichia coli* and *Staphylococcus aureus*. *International Journal of Biological Macromolecules* 52: 85–91.

Huang, R., Y. Du, L. Zheng, H. Liu, and L. Fan. 2004. A new approach to chemically modified chitosan sulfates and study of their influences on the inhibition of *Escherichia coli* and *Staphylococcus aureus* growth. *Reactive and Functional Polymers* 59: 41–51.

Hudson, S. and C. Smith. 1998. Polysaccharides: Chitin and chitosan: Chemistry and technology of their use as structural materials biopolymers from renewable resources. In *Biopolymers from Renewable Resources*, D.L. Kaplan (ed.). Berlin, Germany: Springer, pp. 96–118.

Il'Ina, A.V. and V.P. Varlamov. 2004. Hydrolysis of chitosan in lactic acid. *Applied Biochemistry and Microbiology* 40: 300–303.

Ilium, L. 1998. Chitosan and its use as a pharmaceutical excipient. *Pharmaceutical Research* 15: 1326–1331.

Inoue, K., Y. Baba, and K. Yoshizuka. 1993. Adsorption of metal ions on chitosan and crosslinked copper (II)-complexed chitosan. *Bulletin of the Chemical Society of Japan* 66: 2915–2921.

Inui, H., M. Tsujikubo, and S. Hirano. 1995. Low molecular weight chitosan stimulation of mitogenic response to platelet-derived growth factor in vascular smooth muscle cells. *Bioscience, Biotechnology, and Biochemistry* 59: 2111–2114.

Inui, K., K. Tsukamoto, T. Miyata, and T. Uragami. 1998. Permeation and separation of a benzene/cyclohexane mixture through benzoylchitosan membranes. *Journal of Membrane Science* 138: 67–75.

Izume, M. 1998. The application of chitin and chitosan to cosmetics. *Chitin and Chitosan Research* 4: 12–17.

Izume, M. and A. Ohtakara. 1987. Preparation of D-glucosamine oligosaccharides by the enzymatic hydrolysis of chitosan. *Agricultural and Biological Chemistry* 51: 1189–1191.

Janes, K. and M. Alonso. 2003. Depolymerized chitosan nanoparticles for protein delivery: Preparation and characterization. *Journal of Applied Polymer Science* 88: 2769–2776.

Jayakumar, R., T. Egawa, T. Furuike, S. Nair, and H. Tamura. 2009. Synthesis, characterization, and thermal properties of phosphorylated chitin for biomedical applications. *Polymer Engineering & Science* 49: 844–849.

Jayakumar, R., H. Nagahama, T. Furuike, and H. Tamura. 2008a. Synthesis of phosphorylated chitosan by novel method and its characterization. *International Journal of Biological Macromolecules* 42: 335–339.

Jayakumar, R., N. Nwe, S. Tokura, and H. Tamura. 2007. Sulfated chitin and chitosan as novel biomaterials. *International Journal of Biological Macromolecules* 40: 175–181.

Jayakumar, R., M. Prabaharan, S.V. Nair, and H. Tamura. 2010. Novel chitin and chitosan nanofibers in biomedical applications. *Biotechnology Advances* 28: 142–150.

Jayakumar, R., M. Prabaharan, R.L. Reis, and J. Mano. 2005. Graft copolymerized chitosan—present status and applications. *Carbohydrate Polymers* 62: 142–158.

Jayakumar, R., R. Reis, and J. Mano. 2006. Chemistry and applications of phosphorylated chitin and chitosan. *e-Polymers* 6: 447–462.

Jayakumar, R., N. Selvamurugan, S. Nair, S. Tokura, and H. Tamura. 2008b. Preparative methods of phosphorylated chitin and chitosan-An overview. *International Journal of Biological Macromolecules* 43: 221–225.

Je, J.Y., P.J. Park, and S.K. Kim. 2005. Prolyl endopeptidase inhibitory activity of chitosan sulfates with different degree of deacetylation. *Carbohydrate Polymers* 60: 553–556.

Jeon, Y.J. and S.K. Kim. 2000. Continuous production of chitooligosaccharides using a dual reactor system. *Process Biochemistry* 35: 623–632.

Ješelnik, M. and E. Žagar. 2014. N-functionalization of chitosan with bis-O-glycosylated derivative of 2,2-bis (methylol) propionic acid. *Cellulose* 21: 4145–4156.

Jia, Z. and D. Shen. 2002. Effect of reaction temperature and reaction time on the preparation of low-molecular-weight chitosan using phosphoric acid. *Carbohydrate Polymers* 49: 393–396.

Jia, Z. and W. Xu. 2001. Synthesis and antibacterial activities of quaternary ammonium salt of chitosan. *Carbohydrate Research* 333: 1–6.

Jimtaisong, A. and N. Saewan. 2014. Utilization of carboxymethyl chitosan in cosmetics. *International Journal of Cosmetic Science* 36: 12–21.

Jung, B.O., C.H. Kim, K.S. Choi, Y.M. Lee, and J.J. Kim. 1999. Preparation of amphiphilic chitosan and their antimicrobial activities. *Journal of Applied Polymer Science* 72: 1713–1719.

Kafedjiiski, K., F. Föger, M. Werle, and A. Bernkop-Schnürch. 2005. Synthesis and in vitro evaluation of a novel chitosan–glutathione conjugate. *Pharmaceutical Research* 22: 1480–1488.

Kaifu, K., N. Nishi, T. Komai, S. Tokura, and O. Somorin. 1981. Studies on chitin. V. Formylation, propionylation, and butyrylation of chitin. *Polymer Journal* 13: 241–245.

Kast, C.E. and A. Bernkop-Schnürch. 2001. Thiolated polymers-thiomers: Development and in vitro evaluation of chitosan–thioglycolic acid conjugates. *Biomaterials* 22: 2345–2352.

Kast, C.E. and A. Bernkop-Schnürch. 2002. Polymer–cysteamine conjugates: New mucoadhesive excipients for drug delivery. *International Journal of Pharmaceutics* 234: 91–99.

Kato, Y., H. Onishi, and Y. Machida. 2001a. Biological characteristics of lactosaminated N-succinyl-chitosan as a liver-specific drug carrier in mice. *Journal of Controlled Release* 70: 295–307.

Kato, Y., H. Onishi, and Y. Machida. 2001b. Lactosaminated and intact N-succinyl-chitosans as drug carriers in liver metastasis. *International Journal of Pharmaceutics* 226: 93–106.

Kato, Y., H. Onishi, and Y. Machida. 2002. Depolymerization of N-succinyl-chitosan by hydrochloric acid. *Carbohydrate Research* 337: 561–564.

Kato, Y., H. Onishi, and Y. Machida. 2004. N-succinyl-chitosan as a drug carrier: Water-insoluble and water-soluble conjugates. *Biomaterials* 25: 907–915.

Kenawy, E.R., F.I. Abdel-Hay, M.M. Eldin, T. Tamer, and E.M. Abo-Elghit. 2015. Novel aminated chitosan-aromatic aldehydes schiff bases: Synthesis, characterization and bio-evaluation. *International JournalofAdvanced Research* 3: 563–572.

Khalil, E.S., B. Saad, E.S.M. Negim, and M.I. Saleh. 2015. Novel water-soluble chitosan derivative prepared by graft polymerization of dicyandiamide: Synthesis, characterisation, and its antibacterial property. *Journal of Polymer Research* 22: 1–12.

Kim, C.H., J.W. Choi, H.J. Chun, and K.S. Choi. 1997. Synthesis of chitosan derivatives with quaternary ammonium salt and their antibacterial activity. *Polymer Bulletin* 38: 387–393.

Kim, C.H. and K.S. Choi. 1998. Synthesis and properties of carboxyalkyl chitosan derivatives. *Journal of Industrial and Engineering Chemistry* 4: 19–25.

Kim, C.H. and K.S. Choi. 2002. Synthesis and antibacterial activity of quaternized chitosan derivatives having different methylene spacers. *Journal of Industrial and Engineering Chemistry* 8: 71–76.

Kim, I.Y., S.J. Seo, H.S. Moon, M.K. Yoo, I.Y. Park, B.C. Kim, and C.S. Cho. 2008. Chitosan and its derivatives for tissue engineering applications. *Biotechnology Advances* 26: 1–21.

Kim, J.H., Y.S. Kim, S. Kim, J.H. Park, K. Kim, K. Choi, H. Chung, S.Y. Jeong, R.W. Park, and I.S. Kim. 2006. Hydrophobically modified glycol chitosan nanoparticles as carriers for paclitaxel. *Journal of Controlled Release* 111: 228–234.

Kim, S.K. 2010. *Chitin, Chitosan, Oligosaccharides and Their Derivatives: Biological Activities and Applications.* Boca Raton, FL: CRC Press.

Kim, S.K. and E. Mendis. 2006. Bioactive compounds from marine processing byproducts—a review. *Food Research International* 39: 383–393.

Kim, S.K. and N. Rajapakse. 2005. Enzymatic production and biological activities of chitosan oligosaccharides (COS): A review. *Carbohydrate Polymers* 62: 357–368.

Kim, S.Y., D.H. Shon, and K.H. Lee. 1998. Purification and characteristics of two types of chitosanases from *Aspergillus fumigatus* KH-94. *Journal of Microbiology and Biotechnology* 8: 568–574.

Kittur, F., K.H. Prashanth, K.U. Sankar, and R. Tharanathan. 2002. Characterization of chitin, chitosan and their carboxymethyl derivatives by differential scanning calorimetry. *Carbohydrate Polymers* 49: 185–193.

Knaul, J.Z. and K.A. Creber. 1997. Coagulation rate studies of spinnable chitosan solutions. *Journal of Applied Polymer Science* 66: 117–127.

Kubota, N. and Y. Eguchi. 1997. Facile preparation of water-soluble N-acetylated chitosan and molecular weight dependence of its water-solubility. *Polymer Journal* 29: 123–127.

Kubota, N., N. Tatsumoto, T. Sano, and K. Toya. 2000. A simple preparation of half N-acetylated chitosan highly soluble in water and aqueous organic solvents. *Carbohydrate Research* 324: 268–274.

Kumar, A.V. and R. Tharanathan. 2004. A comparative study on depolymerization of chitosan by proteolytic enzymes. *Carbohydrate Polymers* 58: 275–283.

Kumar, M.N.V.R., R.A. Muzzarelli, C. Muzzarelli, H. Sashiwa, and A.J. Domb. 2004. Chitosan chemistry and pharmaceutical perspectives. *Chemical Reviews* 104: 6017–6084.

Kurita, K. 1986. Chemical modifications of chitin and chitosan. In *Chitin in Nature and Technology*, R.A.A. Muzzarelli, C. Jeuniaux, G.W. Gooday (eds.). Boston, MA: Springer, pp. 287–293.

Kurita, K. 1998. Chemistry and application of chitin and chitosan. *Polymer Degradation and Stability* 59: 117–120.

Kurita, K., H. Akao, M. Kobayashi, T. Mori, and Y. Nishiyama. 1997a. Regioselective introduction of β-galactoside branches into chitosan and chitin. *Polymer Bulletin* 39: 543–549.

Kurita, K., H. Akao, J. Yang, and M. Shimojoh. 2003. Nonnatural branched polysaccharides: Synthesis and properties of chitin and chitosan having disaccharide maltose branches. *Biomacromolecules* 4: 1264–1268.

Kurita, K., H. Ichikawa, S. Ishizeki, H. Fujisaki, and Y. Iwakura. 1982. Studies on chitin, 8. Modification reaction of chitin in highly swollen state with aromatic cyclic carboxylic acid anhydrides. *Die Makromolekulare Chemie* 183: 1161–1169.

Kurita, K., H. Ikeda, Y. Yoshida, M. Shimojoh, and M. Harata. 2002. Chemoselective protection of the amino groups of chitosan by controlled phthaloylation: Facile preparation of a precursor useful for chemical modifications. *Biomacromolecules* 3: 1–4.

Kurita, K., S. Inoue, and Y. Koyama. 1989a. Studies on chitin. XVIII: Preparation of diethyl-aminoethyl-Chitins. *Polymer Bulletin* 21: 13–17.

Kurita, K., Y. Koyama, S. Inoue, and S. Nishimura. 1990. ((Diethylamino) ethyl) chitins: Preparation and properties of novel aminated chitin derivatives. *Macromolecules* 23: 2865–2869.

Kurita, K., Y. Koyama, S.I. Nishimura, and M. Kamiya. 1989b. Facile preparation of water-soluble chitin from chitosan. *Chemistry Letters* 1597–1598.

Kurita, K., T. Sannan, and Y. Iwakura. 1979. Studies on chitin. VI. Binding of metal cations. *Journal of Applied Polymer Science* 23: 511–515.

Kurita, K., K. Shimada, Y. Nishiyama, M. Shimojoh, and S.I. Nishimura. 1998. Nonnatural branched polysaccharides: Synthesis and properties of chitin and chitosan having α-mannoside branches. *Macromolecules* 31: 4764–4769.

Kurita, K., K. Tomita, T. Tada, S. Ishii, S.I. Nishimura, and K. Shimoda. 1993a. Squid chitin as a potential alternative chitin source: Deacetylation behavior and characteristic properties. *Journal of Polymer Science Part A: Polymer Chemistry* 31: 485–491.

Kurita, K., M. Uno, Y. Saito, and Y. Nishiyama. 2000. Regioselectivity in protection of chitosan with the phthaloyl group. *Chitin and Chitosan Research* 6: 43–50.

Kurita, K., H. Yoshino, S.I. Nishimura, and S. Ishii. 1993b. Preparation and biodegradability of chitin derivatives having mercapto groups. *Carbohydrate Polymers* 20: 239–245.

Kurita, K., H. Yoshino, S.I. Nishimura, S. Ishii, T. Mori, and Y. Nishiyama. 1997b. Mercapto-chitins: A new type of supports for effective immobilization of acid phosphatase. *Carbohydrate Polymers* 32: 171–175.

Kuroiwa, T., S. Ichikawa, O. Hiruta, S. Sato, and S. Mukataka. 2002. Factors affecting the composition of oligosaccharides produced in chitosan hydrolysis using immobilized chitosanases. *Biotechnology Progress* 18: 969–974.

Kuroyanagi, Y., A. Shiraishi, Y. Shirasaki, N. Nakakita, Y. Yasutomi, Y. Takano, and N. Shioya. 1994. Development of a new wound dressing with antimicrobial delivery capability. *Wound Repair and Regeneration* 2: 122–129.

Kyzas, G.Z. and D.N. Bikiaris. 2015. Recent modifications of chitosan for adsorption applications: A critical and systematic review. *Marine Drugs* 13: 312–337.

Kyzas, G.Z., M. Kostoglou, and N.K. Lazaridis. 2009. Copper and chromium (VI) removal by chitosan derivatives—equilibrium and kinetic studies. *Chemical Engineering Journal* 152: 440–448.

Lang, G., G. Maresch, and S. Birkel. 1997. Hydroxyalkyl chitosans. In *Chitin Handbook*, R.A.A. Muzzarelli, M.G. Peter (eds.). Grottammare, Italy: European Chitin Society, pp. 61–66.

Lang, G., G. Maresch, and H.R. Lenz. 1990a. O-benzyl-N-hydroxyalkyl derivatives of chitosan and nail polish containing the same. US8680074 B2, July 11, 1988.

Lang, G., G. Maresch, H. Wendel, E. Konrad, H.R. Lenz, and J. Titze.1988. Cosmetic compositions based upon N-hydroxypropyl-chitosans, new N-hyroxypropyl-chitosans, as well as processes for the production thereof. US4780310 A, November 21, 1986.

Lang, G. and H. Wendel. 1990. Macromolecular, surface-active, quaternary, N-substituted chitosan derivatives as well as cosmetic composition based on these new chitosan derivatives. US4976952 A, March 10, 1988.

Lang, G., H. Wendel, and E. Konrad. 1990b. Process for making quaternary chitosan derivatives for cosmetic agents. US4921949, March 8, 1989.

Laus, R., T.G. Costa, B. Szpoganicz, and V.T. Fávere. 2010. Adsorption and desorption of Cu (II), Cd (II) and Pb (II) ions using chitosan crosslinked with epichlorohydrin-triphosphate as the adsorbent. *Journal of Hazardous Materials* 183: 233–241.

Lebouc, F., I. Dez, and P.J. Madec. 2005. NMR study of the phosphonomethylation reaction on chitosan. *Polymer* 46: 319–325.

Lee, E.S., K.H. Park, I.S. Park, and K. Na. 2007. Glycol chitosan as a stabilizer for protein encapsulated into poly (lactide-co-glycolide) microparticle. *International Journal of Pharmaceutics* 338: 310–316.

Lee, Y.M., Y.J. Park, S.J. Lee, Y. Ku, S.B. Han, P.R. Klokkevold, S.M. Choi, and C.P. Chung. 2000. Tissue engineered bone formation using chitosan/tricalcium phosphate sponges. *Journal of Periodontology* 71: 410–417.

Leitner, V.M., G.F. Walker, and A. Bernkop-Schnürch. 2003. Thiolated polymers: Evidence for the formation of disulphide bonds with mucus glycoproteins. *European Journal of Pharmaceutics and Biopharmaceutics* 56: 207–214.

Le Tien, C., M. Lacroix, P. Ispas-Szabo, and M.-A. Mateescu. 2003. N-acylated chitosan: Hydrophobic matrices for controlled drug release. *Journal of Controlled Release* 93: 1–13.

Li, C., J. Hou, J. Gu, Q. Han, Y. Guan, and Y. Zhang. 2015. Synthesis and thermal gelation of hydroxypropyl chitin. *RSC Advances* 5: 39677–39685.

Li, L., X.Y. Xu, and J.P. Zhou. 2007. Preparation and characterization of N-octyl-N'-succinyl chitosan micelles. *Chinese New Drugs Journal* 16: 543.

Li, P., Y.F. Poon, W. Li, H.Y. Zhu, S.H. Yeap, Y. Cao, X. Qi, C. Zhou, M. Lamrani, and R.W. Beuerman. 2011. A polycationic antimicrobial and biocompatible hydrogel with microbe membrane suctioning ability. *Nature Materials* 10: 149–156.

Li, S.D., P.W. Li, Z.M. Yang, Z. Peng, W.Y. Quan, X.H. Yang, L. Yang, and J.J. Dong. 2014. Synthesis and characterization of chitosan quaternary ammonium salt and its application as drug carrier for ribavirin. *Drug Delivery* 21: 548–552.

Li, X., M. Morimoto, H. Sashiwa, H. Saimoto, Y. Okamoto, S. Minami, and Y. Shigemasa. 1999. Synthesis of chitosan–sugar hybrid and evaluation of its bioactivity. *Polymers for Advanced Technologies* 10: 455–458.

Li, X., Y. Tushima, M. Morimoto, H. Saimoto, Y. Okamoto, S. Minami, and Y. Shigemasa. 2000. Biological activity of chitosan–sugar hybrids: Specific interaction with lectin. *Polymers for Advanced Technologies* 11: 176–179.

Lillo, L.E. and B. Matsuhiro. 1997. Chemical modifications of carboxylated chitosan. *Carbohydrate Polymers* 34: 397–401.

Lim, S.H. and S.M. Hudson. 2004. Synthesis and antimicrobial activity of a water-soluble chitosan derivative with a fiber-reactive group. *Carbohydrate Research* 339: 313–319.

Lin, J., Y.M. Wu, and Y.H. Lu. 2014. Study on reactive dye wastewater treatment with quaternary chitosan. In *Advanced Materials Research*, J. Zeng, L. Jiahao, and Z. Hongxi (eds.). Zurich, Switzerland: Trans Tech Publications, pp. 525–528.

Lin, Y., Q. Chen, and H. Luo. 2007. Preparation and characterization of N-(2-carboxybenzyl) chitosan as a potential pH-sensitive hydrogel for drug delivery. *Carbohydrate Research* 342: 87–95.

Lin, Y.H., H.F. Liang, C.K. Chung, M.C. Chen, and H.W. Sung. 2005. Physically crosslinked alginate/N, O-carboxymethyl chitosan hydrogels with calcium for oral delivery of protein drugs. *Biomaterials* 26: 2105–2113.

Liu, L., Y. Li, Y. Li, and Y.E. Fang. 2004. Rapid N-phthaloylation of chitosan by microwave irradiation. *Carbohydrate Polymers* 57: 97–100.

Liu, Y., G. Chen, and K.A. Hu. 2003. Synthesis, characterization and structural analysis of polylactide grafted onto water-soluble hydroxypropyl chitin as backbone. *Journal of Materials Science letters* 22: 1303–1305.

Liu, X.F., Y.L. Guan, D.Z. Yang, Z. Li, and K. De Yao. 2001. Antibacterial action of chitosan and carboxymethylated chitosan. *Journal of Applied Polymer Science* 79: 1324–1335.

Loubaki, E., M. Ourevitch, and S. Sicsic. 1991. Chemical modification of chitosan by glycidyl trimethylammonium chloride. Characterization of modified chitosan by ^{13}C-and ^{1}H-NMR spectroscopy. *European Polymer Journal* 27: 311–317.

Ma, G., D. Yang, J.F. Kennedy, and J. Nie. 2009. Synthesize and characterization of organic-soluble acylated chitosan. *Carbohydrate Polymers* 75: 390–394.

Mao, S., X. Shuai, F. Unger, M. Simon, D. Bi, and T. Kissel. 2004. The depolymerization of chitosan: Effects on physicochemical and biological properties. *International Journal of Pharmaceutics* 281: 45–54.

Maresh, G., T. Clausen, and G. Lang. 1989. Hydroxypropylation of chitosan. In *Chitin and Chitosan*, G. Skjak-Braek, T. Anthonsen, P. Sanford (eds.). New York: Elsevier Science Publishing Co, pp. 389–395.

Martins, A.F., S.P. Facchi, H.D. Follmann, A.G. Pereira, A.F. Rubira, and E.C. Muniz. 2014. Antimicrobial activity of chitosan derivatives containing N-quaternized moieties in its backbone: A review. *International Journal of Molecular Sciences* 15: 20800–20832.

Mawad, D., C. Warren, M. Barton, D. Mahns, J. Morley, B.T. Pham, N.T. Pham, S. Kueh, and A. Lauto. 2015. Lysozyme depolymerization of photo-activated chitosan adhesive films. *Carbohydrate Polymers* 121: 56–63.

McCormick, C. and D.K. Lichatowich. 1979. Homogeneous solution reactions of cellulose, chitin, and other polysaccharides to produce controlled activity pesticide systems. *Journal of Polymer Science: Polymer Letters Edition* 17: 479–484.

Meng, S., Z. Liu, W. Zhong, Q. Wang, and Q. Du. 2007. Phosphorylcholine modified chitosan: Appetent and safe material for cells. *Carbohydrate Polymers* 70: 82–88.

Miretzky, P. and A.F. Cirelli. 2009. Hg (II) removal from water by chitosan and chitosan derivatives: A review. *Journal of Hazardous Materials* 167: 10–23.

Mitani, T., N. Fukumuro, C. Yoshimoto, and H. Ishii. 1991. Effects of counter ions (SO_4^{2-} and Cl$^-$) on the adsorption of copper and nickel ions by swollen chitosan beads. *Agricultural and Biological Chemistry* 55: 2419–2419.

Moedritzer, K. and R.R. Irani. 1966. The direct synthesis of α-aminomethylphosphonic acids. Mannich-type reactions with orthophosphorous acid. *The Journal of Organic Chemistry* 31: 1603–1607.

Mohamed, N.A., M.W. Sabaa, A.H. El-Ghandour, M.M. Abdel-Aziz, and O.F. Abdel-Gawad. 2013. Quaternized N-substituted carboxymethyl chitosan derivatives as antimicrobial agents. *International Journal of Biological Macromolecules* 60: 156–164.

Monier, M., D. Ayad, Y. Wei, and A. Sarhan. 2010. Adsorption of Cu (II), Co (II), and Ni (II) ions by modified magnetic chitosan chelating resin. *Journal of Hazardous Materials* 177: 962–970.

Moore, G.K. and G.A. Roberts. 1980a. Chitosan gels: 1. Study of reaction variables. *International Journal of Biological Macromolecules* 2: 73–77.

Moore, G.K. and G.A. Roberts. 1980b. Chitosan gels: 2. Mechanism of gelation. *International Journal of Biological Macromolecules* 2: 78–80.

Moore, G.K. and G.A. Roberts. 1982. Reactions of chitosan: 4. Preparation of organosoluble derivatives of chitosan. *International Journal of Biological Macromolecules* 4: 246–249.

Morimoto, M., H. Saimoto, H. Usui, Y. Okamoto, S. Minami, and Y. Shigemasa. 2001. Biological activities of carbohydrate-branched chitosan derivatives. *Biomacromolecules* 2: 1133–1136.

Mourya, V.K. and N.N. Inamdar. 2008. Chitosan-modifications and applications: Opportunities galore. *Reactive and Functional Polymers* 68: 1013–1051.

Mourya, V.K. and N.N. Inamdar. 2009. Trimethyl chitosan and its applications in drug delivery. *Journal of Materials Science: Materials in Medicine* 20: 1057–1079.

Mourya, V.K., N.N. Inamdar, and A. Tiwari. 2010. Carboxymethyl chitosan and its applications. *Advanced Materials Letters* 1: 11–33.

Muñoz-Bonilla, A. and M. Fernández-García. 2012. Polymeric materials with antimicrobial activity. *Progress in Polymer Science* 37: 281–339.

Muzzarelli, R.A.A. 1973. *Natural Chelating Polymers; Alginic Acid, Chitin and Chitosan.* New York: Pergamon Press.

Muzzarelli, R.A.A. 1977. *Chitin.* Oxford: Pergamon Press.

Muzzarelli, R.A.A. 1983. Chitin and its derivatives: New trends of applied research. *Carbohydrate Polymers* 3: 53–75.

Muzzarelli, R.A.A. 1988. Carboxymethylated chitins and chitosans. *Carbohydrate Polymers* 8: 1–21.

Muzzarelli, R.A.A., N. Frega, M. Miliani, C. Muzzarelli, and M. Cartolari. 2000. Interactions of chitin, chitosan, N-lauryl chitosan and N-dimethylaminopropyl chitosan with olive oil. *Carbohydrate Polymers* 43: 263–268.

Muzzarelli, R.A.A., P. Ilari, and M. Petrarulo. 1994a. Solubility and structure of N-carboxymethylchitosan. *International Journal of Biological Macromolecules* 16: 177–180.

Muzzarelli, R.A.A., C. Jeuniaux, and G.W. Gooday. 1986a. *Chitin in Nature and Technology.* Boston, MA: Springer.

Muzzarelli, R.A.A., C. Muzzarelli, and M. Terbojevich. 1997. Chitin chemistry, upgrading a renewable resource. *Carbohydrates in Europe* 19: 10–17.

Muzzarelli, R.A.A. and F. Tanfani. 1982. N-(o-carboxybenzyl) chitosan, N-carboxymethyl chitosan and dithiocarbamate chitosan: New chelating derivatives of chitosan. *Pure and Applied Chemistry* 54: 2141–2150.

Muzzarelli, R.A.A., F. Tanfani, M. Emanuelli, E. Chiurazzi, and M. Piani. 1986b. Sulfated N-carboxymethyl chitosans as blood anticoagulants. In *Chitin in Nature and Technology*, R.A.A. Muzzarelli, C. Jeuniaux, G.W. Gooday (eds.). Boston, MA: Springer, pp. 469–476.

Muzzarelli, R.A.A., F. Tanfani, M. Emanuelli, and S. Mariotti. 1982a. N-(carboxymethylidene) chitosans and N-(carboxymethyl) chitosans: Novel chelating polyampholytes obtained from chitosan glyoxylate. *Carbohydrate Research* 107: 199–214.

Muzzarelli, R.A.A., F. Tanfani, M. Emanuelli, D.P. Pace, E. Chiurazzi, and M. Piani. 1984. Sulfated N-(Carboxymethyl) chitosans: Novel blood anticoagulants. *Carbohydrate Research* 126: 225–231.

Muzzarelli, R.A.A., F. Tanfani, S. Mariotti, and M. Emanuelli. 1982b. N-(o-carboxybenzyl) chitosans: Novel chelating polyampholytes. *Carbohydrate Polymers* 2: 145–157.

Muzzarelli, R.A.A., M. Tomasetti, and P. Ilari. 1994b. Deploymerization of chitosan with the aid of papain. *Enzyme and Microbial Technology* 16: 110–114.

Muzzarelli, R.A.A. and O. Tubertini. 1969. Chitin and chitosan as chromatographic supports and adsorbents for collection of metal ions from organic and aqueous solutions and sea-water. *Talanta* 16: 1571–1577.

Muzzarelli, R.A.A., W. Xia, M. Tomasetti, and P. Ilari. 1995. Depolymerization of chitosan and substituted chitosans with the aid of a wheat germ lipase preparation. *Enzyme and Microbial Technology* 17: 541–545.

Nagasawa, K., Y. Tohira, Y. Inoue, and N. Tanoura. 1971. Reaction between carbohydrates and sulfuric acid: Part I. Depolymerization and sulfation of polysaccharides by sulfuric acid. *Carbohydrate Research* 18: 95–102.

Naggi, A.M., G. Torri, T. Compagnoni, and B. Casu.1986. Synthesis and physico-chemical properties of the polyampholyte chitosan 6-sulfate. In *Chitin in Nature and Technology*, R.A.A. Muzzarelli, C. Jeuniaux, G.W. Gooday (eds.). Boston, MA: Springer, pp. 371–377.

Narayanan, D., R. Jayakumar, and K. Chennazhi. 2014. Versatile carboxymethyl chitin and chitosan nanomaterials: A review. *Wiley Interdisciplinary Reviews: Nanomedicine and Nanobiotechnology* 6: 574–598.

Ngah, W.W., C. Endud, and R. Mayanar. 2002. Removal of copper (II) ions from aqueous solution onto chitosan and cross-linked chitosan beads. *Reactive and Functional Polymers* 50: 181–190.

Ngah, W.W., L. Teong, and M. Hanafiah. 2011. Adsorption of dyes and heavy metal ions by chitosan composites: A review. *Carbohydrate Polymers* 83: 1446–1456.

Nishi, N. 1986. Preparation and characterization of phosphorylated chitin and chitosan. In *Chitin in Nature and Technology*, R.A.A. Muzzarelli, C. Jeuniaux, G.W. Gooday (eds.). New York: Plenum Press, pp. 297–299.

Nishi, N., A. Ebina, S.I. Nishimura, A. Tsutsumi, O. Hasegawa, and S. Tokura. 1986. Highly phosphorylated derivatives of chitin, partially deacetylated chitin and chitosan as new functional polymers: Preparation and characterization. *International Journal of Biological Macromolecules* 8: 311–317.

Nishi, N., Y. Maekita, S.I. Nishimura, O. Hasegawa, and S. Tokura. 1987. Highly phosphorylated derivatives of chitin, partially deacetylated chitin and chitosan as new functional polymers: Metal binding property of the insolubilized materials. *International Journal of Biological Macromolecules* 9: 109–114.

Nishi, N., S.I. Nishimura, A. Ebina, A. Tsutsumi, and S. Tokura. 1984. Preparation and characterization of water-soluble chitin phosphate. *International Journal of Biological Macromolecules* 6: 53–54.

Nishimura, K., S. Nishimura, N. Nishi, S. Tokura, and I. Azuma. 1986. Immunological activity of chitin derivatives. In *Chitin in Nature and Technology*, R.A.A. Muzzarelli, C. Jeuniaux, G.W. Gooday (eds.). Boston, MA: Springer, pp. 477–483.

Nishimura, S., O. Kohgo, K. Kurita, and H. Kuzuhara. 1991. Chemospecific manipulations of a rigid polysaccharide: Syntheses of novel chitosan derivatives with excellent solubility in common organic solvents by regioselective chemical modifications. *Macromolecules* 24: 4745–4748.

Nishimura, S.I., H. Kai, K. Shinada, T. Yoshida, S. Tokura, K. Kurita, H. Nakashima, N. Yamamoto, and T. Uryu. 1998. Regioselective syntheses of sulfated polysaccharides: Specific anti-HIV-1 activity of novel chitin sulfates. *Carbohydrate Research* 306: 427–433.

Nishimura, S.I., O. Kohgo, K. Kurita, C. Vittavatvong, and H. Kuzuhara. 1990. Synthesis of novel chitosan derivatives soluble in organic solvents by regioselective chemical modifications. *Chemistry Letters* 2: 243–246.

No, H.K. and S.P. Meyers. 1995. Preparation and characterization of chitin and chitosan-a review. *Journal of Aquatic Food Product Technology* 4: 27–52.

Ogawa, K., K. Oka, and T. Yui. 1993. X-ray study of chitosan-transition metal complexes. *Chemistry of Materials* 5: 726–728.

Ohga, K., H. Oyama, and Y. Muta. 1991. Chromatographic optical resolution on phenylcarbamates of N-arylidenechitosans. *Analytical Sciences* 7: 653–656.

Olteanu, M., I. Mandru, M. Dudau, S. Peretz, and O. Cinteza. 2003. The aqueous liquid/liquid interphases formed by chitosan-anionic surfactant complexes aqueous polymer-cosolute systems. In *Progress in Colloid & Polymer Science*, Vol. 122, D.F. Anghel (ed.). Berlin, Germany: Springer, pp. 87–94.

Omari, K.W., J.E. Besaw, and F.M. Kerton. 2012. Hydrolysis of chitosan to yield levulinic acid and 5-hydroxymethylfurfural in water under microwave irradiation. *Green Chemistry* 14: 1480–1487.

Onishi, H., H. Takahashi, M. Yoshiyasu, and Y. Machida. 2001. Preparation and in vitro properties of N-succinylchitosan–or carboxymethylchitin–mitomycin C conjugate microparticles with specified size. *Drug Development and Industrial Pharmacy* 27: 659–667.

Oshita, K., Y.H. Gao, M. Oshima, and S. Motomizu. 2001. Adsorption behavior of mercury in aqueous solution on cross-linked chitosan. *Analytical Sciences/Supplements* 17: a317–a320.

Park, I.K. and Y.H. Park. 2001. Preparation and structural characterization of water-soluble O-hydroxypropyl chitin derivatives. *Journal of Applied Polymer Science* 80: 2624–2632.

Park, J.H., Y.W. Cho, H. Chung, I.C. Kwon, and S.Y. Jeong. 2003. Synthesis and characterization of sugar-bearing chitosan derivatives: Aqueous solubility and biodegradability. *Biomacromolecules* 4: 1087–1091.

Park, J.H., S. Kwon, M. Lee, H. Chung, J.H. Kim, Y.S. Kim, R.W. Park, I.S. Kim, S.B. Seo, and I.C. Kwon. 2006. Self-assembled nanoparticles based on glycol chitosan bearing hydrophobic moieties as carriers for doxorubicin: In vivo biodistribution and anti-tumor activity. *Biomaterials* 27: 119–126.

Patrulea, V., L.A. Applegate, V. Ostafe, O. Jordan, and G. Borchard. 2015. Optimized synthesis of O-carboxymethyl-N,N,N-trimethyl chitosan. *Carbohydrate Polymers* 122: 46–52.

Peng, Y., B. Han, W. Liu, and X. Xu. 2005. Preparation and antimicrobial activity of hydroxypropyl chitosan. *Carbohydrate Research* 340: 1846–1851.

Peng, Z.X., L. Wang, L. Du, S.R. Guo, X.Q. Wang, and T.T. Tang. 2010. Adjustment of the antibacterial activity and biocompatibility of hydroxypropyltrimethyl ammonium chloride chitosan by varying the degree of substitution of quaternary ammonium. *Carbohydrate Polymers* 81: 275–283.

Peniche-Covas, C., L. Alvarez, and W. Argüelles-Monal. 1992. The adsorption of mercuric ions by chitosan. *Journal of Applied Polymer Science* 46: 1147–1150.

Peniche-Covas, C., M. Jimenez, and A. Nunez. 1988. Characterization of silver-binding chitosan by thermal analysis and electron impact mass spectrometry. *Carbohydrate Polymers* 9: 249–256.

Peniston, Q.P. and E.L. Johnson. 1980. Deacetylation of chitin at reduced temperatures. Patent number US4195175 A, January 03, 1978.

Pillai, C., W. Paul, and C.P. Sharma. 2009. Chitin and chitosan polymers: Chemistry, solubility and fiber formation. *Progress in Polymer Science* 34: 641–678.

Prabaharan, M. 2008. Review paper: Chitosan derivatives as promising materials for controlled drug delivery. *Journal of Biomaterials Applications* 23: 5–36.

Prashanth, K.H. and R. Tharanathan. 2007. Chitin/chitosan: Modifications and their unlimited application potential—an overview. *Trends in Food Science & Technology* 18: 117–131.

Qian, G., J. Zhou, J. Ma, and D. Wang. 1996. The chemical modification of *E. coli* L-asparaginase by N, O-carboxymethyl chitosan. *Artificial Cells, Blood Substitutes and Biotechnology* 24: 567–577.

Qu, G., Z. Yao, C. Zhang, X. Wu, and Q. Ping. 2009. PEG conjugated N-octyl-O-sulfate chitosan micelles for delivery of paclitaxel: In vitro characterization and in vivo evaluation. *European Journal of Pharmaceutical Sciences* 37: 98–105.

Rabea, E.I., M.E. Badawy, T.M. Rogge, C.V. Stevens, M. Höfte, W. Steurbaut, and G. Smagghe. 2005. Insecticidal and fungicidal activity of new synthesized chitosan derivatives. *Pest Management Science* 61: 951–960.

Rabea, E.I., M.E. Badawy, T.M. Rogge, C.V. Stevens, W. Steurbaut, M. Höfte, and G. Smagghe. 2006. Enhancement of fungicidal and insecticidal activity by reductive alkylation of chitosan. *Pest Management Science* 62: 890–897.

Rabea, E.I., M.E. Badawy, C.V. Stevens, G. Smagghe, and W. Steurbaut. 2003. Chitosan as antimicrobial agent: Applications and mode of action. *Biomacromolecules* 4: 1457–1465.

Ramírez-Coutiño, L., M. del Carmen Marín-Cervantes, S. Huerta, S. Revah, and K. Shirai. 2006. Enzymatic hydrolysis of chitin in the production of oligosaccharides using Lecanicillium fungicola chitinases. *Process Biochemistry* 41: 1106–1110.

Ramos, V., A. Heras, and E. Agullo. 2003a. Modified chitosan carrying phosphonic and alkyl groups. *Carbohydrate Polymers* 51: 425–429.

Ramos, V., N. Rodríguez, M. Díaz, M. Rodríguez, A. Heras, and E. Agullo. 2003b. N-methylene phosphonic chitosan. Effect of preparation methods on its properties. *Carbohydrate Polymers* 52: 39–46.

Ren, D., H. Yi, W. Wang, and X. Ma. 2005. The enzymatic degradation and swelling properties of chitosan matrices with different degrees of N-acetylation. *Carbohydrate Research* 340: 2403–2410.

Rhazi, M., J. Desbrieres, A. Tolaimate, M. Rinaudo, P. Vottero, A. Alagui, and M. El Meray. 2002. Influence of the nature of the metal ions on the complexation with chitosan: Application to the treatment of liquid waste. *European Polymer Journal* 38: 1523–1530.

Rinaudo, M. 2006. Chitin and chitosan: Properties and applications. *Progress in Polymer Science* 31: 603–632.

Rinaudo, M., R. Auzely, C. Vallin, and I. Mullagaliev. 2005. Specific interactions in modified chitosan systems. *Biomacromolecules* 6: 2396–2407.

Rinaudo, M., P. Le Dung, C. Gey, and M. Milas. 1992. Substituent distribution on O, N-carboxymethylchitosans by ^{1}H and ^{13}C NMR. *International Journal of Biological Macromolecules* 14: 122–128.

Rodrigues, C.A., M.C. Laranjeira, V.T. de Fávere, and E. Stadler. 1998. Interaction of Cu (II) on N-(2-pyridylmethyl) and N-(4-pyridylmethyl) chitosan. *Polymer* 39: 5121–5126.

Rodrigues, M.R. 2005. Synthesis and investigation of chitosan derivatives formed by reaction with acyl chlorides. *Journal of Carbohydrate Chemistry* 24: 41–54.

Roldo, M., M. Hornof, P. Caliceti, and A. Bernkop-Schnürch. 2004. Mucoadhesive thiolated chitosans as platforms for oral controlled drug delivery: Synthesis and in vitro evaluation. *European Journal of Pharmaceutics and Biopharmaceutics* 57: 115–121.

Ronghua, H., D. Yumin, and Y. Jianhong. 2003. Preparation and anticoagulant activity of carboxybutyrylated hydroxyethyl chitosan sulfates. *Carbohydrate Polymers* 51: 431–438.

Roseman, S. and J. Ludowieg. 1954. N-acetylation of the hexosamines. *Journal of the American Chemical Society* 76: 301–302.

Roy, I., M. Sardar, and M.N. Gupta. 2003. Hydrolysis of chitin by Pectinex™. *Enzyme and Microbial Technology* 32: 582–588.

Ruiz, M., A. Sastre, and E. Guibal. 2002. Pd and Pt recovery using chitosan gel beads. II. Influence of chemical modifications on sorption properties. *Separation Science and Technology* 37: 2385–2403.

Rúnarsson, Ö.V., J. Holappa, T. Nevalainen, M. Hjálmarsdóttir, T. Järvinen, T. Loftsson, J. M. Einarsson, S. Jónsdóttir, M. Valdimarsdóttir, and M. Másson. 2007. Antibacterial activity of methylated chitosan and chitooligomer derivatives: Synthesis and structure activity relationships. *European Polymer Journal* 43: 2660–2671.

Rwei, S.P., Y.M. Chen, W.Y. Lin, and W.Y. Chiang. 2014. Synthesis and rheological characterization of water-soluble glycidyltrimethylammonium-chitosan. *Marine Drugs* 12: 5547–5562.

Sahariah, P., B.E. Benediktssdóttir, M.Á. Hjálmarsdóttir, O.E. Sigurjonsson, K.K. Sørensen, M.B. Thygesen, K.J. Jensen, and M. Másson. 2015. Impact of chain length on antibacterial activity and hemocompatibility of quaternary N-alkyl and N,N-dialkyl chitosan derivatives. *Biomacromolecules* 16: 1449–1460.

Sahin, M., N. Kocak, G. Arslan, and H.I. Ucan. 2011. Synthesis of crosslinked chitosan with epichlorohydrin possessing two novel polymeric ligands and its use in metal removal. *Journal of Inorganic and Organometallic Polymers and Materials* 21: 69–80.

Sajomsang, W. 2010. Synthetic methods and applications of chitosan containing pyridylmethyl moiety and its quaternized derivatives: A review. *Carbohydrate Polymers* 80: 631–647.

Sajomsang, W., P. Gonil, and S. Saesoo. 2009a. Synthesis and antibacterial activity of methylated N-(4-N,N-dimethylaminocinnamyl) chitosan chloride. *European Polymer Journal* 45: 2319–2328.

Sajomsang, W., P. Gonil, S. Saesoo, and C. Ovatlarnporn. 2012. Antifungal property of quaternized chitosan and its derivatives. *International Journal of Biological Macromolecules* 50: 263–269.

Sajomsang, W., P. Gonil, and S. Tantayanon. 2009b. Antibacterial activity of quaternary ammonium chitosan containing mono or disaccharide moieties: Preparation and characterization. *International Journal of Biological Macromolecules* 44: 419–427.

Sajomsang, W., U.R. Ruktanonchai, P. Gonil, and C. Warin. 2010. Quaternization of N-(3-pyridylmethyl) chitosan derivatives: Effects of the degree of quaternization, molecular weight and ratio of N-methylpyridinium and N,N,N-trimethyl ammonium moieties on bactericidal activity. *Carbohydrate Polymers* 82: 1143–1152.

Sajomsang, W., S. Tantayanon, V. Tangpasuthadol, and W.H. Daly. 2008a. Synthesis of methylated chitosan containing aromatic moieties: Chemoselectivity and effect on molecular weight. *Carbohydrate Polymers* 72: 740–750.

Sajomsang, W., S. Tantayanon, V. Tangpasuthadol, M. Thatte, and W.H. Daly. 2008b. Synthesis and characterization of N-aryl chitosan derivatives. *International Journal of Biological Macromolecules* 43: 79–87.

Sakaguchi, T. and A. Nakajima. 1982. Recovery of uranium by chitin phosphate and chitosan phosphate. In *2nd Proceedings of International Conference on Chitin and Chitosan*, S. Hirano, S. Tokura (eds.). Sapporo, Japan, pp. 177–182.

Sakamoto, M., H. Tseng, and K.I. Furuhata. 1994. Regioselective chlorination of chitin with N-chlorosuccinimide-triphenylphosphine under homogeneous conditions in lithium chloride-N,N-dimethylacetamide. *Carbohydrate Research* 265: 271–280.

Sandford, P.A. 1989. Chitosan: Commercial uses and potential applications. In *Chitin and Chitosan*, G.S. Brack, T. Anthonsen, and P. Sandford (eds.). New York: Elsevier Applied Science, 51–69.

Sandford, P.A. 2003. Commercial sources of chitin and chitosan and their utilization. *Advances in Chitin Sciences* 6: 35.

Sarti, F. and A. Bernkop-Schnürch. 2011. Chitosan and thiolated chitosan. In *Chitosan for BiomaterialsI*, R. Jayakumar, M. Prabaharan, R.A.A. Muzzarelli (eds.). Berlin, Germany: Springer, pp. 93–110.

Sashiwa, H., H. Saimoto, Y. Shigemasa, and S. Tokura. 1993. N-Acetyl group distribution in partially deacetylated chitins prepared under homogeneous conditions. *Carbohydrate Research* 242: 167–172.

Sashiwa, H., N. Kawasaki, A. Nakayama, E. Muraki, H. Yajima, N. Yamamori, Y. Ichinose, J. Sunamoto, and S.I. Aiba. 2003. Chemical modification of chitosan. Part 15: Synthesis of novel chitosan derivatives by substitution of hydrophilic amine using N-carboxyethylchitosan ethyl ester as an intermediate. *Carbohydrate Research* 338: 557–561.

Sashiwa, H., N. Kawasaki, A. Nakayama, E. Muraki, N. Yamamoto, and S.I. Aiba. 2002a. Chemical modification of chitosan. 14:1 Synthesis of water-soluble chitosan derivatives by simple acetylation. *Biomacromolecules* 3: 1126–1128.

Sashiwa, H., N. Kawasaki, A. Nakayama, E. Muraki, N. Yamamoto, I. Arvanitoyannis, H. Zhu, and S.I. Aiba. 2002b. Chemical modification of chitosan 12:1 synthesis of organo-soluble chitosan derivatives toward palladium absorbent for chemical plating. *Chemistry Letters* 6: 598–599.

Sashiwa, H., N. Kawasaki, A. Nakayama, E. Muraki, N. Yamamoto, H. Zhu, H. Nagano. et al. 2002c. Chemical modification of chitosan. Synthesis of organosoluble, palladium adsorbable, and biodegradable chitosan derivatives toward the chemical plating on plastics. *Biomacromolecules* 3: 1120–1125.

Sashiwa, H., Y. Makimura, Y. Shigemasa, and R. Roy. 2000a. Chemical modification of chitosan: Preparation of chitosan-sialic acid branched polysaccharide hybrids. *Chemical Communications* 11: 909–910.

Sashiwa, H. and Y. Shigemasa. 1999. Chemical modification of chitin and chitosan 2: Preparation and water soluble property of N-acylated or N-alkylated partially deacetylated chitins. *Carbohydrate Polymers* 39: 127–138.

Sashiwa, H., Y. Shigemasa, and R. Roy. 2000b. Chemical modification of chitosan. 3. Hyperbranched chitosan-sialic acid dendrimer hybrid with tetraethylene glycol spacer. *Macromolecules* 33: 6913–6915.

Sashiwa, H., Y. Shigemasa, and R. Roy. 2000c. Homogeneous N, O-acylation of chitosan in dimethyl sulfoxide with cyclic acid anhydrides. *Chemistry Letters* 10: 1186–1187.

Sashiwa, H., Y. Shigemasa, and R. Roy. 2001a. Chemical modification of chitosan. 10. 1 synthesis of dendronized chitosan-sialic acid hybrid using convergent grafting of preassembled dendrons built on gallic acid and tri (ethylene glycol) backbone. *Macromolecules* 34: 3905–3909.

Sashiwa, H., Y. Shigemasa, and R. Roy. 2001b. Chemical modification of chitosan. Part 7. Preparation and lectin binding property of chitosan-carbohydrate conjugates. *Bulletin of the Chemical Society of Japan* 74: 937–943.

Sashiwa, H., Y. Shigemasa, and R. Roy. 2002d. Chemical modification of chitosan 11: Chitosan–dendrimer hybrid as a tree like molecule. *Carbohydrate Polymers* 49: 195–205.

Satoh, T., L. Vladimirov, M. Johmen, and N. Sakairi. 2003. Preparation and thermal dehydration of N-(Carboxy) acyl chitosan derivatives with high stereoregularity. *Chemistry Letters* 32: 318–319.

Seo, T., Y. Ikeda, K. Torada, Y. Nakata, and Y. Shimomura. 2001. Synthesis of N,O-acylated chitosan and its sorptivity. *Chitin and Chitosan Research* 7: 212–213.

Shelma, R. and C.P. Sharma. 2010. Acyl modified chitosan derivatives for oral delivery of insulin and curcumin. *Journal of Materials Science: Materials in Medicine* 21: 2133–2140.

Shelma, R. and C.P. Sharma. 2011. Development of lauroyl sulfated chitosan for enhancing hemocompatibility of chitosan. *Colloids and Surfaces B: Biointerfaces* 84: 561–570.

Shibano, M., S. Nishida, Y. Saito, H. Kamitakahara, and T. Takano. 2014. Facile synthesis of acyl chitosan isothiocyanates and their application to porphyrin-appended chitosan derivative. *Carbohydrate Polymers* 113: 279–285.

Shigemasa, Y., A. Ishida, H. Sashiwa, H. Saimoto, Y. Okamoto, and S. Minami. 1995. Synthesis of a new chitin derivative (1-carboxyethyl) chitosan. *Chemistry Letters* 1995: 623–624.

Shigemasa, Y., H. Usui, M. Morimoto, H. Saimoto, Y. Okamoto, S. Minami, and H. Sashiwa. 1999. Chemical modification of chitin and chitosan 1: Preparation of partially deacetylated chitin derivatives via a ring-opening reaction with cyclic acid anhydrides in lithium chloride/N, N-dimethylacetamide. *Carbohydrate Polymers* 39: 237–243.

Shim, S.K. and J.J. Ryu. 1998. Synthesis of chelating adsorbent (2, 2'-iminodibenzoic acid-crosslinked chitosan) and adsorptivity of Pb (II), Cu (II), Cd (II). *Analytical Science and Technology* 11: 452–459.

Sieval, A., M. Thanou, A. Kotze, J. Verhoef, J. Brussee, and H. Junginger. 1998. Preparation and NMR characterization of highly substitutedN-trimethyl chitosan chloride. *Carbohydrate Polymers* 36: 157–165.

Somorin, O., N. Nishi, S. Tokura, and J. Noguchi. 1979. Studies on chitin. II. Preparation of benzyl and benzoylchitins. *Polymer Journal* 11: 391–396.

Spinelli, V.A., M. Laranjeira, and V.T. Fávere. 2004. Preparation and characterization of quaternary chitosan salt: Adsorption equilibrium of chromium (VI) ion. *Reactive and Functional Polymers* 61: 347–352.

Sreenivas, S. and K. Pai. 2008. Thiolated chitosans: Novel polymers for mucoadhesive drug delivery–a review. *Tropical Journal of Pharmaceutical Research* 7: 1077–1088.

Sugano, M., S. Watanabe, A. Kishi, M. Izume, and A. Ohtakara. 1988. Hypocholesterolemic action of chitosans with different viscosity in rats. *Lipids* 23: 187–191.

Sugita, K., Y. Tanabe, N. Kodaira, M. Hirakawa, S. Yamaguchi, A. Shibata, M. Shimojoh, and K. Kurita. 2014. Facile synthesis of branched chitin by glycosylation of fully tri-methylsilylated chitin with a glucosamine-derived oxazoline. *Polymer Bulletin* 71: 965–976.

Sun, L., Y. Du, L. Fan, X. Chen, and J. Yang. 2006a. Preparation, characterization and anti-microbial activity of quaternized carboxymethyl chitosan and application as pulp-cap. *Polymer* 47: 1796–1804.

Sun, S. and A. Wang. 2006. Adsorption kinetics of Cu (II) ions using N,O-carboxymethyl-chitosan. *Journal of Hazardous Materials* 131: 103–111.

Sun, S., L. Wang, and A. Wang. 2006b. Adsorption properties of crosslinked carboxymethyl-chitosan resin with Pb (II) as template ions. *Journal of Hazardous Materials* 136: 930–937.

Swain, P.K., M. Dash, and P. Nayak. 2015. Synthesis and characterization of chitosan-based novel superabsorbent hydrogel. *Middle-East Journal of Scientific Research* 23: 259–276.

Tajima, M., M. Izume, T. Fukuhara, T. Kimura, and Y. Kuroyanagi. 2000. Development of new wound dressing composed of N-succinyl chitosan and gelatin. *Journal-Japanese Society for Biomaterials* 18: 220–226.

Tan, H., R. Ma, C. Lin, Z. Liu, and T. Tang. 2013. Quaternized chitosan as an antimicro-bial agent: Antimicrobial activity, mechanism of action and biomedical applications in orthopedics. *International Journal of Molecular sciences* 14: 1854–1869.

Tang, L.G. and D.N.S. Hon. 2001. Chelation of chitosan derivatives with zinc ions. II. Association complexes of Zn^{2+} onto O,N-carboxymethyl chitosan. *Journal of Applied Polymer Science* 79: 1476–1485.

Terbojevich, M., C. Carraro, A. Cosani, and E. Marsano. 1988. Solution studies of the chitin-lithium chloride-N,N-di-methylacetamide system. *Carbohydrate Research* 180: 73–86.

Thanou, M., B. Florea, M. Geldof, H. Junginger, and G. Borchard. 2002. Quaternized chito-san oligomers as novel gene delivery vectors in epithelial cell lines. *Biomaterials* 23: 153–159.

Thanou, M., A. Kotze, T. Scharringhausen, H. Luessen, A. De Boer, J. Verhoef, and H. Junginger. 2000. Effect of degree of quaternization of N-trimethyl chitosan chloride for enhanced transport of hydrophilic compounds across intestinal Caco-2 cell monolayers. *Journal of Controlled Release* 64: 15–25.

Tharanathan, R.N. and F.S. Kittur. 2003. Chitin—The undisputed biomolecule of great potential. *Critical Review in Food Science and Nutrition* 43: 61–87.

Tian, F., Y. Liu, K. Hu, and B. Zhao. 2003. The depolymerization mechanism of chitosan by hydrogen peroxide. *Journal of Materials Science* 38: 4709–4712.

Tian, F., Y. Liu, K. Hu, and B. Zhao. 2004. Study of the depolymerization behavior of chitosan by hydrogen peroxide. *Carbohydrate Polymers* 57: 31–37.

Tikhonov, V.E., L.A. Radigina, and Y.A. Yamskov. 1996. Metal-chelating chitin derivatives via reaction of chitosan with nitrilotriacetic acid. *Carbohydrate Research* 290: 33–41.

Toffey, A., G. Samaranayake, C.E. Frazier, and W.G. Glasser. 1996. Chitin derivatives. I. Kinetics of the heat induced conversion of chitosan to chitin. *Journal of Applied Polymer Science* 60: 75–85.

Tokura, S., S. Baba, Y. Uraki, Y. Miura, N. Nishi, and O. Hasegawa. 1990. Carboxymethylchitin as a drug carrier of sustained release. *Carbohydrate Polymers* 13: 273–281.

Tokura, S., K. Itoyama, N. Nishi, S.I. Nishimura, I. Saiki, and I.A. Nishimura. 1994. Selective sulfation of chitin derivatives for biomedical functions. *Journal of Macromolecular Science, Part A* 31: 1701–1718.

Tokura, S., N. Nishi, A. Tsutsumi, and O. Somorin. 1983. Studies on chitin VIII. Some properties of water soluble chitin derivatives. *Polymer Journal* 15: 485–489.

Tømmeraas, K., K.M. Vårum, B.E. Christensen, and O. Smidsrød. 2001. Preparation and characterisation of oligosaccharides produced by nitrous acid depolymerisation of chitosans. *Carbohydrate Research* 333: 137–144.

Tong, P., Y. Baba, Y. Adachi, and K. Kawazu. 1991. Adsorption of metal ions on a new chelating ion-exchange resin chemically derived from chitosan. *Chemistry Letters* 9: 1529–1532.

Trujillo, R. 1968. Preparation of carboxymethylchitin. *Carbohydrate Research* 7: 483–485.

Tseng, H., K.I. Furuhata, and M. Sakamoto. 1995a. Bromination of regenerated chitin with N-bromosuccinimide and triphenylphosphine under homogeneous conditions in lithium bromide-N,N-dimethylacetamide. *Carbohydrate Research* 270: 149–161.

Tseng, H., R.S. Lee, K.I. Furuhata, and M. Sakamoto. 1995b. Bromination of chitin with tribromoimidazole and triphenylphoshine in LiBr-dimethylacetamide. *Sen'i Gakkaishi* 51: 540–543.

Tseng, H., K. Takechi, and K.I. Furuhata. 1997. Chlorination of chitin with sulfuryl chloride under homogeneous conditions. *Carbohydrate Polymers* 33: 13–18.

Uchegbu, I.F., L. Sadiq, M. Arastoo, A.I. Gray, W. Wang, R.D. Waigh, and A.G. Schätzleinä. 2001. Quaternary ammonium palmitoyl glycol chitosan-a new polysoap for drug delivery. *International Journal of pharmaceutics* 224: 185–199.

Uchida, Y., M. Izume, and A. Ohtakara. 1989. Preparation of chitosan oligomers with purified chitosanase and its application. In *Proceedings of 4th International Conference on Chitin/Chitosan*. Essex, UK: Elsevier Applied Science, pp. 372–382.

Uragami, T., K. Tsukamoto, K. Inui, and T. Miyata. 1998. Pervaporation characteristics of a benzoylchitosan membrane for benzene-cyclohexane mixtures. *Macromolecular Chemistry and Physics* 199: 49–54.

Uryash, V., N.Y. Kokurina, V. Larina, V. Varlamov, A. Ilina, and N. Grishatova. 2007. Gruzdeva AE: Influence of acidic hydrolysis on heat capacity and physical transitions of chitin and chitosan. *Bulletin of Lobachevsky NIzhegorodsky University, Nizhny Novgorod* 3: 98–104.

Varma, A., S. Deshpande, and J. Kennedy. 2004. Metal complexation by chitosan and its derivatives: A review. *Carbohydrate Polymers* 55: 77–93.

Vårum, K., M. Ottøy, and O. Smidsrød. 2001. Acid hydrolysis of chitosans. *Carbohydrate Polymers* 46: 89–98.

Venditti, R.A., J.J. Pawlak, A. Salam, and K.F. El-Tahlawy. 2015. Modified carbohydrate-chitosan compounds, methods of making the same and methods of using the same. Patent number US 8,975,387 B1, March 10, 2015.

Verbych, S., M. Bryk, A. Alpatova, and G. Chornokur. 2005. Ground water treatment by enhanced ultrafiltration. *Desalination* 179: 237–244.

Verheul, R.J., M. Amidi, S. van der Wal, E. van Riet, W. Jiskoot, and W.E. Hennink. 2008. Synthesis, characterization and in vitro biological properties of O-methyl free N,N, N-trimethylated chitosan. *Biomaterials* 29: 3642–3649.

Vikhoreva, G., V. Babak, E. Galich, and L. Gal'braikh. 1997. Complex formation in the sodium dodecyl sulfate-chitosan system. *Polymer Science Series A* 39: 617–622.

Vikhoreva, G., G. Bannikova, P. Stolbushkina, A. Panov, N. Drozd, V. Makarov, V. Varlamov, and L. Gal'braikh. 2005. Preparation and anticoagulant activity of a low-molecular-weight sulfated chitosan. *Carbohydrate Polymers* 62: 327–332.

Vincendon, M. 1993. Xylan derivatives: Aromatic carbamates. *Die Makromolekulare Chemie* 194: 321–328.

Vold, I.M., K.M. Vårum, E. Guibal, and O. Smidsrød. 2003. Binding of ions to chitosan-selectivity studies. *Carbohydrate Polymers* 54: 471–477.

Vongchan, P., W. Sajomsang, D. Subyen, and P. Kongtawelert. 2002. Anticoagulant activity of a sulfated chitosan. *Carbohydrate Research* 337: 1239–1242.

Wan Ngah, W. and K. Liang. 1999. Adsorption of gold (III) ions onto chitosan and N-carboxymethyl chitosan: Equilibrium studies. *Industrial & Engineering Chemistry Research* 38: 1411–1414.

Wan, Y., K.A. Creber, B. Peppley, and V.T. Bui. 2003. Synthesis, characterization and ionic conductive properties of phosphorylated chitosan membranes. *Macromolecular Chemistry and Physics* 204: 850–858.

Wang, K. and Q. Liu. 2014. Chemical structure analyses of phosphorylated chitosan. *Carbohydrate Research* 386: 48–56.

Wang, L., X. Xu, S. Guo, Z. Peng, and T. Tang. 2011. Novel water soluble phosphonium chitosan derivatives: Synthesis, characterization and cytotoxicity studies. *International Journal of Biological Macromolecules* 48: 375–380.

Wang, X., Y. Du, L. Fan, H. Liu, and Y. Hu. 2005. Chitosan-metal complexes as antimicrobial agent: Synthesis, characterization and structure-activity study. *Polymer Bulletin* 55: 105–113.

Wang, X., Y. Du, and H. Liu. 2004. Preparation, characterization and antimicrobial activity of chitosan–Zn complex. *Carbohydrate Polymers* 56: 21–26.

Wang, X., J. Ma, Y. Wang, and B. He. 2001. Structural characterization of phosphorylated chitosan and their applications as effective additives of calcium phosphate cements. *Biomaterials* 22: 2247–2255.

Webster, A., M.D. Halling, and D.M. Grant. 2007. Metal complexation of chitosan and its glutaraldehyde cross-linked derivative. *Carbohydrate Research* 342: 1189–1201.

Werle, M. and A. Bernkop-Schnürch. 2008. Thiolated chitosans: Useful excipients for oral drug delivery. *Journal of Pharmacy and Pharmacology* 60: 273–281.

Woraphatphadung, T., W. Sajomsang, P. Gonil, S. Saesoo, and P. Opanasopit. 2015. Synthesis and characterization of pH-responsive N-naphthyl-N,O-succinyl chitosan micelles for oral meloxicam delivery. *Carbohydrate Polymers* 121: 99–106.

Wu, F.C., R.L. Tseng, and R.S. Juang. 2001. Kinetic modeling of liquid-phase adsorption of reactive dyes and metal ions on chitosan. *Water Research* 35: 613–618.

Xie, W., P. Xu, W. Wang, and Q. Liu. 2002. Preparation and antibacterial activity of a water-soluble chitosan derivative. *Carbohydrate Polymers* 50: 35–40.

Xie, Y., X. Liu, and Q. Chen. 2007. Synthesis and characterization of water-soluble chitosan derivate and its antibacterial activity. *Carbohydrate Polymers* 69: 142–147.

Xing, R., S. Liu, H. Yu, Z. Guo, P. Wang, C. Li, Z. Li, and P. Li. 2005a. Salt-assisted acid hydrolysis of chitosan to oligomers under microwave irradiation. *Carbohydrate Research* 340: 2150–2153.

Xing, R., S. Liu, H. Yu, Q. Zhang, Z. Li, and P. Li. 2004. Preparation of low-molecular-weight and high-sulfate-content chitosans under microwave radiation and their potential anti-oxidant activity in vitro. *Carbohydrate Research* 339: 2515–2519.

Xing R., H. Yu, S. Liu, W. Zhang, Q. Zhang, Z. Li, and P. Li. 2005b. Antioxidant activity of differently regioselective chitosan sulfates in vitro. *Bioorganic & Medicinal Chemistry* 13: 1387–1392.

Xu, T., M. Xin, M. Li, H. Huang, and S. Zhou. 2010. Synthesis, characteristic and antibacterial activity of N,N,N-trimethyl chitosan and its carboxymethyl derivatives. *Carbohydrate Polymers* 81: 931–936.

Xu, T., M. Xin, M. Li, H. Huang, S. Zhou, and J. Liu. 2011. Synthesis, characterization, and antibacterial activity of N, O-quaternary ammonium chitosan. *Carbohydrate Research* 346: 2445–2450.

Xu, Y., Y. Du, R. Huang, and L. Gao. 2003. Preparation and modification of N-(2-hydroxyl) propyl-3-trimethyl ammonium chitosan chloride nanoparticle as a protein carrier. *Biomaterials* 24: 5015–5022.

Yalpani, M. 1992. Synthesis of some sulfur-and phosphorus-containing carbohydrate polymer derivatives. *Carbohydrate Polymers* 19: 35–39.

Yalpani, M. and L.D. Hall. 1984. Some chemical and analytical aspects of polysaccharide modifications. III. Formation of branched-chain, soluble chitosan derivatives. *Macromolecules* 17: 272–281.

Yamaguchi, R., Y. Arai, T. Itoh, and S. Hirano. 1981. Preparation of partially N-succinylated chitosans and their cross-linked gels. *Carbohydrate Research* 88: 172–175.

Yang, J., H. Akao, M. Shimojoh, and K. Kurita. 2004. Efficient introduction of β-maltoside branches into chitin and chitosan. *Chitin and Chitosan Research* 10: 51–56.

Yang, T.C., C.C. Chou, and C.F. Li. 2002. Preparation, water solubility and rheological property of the N-alkylated mono or disaccharide chitosan derivatives. *Food Research International* 35: 707–713.

Yang, X., C. Zhang, C. Qiao, X. Mu, T. Li, J. Xu, L. Shi, and D. Zhang. 2015. A simple and convenient method to synthesize N-[(2-hydroxyl)-propyl-3-trimethylammonium] chitosan chloride in an ionic liquid. *Carbohydrate Polymers* 130: 325–32

Yao, D.R., M.Q. Zhou, S.J. Wu, and S.K. Pan. 2014. Depolymerization of chitosan by enzymes from the digestive tract of sea cucumber *Stichopus japonicus*. *African Journal of Biotechnology* 11: 423–428.

Zhang, C., Q. Ping, H. Zhang, and J. Shen. 2003a. Preparation of N-alkyl-O-sulfate chitosan derivatives and micellar solubilization of taxol. *Carbohydrate Polymers* 54(2): 137–141.

Zhang, C., Q. Ping, H. Zhang, and J. Shen. 2003b. Synthesis and characterization of water-soluble O-succinyl-chitosan. *European Polymer Journal* 39: 1629–1634.

Zhang, C., G. Qu, Y. Sun, X. Wu, Z. Yao, Q. Guo, Q. Ding, S. Yuan, Z. Shen, and Q. Ping. 2008a. Pharmacokinetics, biodistribution, efficacy and safety of N-octyl-O-sulfate chitosan micelles loaded with paclitaxel. *Biomaterials* 29: 1233–1241.

Zhang, C., G. Qu, Y. Sun, T. Yang, Z. Yao, W. Shen, Z. Shen, Q. Ding, H. Zhou, and Q. Ping. 2008b. Biological evaluation of N-octyl-O-sulfate chitosan as a new nano-carrier of intravenous drugs. *European Journal of Pharmaceutical Sciences* 33: 415–423.

Zhang, L., B. Li, X. Meng, L. Huang, and D. Wang. 2015. Degradation of four organophosphorous pesticides catalyzed by chitosan-metal coordination complexes. *Environmental Science and Pollution Research* 1–9.

Zhang, M. and S. Hirano. 1995. Novel N-unsaturated fatty acyl and N-trimethylacetyl derivatives of chitosan. *Carbohydrate Polymers* 26: 205–209.

Zhang, Y., C. Xue, Z. Li, Y. Zhang, and X. Fu. 2006. Preparation of half-deacetylated chitosan by forced penetration and its properties. *Carbohydrate Polymers* 65: 229–234.

Zhao, Y., W.T. Ju, G.H. Jo, W.J. Jung, and R.D. Park. 2011. Perspectives of chitin deacetylase research. In *Biotechnology of Biopolymers*, M. Elnashar (ed.), pp. 131–144.

Zhao, Y., W.T. Ju, and R.D. Park. 2010. Enzymatic modifications of chitin and chitosan (chapter 14). In *Chitin, Chitosan, Oligosaccharides and Their Derivatives: Biological Activities and Applications*, S.-K. Kim (ed.). Boca Raton, FL: CRC Press.

Zhou, L., Y. Wang, Z. Liu, and Q. Huang. 2009. Characteristics of equilibrium, kinetics stud-
  ies for adsorption of Hg (II), Cu (II), and Ni (II) ions by thiourea-modified magnetic
  chitosan microspheres. *Journal of Hazardous Materials* 161: 995–1002.
Zikakis, J. 2012. *Chitin, Chitosan, and Related Enzymes.* Burlington, MA: Elsevier Science.
Zikakis, J., W. Saylor, P. Austin, S. Hirano, and S. Takura. 1982. *Chitin and Chitosan.* Tottori,
  Japan: The Japanese Society of Chitin and Chitosan, p. 233.
Zong, Z., Y. Kimura, M. Takahashi, and H. Yamane. 2000. Characterization of chemical and
  solid state structures of acylated chitosans. *Polymer* 41: 899–906.

Section II

Biological and Agriculture Application of the Marine Biopolymers

6 Biological Activities of Marine Biopolymers

K. Kamala and P. Sivaperumal

CONTENTS

6.1 INTRODUCTION

Biopolymers are usually produced naturally by living organisms. Their molecular backbones are made of repeating units of saccharides, amino acids, or nucleic acids, and occasionally different additional chemical side chains contribute to their various functions. Nowadays, the largest part of marine biopolymers is extracted from biomass, such as marine polysaccharides from cellulose and marine proteins from collagen; marine biopolymers can also be formed from biomonomers using traditional chemical processes as polylactic acid, directly in marine microorganisms and genetically modified marine micro/macroorganisms. Especially, the genetic manipulation of marine organisms biopolymers are carries an enormous biotechnological and quite appropriate for high-value biomedical applications such as tissue engineering and drug delivery system. In addition, the biodegradability of biopolymers gives them a specific advantage in many opportunities areas such as industrial, pharmaceutical, and marine drug production (Johansson et al. 2012). The extraordinary flexibility of these new biodegradable materials comes from the large choice of marine biopolymers such as cellulose whiskers, clays, and metal nanoparticles. These new biopolymer materials have been expanded through new powerful techniques such as electrospinning (Schiffman and Schauer 2008). Furthermore, such products would also contribute to a more sustainable utilization of natural resources in all areas, particularly in marine resources.

Marine organisms still remain a mostly unexploited resource in biotechnological applications. Many marine organisms are composed of molecules and materials showing interesting characteristics and properties, which create an exciting reserve for the development of novel medical products. An increasing number of compounds are currently being isolated from aquatic organisms and suggested as potential novel products for biomedical applications ranging from bioactive ingredients to medical devices. The exploration of many molecules takes led to broad preclinical studies, which have justified, in some cases, clinical trials in several biomedical applications as well as cancer (Urban et al. 2000; Newman and Cragg 2004; Dembitsky et al. 2005). Biopolymers produced by marine organisms are being increasingly investigated for several biomedical applications (Rinaudo 2006a; d'Ayala et al. 2008; Silva et al. 2012). This chapter addresses marine biopolymers and their biological activities mostly carried out during the past few decades. Different aspects are covered, namely, classification, biopolymers sources, and advanced technology-related biomedical applications, with a special emphasis on drug delivery applications.

6.2 MARINE BIOPOLYMERS AND THEIR CLASSIFICATION

Biopolymers are organic chemical compounds obtained from living organisms. These biopolymers have a well-defined structure and are composed of carbon dioxide and water molecules. During the cell growth within the cells, biopolymers are formed by multifaceted processes. A wide range of biopolymers are produced by living organisms in their cytoplasm by enzymatic processes. Other than the cytoplasm, various cell organelles, cell surface, and cytoplasmic membrane, generally the biopolymer synthesis is initiated in any part of the cell and other parts may carry on the processes (Asada et al. 1999; Madigan et al. 1999). Intracellular biopolymers such as polyphosphate, poly-hydroxy-alkanoates, glycogen, cyanopycin, and starch are produced in the limited space of the cytoplasm and by the fermentation process of microorganisms. Thus, the biopolymer production is limited, and it can be determined by the cell density. In addition, the extracellular biopolymers of alginate, dextran, xanthan, and chitosan take place in the outside of the cell. These extracellular biopolymers are easy to differentiate, cell lyses are not essential, and large-scale production is also possible (Alexander et al. 2001). Moreover, biopolymers play various functions in the organisms as follows: conserving and expressing the genetic information in the cell, catalyzing the reactions, storage of carbon and energy in the cell, mediation of adhesion on nonliving things, and communication with environment and other organisms.

Various organisms may produce different types of biopolymers depending on their input units: sugar-based biopolymers have sucrose as an input material. These are conflict to water and can be manufactured by vacuum forming, blowing and injection methods. Starch-based biopolymers have starch as an input unit; these polymers are not present in the animal tissue, but stored in plants as simple carbohydrates. Cellulose-based biopolymers has glucose as an input material, and synthetic biopolymers are produced from synthetic compounds that are entirely biodegradable (e.g., petroleum). Based on the monomeric (simple building blocks) unit, biopolymers are classified into three types: polynucleotides having a minimum of 13 nucleotides, polypeptides which are short polymers comprising amino acids, and polysaccharides composed of linear bonded polymeric carbohydrates. All these biopolymers have a similar kind of sequences and monomers; thus, the mass of all these biopolymers is almost the same, which is called monodispersity.

6.3 MARINE POLYMER SOURCES

One-third of the earth covered by ocean holds 10%–25% of total oceanic dissolved organic matter (DOM) which is present as a biopolymer (Verdugo 1994; Chin et al. 1998; Hansell and Carlson 1998); it goes through conversion among colloidal and dissolved phases (Verdugo 1994; Chin et al. 1998). The total pool of DOM in the ocean was contributed by the extracellular polymeric substances (EPSs) obtained from bacteria (Azam 1998) serve as binding and fate of cationic species and the solubilization of hydrophobic organic chemicals (Decho 1990; Santschi et al. 1998). Negatively charged marine microbial biopolymers are accredited with various amino groups having higher level of uronic acids, such as $C-O^-$, SO_4, and COO^- (Bhaskar and Bhosle 2005). Marine microbial biopolymers are connected with proteins and amino acids, which give both the hydrophobic and hydrophilic nature to the macromolecules (Belsky et al. 1979; Gutierrez et al. 2008). *Actinomycetes*, *Neptunomonas*, and *Cycloclasticus* are the active genera for aromatic hydrocarbon degradation (Head et al. 2006). Bacterial and algal association may actively translocate the hydrocarbons to the algal cell wall, where the bacteria degrade the hydrocarbon to produce a novel biosurfactant (Pastuska 1961; Golman et al. 1973; Gunnison and Alexander 1975; Zelibor et al. 1988). As mentioned previously, the aromatic hydrocarbons are degraded by *Roseobacter clade* found in the phycosphere of *Pseudonitzschia* (Buchan et al. 2000, 2004; Moran et al. 2007; Makkar et al. 2011). Recently, graphite anode has been replaced by silicon with biopolymer alginate in researchable batteries, which is 8 times greater than the ability of graphite-based anodes (Rachel 2011; Ryou et al. 2013). Agar polymer extracted from the red seaweed *Gracilaria dura* shows lesser methoxyl and enough pyruvate content. The rheological properties, molecular weight, and chemical structure will change based on the algal sources (Murano et al. 1992). Biopolymers from the seaweeds are stable, thick, and good emulsifying agents. The heteropolysaccharide algin/alginate made up of linear sequences of D-mannuronic acid and C_3 epimer L-gluronic acid. The interchain linkage of monomers in the presence of calcium leads to form hydrated gels from alginate (Kaplan 1998). Starch is a heterogeneous biodegradable material made up of amylose and amylopectin polymers. It is present in a granular form with low mechanical properties and widely available in nature. Biopolymers have numerous applications such as wound healing, biodegradable capsule, replacement of human tissue, and staple clips. In the tissue engineering application, starch has been used as a drug delivery carrier in the form of microcellular foam.

6.4 BIOLOGICAL ACTIVITIES OF MARINE BIOPOLYMERS

6.4.1 POLYSACCHARIDE

Marine organisms produce an important variety of biopolymers, which can be assembled in three main classes: polysaccharides, proteins, and nucleic acids (McNaught and Wilkinson 1997). Within polysaccharides, a particular group of sulfated polymer glycosaminoglycans will be delivered in a different section. These typically sulfated polymers will be constituted by a hexose and a hexamine unit, and synthesized proteins will form proteoglycans within the organism (Hardingham and Fosang 1992). Hyaluronic acid does not accept sulfate groups nor form proteoglycans (Laurent and Fraser 1992). In addition, polysaccharides are biopolymers made up of carbohydrate monomers linked by glycosidic bonds. The greatest typical polysaccharides in the marine environment are alginate, agar, carrageenans, and chitin. The second most abundant biopolymer is chitin just after cellulose. All polysaccharides have a parallel chemical structure, but the seemingly small differences are answerable for distinct properties of the polymers. In this view, depending on the application predicted for the polymer, one or many other polymers might be selected. In fact, the search for new natural sulfated polysaccharides with significant antithrombotic action and anticoagulant is an attractive alternative for the traditional heparin usage in medicine, and there are many reports of other sulfated compounds from marine origin, such as heparin and fucans, being investigated. Venkata Rao and Sri Ramana (1991) reported the structural studies of polysaccharides extracted from the green seaweed *Chaetomorpha anteninna* of Indian waters. Antiviral polysaccharides have been reported from the red seaweed *Gracilaria corticata* as well as the brown seaweed *Stoechospermum marginatum* of Indian waters (Adhikari et al. 2005; Chattophadhyay and Ray 2005). Seaweed polysaccharides including the sulfated ones have been extensively reported to be exhibiting various bioactivities, for example, antiviral and anticoagulant (Siddhanta and Sai Krishnamurthy 2001). Partially reduced sulfated alginic acid was reported to exhibit the antithrombic activity (Shanmugam and Mody 2000).

The sulfated polymer GAGs are linear, multifaceted, and polydisperse natural polysaccharides, classically bearing a repeating disaccharide unit organized by a hexose and a hexosamine. The presence of sulfated GAG in a wide diverse marine phyla-like sponges such as Porifera (Zierer and Mourao 2000) and several classes of fishes, particularly in commercially related species such as skate, codfish, sharks, salmon, and trout, (Tingbo et al. 2005, 2006; Im et al. 2009) is now well recognized, and an increasing interest is being shown by diverse sectors such as research, biochemical, nutraceutical, biomedical, and biopharmaceutical applications. Due to their unusual chemistry, marine-derived GAGs are being widely documented because of their pharmaceutical activities (antipathogenic, antitumor, and anticoagulant) and as new biomaterials potential in different areas such as biomedical/bioengineered biomaterial applications, *that is*, tissue engineering, bioadhesive molecules and regenerative medicine research.

6.4.2 ALGINATE

Alginate is another important biopolymer, and it was discovered by Stanford in 1881, followed by a patent where Stanford claims the application of alginate as a pharmaceutical agent. Later, in 1929, Kelco Co. Big lake, MN, started to commercialize these polysaccharides extracted from the giant brown seaweed *Macrocystis pyrifera*. In 1959, the production of alginate had been developed worldwide (d'Ayala et al. 2008). In addition, alginate is widely used as a gelling agent for different pharmaceutical and biomedical applications, and personal care purposes (Hernandez-Carmona et al. 1998; Tonnesen and Karlsen 2002; Brownlee et al. 2005). The achievement of profitable development of alginate lies in its capability to retain water and in its gelling, viscosifying, and stabilizing assets, in certain fact that it increases the viscosity of aqueous solutions and forms gels without temperature dependence, in contrast with other polysaccharides of agar and carrageenan (Gomez et al. 2009). Other biotechnological applications can take the benefit of the specific biological effects of alginate, such as hypolipidemic and hypocholesterolemic effects (Smit 2004). It is supported that prospect of the expansion of alginate market will be through more knowledge-demanding areas of biotechnology, pharmacy, and biomedicine.

6.4.3 CHITOSAN

Chitosan has profound applications in the fields of pharmaceuticals and biomedicines because it has antibacterial, fungistatic, haemostatic, antitumoral, and anticholesteremic properties (Krajewska 2005). It also has the ability to prevent the liver damage. Earlier, Sugiyama et al. (1999) reported that chitosan suppresses the plasma liver marker enzyme activities. Chitin, chitosan, and their by-products are widespread in economic sectors, being used in different pharmaceutical and veterinary medicine fields (Senel and McClure 2004; Baldrick 2010). Chitosan and alginate have been probably the greatest used marine-derived biopolymers in the preparation of drug delivery particles (Prabaharan and Mano 2005; Liew et al. 2006; Oh et al. 2008). Chitosan itself may be chemically modified to control the interaction with drug-loaded molecules. The chemical attachment of cyclodextrins or amphiphilic molecules to chitosan-based macromolecules might enhance the affinity of the polysaccharide with hydrophobic drugs (Prabaharan et al. 2007). The antimicrobial activity, film-forming ability, high adsorption, excellent chelation behavior, biocompatibility, and nontoxicity activities have been pointed out as the main answerable by performance of chitosan on the cited applications (Rinaudo 2006b; Honarkar and Barikani 2009; Silva et al. 2010). For example, antimicrobial chitosan films have been used as a packaging material for protection of a different variety of foods and an antioxidant in sausages (Campaniello et al. 2008; Aider 2010). Recently Ramasamy et al. (2014) have found out the protective effect of chitosan from the cuttlebone of *Sepia kobiensis* on carbon tetrachloride-induced hepatic damage in male Wistar rats.

6.4.4 HYALURONIC ACID

Hyaluronic acid is commonly present in the human body, namely, in the intercellular matrix of most connective tissues; thus, it has created applications mainly in the biomedical field. In particular, it is used as a surgical aid in ophthalmology and show an important therapeutic potential in wound healing and joint disease (Goa and Benfield 1994; Lee et al. 2003). Its ophthalmological use is based on the semiflexible assets of the high-molecular-weight chains and the connections between them, which reduce solutions with distinctive viscoelastic properties (Lapcik et al. 1998). Hyaluronic acid has also further clinical medicine uses, such as a diagnostic marker for diseases such as rheumatoid arthritis, cancer, and liver pathologies (Kogan et al. 2007), but also possibilities application in the surface modification of titanium orthopedic implants and aiming to enhance cell adhesion and reduce bacterial infection (Chua et al. 2008).

6.4.5 COLLAGEN AND NANOPARTICLES

Collagen is an important component for health-related applications. Nowadays, this animal-based collagen is widely used in the field of biomedical applications such as skin regeneration templates, dental composites, biodegradable matrices, plastic surgery and shields in ophthalmology, cardiovascular surgery, orthopedics, neurology, and urology (Meena et al. 1999). Marine collagen is currently being studied to be used in all the traditional areas where mammal collagen discoveries application to overcome the disease-related issues, as well as in innovative methodologies for tissue engineering, artificial organs, and drug delivery applications (Swatschek et al. 2002; Song et al. 2006; Jeong et al. 2007). Nanoparticles are particularly adequate to act as injectable delivery systems for a variety of healing molecules. Polysaccharide-based nanoparticles can be produced by different chemical and biological methods, including ionic cross-linking, covalent cross-linking, polyelectrolyte complex, and the self-assembly of hydrophobically modified polysaccharides (Liu et al. 2008). Low-generation poly(amidoamine) dendrimers are chemically modified with carboxymethyl chitosans such as rendering dendritic nanoparticles. These nanoparticles are shown to be internalized by cells and thus used in intracellular drug delivery strategies (Oliveira et al. 2008). Moreover, using a rationale of electrostatic interactions, carrageenan/chitosan nanoparticles are created in mild conditions and showed to permit the encapsulation and latter release of proteins (Grenha et al. 2010).

6.5 MARINE POLYMERS IN TISSUE ENGINEERING APPLICATIONS

In the overall tissue engineering approach, matrices are developed to support cells, stimulating their differentiation and proliferation to form a novel new and functional tissue (Langer and Vacanti 1993). Such approaches are allowed to produce hybrid constructs that can be implantable in patients to induce the redevelopment of tissues or replace malfunctioning or failing organs. Diverse materials have been recommended to be used in the processing of scaffolds, namely, biodegradable biopolymers derived from marine sources. Natural-based biopolymers suggested the advantage similar to biological macromolecules, in which the biological environment is prepared to identify and easily deal with metabolic activities. Due to their resemblance to natural polymers and extracellular matrices may also evade the stimulation of immunological reactions or chronic inflammation and toxicity, often discovered with synthetic polymers. The ocean may be an important source of materials to be used in different applications, in which diverse polysaccharides with different chemical natures, minerals, and proteins could be found. An important aspect is the processing of such kind of materials into porous matrices, a task that usually essentials other technologies than those frequently employed in the processing of conventional synthetic polymers that frequently suggests the use of organic solvents or melting of the materials (Hutmacher 2000).

Warm techniques have been extensively used to process marine-derived polymers that may also be attractive by the fact that cells or unstable proteins can be combined during the fabrication of the device. Freeze–drying has been extensively used to develop natural polymers, including marine-derived polysaccharides. A typical example is the production of scaffolds from chitosan (Madihally and Matthew 1999): Acidic aqueous solutions are frozen and lyophilized, and the final scaffold is neutralized and stabilized in an alkaline solution and water. The structure of the final scaffold will essentially depend on the initial chitosan concentration and the shape and size of the ice crystals generated during the freezing step. Cross-linking or the combination of other biomacromolecules could also be combined with different method (Silva et al. 2008). In case of orthopedic application, scaffolds could be incorporated into more stiff prefabricated scaffolds (Prabaharan et al. 2007).

Among other marine-derived biopolymers of polysaccharides, collagen is also used in tissue engineering strategies. Being the foremost protein in the body, marine-derived collagen is a biomaterial for excellence and a relevant choice when one wants to develop a tissue engineering micro/nanoscaffold. In this view, marine-derived collagen scaffolds were developed by jellyfish collagen, and further cross-linked, which did not prompt a significant cytotoxic effect and had higher cell proliferation than other biomaterials, including bovine collagen. Moreover, *in vivo* examinations confirmed that jellyfish collagen induced a similar immune response to that induced by bovine collagen (Song et al. 2006). Jellyfish collagen has also been combined with poly(lactic-*co*-glycolic acid) and processed by freeze–drying and electrospinning to obtain tubular nanoscaffolds, in which smooth muscle cells and endothelial cells were shown to proliferate the effect (Jeong et al. 2007). The above-mentioned finding supported the great potential of marine origin collagen for tissue engineering applications.

Electrospun scaffolds from collagen (Rho et al. 2006), poly(ethylene-*co*-vinyl alcohol) (Kenawy et al. 2003), collagen-poly-(ethylene oxide) (PEO) (Huang et al. 2001), and polyurethane (Khil et al. 2003) have been examined for prospective applications such as as wound healing. There also has been increasing concern in the combination of drugs using electrospun fibers in areas except wound dressing. Few studies have been performed in the areas of cancer therapy and heart disorders (Verreck et al. 2003; Zeng et al. 2003, 2005; Brewster et al. 2004; Jiang et al. 2004, 2005). In addition, infection is usually encountered in wounds due to the microorganisms, which are from the internal resources, hospitalized patients, and the surrounding skin, and can colonize and affect the wound healing (Siddiqui and Bernstein 2010).

6.6   CONCLUSION

The ocean has been confirmed to be a huge source of bioactive materials, even though the accessible knowledge of marine biomaterials and their mechanism are still in their infancy. In addition, the marine environment shields a wide diversity of natural products and indeed can be a treasure chest for pharmaceutical purposes. Especially, marine biopolymeric bioactive molecules are emphasized for many interests in search of new beneficial drugs. It is envisaged that biomedical field will be an area in which marine-derived polymers will have a part of major relevance, in particular with their use on tissue regeneration and tissue repair. These multidisciplinary methods are aimed to go from engineered nanoscaffolds to the clinic applications that enhanced regeneration of injured or damaged tissues/organs is not that's reasonable to achieve its goals and marine-derived polymers are being increased Studied. However, a strong determination is still necessary to get medical-grade biopolymers from marine sources, in a reproducible way, for allow their use in the development of scaffolds in which different cells can be scattered and then proliferate, rendering a new tissue that could be embedded in the patient. In addition, the use of marine-origin biopolymers in tissue engineering approaches, in particular their success in *in vivo* analysis, is still needed to boost their potential in this particular area. However, basic and applied research efforts in this marine-synthesized biomedical field require a close collaboration between biologists and chemists and expertise in marine microbiology, biology, biochemistry, chemistry, and computational sciences to fulfill screening, structural characterization, and bioactivities studies. Due to a diverse chemical ecology in the marine organisms have a great promise of providing effective, low-cost and safer therapeutic drugs, which deserve a broad exploration.

ACKNOWLEDGMENT

The authors are grateful to SRM University, Tamil Nadu, India, and to Dr. R. Rajaram, department of marine science, Bharathidasan University, Tamil Nadu, India, for giving his valuable suggestion while drafting this chapter.

REFERENCES

Adhikari, U., C. Mateu, E.B. Damonte, and B. Ray. 2005. *Proceedings of CARBO XX Carbohydrate Conference*, November 24–26, Lucknow, India: Lucknow University, p. 12.
Aider, M. 2010. Chitosan application for active bio-based films production and potential in the food industry: Review. *LWT–Food Science Technology* 43: 837–842.
Alexander, S. 2001. Thermo responsive polymer colloids for drug delivery and cancer therapy. *Macromolecule Bioscience* 11: 1722–1734.
Asada, Y., J. Miyake, M. Miyake, R. Kurane, and Y. Tokiwa. 1999. Polysynthetic accumulation of poly-(hydroxybutyratae) by cyanobacteria—the metabolism and potential for CO_2 recycling. *International Journal of Biological Macromolecules* 25: 37–42.
Azam, F. 1998. Microbial control of oceanic carbon flux: The plot thickens. *Science* 280: 694–696.
Baldrick, P. 2010. The safety of chitosan as a pharmaceutical excipient. *Regulatory Toxicology and Pharmacology* 56(3): 290–299.
Belsky, I., D.L. Gutnick, and E. Rosenberg, 1979. Emulsifier of *Arthrobacter* RAG-1: Determination of emulsifier-bound fatty acids. *FEBS Letter* 101: 175–178.
Bhaskar, P.V. and N.B. Bhosle. 2005. Microbial extracellular polymeric substances in marine biogeochemical processes. *Current Science* 88: 45–53.

Brewster, M.E., G. Verreck, I. Chun, J. Rosenblatt, J. Mensch, A. Van Dijck, M. Noppe, A. Arien, M. Bruining, and J. Peeters. 2004. The use of polymer-based electrospun nanofibers containing amorphous drug dispersions for the delivery of poorly water-soluble pharmaceuticals. *Die Pharmazie* 59: 387–391.

Brownlee, I.A., A. Allen, J.P. Pearson, P.W. Dettmar, M.E. Havler, M.R. Atherton, and E. Onsoyen. 2005. Alginate as a source of dietary fiber. *Critical Review on Food Science and Nutrition* 45: 497–510.

Buchan, A., L.S. Collier, E.L. Neidle, and M.A. Moran. 2000. Key aromatic-ring-cleaving enzyme, protocatechuate 3,4-dioxygenase, in the ecologically important marine *Roseobacter* lineage. *Applied Environmental Microbiology* 66: 4662–4672.

Buchan, A., E.L. Neidle, and M.A. Moran. 2004. Diverse organization of genes of the β-ketoadipate pathway in members of the marine *Roseobacter* lineage. *Applied Environmental Microbiology* 70: 1658–1668.

Campaniello, D., A. Bevilacqua, M. Sinigaglia, and M.R. Corbo. 2008. Chitosan: Antimicrobial activity and potential applications for preserving minimally processed strawberries. *Food Microbiology* 25(8): 992–1000.

Chattophadhyay, K. and B. Ray. 2005. *Proceedings of CARBO XX Carbohydrate Conference*, November 24–26, Lucknow, India: Lucknow University, p. 9.

Chin, W.C., M.V. Orellana, and P. Verdugo. 1998. Formation of micro gels by spontaneous assembly of dissolved marine polymers. *Nature* 391: 568–572.

Chua, P.H., K.G. Neoh, E.T. Kang, and W. Wang. 2008. Surface functionalization of titanium with hyaluronic acid/chitosan polyelectrolyte multilayers and RGD for promoting osteoblast functions and inhibiting bacterial adhesion. *Biomaterials* 29(10): 1412–1421.

d'Ayala, G.G., M. Malinconico, and P. Laurienzo. 2008. Marine derived polysaccharides for biomedical applications: Chemical modification approaches. *Molecules* 13(9): 2069–2106.

Decho, A.W. 1990. Microbial exopolymer secretions in ocean environments: Their role(s) in food webs and marine processes. In *Oceanography Marine Biology Annual Review*, M. Barnes (ed.). Aberdeen, Scotland: Aberdeen University Press, pp. 73–153.

Dembitsky, V.M., T.A. Gloriozova, and V.V. Poroikov. 2005. Novel antitumor agents: Marine sponge alkaloids, their synthetic analogs and derivatives. *Mini Reviews in Medical Chemistry* 5: 319–336.

Goa, K.L. and P. Benfield. 1994. Hyaluronic-acid—A review of its pharmacology and use as a surgical aid in ophthalmology, and its therapeutic potential in joint disease and wound-healing. *Drugs* 47:536–566.

Golman, L.P., M.F. Mikhaseva, and V.M. Reznikov. 1973. Infrared spectra of lignin reparations of pteridophytes and seaweeds. *Doklady Akadameii Nauk BSSR* 17: 1031–1033.

Gomez, C.G., M.V.P. Lambrecht, J.E. Lozano, M. Rinaudo, and M.A. Villar. 2009. Influence of the extraction–purification conditions on final properties of alginates obtained from brown algae (*Macrocystis pyrifera*). *International Journal of Biological Macromolecules* 44: 365–371.

Grenha, A., M.E. Gomes, M. Rodrigues, V.E. Santo, J.F. Mano, N.M. Neves, and R.L. Reis. 2010. Development of new chitosan/carrageenan nanoparticles for drug delivery applications. *Journal Biomedical Material Research Part A* 92: 1265–1272.

Gunnison, D. and M. Alexander. 1975. Basis for the resistance of several algae to microbial decomposition. *Applied Microbiology* 29: 729–738.

Gutierrez, T., T. Shimmield, C. Haidon, K. Black, and D.H. Green. 2008. Emulsifying and metal ion binding activity of a glycoprotein exopolymer produced by *Pseudoalteromonas* species TG12. *Applied Environmental Microbiology* 74: 4867–4876.

Hansell, D.A. and C.A. Carlson. 1998. Deep-ocean gradients in the concentration of dissolved organic carbon. *Nature* 395: 263–268.

Hardingham, T.E. and A.J. Fosang, 1992. Proteoglycans: Many forms and many functions. *FASEB Journal* 6(3): 861–870.

Head, I.M., M.D. Jones, and W.F.M. Roling. 2006. Marine microorganisms make a meal of oil. *Nature* 4: 173–182.

Hernandez-Carmona, G., D.J. McHugh, D.L. Arvizu-Higueraand, Y.E. Rodriguez-Montesinos. 1998. Pilot plant scale extraction of alginate from *Macrocystis pyrifera*. 1. Effect of pre-extraction treatments on yield and quality of alginate. *Journal of Applied Phycology* 10(6): 507–513.

Honarkar, H. and M. Barikani. 2009. Applications of biopolymers I: Chitosan. *Chemical Monthly* 140(12): 1403–1420.

Huang, L., K. Nagapudi, R.P. Apkarian, E.L. Chaikof. 2001. Engineered collagen-PEO nanofibers and fabrics. *Journal of Biomaterials Science Polymer Edition* 12: 979–993.

Hutmacher, D.W. 2000. Scaffolds in tissue engineering bone and cartilage. *Biomaterials* 21(24): 2529–2543.

Im, A.R., J.S. Sim, Y. Park, B.S. Hahn, T. Toida, and Y.S. Kim. 2009. Isolation and characterization of chondroitin sulfates from the by-products of marine organisms. *Food Science and Biotechnology* 18(4): 872–877.

Jeong, S.I., S.Y. Kim, S.K. Cho, M.S. Chong, K.S. Kim, H. Kim, S.B. Lee, and Y.M. Lee. 2007. Tissue-engineered vascular grafts composed of marine collagen and PLGA fibers using pulsatile perfusion bioreactors. *Biomaterials* 28(6): 1115–1122.

Jiang, H.L., D.F. Fang, B.S. Hsiao, B. Chu, and W.L. Chen. 2004. Optimization and characterization of dextran membranes prepared by electro spinning. *Biomacromolecules* 5: 326–333.

Jiang, H., Y. Hu, Y. Li, P. Zhao, K. Zhu, and W. Chen. 2005. A facile technique to prepare biodegradable coaxial electrospun nanofibers for controlled release of bioactive agents. *Journal of Control Release* 108: 237–243.

Johansson, C., J. Bras, I. Mondragon, P. Nechita, D. Plackett, P. Simon, D.G. Svetec, S. Virtanen, M.G. Baschetti, C. Breen, and S. Aucejo. 2012. Renewable fibers and bio-based materials for packaging applications—A review of recent developments. *Bioresources* 7(2): 2506–2552.

Kaplan, D.L. (ed.) 1998. *Biopolymers from Renewable Resources* (Macromolecular Systems - Materials Approach). Medford, MA: Tufts University. Eds.: Springer-Verlag Berlin and Heidelberg GmbH & Co. K, Springer-Verlag Berlin and Heidelberg GmbH & Co. pp 420.

Kenawy, R., J.M. Layman, J.R. Watkins, G.L. Bowlin, J.A. Matthews, D.G. Simpson and G.E. Wnek. 2003. Electro spinning of poly (ethylene-co-vinyl alcohol) fibers. *Biomaterials* 24: 907–913.

Khil, M.S., D.I. Cha, H.Y. Kim, I.S. Kim, and N. Bhattara. 2003. Electrospun nanofibrous polyurethane membrane as wound dressing. *Journal of Biomedical Material Research* 67(2) 675–679.

Kogan, G., L. Soltes, R. Stern, and P. Gemeiner. 2007. Hyaluronic acid: A natural biopolymer with a broad range of biomedical and industrial applications. *Biotechnology Letters* 29(1): 17–25.

Krajewska, B. 2005. Membrane based process performed with use of chitin/chitosan materials. *Separation and Purification Technology* 41: 305–312.

Langer, R. and J.P. Vacanti. 1993. Tissue engineering. *Science* 260: 920–926.

Lapcik, L., L. Lapcik, S. de Smedt, J. Demeester, and P. Chabrecek. 1998. Hyaluronan: Preparation, structure, properties, and applications. *Chemical Reviews* 98(8): 2663–2684.

Laurent, T.C. and J.R. Fraser. 1992. Hyaluronan. *FASEB Journal* 6(7): 2397–2404.

Lee, S.B., Y.M. Lee, K.W. Song, and M.H. Park. 2003. Preparation and properties of polyelectrolyte complex sponges composed of hyaluronic acid and chitosan and their biological behaviors. *Journal of Applied Polymer Science* 90(4): 925–932.

Liew, C.V., L.W. Chan, A.L. Ching, and P.W.S. Heng. 2006. Evaluation of sodium alginate as drug release modifier in matrix tablets. *International Journal of Pharmaceutics* 309: 25–37.

Liu, Z.H., Y.P. Jiao, Y.F. Wang, C.R. Zhou, and Z.Y. Zhang, 2008. Polysaccharides-based nanoparticles as drug delivery systems. *Advanced Drug Delivery Reviews* 60(15): 1650–1662.

Madigan, M.T., J.M. Martinko, and J. Parker. 1999. *Brock Biology of Microorganisms*, 9th edition. Upper Saddle River, NJ: Prentice Hall.

Madihally, S.V. and H.W.T. Matthew. 1999. Porous chitosan scaffolds for tissue engineering. *Biomaterials* 20(12): 1133–1142.

Makkar, R.S., S.S. Cameotra, and I.M. Banat. 2011. Advances in utilization of renewable substrates for biosurfactant production. *AMB Express* 1: 1–5.

McNaught, A.D. and A. Wilkinson. 1997. *Compodium of Chemical Terminology, IUPAC*. Oxford: Black Well Scientific Publications.

Meena, C., S. Mengi, and S. Deshpande. 1999. Biomedical and industrial applications of collagen. *Journal of Chemical Science* 111(2): 319–329.

Moran, M.A., R. Belas, M.A. Schell, J.M. Gonzalez, F. Sun, S. Sun, B.J. Binder et al. 2007. Ecological genomics of marine *Roseobacters*. *Applied Environmental Microbiology* 73: 4559–4569.

Murano, E., R. Toffanin, and F. Zanetti. 1992. Chemical and macromolecular characterization of agar polymers from *Gracilaria dura* (C. Agardh) J. Agardh (Gracilariacea, Rhodophyta). *Carbohydrate Polymers* 18(3): 171–178.

Newman, D.J. and G.M. Cragg. 2004. Marine natural products and related compounds in clinical and advanced preclinical trials. *Journal of Natural Products* 67(8): 1216–1238.

Oh, J.K., R. Drumright, D.J. Siegwart, and K. Matyjaszewski. 2008. The development of microgels/nanogels for drug delivery applications. *Progress in Polymer Science* 33(4): 448–477.

Oliveira, J.M., N. Kotobuki, A.P. Marques, R.P. Pirraco, J. Benesch, M. Hirose, S.A. Costa, J.F. Mano, H. Ohgushi, and R.L. Reis. 2008. Surface engineered carboxymethyl chitosan/poly (amidoamine) dendrimer nanoparticles for intracellular targeting. *Advanced Functional Materials* 18(12): 1840–1853.

Pastuska, G. 1961. Die Kieselgelschicht-Chromatographie von Phenolen and Phenol carbensiuren. *Analytical Chemistry* 179: 355–358.

Prabaharan, M. and J.F. Mano. 2005. Chitosan-based particles as controlled drug delivery systems. *Drug Delivery* 12(1): 41–57.

Prabaharan, M., M.A. Rodriguez-Perez, J.A. de Saja, and J.F. Mano. 2007. Preparation and characterization of poly (L-lactic acid)-chitosan hybrid scaffolds with drug release capability. *Journal of Biomedical Material Research Part B: Applied Biomaterials* 81B(2): 427–434.

Rachel, P. 2011. Seaweed polymer can improve battery storage. Polymer solutions, November 14, https://www.polymersolutions.com/blog/seaweed-polymer-can-improve-battery-storage/.

Ramasamy, P., N. Subhapradha, S. Vairamani, and A. Shanmugam. 2014. Protective effect of chitosan from *Sepia kobiensis* (Hoyle 1885) cuttlebone against CCl_4 induced hepatic injury. *International Journal of Biological Macromolecules* 65: 559–563.

Rao, E.V. and K. Sri Ramana. 1991. Structural studies of a polysaccharide isolated from the green seaweed *Chaetomorpha anteninna*. *Carbohydrate Research* 217: 163–170.

Rho, K.S., L. Jeong, G. Lee, B.M. Seo, Y.J. Park, S.D. Hong, S. Rho, J.J. Cho, W.H. Park, and B.M. Min. 2006. Electrospinning of collagen nanofibers: Effects on the behavior of normal human keratinocytes and early-stage wound healing. *Biomaterials* 27: 1452–1461.

Rinaudo, M. 2006a. Properties and applications. *Progresses Polymeric Science* 31: 603–632.

Rinaudo, M. 2006b. Chitin and chitosan: Properties and applications. *Progresses Polymeric Science* 31(7): 603–632.

Ryou, M.H., S. Hong, M. Winter, H. Lee, and J.W. Choi. 2013. Improved cycle lives of LiMnO$_4$ cathodes in lithium ion batteries by an alginate biopolymer from seaweed. *Journal of Material Chemistry A* 1: 15224–15229.

Santschi, P.H., L. Guo, J.C. Means, and M. Ravichandran. 1998. Natural organic matter binding of trace metal and trace organic contaminants in estuaries. In *Biogeochemistry of Gulf of Mexico Estuaries*, T.S. Bianchi, J.R. Pennock, R. Twilley (eds.). New York: Wiley, pp. 347–380.

Schiffman, J.D. and C.L. Schauer. 2008. A review: Electrospinning of biopolymer nanofibers and their applications. *Polymer Reviews* 48(2): 317–352.

Senel, S. and S.J. McClure. 2004. Potential applications of chitosan in veterinary medicine. *Advanced Drug Delivery Reviews* 56(10): 1467–1480.

Shanmugam, M. and K.H. Mody. 2000. Heparinoid-active sulphated polysaccharides from marine algae as potential blood anticoagulant agents. *Current Science* 79: 1672–1683.

Siddhanta, A.K. and A.S. Krishnamurthy. 2001. Sterols from marine green algae of Indian waters. *Journal of Indian Chemical Society* 78: 431–437.

Siddiqui, A.R. and J.M. Bernstein. 2010. Chronic wound infection: Facts and controversies. *Clinics in Dermatology* 28: 519–526.

Silva, F.R.F., C.M.P.G. Dore, C.T. Marques, M.S. Nascimento, N.M.B. Benevides, H.A.O. Rocha, S.F. Chavante, and E.L. Leite. 2010. Anticoagulant activity, paw edema and pleurisy induced carrageenan: Action of major types of commercial carrageenans. *Carbohydrate Polymers* 79(1): 26–33.

Silva, S.S., A. Motta, M.T. Rodrigues, A.F.M. Pinheiro, M.E. Gomes, J.F. Mano, R.L. Reis, and C. Migliaresi. 2008. Novel genipin cross-linked chitosan/silk fibroin sponges for cartilage engineering strategies. *Biomacromolecules* 9(10): 2764–2774.

Silva, T.H., A. Alves, B.M. Ferreira, M. Oliveira, L.L. Reys, R.J.F. Ferreria, R.A. Sousa, S.S. Silva, J.F. Mano, and R.L. Reis. 2012. Materials of marine origin: A review on polymers and ceramics of biomedical interest. *International Material Reviews Vol 57,* 1–32.

Smit, A.J. 2004. Medicinal and pharmaceutical uses of seaweed natural products: A review. *Journal of Applied Phycology* 16(4): 245–262.

Song, E., S.Y. Kim, T. Chun, H.J. Byun, and Y.M. Lee. 2006. Collagen scaffolds derived from a marine source and their biocompatibility. *Biomaterials* 27(15): 2951–2961.

Sugiyama, K., P. He, S. Wada, and S. Saeki. 1999. Teas and other beverages suppress D-Galactosamine-induced liver injury in rats. *Journal of Nutrition* 129: 1361–1367.

Swatschek, D., W. Schatton, W.E.G. Muller, and J. Kreuter. 2002. Micro particles derived from marine sponge collagen (SCMPs): Preparation, characterization and suitability for dermal delivery of all-trans retinol. *European Journal of Pharmaceutics and Biopharmaceutics* 54(2): 125–133.

Tingbo, M.G., S.O. Kolset, R. Ofstad, G. Enersen, and K.O. Hannesson. 2005. Sulfated glycosaminoglycans in the extracellular matrix of muscle tissue in Atlantic cod (*Gadus morhua*) and Spotted wolffish (*Anarhichas minor*). *Comparative Biochemistry and Physiology Part B: Biochemistry and Molecular Biology* 140B(3): 349–357.

Tingbo, M.G., S.O. Kolset, R. Ofstad, G. Enersen, and K.O. Hannesson. 2006. Identification and distribution of heparan sulfate proteoglycans in the white muscle of Atlantic cod (*Gadus morhua*) and spotted wolffish (*Anarhichas minor*). *Comparative Biochemistry and Physiology Part B: Biochemistry and Molecular Biology* 143B(4): 441–452.

Tonnesen, H.H. and J. Karlsen. 2002. Alginate in drug delivery systems. *Drug Development and Industrial Pharmacy* 28(6): 621–630.

Urban, S., S.J.H. Hickford, J.W. Blunt, and M.H.G. Munro. 2000. Bioactive marine alkaloids. *Current Organic Chemistry* 4: 765–807.

Verdugo, P. 1994. Polymer gel phase transition in condensation-decondensation of secretory products. *Advance Polymeric Science* 110: 145–156.

Verreck, G., I. Chun, J. Rosenblatt, J. Peeters, A.V. Dijck, J. Mensch, M. Noppe, and M.E. Brewster. 2003. Incorporation of drugs in an amorphous state into electrospun nanofibers composed of a water-insoluble, non-biodegradable polymer. *Journal of Controlled Release* 92: 349–360.

Zelibor, J.L., L. Romankiw, P.G. Hatcherm, and R.R. Colwell. 1988. Comparative analysis of the chemical composition of mixed and pure cultures of green algae and their decomposed residues by ^{13}C nuclear magnetic resonance. *Applied Environmental Microbiology* 54: 1051–1060.

Zeng, J., X. Xu, X. Chen, Q. Liang, X. Bian, L. Yang, and X. Jing, 2003. Biodegradable electrospun fibers for drug delivery. *Journal of Controlled Release* 92: 227–231.

Zeng, J., L. Yang, Q. Liang, X. Zhang, H. Guan, X. Xu, X. Chen, and X. Jing, 2005. Influence of the drug compatibility with polymer solution on the release kinetics of electrospun fiber formulation. *Journal of Controlled Release* 105: 43–51.

Zierer, M.S. and P.A. Mourao. 2000. A wide diversity of sulfated polysaccharides are synthesized by different species of marine sponges. *Carbohydrate Research* 328: 209–216.

7 Sulfated Chitosan as a Modified Marine Polysaccharides
From Synthesis to Applications

Nazma Inamdar and V.K. Mourya

CONTENTS

7.1 INTRODUCTION

Chitin and chitosan, the biorenewable marine polysaccharides, are currently explored extensively for their myriad of applications such as pharmaceutical, cosmetic, biomedical, veterinary medicine, biotechnological, agricultural, food industries, paper, and textile industries as well as in water treatment. These polymers have now been considered as an important class of physiological materials due to their unique sets of properties such as cationic nature, versatile biological activity, excellent biocompatibility, complete biodegradability, and low toxicity. To employ these properties and to appreciate the full potential of these multitalented polysaccharides, attempts are continuously being made to modify them (Mourya and Inamdar 2008).

Chitin is a linear heteropolymer of randomly distributed N-acetylglucosamine and glucosamine residues with β-1,4-linkage, mostly derived from the exoskeleton of crustaceans. The degree of deacetylation (DDA) of chitin ranges from 5% to 10%, and the molecular weight (MW) can be upto $1-2 \times 10^6$ Da, corresponding to the degree of polymerization of ~5,000–10,000. Chitosan is derived from alkaline N-deacetylation of chitin. In chitosan, the DDA is >60% and the MW ranges from 2000 Da (oligomers) to $10^4–2 \times 10^6$ Da (Ravi Kumar et al. 2004). With multiplicity in the properties of chitosan arising with the combination of DDA and MW, a variety of applications can be designed. The properties can be further modulated with chemical modifications. One can chemically modify chitinous polymers, especially the acid-soluble chitosan, because monomers provide functional groups such as primary amine, primary hydroxyl, and secondary hydroxyl groups (Figure 7.1). The chemical modification of chitin and chitosan is of primary interest because depending on the nature of the group(s) introduced, the resultant polysaccharides retain their fundamental skeleton and also many of their original physicochemical and biochemical properties (Illum 1998).

Sulfated chitosans represent a very important family of such derivatives of chitosan, which can demonstrate a gamut of biological activities. The site-specific chemical modification of the amino and hydroxyl groups in chitin and chitosan, with sulfate, can generate products for pharmaceutical applications, because the structure of sulfated chitin and chitosan serves as the nearest structural analogs of the natural blood anticoagulant, heparin, and demonstrate the biomolecular mechanism of anticoagulant, antisclerotic, and antiviral activities. The sulfated derivatives also exhibit enzyme inhibitory, antioxidant, antitumor, and wound healing properties. These derivatives also have been found useful in drug delivery.

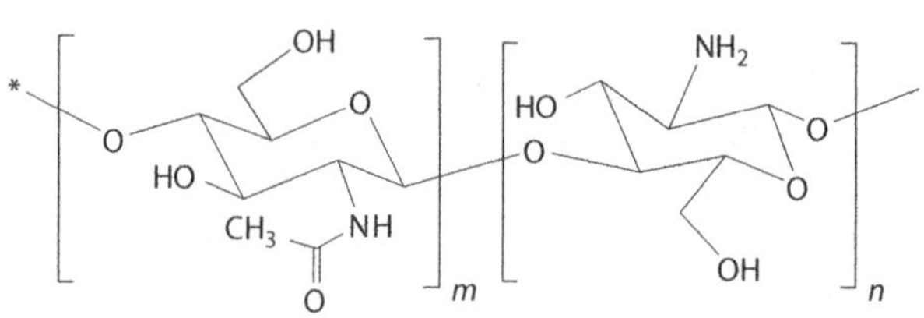

FIGURE 7.1 Chitin and chitosan: Chitin is composed predominantly of m units and chitosan is composed predominantly of n units distributed in a random fashion.

7.2   SYNTHESIS

Introduction of $-SO_3^-$ group on the chitosan backbone can be achieved by various methods, which involve combinations of sulfating reagents and reaction media as used for the sulfation of other polysaccharides (Gilbert 1962). Similar to sulfation reactions of multifunctional polysaccharides, sulfation of chitosan is accompanied by structural heterogeneity in the product. The $-SO_3^-$ group can get substituted at N-2, O-3, and/or O-6 position of the chitosan monomer unit. The chitosan sulfates thus obtained are not monosubstituted, but often disubstituted and may also be partially trisubstituted. This means that chitosan sulfates may be considered as copolymers composed of random mono-, di-, and trisubstituted units of chitosan. A structural variety of products are related to the various reactivities of the three functional groups of chitosan, leading to different degrees of substitution in the individual groups. The sulfation conditions of chitosan essentially affect the position and degree of substitution with sulfate in chitosan, and the factors influencing the sulfation process include the acetylation state of chitosan, sulfation agent, solvents, reaction time, and temperature (Nagasawa et al. 1972).

For sulfation, the polymer is reacted with a sulfating agent, and after completion of the reaction, the product is desalted, precipitated with solvents, or lyophilized. The sulfating reagents being used include concentrated sulfuric acid, oleum, sulfur trioxide, trimethylamine-sulfur trioxide, pyridine-sulfur trioxide, chlorosulfonic acid-sulfuric acid, and the most commonly used chlorosulfonic acid ($ClSO_3H$) in solvents such as pyridine, N,N-dimethyl formamide (DMF), and dichloroacetic acid (DCAA). Sulfuric acid causes extensive degradation, even when employed under controlled conditions, as do $ClSO_3H$ and sulfur trioxide when applied alone. When combined with Lewis bases, these two reagents cause less degradation, and they have been widely used.

Nagasawa et al. (1971) prepared sulfated chitin and chitosan by using sulfuric acid, tetrahydrofuran, and phosphorus pentoxide at $-20°C$. The average MW and yield of sulfated chitin and chitosan showed the extent of degradation of the polysaccharide structure by concentrated sulfuric acid where the reaction temperature and time influenced the depolymerization of polymer. Xu and Xiao (1994) reported that chitosan was sulfated in sulfuric acid (95%, 90%, and 80%) at $-10°C–0°C$ for 3 hours, and the MW of the resulting product was 2.51×10^4 Da.

Vikhoreva et al. (2005) prepared a sulfating complex by adding small portions of oleum to a DMF excess (3–4 mol oleum and 29 mol DMF per mole of chitosan at $0°C–5°C$) and reacted it with DMF-activated chitosan at $60°C$ with stirring for 1–3 hours. Heating 30% oleum over phosphoric anhydride generates sulfur trioxide, which with DMF forms solid complex soluble in excess DMF.

Trimethylamine-sulfur trioxide (Me_3N-SO_3), which is known to achieve selective N-sulfation of amino alcohols, has been employed for sulfation of chitosan (Warner 1958). Lyophilized chitosan dispersed in sufficient dilute sodium carbonate solution pH ~9 was heated at $55°C–65°C$ with $Me_3N:SO_3$ (~3:1) until a clear viscous solution or gel was formed (4–12 hours) to achieve N-sulfation (Holme and Perlin 1997; Je et al. 2005). Isolation at that point provided low degree of sulfation (DS) products (~0.50), whereas continued heating resulted in the formation of the additional range of DS 0.4–0.86 (±0.05). Attempts to prepare similar products by pre-dissolving the chitosan in aqueous acetic acid, then neutralizing, and introducing the Me_3N-SO_3 without isolation of the dispersed material were unsuccessful. The low-MW sulfated chitosan was prepared by dissolving chitosan in an aqueous medium and reacting with pyridine-SO_3 complex for 1 hour maintaining the pH at 9 and neutralizing with sulfuric acid on completion of the reaction (Gamzazade et al. 1997a).

$ClSO_3H$ is the most commonly used sulfating reagent. Naggi et al. (1986) used a precooled mixture of sulfuric acid-$ClSO_3H$ (2:1) in the ratio of polymer:total sulfating agent as 1 gm:24–60 mL. The reaction was carried out for 1 hour at room temperature and terminated by pouring the reaction mixture in dimethyl ether to get chitosan 6-sulfate.

The conventional process of sulfation of chitosan by heating polymer with pyridine-$ClSO_3H$ however has its difficulties as a lack of reproducibility and a very poor color of the finished product due to the interaction of pyridine with the polysaccharide at the elevated temperature. To avoid these difficulties, Cushing et al. (1954) used dichloroethane as a solvent for reaction of chitin with $ClSO_3H$ and solvents such as water, triethylamine, ethyl alcohol, and isopropyl alcohol for isolation of sulfated product.

Gamzazade et al. (1997a) expounded the action of DCAA as an acid solvent. Chitosan sulfates were prepared under different conditions such as pseudo-homogeneous, homogeneous, and semi-heterogeneous (swollen) with the use of a sulfating reagent such as $ClSO_3H$ or oleum (30% sulfur trioxide) in DMF at 0°C–4°C. DCAA was used as a solvent for pseudo-homogeneous and homogeneous methods. In the pseudo-homogeneous method, sulfated chitosan was prepared by reacting 2% chitosan solution in an anhydrous solvent of DMF:DCAA (60:1 w/w) with $ClSO_3H$ reagent. The reaction was run at room temperature for 4 hours, which resulted in the gel formation. At the end of the reaction, the gel was diluted with water, neutralized by sodium hydroxide, and precipitated with methanol. The homogeneous method of sulfated chitosan was followed by using 3% chitosan solution and the anhydrous mixture of DMF:DCAA (40:1 w/w) with $ClSO_3H$. The reaction was run at 50°C for 1 hour. The solvent DCAA however is expensive and noxious; therefore, Xing et al. (2005a) tried cheap and non-noxious formic acid (88%) in its place. With $ClSO_3H$-DMF, sulfation of chitosan under homogeneous conditions using formic acid as the solvent presented satisfying results in the form of higher yield and equivalent sulfur contents compared to the DCAA solvent. In the semi-heterogeneous method, chitosan was activated by dissolving it in acetic acid, precipitating with sodium hydroxide, and washing with methanol and DMF for 12 hours. This solvated chitosan was reacted with a sulfating reagent at room temperature for 1 hour to get to a swollen state and then neutralized. To improve the substitution, chitosan was reacted (solvated over a period of 1 hour) with $ClSO_3H$ in cold DMF at room temperature for 5 hours (Vongchan et al. 2002). Sulfated products obtained under homogeneous conditions displayed more heterogeneity and were considered as copolymers of chitosan 6-monosulfate and 3,6-disulfate, whereas those produced by semi-heterogeneous synthesis were considered preferentially as chitosan 3,6-disulfate.

For sulfation of highly acetylated chitosan or chitin, the solvent system used was LiCl/DMA to get homogeneous conditions (Terbojevich et al. 1989). Zou and Khor

(2009) have reported recently the temperature-dependent regioselectivity of sulfation using sulfur trioxide-pyridine complex as a sulfating agent at 8°C or room temperature. It was selective for the O-6 position with the DS ranging from 0.53 to 1.00, depending on the reaction time. At elevated temperatures, DS at O-6 position was elevated, as also sulfation at O-3 position. The extent of sulfation at the O-3 position was a function of the concentration of sulfating reagent, reaction time, and temperature. (Zou and Khor 2009).

Selective substitution of –SO3⁻ group at N-2, O-3, and O-6 positions in chitosan is possible with combination of protection of hydroxyl group by tritylation and of amino group by acetylation or phathaloylation, followed by sulfation and then deprotection of added groups. Baumann and Faust (2001) reported the synthesis of 3-sulfated chitosan by 6-desulfation of 3,6-di-sulfated chitosan (Figure 7.2). For desulfation, the pyridinium salt of this 3,6-disulfated chitosan

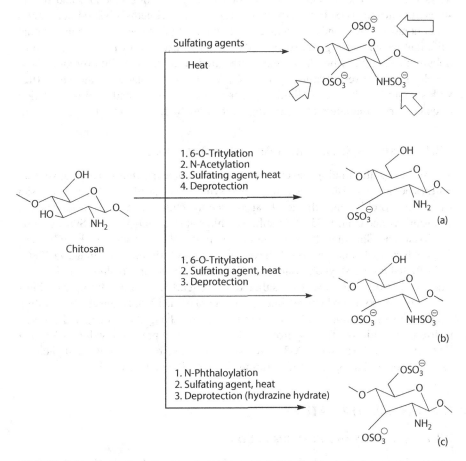

FIGURE 7.2 Synthesis of sulfated chitosan. 6-O-Tritylation includes treatment with (a) phthalic anhydride, ethylene glycol, DMF, 130°C; (b) trityl chloride, pyridine-4-dimethyl-aminopyridine, 90°C; and (c) NH₂-NH₂. H₂O, 100°C. N-Acetylation includes treatment with acetic anhydride and DMF-MeOH.

was treated with N-methyl-N-(trimethylsilyl)trifluoroacetamide in pyridine solvent (Baumann and Faust 2001).

The sulfation of chitosan was performed in a microwave oven using SO_3-DMF reagent at a power of 480–800 W for 70–120 seconds conveniently to get a wide range of products of different DSs by changing the reaction time or/and the radiation power. However, microwave radiation accelerated the degradation of sulfated chitosan, and the MW of sulfated chitosan was considerably lower than that obtained by traditional heating (chitosan with an MW of 1.25×10^5 Da gave sulfated chitosans in the range of $4.41 \times 10^3 – 34.6 \times 10^3$ Da) (Xing et al. 2004).

Recently, silylation reaction has been used to improve the solubility of chitin and chitosan in organic solvents. This provides a new approach to modify the chitinous compounds (Kurita et al. 2005). Sulfation of silylated chitin and chitosan has also been reported in the work of Yang et al. (2013), where chitosans of different MWs (51.5–112.4 kDa) were selected for trimethylsilylation reaction, and highly sulfated chitosans (DS 1.65–2.46) were prepared via trimethylsilylated derivatives under homogeneous conditions with conventional sulfating agents. The conventional sulfating agents and organic solvents can result in extreme hydrolyzation, serious pollution and security problems, and degradation of the reactant. To overcome these drawbacks, the novel sulfating agent $N(SO_3Na)_3$ was synthesized by Fan et al. (2012) with sodium bisulfite and sodium nitrite in aqueous solution and used for sulfation of quaternary ammonium chitosans and carboxymethytl chitosans (Tao et al. 2013).

7.2.1 CHITOSAN SULFATES WITH ADDITIONAL FUNCTIONS

The reaction with sulfating reagents can be carried out using chitosan derivatives too. Sulfur trioxide with DMF was employed to synthesize O-sulfated N-acetyl chitosan from N-acetyl chitosan, sulfated O-carboxymethyl chitosan from O-carboxymethyl chitosan (Hirano et al. 1985), N,O-sulfated chitosan from SO_3-DMF or SO_3-pyridine (Wolfrom and Shienhan 1959; Hirano et al. 1985; Whistler and Kosik 1971), sulfated N-hexanoyl chitosan from N-hexanoyl chitosan (Hirano and Kinugawa 1986), and sulfated N-myristoyl chitosan from N-myristoyl chitosan (Yoshioka et al. 1993). The sulfated derivatives such as sulfated-3, 6-O-carboxymethyl chitin, and chitosan from carboxymethyl chitin/chitosan (Ishihara et al. 1995; Hagiwara et al. 1999), N-alkyl-O-sulfated chitosan from N-alkyl-chitosan (Zhang et al. 2003), and sulfated hydroxyethyl chitosan from hydroxyethyl chitosan were prepared with $ClSO_3H$ and DMF. The N-carboxymethyl N-3,6-chitosan trisulfate from N-carboxymethyl chitosan was prepared using $ClSO_3H$-pyridine (Muzzarelli and Giacomelli 1987).

7.3 CHARACTERIZATION

7.3.1 SOLUBILITY AND BEHAVIOR IN SOLUTION

Unlike chitosan that is soluble only in acidic pH (<6.5), the sulfonated derivative was soluble over a wide pH range. Holme and Perlin (1997) synthesized sulfated chitosan derivatives with DS ranging from 0.4 to 0.86 (± 0.05) from chitosans with DDA of 96%, 90%, and 78%. All were soluble in water. The initial N-acetyl content of the chitosan had bearing on the solubility and *N*-sulfation reaction, that is, the sample having fewer *N*-acetyl groups required longer reaction periods to become fully solubilized, which occurred when the DS level reached about one-half its final value. With the most highly acetylated material, by contrast, dissolution of the solids occurred at relatively lower DS levels. The qualitative observations too suggested that the solubility of the isolated products was dependent upon DDA for materials having similar DS values. These observations suggest that not only the sulfoamino substituents but also the co-occurrence of a substantial proportion of acetamido groups are important for efficient disruption of interchain associations within a chitosan suspension, and that solubility is imparted more readily by a specific combination of the two substituents, for example, 4:1 *N*-sulfate-*N*-acetyl. Presumably, an initially broad distribution of acetamido groups also contributes to a more favorable overall substitution pattern.

The synthesized derivatives, isolated as sodium salts, on solubilization in water at 0.5% concentration had pH ~8 and were pseudoplastic. They were less soluble in aqueous acidic media, giving higher viscosity solutions, gels, or precipitates, depending on the DS and DDA.

The effect of alteration of pH on the behavior of the solution of sulfated chitosan polymeric chains was studied. For this, the acidification of aqueous solutions of chitosan sulfate having a DDA of 76% and a DS of 34 or 56 was followed stepwise by turbidimetry, dynamic light scattering, and electrophoresis (Schatz et al. 2005). With the highest sulfated chitosan, no turbidity was recorded between pH 7.8 and 2.0, traducing a high apparent solubility of the polymer chains in this domain of pH. With the lowest sulfated chitosan, a steady increase in turbidity was monitored from pH 6.90 to 6.15 followed by the flocculation of the polymer at pH ~6.0. In this range of pH, the polymer phase separated to yield particles having hydrodynamic diameters decreasing from 350 to 260 nm and an almost constant negative charge. The particles could be separated from the reaction medium and concentrated by centrifugation–redispersion cycles without alteration of their structure. A spontaneous phase separation observed at low levels of sulfation and pH above the isoelectric point was due to self-association of the polymer chains by electrostatic interactions between the protonated amino residues and the sulfate functions. At high sulfation, electrostatic repulsion forces prevented macromolecules from aggregating into colloidal particles at any pH.

7.3.2 MOLECULAR WEIGHT

The MWs of chitin heparinoids were estimated from viscosity measurements using Ubbelohde-type viscometer (ASTM D 445 and ISO 3104) by applying Mark–Houwink equation $[\eta] = KM_v^a$. Where K and a are constants, M_v is viscosity average molecular weight. The equation was $[\eta] = 1.75 \times 10^{-5} M_v^{0.98}$ or $[\eta] = 4.97 \times 10^{-5} M_v^{0.77}$ in the solvent 0.1 M NaCl at 25°C (Noreyka et al. 1895; Nishimura and Tokura 1987; Drozd et al. 2001). In the solvent 0.1 M CH_3COOH/0.2 M NaCl, the Mark–Houwink parameters were $a = 0.96$, and $K = 1.424$ at 25°C when the intrinsic viscosity was expressed in mL/g.

7.3.3 FOURIER TRANSFORM INFRARED SPECTROSCOPY

The basic characteristic peaks of chitosan are at 3455 cm^{-1} (O–H stretch), 2923–2867 cm^{-1} (C–H stretch), 1598–1600 cm^{-1} (N–H bend), 1154 cm^{-1} (bridge-O stretch), and 1094 cm^{-1} (C–O stretch) (Shigemasa et al. 1996; Brugnerotto et al. 2001). In addition to the peaks of chitosan, the sulfated chitosan infrared (IR) spectrum shows the characteristic absorption bands of S=O, C–O–S, and –N–S bonds (Figure 7.3). There are specific absorption bands of sulfate groups in the area of 1200–1260 cm^{-1}, representing asymmetric valence fluctuations of SO$_2$ and the band of symmetric valence fluctuations at 1060 cm^{-1}; there are also bands of S–O bonds in the area of 580–625 cm^{-1} and valence fluctuations of C–O–S in the area of 800 cm^{-1}.

7.3.4 PROTON NUCLEAR MAGNETIC RESONANCE

For proton nuclear magnetic resonance (^{1}H NMR), the samples were dissolved in deuterium oxide (D$_2$O) that contained Na$_2$CO$_3$ (pD ~9), and were repeatedly evaporated (3–4 times) and redissolved in D$_2$O, to give a final concentration of ~2% w/v 70°C, and were referenced to internal sodium 2,2,3,3-tetradeuterio-4,4-dimethyl-4-silapentanoate. Otherwise, the recording of ^{1}H NMR spectra was done with D$_2$O as the solvent and sodium 2,2-dimethyl-2-silapentane-5-sulfonate as the internal reference (Vongchan et al. 2003).

The major peaks observed in ^{1}H NMR (4,4-dimethyl-4-silapentane-1-sulfonic acid, D$_2$O) were: δ 4.98 (d, 1H, H-1), 4.60 (br t, 1H, H-3S), 4.35–4.25 (m, 2H, H-4, H-5), 4.00 (br d, 2H, H-6S), 3.41 (br t, 1H, H-2S), 3.18 (br t, 1H, H-2), and 2.08 (s, 3H, CH3). The major peak at δ 3.41 and the minor one at δ 3.18 indicated the substitution of H-2S and also confirmed the decrease of free amino groups compared to the starting chitosan. Separation of the 1H signals for H-6S, H-3S, and H-2S was enhanced by recording the spectra at pD ~9, rather than at neutrality (Figure 7.4). The data are comparable to those reported by Holme and Perlin (1997).

7.3.5 CARBON-13 NUCLEAR MAGNETIC RESONANCE

Samples for carbon-13 nuclear magnetic resonance (^{13}C NMR) were typically 5%–10% w/v in D$_2$O containing Na$_2$CO$_3$ (pD ~9); their spectra were recorded at 70°C and referenced with respect to external tetramethylsilane.

Naggi et al. (1986) reported the ^{13}CNMR of chitosan-6-sulfate that essentially consisted of six major signals as given in Table 7.1. Signals were shifted to different extents with respect to chitosan. Shifts for carbon 1–5 were relatively small, whereas the C6 signal was shifted to downfield by ~6 ppm due to sulfation at this carbon. These major peaks are accompanied by minor signals of N-acetylglucosamine units (Figure 7.5).

For accounting the structural features of sulfated chitosan, Gamzazade et al. (1997a) recorded the NMR spectra of sulfated chitosan prepared under differing conditions at 80°C in D$_2$O with acetone as the internal reference (δ$_H$ ~2.23 and δ$_C$ ~31.45 ppm). The spectrum of chitosan 3,6-disulfate prepared under pseudo-homogeneous

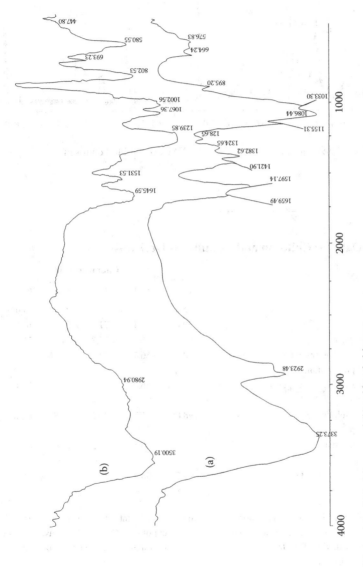

FIGURE 7.3 IR spectra of (a) chitosan and (b) sulfated chitosan.

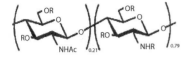

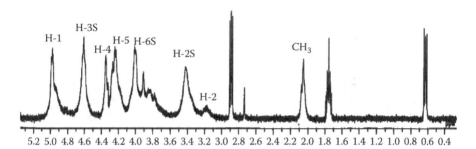

FIGURE 7.4   The major peaks observed in ^{1}H NMR of sulfated chitosan.

TABLE 7.1
^{13}CNMR Data for Chitosan and Its Sulfated Derivatives

Compound	Chemical Shift					
	C-1	C-2	C-3	C-4	C-5	C-6
β-D-Glucosamine	95.2	59.5	74.5	74.2	78.6	63.1
Chitosan	99.0	57.1	71.6	78.7	76.1	61.7
Chitosan 6-sulfate[a]	98.0	56.8	74.3	77.5	74.8	68.2
Chitosan 3,6-disulfate (pseudohomogeneous condition of preparation)[b]	98.1	56.7	77.3	75.1	74.3	68.2
Chitosan 3,6-disulfate (homogeneous condition of preparation)[b]	97.8	56.7	77.0	75.1	74.4	68.2
Chitosan 3,6-disulfate (semiheterogeneous condition of preparation)[b]	98.0	56.7	77.2	74.9	74.4	68.4
High-MW N,3,6-trisulfated chitosan[b,c]	97.8	56.5	77.2	74.6	74.1	67.9
	99.7	—	—	—	—	—
Low-MW N,3,6-trisulfated chitosan[c,d]	99.7	56.5	71.7	77.2	73.7	67.9
	97.8	—	—	—	—	—

[a] Data are given with additive correction by −1 ppm due to different references in the works of Naggi et al. (1986) and Gamzazade et al. (1997b). The assignment of C-3, C-4, and C-5 must be corrected in accordance with data for chitosan 3,6-disulfate (pseudo-homogeneous condition of preparation of chitosan-3,6-disulfate.

[b] Data for glucosamine-3,6-disulfate residue.

[c] The first and second values of C-1 chemical shift belong to the residues glycosylating 3,6-di- and 6-mono-sulfated residues, respectively.

[d] Data for glucosamine-6-sulfate residue.

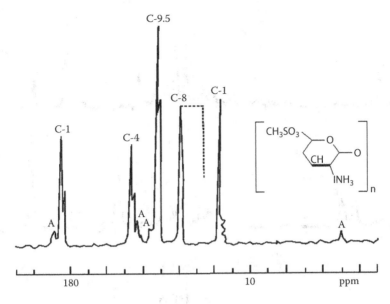

FIGURE 7.5 ^{13}C NMR spectrum (75 MHz) of chitosan-6-sulfate in D2O (pD 8). Signal A represents N-acetylated residues. The arrow shows the shift of the C-6 signal from its typical position of native chitosan.

condition in DMF:DCAA (60:1) at 22°C for 4 hours with ClSO$_3$H (Figure 7.6a) was very similar to that of chitosan 6-sulfate reported by Naggi et al. (1986). The unusual low-field signal of H3 at 4.6 ppm in the ^{1}H NMR spectrum of the polymer (instead of that characteristic of chitosan 6-sulfate at ~4 ppm) is correlated with C3 with a chemical shift at 77.3 ppm in the presence of an electronegative sulfate substituent at this carbon atom. Additional ^{13}C NMR experiments with variation of the pD of the samples in the interval 1–13 confirmed the assignment of the signal at 77.3 ppm to C3. This signal (as well as the signal for the anomeric carbon) showed the sharpest dependence on pD, which is the characteristic of carbons neighboring CHNH$_2$ in amino sugars. The change in pD from 1 to 13 provided a downfield shift of these signals by 4–5 ppm, whereas the other signals shifted by no more than 1.5 ppm. The comparison of chemical shifts for the corresponding carbon atoms in the ^{13}C NMR spectra of chitosan and chitosan 3,6-disulfate shows the typical α and β effects of sulfation for pyranoses (Archibald et al. 1981). The ^{13}C NMR spectrum of high-MW chitosan 3,6-disulfate (prepared under homogeneous condition in DMF:DCAA (40:1) at 50°C for 1 hour with oleum:DMF) is practically identical to the spectrum of chitosan 3,6-disulfate. Minor signals at 62, 72, and 102 ppm are additionally observed with residues that are not sulfated at C3 and/or C6 positions as with sulfated chitosan prepared under semi-heterogeneous or swollen condition with oleum:DMF. The first two signals belong to C6 and C3 of the residues without sulfate at these positions, and the third is probably C1 of the residues with N-acetyl groups.

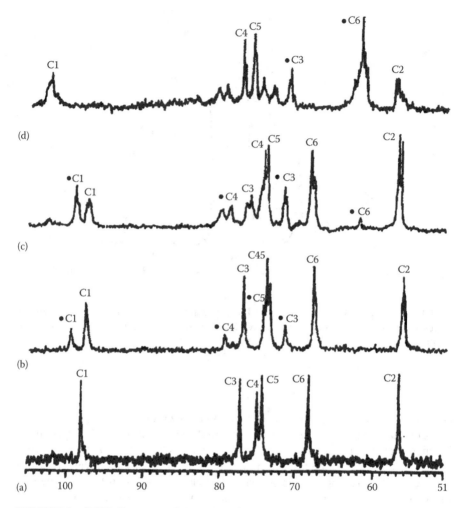

FIGURE 7.6 ^{13}C NMR spectra of chitosan sulfates: (a) chitosan-3,6-disulfate; (b) high-MW chitosan-*N*,3,6–trisulfate; (c) low-MW chitosan-*N*,3,6–trisulfate; (d) chitosan-*N*,3-disulfate. *C, signals of unmodified groups.

The spectrum of high-MW *N*,3,6-trisulfated chitosan obtained from sulfation of high-MW chitosan at 22°C under homogeneous condition with DMF:DCAA (40:1) appeared to be slightly more complicated (Figure 7.6b). It contains minor peaks of 6-substituted residues with diagnostic signals at 67.9 (C6) and 71.7 (C3) ppm, together with the set of main signals belonging to 3,6-di-substituted residues (Hirano et al. 1991). The integral intensity ratio of the major and minor peaks is close to 2:1. The signal with very small intensity at 79.6 ppm may relate to C3 of 2,3,6-tri- or 2,3-disubstituted residues because N-sulfation and N-acetylation shift the C3 signal to low field.

The spectrum of low-MW *N*,3,6-trisulfate chitosan obtained from low-MW chitosan at 22°C under homogeneous condition with DMF:DCAA (40:1) and oleum:DMF complex proved to be the most complicated (Figure 7.6c). Like the spectrum of high-MW *N*,3,6-trisulfated chitosan, it contains two sets of signals belonging to 6- and 3,6-O-sulfated sugar residues. In addition, all but a few signals in both sets are split. The splitting is presumably connected with partial N-sulfation and/or with the influence of neighboring residues with different structures. Additional irregularity may be caused by the presence of residues that are not sulfated at C6 position.

Sulfated chitosan produced in the aqueous medium with pyridine-SO_3 did not bear 6-O-sulfates but had $-SO_3^-$ only at N2 and O3 positions (Figure 7.6d). The absence of a signal at ~68 ppm and the presence of an intense signal at 62 ppm are confirming that signals cannot be excluded. The irregularity and the complexity of this spectrum may be attributed to the presence of 3-O-sulfate groups and the presence of a nonstoichiometrical amount of N-acetylated and N-sulfated groups. The absence of C1 signals at 95–99 ppm, the characteristic signal for chitosan and its O-sulfates, suggests the total substitution of amino groups (Table 7.1).

7.3.6 X-RAY DIFFRACTION

Changes in the X-ray diffraction diagrams of the product, in contrast with native crab chitin and chitosan, were evident (Figure 7.7). The original chitin powder showed three major crystalline peaks at $2\theta = 38.3°$, $23.1°$, and $19°$, and two major peaks were observed at $2\theta = 19.9°$ and $11.1°$ in case of chitosan with a DDA of 89%. However, the peaks in the X-ray diffraction diagrams of chitosan polysulfate were apparently broader than those of chitin and chitosan, suggesting lower crystallinity or a less

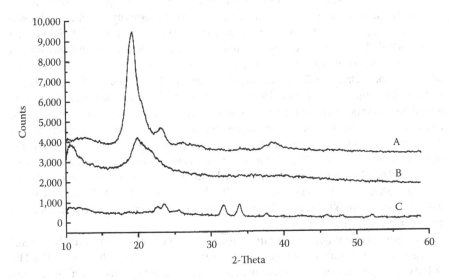

FIGURE 7.7 X-ray powder diffraction patterns of marine crab shell chitin and its derivatives: A—chitin, B—chitosan, and C—chitosan polysulfate.

ordered structure. These results indicated that destruction of the rigid crystalline structure of chitin and chitosan is of great importance for successful solubilization (Vongchan et al. 2003).

7.4   BIOLOGICAL ACTIVITIES AND APPLICATIONS

7.4.1   ANTICOAGULANT ACTIVITY

Chitosan sulfate is structurally similar to the direct action anticoagulant heparin and possesses similar properties. Nonfractionated heparin with an average MW of 5,000–25,000 Da equally inhibits the key enzymes of the blood coagulation cascade, namely, serine proteases, such as thrombin (IIa factor) and Xa factor, whereas low MW heparins (MW 5000–7000) exhibit a higher anti-factor Xa activity (anti-Xa). Sulfated chitosan derivatives too accelerate the inactivation of thrombin (factor IIa) and inhibit Xa factor forming an equimolar complex with antithrombin III (Nishimura et al. 1986).

It had been of interest to study the influence of a chitosan sulfate MW onto its anticoagulant activity. N,O-Chitosan sulfates with an MW of 12,000 do not have the anti-Xa activity, whereas N,O-chitosan sulfates with a little bit higher MW (19,000–71,000) do have this activity. Varying MWs within this range does not influence its level. Study with 3,6-chitosan sulfates with low MW (9000–35,000 Da, DS = 1.10–1.63) demonstrated regular increase of the anti-Xa activity like heparin on lowering of the MW of chitosan sulfates (Vikhoreva et al. 2005). However, it could not be established whether the correlation of a sulfated chitosan MW and the ratio of anti-Xa/anti-IIa activity is analogous to that of heparin.

Drozd et al. (2001) investigated the anticoagulant activity of sulfated chitosan with an average MW of 20–130 kDa and sulfur amounts of 8.8%–16.9% in *in vitro and in vivo* models. In the *in vitro* system, the maximal antithrombin activity of sulfated chitosan was 40.3 ± 2.2 IU/mg. The clear dependence of the specific activity on MWs had not been marked. The specific activity was found to increase with increasing amounts of sulfur. The team demonstrated that sulfated chitosan with a degree of polymerization of 71–547 and a DS of 0.62–1.86 exhibited a nonlinear disappearance of the anticoagulant activity in the *in vivo* model. The IIa activity in the *in vivo* system was from 0.5 to 52.0 IU/mg, had positive correlation with sulfation degree, and had a moderate negative connection with the polymerization degree. Sulfated chitosans with a polymerization degree of <188 and >252 did not have a great antithrombin activity. Low-MW and high sulfation samples of sulfated chitosans were slowly removed and had a longer time of action. The elimination constant increased with decreasing sulfation degree; that is, patterns with lesser sulfation degree (0.62–0.75) were rather of short duration of action with elimination for 60 minutes. The correlation between degree of polymerization and elimination constant was not found.

The anticoagulant activity of chitosan sulfate largely results from its high level of negative charge density produced by the sulfate groups (Huynh et al. 2001). The orderly arrangement of the sulfate groups is more beneficial to thrombin clotting time (TCT) anticoagulant activity of the sulfated polysaccharides in comparison with that of activated partial thromboplastin time (APTT). The higher DS yielded the better anticoagulant activity.

The regioselective introduction of sulfate group(s) at N_2 and/or O_3 had little effect on generating the anticoagulant activity, whereas 6-O-sulfated chitin strongly inhibited blood coagulation (Nishimura et al. 1998). The O6 sulfate group is essential for activity as its desulfation leads to lack of anticoagulant activity. It should be preferably accompanied by sulfation at other positions. Zou and Khor (2009) stated the significance of continuous sequence of 3,6 S units for getting high anticoagulation activity. The N-sulfate group need not be present to a high degree of substitution. Warner and Coleman (1958) selectively N-sulfated all the amino groups of chitosan but obtained a product possessing no anticoagulant activity. However, a further increase in the sulfation to 18.3% sulfur, wherein a number of O-sulfate groups were present in the product, caused it to show an anticoagulant activity of 60 IU/mg. This activity is still much less than the 134 IU/mg exhibited by heparin, which has a sulfur content of only 12%–13%. The observation suggests that uronic carboxyl groups contribute significantly to the anticoagulant activity of heparin. Keeping this in mind, uronic acid carboxyl groups were introduced into N-sulfated and N-sulfated-partly-O-sulfated chitosan oxidized by dinitrogen tetraoxide or by oxygen over Adams platinum catalyst. The degree of substitution of uronic acid carboxyl was 0.24 (compared to the 0.5 of heparin, where every other sugar unit in the chain was a uronic acid). Introduction of uronic acid groups still further increased the anticoagulant activity by about 10 units at all sulfate levels (Whistler and Kosik 1971).

Generally, 6-O-sulfate groups was a prerequisite for the anticoagulant activity, but Horton and Just (1973) reported that complete 6-O-carboxylated and N-sulfated chitosan derivatives showed an anticoagulant activity of 25.8 IU/mg. The carboxymethyl groups increase cooperative effect of sulfate groups and add the anticoagulant activity of sulfated chitosan (Muzzarelli et al. 1984, 1986). Carboxymethyl chitosan sulfate was demonstrated to have greater inhibition on the transformation of fibrinogen to fibrin than chitosan sulfate. Carboxymethylation seems to impart activity if directed to the amino group rather than to the C6. However, Hirano et al. (1991) reported that O-carboxylated chitosan sulfate gave poor delaying effect of heparin on APTT and TT, but provided better inhibition of the complexation of thrombin and antithrombin III. According to Muzzarelli (1986), N-carboxymethyl chitosan trisulfate behavior was distinctly different from heparin that this compound showed an action on the factors participating in the intrinsic pathways, whereas the factors of the extrinsic and common pathways of the coagulation process were unaffected.

The anticoagulant activity of carboxybutyrylated hydroxyethyl chitosan sulfate was studied by Huang et al. (2003a). The introduction of carboxyl groups (carboxybutyryl) to amino groups greatly prolonged the APTT and TT. However, carboxylation at N and O positions gave better results than that at only N positions. The best result occurred when the degree of substitution of the carboxyl groups was ~0.4/unit that prolonged APTT and TT ~5 and 1.5 times compared to that of the uncarboxylated hydroxyethyl chitosan sulfates. Chitosan sulfate with low sulfur content and 6-O-desulfated chitosan sulfate showed little anticoagulant activity, but their N,O-carboxybutyrylated derivatives (0.6/unit degree of substitution) showed an increased APTT or TT, whereas their N-carboxybutyrylated derivatives (0.6/unit degree of substitution) gave no improvement. The introduction of carboxyl groups could not increase the prothrombin time in spite of the position introduced.

To study the effect of acetyl or acyl group content on the anticoagulant activity of sulfated chitosan, two types of hydrophobic groups were introduced onto the amino groups of the chitosan sulfate: *N*-propanoyl and *N*-hexanoyl. Another reason for the introduction of acyl groups was to improve the hydrophobicity of the chitosan sulfate, which had been confirmed to enhance the anticoagulant activity in dextran sulfate. The propanoyl and hexanoyl groups increased the APTT activity, and the propanoyl groups also increased the TT anticoagulant activity slightly (Huang et al. 2003b). In addition, N,O-quaternary substituted chitosan sulfates were also studied to verify that the anticoagulant activity of the sulfates was largely dependent on the density of negative groups. Here the quaternary nitrogen-containing group was $-CH_2CH(OH)CH_2N^+(CH_3)_3Cl^-$ introduced on the reaction with glycidyltrimethylammonium chloride.

In an attempt to bestow the biocompatibility to single-walled carbon nanotubes, *N*-octyl-*O*-sulfate chitosan was used for wrapping of nanotubes. The anticoagulant activity of polymer-wrapped nanotubes was similar to tha of polymer alone. This property of *N*-octyl-*O*-sulfate chitosan would eliminate the coagulation risk displayed by unwrapped single-walled carbon nanotubes (Roldo et al. 2009).

7.4.2 Activity on Red Blood Cells and Hemagglutination Inhibition

In hemagglutination inhibition assay developed to analyze the adhesion property of *Theileria sergenti* merozoites to bovine red blood cells (RBCs) (Bo-RBCs), a 3,6-O-sulfated derivative of carboxymethyl chitin showed a potent inhibitory activity. 6-*O*-Carboxymethyl chitin and N-sulfated derivative of N-deacetylated carboxymethyl chitin, however, were not effective. It is likely that the (1–4)-linked units composed of *N*-acetyl,3,6-O-sulfated glucosamine in the structure preferentially interfere with the merozoite–Bo-RBC interaction (Hagiwara et al. 1999).

In severe combined immunodeficient mouse model where circulating RBCs are entirely substituted with human RBCs (Hu-RBCs), Hu-RBCs show relatively short life span probably due to their rapid clearance by reticulo-endothelial system. When Hu-RBCs were transfused simultaneously with sulfated carboxymethyl chitin, their lifetime in the blood circulation was prolonged significantly. Sulfated chitosan showed only a weak decelerating activity on the clearance of Hu-RBCs, whereas carboxymethyl chitin, which was used as an unsulfated control compound, had no effect on the Hu-RBC clearance. Clearance deceleration by this sulfated polysaccharide was primarily attributed to the inhibition of phagocytosis of the reticuloendothelial system.

7.4.3 Wound Repair

The migration phase of wound repair involves the movement of epithelial cells and fibroblasts to the injured area to replace damaged and lost tissue. Soon after the injury, hyaluronan is predominant in granulation tissue. As hyaluronan wanes, sulfated glycosoaminoglycans predominate. The temporal relationship between the transition from unsulfated to sulfated glycosoaminoglycans and the phenotypic changes in fibroblasts in the wound bed suggest that these two events are interrelated. This possibility was investigated and confirmed by using chitosan and sulfated chitosan (Mariappan et al. 1997). The ability of cultured human foreskin fibroblast to bind and to contact lattices of collagen, collagen-chitosan, and collagen-sulfated chitosan was determined. The results show that chitosan sulfation markedly enhances fibroblast adhesion and promotes contraction of collagen lattice compared to the unsulfated material.

However, the sulfation of chitosan reduced the platelet adhesion as observed in *in vitro* platelet adhesion assay (Lin and Lin 2001). For the observation, the chitosan membrane was directly surface treated by SO_3-pyridine in aqueous acidic and aqueous alkaline media and by SO_3-DMF in DMF in acidic medium. Surface characterization study was carried out using electron spectroscopy for chemical analysis, FTIR, and contact angle measurement. The surface reaction of SO_3-pyridine in aqueous acid medium generated *N,O*-sulfated chitosan with cationic $-NH_3^+$ groups. After neutralization, this surface had shown to induce a low degree of platelet adhesion and activation. Although the DS was lower in alkaline medium than in aqueous medium, the N-sulfated chitosan significantly reduced the adhesion and activation of platelets. Reaction of SO_3-DMF in acidic medium yielded high DS with cationic $-NH_3^+$ groups. On this surface, fully spread platelets and some platelet aggregates were found instead. This may be attributed to the ionic interactions between the platelet membrane surface and the cationic groups on the modified chitosan membrane.

7.4.4 ANTIOXIDANT ACTIVITY

Xing et al. (2005b) established the antioxidant activity of high sulfate containing chitosans and studied the antioxidant potential of differently substituted sulfated chitosans in *in vitro* models (Xing et al. 2005b). The antioxidant potencies were investigated employing various established *in vitro* systems, such as 1,1′-diphenyl-2-picrylhydrazyl (DPPH)/superoxide/hydroxyl radical scavenging, reducing power, iron ion chelation, and total antioxidant activity. The data obtained by *in vitro* models clearly established the antioxidant potency and free radical scavenging activities of all kinds of sulfated chitosans. All kinds of sulfated chitosans (*N*,3,6-sulfated chitosan [HCTS], 3,6-sulfated chitosan [TSCTS], 6-sulfated chitosan [SCTS], 3-sulfated chitosan [TCTS]) showed a strong inhibitory activity toward superoxide radical by the phenazine methosulfate-NADH system compared to ascorbic acid. According to the aforementioned order, their half maximal inhibitory concentration (IC50) values were 0.012, 0.040, 0.015, and 0.022 mg/mL, respectively; however, the scavenging activity of ascorbic acid on superoxide radical was 68.19% at 2.0 mg/mL. The scavenging activity of superoxide radical was found to be on the order of HCTS > SCTS > TCTS > TSCTS > ascorbic acid. Furthermore, all kinds of sulfated chitosans exhibited a strong concentration-dependent inhibition of deoxyribose oxidation. Except for HCTS, others had a stronger scavenging activity on hydroxyl radical than ascorbic acid. The scavenging effect of TSCTS on DPPH radical was little lower than that of butyl hydroxyl anisole, but better than that of others. All kinds of sulfated chitosans were efficient in the reducing power, especially TSCTS. The TSCTS and TCTS showed a considerable ferrous ion chelating potency.

Growing evidence indicates that oxidized low-density lipoprotein (LDL) may promote atherogenesis. Therefore, inhibition of LDL oxidation may impede this process. The effect of chitin sulfate on the susceptibility of human LDL to macrophage-induced oxidation was investigated by monitoring a thiobarbituric acid reactive substance (TBARS). Chitin sulfate inhibited LDL oxidation by macrophages in a dose-dependent manner, with a 50–100 µM, as assessed by TBARS assay. Chitin sulfate, at 100 µM, almost completely inhibited the macrophage-induced increase in the electrophoretic mobility of LDL. Also, chitin sulfate almost completely inhibited O_2^- at a concentration of 100 µM (Ryu et al. 2001).

The result of studies with hydroxyethyl chitosan sulfate showed different results in direct spin trapping techniques and in linoleic acid model system (Huang et al. 2005). Hydroxyethyl chitosan sulfate was an effective scavenger of DPPH (33.78%, 2.5 mg/mL) and carbon-centered radical (67.74%, 0.25 mg/mL). However, it did not exhibit any scavenging activity against hydroxyl radicals. This was different from the published literature and was presumed due to the loss of chelating ability on Fe^{2+}. This assumption was further confirmed from the results obtained for Fe^{2+}-ferrozine method that upon sulfation chitooligosaccharide lost its chelation properties. Therefore, hydroxyethyl chitosan sulfate could be identified as an antioxidant that effectively scavenges carbon-centered radicals to retard lipid peroxidation.

The antioxidative capacity and the blockade of the nuclear factor (NF)-κB signaling pathway by sulfated chitooligosaccharides were shown to be responsible for generating protective effects against H_2O_2-induced apoptosis in pancreatic MIN6 cells (Lu et al. 2013).

7.4.5 ANTITUMOR ACTIVITY

Murata et al. (1989) reported that 6-O-sulfated chitin, 6-O-sulfated-carboxymethyl chitin, and sulfated carboxymethyl chitin (SCM-chitin) with a high DS significantly inhibited the lung tumor colonization of B16-BL6 melanoma in experimental and spontaneous lung metastasis model (Murata et al. 1989). The mechanism responsible for the inhibition of lung metastasis by SCM-chitin probably was through inhibition of tumor cell adhesion to subendothelial matrix (Murata et al. 1990). Saiki et al. (1990) further investigated the effects of sulfated chitin derivatives and heparin on the invasion of B16-BL6 melanoma cells through reconstituted basement membrane. Matrigel containing adhesion molecules such as laminin, type IV collagen, heparan sulfate proteoglycan, and entactin serve as substrates *in vitro* to promote the adhesion, spreading, and migration of tumor cells. 6-O-Sulfated chitin and 6-O-sulfated and carboxymethyl chitin significantly inhibited the penetration of tumor cells through Matrigel in parallel with the increased DS. However, 6-O- and N-sulfated chitosan derivative and carboxymethyl chitin had no effect irrelevant to DS, whereas SCM-chitin was more effective than intact heparin. SCM-chitin and heparin were also shown to block the attachment and migration of tumor cells to laminin-coated substrates. The inhibition of cell attachment and migration by SCM-chitin and heparin is probably due to their specific binding to laminin molecules (possibly the heparin-binding domain). It also may not be due to the inhibition of platelet aggregation and blood coagulation induced by tumor cells because SCM-chitin exhibited fairly low levels of the anticoagulant activity and antiplatelet aggregation activity than heparin. The team further explored the effect of SCM-chitin on angiogenesis induced by B16-BL6 cells in syngeneic mice. SCM-chitin caused a marked decrease in the number of vessels toward tumor mass (angiogenic response) without affecting the tumor cell growth when coinjected with tumor cells (on day 0), or injected into the tumor site on day 1 or 3 after tumor inoculation. The inhibition of tumor angiogenesis in mice may mainly be due to the inhibition of endothelial cell migration to extracellular matrix components, including fibronectin. Along with these, SCM-chitin and heparin inhibited enzymes such as heparanase and type IV collagenase catalyzing the degradation of extracellular matrix. SCM-chitin could inhibit type IV collagenolytic activity of tumor cells more potently than heparin.

The chemically modified sulfated chitosan derivatives and oligomers too were evaluated for the antitumor activity. The sulfated chitosan and Schiff base of sulfated chitosan with benzaldehyde significantly inhibited cell proliferation, induced apoptosis, and blocked the fibroblast growth factor-2-induced phosphorylation of extracellular signal-regulated kinases in breast cancer MCF-7 cells. The benzaldehyde Schiff base of sulfated chitosan had better inhibitory effects and lower IC50 compared to sulfated chitosan (Jiang et al. 2011).With randomly sulfated derivatives of chitooligosaccharide (3–5 kDa), inhibition of the expressions of collagenases 1 and 3 via suppressing tumor necrosis factor (TNF)-α-induced NF-κB signaling was seen in human chondrosarcoma cells (SW-1353) (Ryu et al. 2012).

The low-MW sulfated chitosan oligosaccharides also displayed the anti-inflammatory activity by suppressing the pro-inflammatory mediators such as NO and inducible NO synthase in lipopolysaccharide (LPS)-stimulated murine macrophage RAW264.7cells. The probable molecular mechanisms behind this bioactivity might be due to the inhibition of LPS-induced interleukin-6 and TNF-α release, by downregulating the phosphorylation levels of mitogen-activated protein kinases (MAPK) signaling pathways, decreasing inhibitor of NF-κB (IκBα) degradation and subsequent NF-κB activation in RAW264.7 cells (Kim et al. 2014).

7.4.6 ENZYME INHIBITION ACTIVITIES

Prolyl endopeptidase (PEP, EC 3.4.21.26) is a proline-specific endopeptidase with a serine-type mechanism, which digests small peptide-like hormones, neuroactive peptides, and various cellular factors. It has been involved in neurodegenerative disorders; therefore, the discovery of PEP inhibitors can revert memory loss caused by amnesic compounds.

PEP inhibitory activities of sulfated chitosans with different DDAs (90%, 75%, and 50%) and sulfated derivatives of hetero-chitooligosaccharides with MWs of <1, 1–5, and 5–10 kDa prepared from the chitosans with DDAs of 90%, 75% and 50%, were investigated by Je et al. (2007). Chitosan sulfate with a DDA of 50% exhibited the highest inhibitory activity, and the inhibition rate was dose dependent. Dixon plots suggested that action was as competitive inhibitor, and the inhibition constant (K_i) was 2.6 mg/mL. The sulfated derivative of 1–5 kDa hetero-chitooligosaccharides obtained from chitosan with a DDA of 50% exhibited higher PEP inhibitory activities than the sulfated derivative of <1 and 5–10 kDa hetero-chitooligosaccharides obtained from chitosans with DDAs of 90% and 75%. The IC50 value was 0.38 mg/mL, and the inhibition constant K_i was 0.78 mg/mL.

7.4.7   Anti-Human Immunodeficiency Virus Type 1 Activity

At present, the sulfated polysaccharide for example, curdlan sulfate, is regarded as a potent and practical antiretroviral polysaccharide reagent (Yoshida et al. 1990). Among the sulfated derivatives of polysaccharide chitosan, Sosa et al. (1991) reported that the randomly sulfated N-carboxymethyl chitosan (N,O-sulfate carboxymethyl chitosan) inhibited the propagation of the human immunodeficiency virus type 1 (HIV-1) in human CD4+ cells and that of Rauscher murine leukemia virus in murine fibroblasts. The activity was suggested due to blocking of the interactions of viral coat glycoprotein receptors to target proteins on lymphocytes and competitive inhibition of HIV-1 reverse transcriptase. The randomly sulfated chitooligosaccharides (3–5 kDa) too possess anti-HIV-1 activity (Artan et al. 2010). At nontoxic concentrations, sulfated chitooligosaccharides significantly inhibited HIV-1-induced syncytia formation and the lytic effect at EC50 values of 2.19 and 1.43 μg/mL, respectively. In addition, the production of p24 antigen was suppressed at EC50 values of 4.33 and 7.76 μg/mL for HIV-1RF and HIV-1Ba-L, respectively. Moreover, sulfated chitooligosaccharides exhibited inhibitory activities on viral entry and virus cell fusion via the blockade of binding between HIV-1 gp120 and CD4+ cell surface receptor. These observations indicate that sulfated chitooligosaccharides might be used as a novel candidate for the development of anti-HIV-1 agents (Vo and Kim 2010).

However, anti-HIV activities of sulfated chitin were found to be controllable by changing the position of the sulfate groups at N2, O3 and O6 positions of chitin/ chitosan. A regioselective sulfation of groups at N2 and/or O3 positions of chitin showed a much higher inhibitory effect on the infection of acquired immunodeficiency syndrome (AIDS) virus *in vitro* than the 6-O-sulfated derivatives. Moreover, the product with sulfation at both 2 and 3 positions completely inhibited the infection of AIDS virus to T lymphocytes at a concentration of 0.28 μg/mL without significant cytotoxicity. These results suggest that the specific interaction of these chitin sulfates with positively charged V3-loop in the gp120 molecule of the AIDS virus preventing the fusion of the virus and host cell membrane. The interaction depends significantly on the sites of sulfation rather than on the total degree of substitution on sugar residues.

7.4.8   Antimicrobial Agents

The antibacterial mechanism of chitosan has suggested that the trace metal cations selectively chelated by the chitosan could be necessary for the growth of microorganisms and therefore could inhibit the proliferation of the microbes (Huang et al. 2004). The sulfated derivatives of polysaccharides possess negative charges making them an excellent chelating host for metal cation substrates. Hence, chitosan sulfate and its derivatives were explored for antimicrobial action. To get derivatives, N-acyl or N,O-quaternary ammonium groups were introduced on chitosan sulfate by its reaction with caproic anhydride, propanoic anhydride, or 2,3-epoxypropyl trimethylammonium. It was found that the chitosan sulfate showed no inhibition against *Escherichia coli*, whereas at a concentration below 102 μg/mL, its inhibition against *Staphylococcus aureus* was higher than phenic acid, a widely used biocide. The quaternized derivatives of the chitosan sulfate also showed *S. aureus* inhibition but no *E. coli* inhibition. The acylated chitosan sulfates were found to be not only increasing the *S. aureus* inhibition activities but also exhibiting some inhibition toward the growth of *E. coli* slightly. The activities of N-acyl chitosan sulfates seem to be related to the structures of the covalently bonded acyl moieties, among which the N-hexanoyl moiety was more effective in enhancing the *E. coli* inhibition activities. In contrast, chitosan could inhibit the growth of *E. coli* and *S. aureus* significantly (Jeon and Kim 2000; Muhannad et al. 2002). Probably, the antibacterial mechanism of the chitosan sulfate and its derivatives are different from that of chitosan.

7.4.9 DRUG DELIVERY APPLICATIONS

Chitosan and chitosan sulfates are polyelectrolytes without the amphiphilic character and cannot congregate to micelles in water. The derivatives such as N-alkyl or N-acyl-O-sulfate chitosans have amphiphilicity because they carry long-chain alkyl groups such as hydrophobic and $-SO_3^-$ groups such as hydrophilic ones. Chitosan with 92% DD and average MW of 65 kDa, Zhang et al. (2003) synthesized a series of N-alkyl sulfate chitosans with long-chain alkyl groups of 8, 10, or 12 carbons. These derivatives were self-assembled in water to form polymeric micelles of size around 100–400 nm.

Further studies revealed that the critical micelle concentration (CMC) of the N-octyl-O-sulfate chitosan (NOSC) was found to be 0.45 mg/mL. The micelles of NOSC prepared by dialysis method were employed to solubilize water-insoluble drug paclitaxel (PTX) by its physical entrapment (Zhang et al. 2004). The polymeric micelle formation and the loading of drug occurred simultaneously in the dialysis process when ethanol and water were used as solvents for PTX and the polymer, respectively. The results showed that PTX concentration in NOSC micellar solution was 2.01 mg/mL, which was much higher than that in water (<0.001 mg/mL). Compared with the amount of NOSC, the PTX loading amount in the system was up to 25% (w/w), depending on the solvents used in dialysis and the feed weight ratio of PTX to the derivative. The characterization of PTX-loaded NOSC micelles (PTX-M) by transmission electron microscopy revealed that PTX existed as the colloid particulates in ethanol before loading and in the cores of the spherical polymeric micelles after loading. The characterization of differential scanning calorimeter (DSC) and wide-angle X-ray diffraction (WXRD) indicated that PTX was transferred from the crystalline state to the amorphous state after loading. The lyophilized powder of the micellar system (25% [w/w] loading) could be reconstituted easily in aqueous media even after 2-month storage at 4°C without the change of PTX entrapment and micelle size. The reconstituted solution (2.1 mg PTX/mL) also showed good stability. The dilution with saline may decrease the loading and physical stability based on the dilution times, which was related with CMC of the polymer. *In vitro* tests showed that PTX was slowly released from micellar solution, and the release lasted up to 220 hours by means of the dialysis method. The pharmacokinetics, efficacy, and safety of PTX-M showed that PTX-M had the similar antitumor efficacy as Taxol® (Bristol-Myers Squibb Company), but significantly reduced the toxicity and improved the bioavailability of PTX (Zhang et al. 2008). Biodistribution study of PTX-M indicated that most of the PTX were distributed in the liver, kidney, spleen, and lung, and the longest retention effect was observed in the lung.

Zhang et al. (2003) further demonstrated that oral absorption of PTX with PTX-M *in vivo* and *in vitro* was enhanced. *In vivo*, the oral bioavailability of PTX-M was improved sixfold in comparison with that of an orally dosed Taxol. In *in vitro* uptake studies in Caco-2, PTX accumulation in cells was found to be significantly higher. It was further demonstrated that the effect of NOSC micelles on enhancing the absorption of PTX was resulted from P-gp inhibition by NOSC and the transport of PTX-M in a P-gp-independent way. Moreover, the mechanism of P-gp inhibition by NOSC was proved in relation to the interference with the P-gp ATPase rather than the reduction in the P-gp expression (Mo et al. 2011).

The micelle formation was facilitated when NOSCs were conjugated with polyethylene glycol (PEG) 1100, 2000, and 5000. The CMC values were 0.011–0.079 mg/mL (Yao et al. 2007). The log CMC was linearly related to four structure parameters: DS of chitosan unit, sulfate group, PEG unit, and octyl group by mole per kilogram. PTX was solubilized into the polymeric micelles of PEGylated NOSC utilizing physical entrapment method, with a micellar size around 100–130 nm. The solubility of PTX in micellar solution was significantly improved by 4000 times, in comparison with that of free PTX in water (3.94 mg/mL PTX in PTX-PEG conjugated N-octyl-O-sulfate chitosan (mPEGOSC) and <0.001 mg/mL in water). The introduction of mPEG block decreased the adhesion of plasma proteins to micelles and also decreased phagocytosis by the reticuloendothelial system and increased the circulation time of micelles after intravenous administration.

PTX-mPEOSC could be targeted passively to the uterus, and its targeting efficacy was 2.27 times higher than that of Taxol (Qu et al. 2009). With the observations of selective tissue accumulation of sulfated chitosan derivatives, the group designed glycyrrhetinic acid-modified sulfated chitosan primarily by sulfation of hydroxyl groups and then hydrophobic modification with glycyrrhetinic acid to amino groups on chitosan molecules. In this amphiphilic polymer with self-assembly property, the sulfate groups provided the hydrophilic moieties, and the glycyrrhetinic acid (GA) molecules offered both the hydrophobic and liver-targeting ligands (Tian et al. 2012). Doxorubicin (DOX)-loaded glycyrrhetinic acid-sulfated chitosan micelles could target specifically the liver cancer cells. They had nearly 2.18-fold higher affinity for the liver cancer cells, that is, HepG2 cells than for the normal liver cells, that is, Chang liver cells. The IC50 for DOX-loaded GA-SCTS micelles against HepG2 cells was 54.7 ng/mL, which was extremely lower than the amount of no-GA-modified DOX-loaded micelles.

The impact of sulfated and nonsulfated N-octyl-chitosans on the release profiles of model drugs was evaluated in calcium phosphate implant by monitoring the rate and extent of calcein (MW 650 Da) and fluorescein isothiocyanate (FITC-dextran (MW 40 kDa) *in vitro* release by fluorescence spectroscopy (Green et al. 2009).

A higher percentage of model drug was released from tablet with hydrophilic polymer, that is, NOSC, compared with the tablets containing hydrophobic polymer, that is, *N*-octyl-chitosan. The release profile of calcein or FITC-dextran from tablets containing NOSC revealed a complete release for FITC-dextran after 120 hours compared with calcein where 20% of the drug was released over the same time period, suggesting the possibility of drug release dependent on the MW of the model drugs.

When used in the implants of bone morphogenic protein-2 (BMP-2), the 2-N,6-O-sulfated chitosan at low dose markedly enhanced protein bioactivity to induce osteoblastic differentiation *in vitro* and *in vivo* by promoting BMP-2 signaling pathway (Zhou et al. 2009). In C2C12 myoblast cells, as *in vitro* models, sulfated chitosan showed a significant enhancement on the alkaline phosphatase activity and the mineralization induced by BMP-2, as well as the expression of alkaline phosphatase and osteocalcin mRNA. Simultaneous administration of BMP-2 and sulfated chitosan *in vivo* dose-dependently induced larger amounts of ectopic bone formation compared with BMP-2 alone. The enhancement in osteogenic activity of BMP-2 and its prolonged release were observed in 2-N,6-O-sulfated chitosan-immobilized poly(lactide-*co*-glycolide) scaffolds (Kong et al. 2014). For this, the surface of scaffolds was initially aminolyzed by ethylenediamine and immobilized with 2-N,6-O-sulfated chitosan via electrostatic assembly. Upon the presence of sulfated chitosan, the system displayed improved BMP-2 adsorption and prolonged the release process *in vitro* due to the high affinity of BMP-2 with sulfated chitosan. However, because of the incorporation of sulfated chitosan, the system appeared to be more hydrophilic and provided a better environment for cell attachment.

Cao et al. (2014a) developed BMP-2-loaded nanoparticles with 2-N,6-O-sulfated chitosan, which showed a dose-dependent enhancement on angiogenesis *in vitro*.

From the studies on 2-N,6-O-sulfated chitosan, Cao et al. (2014b) put forth a hypothesis that if 2-N,6-O-sulfated chitosan is fabricated as a carrier for rhBMP-2 loading, it could serve as a delivery vehicle and a specific enhancer of rhBMP-2 activity. For the study, they prepared rhBMP-2-loaded 2-N,6-O-sulfated chitosan nanoparticles (rhBMP-2/NPs) and a composite hydrogel of photopolymerizable gelatin incorporating rhBMP-2/NPs (PH/rhBMP-2/NPs). The intrinsically protective sulfated chitosan nanoparticles that are further encapsulated within a controlled photo-cross-linkable hydrogel presented clear advantages for sustained growth factor delivery. The utility of the PH/rhBMP-2/NP gel as an effective controlled delivery vehicle was assessed in *in vivo* bone repair using an ectopic model of new bone formation and an orthotopic critical size defect model in the rabbit radius.

Sulfated *N*-myristoyl chitosan was used to modify liposome surface. The effect of the treatment of an aqueous sulfated *N*-myristoyl chitosan was examined on the liposomes prepared from hydrogenated egg yolk lecithin. The precipitation of suspension of liposome was restrained on standing or freeze–thaw cycle or dilution due to the development of negative charge and hence stabilizing repulsive forces (Yoshioka et al. 1993).

N-Sulfonato-*N,O*-carboxymethyl chitosan (SNOCC) has been assessed as a potential intestinal absorption enhancer of Reviparin (low-MW heparin), mannitol, and FITC-dextran (MW 4400 Da) (Thanou et al. 2007). SNOCC was prepared at three different viscosity grades: 20, 40, and 60 cps (SNOCC-20, SNOCC-40, and

SNOCC-60, respectively); it was tested *in vitro* for their ability to decrease the transepithelial electrical resistance (TEER) of Caco-2 cell monolayers. *In vitro* studies showed that SNOCC materials were able to induce a concentration-dependent decrease in the TEER of the Caco-2 monolayers. SNOCC-40 and SNOCC-60 were shown to decrease resistance more readily compared to the low-viscosity SNOCC-20. ^{14}C-Mannitol permeation data across intestinal epithelia were in agreement with the observed decrease in the TEER; the higher viscosity SNOCC-60 was the most effective, demonstrating a 51-fold enhancement of the permeation of the radio-labeled marker. Studies with both FITC-dextran and Reviparin demonstrated significantly increased permeation across Caco-2 cell monolayers when they were co-incubated at the apical side of the monolayer. For *in vivo* evaluation, solutions of Reviparin, with or without SNOCC, were administered intraduodenally in rats, and the absorption of the drug was assessed by measuring the anti-Xa levels in rat plasma. Intestinal absorption of Reviparin in rats was increased when it was coadministered with SNOCC-40 and SNOCC-60, in agreement with *in vitro* data. Anti-Xa levels were elevated to and above the antithrombotic levels, and were sustained for at least 6 hours, giving an 18.5-fold increase in the area under the curve (AUC) of Reviparin in rats.

Jordan et al. (2007) have presented data showing that use of N-sulfated-*N,O*-carboxymethyl chitosan combined with the anti-inflammatory agent 5-aminosalicylic acid (5-ASA) reduced inflammation and urinary frequency in a rat model of bladder inflammation. This effect was not seen while using polymer alone. It was suggested most likely that the primary effect of polymer was to allow a close approximation of the 5-ASA with the epithelium, enhancing an efficient transepithelial transport of 5-ASA into the bladder lamina propria.

Sulfated chitosan with its acquired anionic centers can play a role of partner in the polyelectrolyte complex (PEC) formation with positively charged polyelectrolyte like native chitosan (Berth et al. 2002). PEC formation between chitosans of various MWs or degree of acetylation with chitosan sulfate in dilute solution was studied by static light scattering at various ionic strengths. Unlike the MW, the degree of acetylation was found to have a significant effect on the resultant structural densities of the complexes. The same system was applied to the preparation of micrometer-sized hollow shells by means of a layer-by-layer technique (in total eight layers). Their behavior toward fluorescent probes such as fluorescein and rhodamin 6G or fluorescein isothiocyanate-labeled dextrans at various ionic strengths and pH (observed by confocal laser light scanning microscopy) could be related to electrostatic forces between the highly charged shells and the probes. At an ionic strength of ≥ 0.1 M, charge effects were largely suppressed (screening effect) and a size-dependent "cutoff" for the permeation of the macromolecular fluorophore was observed and the preparation and behavior of hollow capsules made of these materials.

7.4.10 SORPTION PROPERTIES

The possibility of deposition of lipoproteins from blood plasma by different chitosan sulfo derivatives has been demonstrated by evaluating chitosan-*N*-sulfosuccinate of different MWs immobilized on silica matrixes (Gamzazade et al. 1997b). The sulfo derivatives of chitosan as affinity ligands revealed high specificity in relation to LDL and did not cause essential changes in blood count during contact with the blood.

The protein adsoption on chitosan sulfate was demonstrated with 6-sulfated, 3,6-O-sulfated, and N,6-O-sulfated chitosans (Yuan et al. 2009). All exhibited the lysozyme binding activity, but the maximum binding ratios of lysozyme/polysaccharide were significantly different. Although 6-sulfated chitosan possessed the lowest sulfur content among the derivatives, it displayed the highest binding activity with lysozyme and the highest selective binding activity with lysozyme in the presence of γ-globulin and bovine serum albumin. The results indicated that 6-O-sulfate groups may be responsible for the high affinity and specific interaction of sulfated chitosan with lysozyme, whereas 2-O-sulfate and 3-O-sulfate groups are unfavorable to this interaction.

7.4.11 CHITOSAN WITH SPACED SULFONIC GROUPS

Rather than introducing the sulfate group on hydroxyl or amine functions, the groups such as alkyl aryl acyl bearing sulfate can be introduced to get the spaced sulfur-containing groups on a chitinous polymer (Figure 7.8).

The sulfonic acid function can also be introduced into chitosan by reacting it with sulfonic function bearing formyl aromatic derivatives such as 5-formyl-2-furansulfonic acid sodium salt to get Schiff's base for further reduction (Figure 7.9). This gave derivatives as N-sulfofurfuryl chitosan derivative of chitosan (Muzzarelli 1992). An analogous preparation of benzyl sulfonated chitosan was carried with 2-formyl benzenesulfonic acid or 4-formyl-1,3-benzene sodium disulfonic acid (Crini et al. 1997a).

Reaction of chitosan and 5-formyl-2-furansulfonic acid sodium salt and hydrogenation yielded N-sulfofurfuryl chitosan sodium salt dodging polymer degradation and O-substitution along with the introduction of spacer in between the chitosan backbone and the sulfonate group. For this, chitosan or activated chitosan (by dissolving in acetic acid, precipitated in 1% v/v triethanolamine in methanol and swollen) is reacted with N-sulfofurfuryl chitosan sodium salt at room temperature for 12–18 hours, reduced by slow addition of $NaBH_4$ and precipitated at high pH in methanol/ acetone (Amiji et al. 1998). The concentration of the sulfonic acid groups in modified chitosan increased as the feeding ratio of 5-formyl-2-furansulfonic acid increased (Liu et al. 2004).

The presence of a sulfonic acid group on the furan ring is expected to impart solubility and polyampholyte behavior to chitosan and to affect the biological activity. N-Sulfofurfuryl chitosan displayed reduced platelet adhesion and activation properties, and may prove to be suitable for some blood-contacting applications. In contrast to an average of 73 fully activated platelets on unmodified chitosan, only 4.50 contact-adherent platelets were found on N-sulfofurfuryl chitosan surface per 25,000 μm^2 (Amiji et al. 1998). Circular dichroism demonstrated that N-sulfofurfuryl chitosan significantly altered the conformation of thrombin, whereas no obvious variation in the conformation of thrombin was observed with the addition of chitosan. APTT of N-sulfofurfuryl chitosan membrane was prolonged in comparison with that of its chitosan counterpart and showed a rising trend with an increasing concentration of the sulfonic acid moieties. However, PT and TT were not markedly affected.

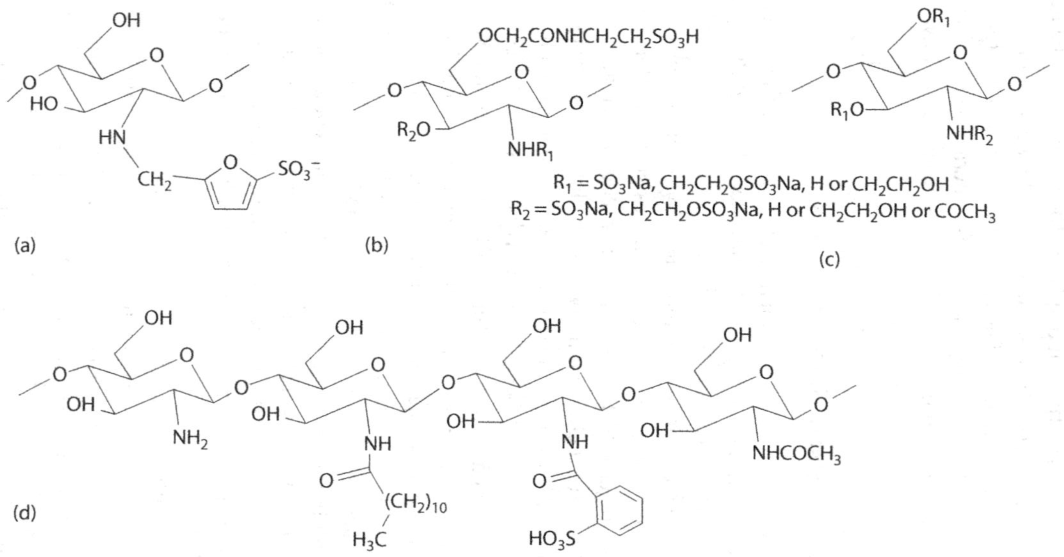

FIGURE 7.8 Spaced sulfated chitosan: (a) *N*-sulfofurfuryl chitosan, (b) sulfoethyl-*N*-carboxymethyl chitosan, (c) sulfoethyl chitosan, and (d) lauryl sulfated chitosan.

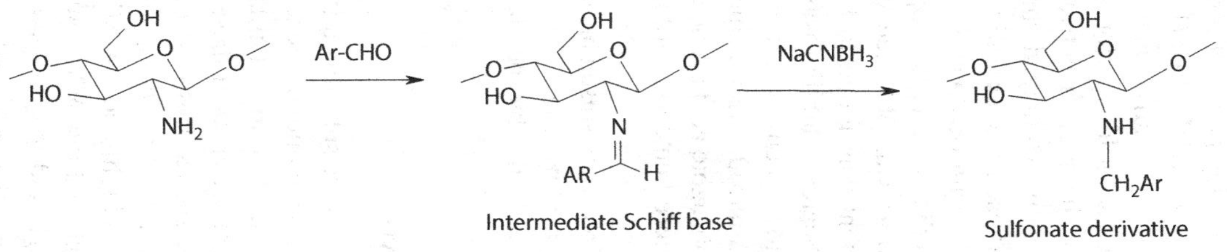

FIGURE 7.9 Synthesis of *N*-(sulfonated aryl)methyl chitosan derivative. Ar is with sulfo group.

The anticoagulant mechanism of the *N*-sulfofurfuryl chitosan membranes supposedly originated from an intrinsic pathway to the inhibition of coagulation enzymes.

The chelating ability of a parent polymer was improved with the presence of sulfofurfuryl group. Solutions of *N*-sulfofurfuryl chitosan, when treated with 0.1–5.0 mM Ni(II), Cu(II), and Pb(II) solutions, yielded insoluble metal chelates, whereas dilute solutions of Cr(III), up to 0.5 mM, and solutions of Co(II) up to 5 mM did not produce precipitates. The metal chelation power of *N*-sulfofurfuryl chitosan was on the order: Cu(II) > Pb(II) > Ni(II) > Cr(III) > Co(II). However, the benzyl sulfonated chitosans such as *N*-2-sulfobenzyl chitosan and *N*-2,4-disulfobenzyl chitosan, especially the former, displayed apparent low performances for metal ion sorption. This might be due to electrostatic interaction between ammonium ion sulfonate groups. As a consequence, the negatively charged character of sulfonate groups is reduced and the adsorption properties of the derivatives are weakened.

Sulfoethyl-*N*-carboxymethyl chitosan was synthesized from 2-chloroethane sulfonic acid in alkaline organic media such as isopropanol or *tert*-butanol (Nudga et al. 2001). The sulfoethyl chitosan was obtained with a degree of substitution of 0.11–0.35, and the sulfur content was found to be 1.39%–5.32%. Substitution involved O-6 and N-2 positions. Scarce solubility was observed for the degrees of substitution higher than 0.30. Sulfoethyl chitosan films had good antithrombogenic properties. The sulfate group was introduced specifically on N along with spacer of with phenyl ring by using sulfobenzoic acid cyclic anhydride. Such sulfated chitosan after its lauroylation was more hemocompatible than chitosan (Shelma and Sharma 2011).

Jaykumar et al. (2008) synthesized water-insoluble sulfated carboxymethyl chitin by grafting 2-aminoethyl sulfonic acid by using 1-ethyl-3-(3-dimethylaminopropyl) carbodiimide (EDC) catalyst to study the biospecific degradation behavior of its cross-linked membrane by lysozyme.

7.4.12 Sulfonamido Derivatives

The sulfa group added to chitosan can be substituted further (Figures 7.10 and 7.11). For example, a sulfonating agent 4-acetamidobenzene sulfonyl chloride reacts with –NH$_2$ or –OH (C6 position) group leading to sulfanilamide derivatives of chitosan (Zhong et al. 2007). The antioxidant activities of these derivatives were investigated employing various *in vitro* systems, such as hydroxyl-radical, superoxide anion scavenging, and reducing power. All kinds of the compounds (high-MW [20 kDa] and low-MW [4 kDa] chitosans, sulfated high- and low-MW chitosans, 2-(4-acetamido-2-sulfanilamide)-chitosan with high and low MWs, and 6-sulfated 2-(4-acetamido-2-sulfanilamide)-chitosan with high and low MWs showed a stronger scavenging activity on hydroxyl radical than ascorbic acid. All of the derivatives were efficient in the reducing power, whereas the superoxide radical scavenging effect of sulfanilamide derivatives of chitosan and chitosan sulfates was stronger than that of original chitosan and chitosan sulfates.

The derivatives of chitosan prepared with analogous reactions with substituted benzene disulfonyl chloride were 2-(4(or2)-hydroxyl-5-chloride-1,3-benzene-disulfanimide)-chitosan (Zhong et al. 2008). These derivatives also displayed the

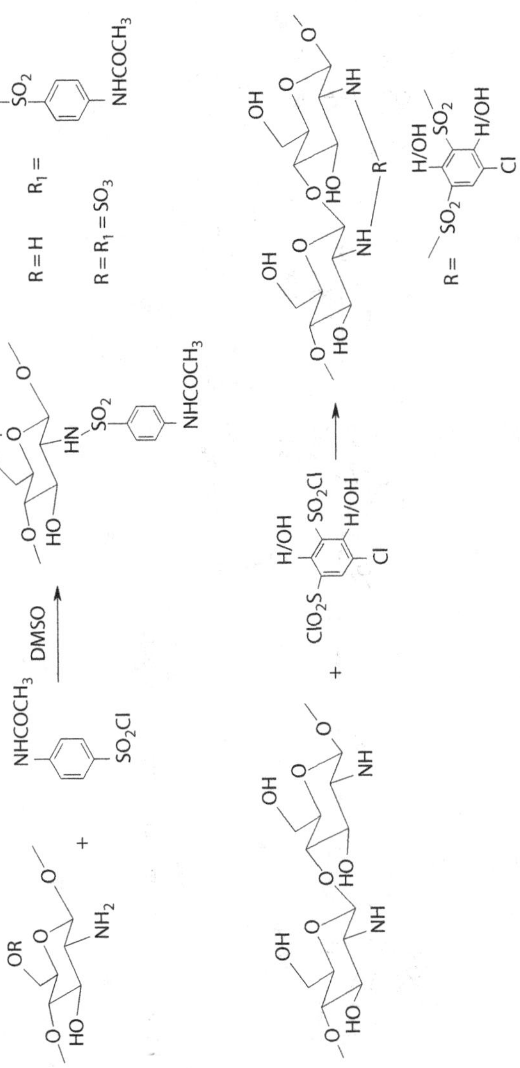

FIGURE 7.10 Synthesis of sulfonamide derivatives of chitosan such as 2-(4-acetamido-2-sulfanilamide)-chitosan, 6-sulfated 2-(4-acetamido-2-sulfanilamide)-chitosan, and 2-(4(or2)-hydroxyl-5-chloride-1,3-benzene-di-sulfanimide)-chitosan.

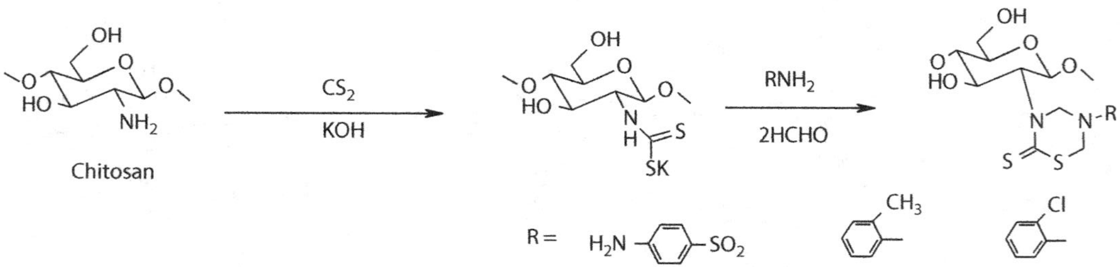

FIGURE 7.11   1,3,5-Thiadiazine-2-thione derivatives of chitosan.

antioxidant activity probably supported by the presence of active hydroxyl group of aromatic ring and the disruption of intramolecular hydrogen bonds between amine and hydroxyl groups.

The preparation of 1,3,5-thiadiazine-2-thione derivatives of chitosan and their potential antioxidant activity *in vitro* has been published (Ji et al. 2007). The sulfur-containing derivatives were obtained by reacting chitosan with CS_2, formaldehyde, and primary amine.

7.5   CONCLUSION

In this chapter, different methods of preparation of chitosan and its characterization and properties have been summarized. The role of their derivatives as blood anticoagulant, antioxidant, antitumor, and antimicrobial anti-HIV-1 and in hemagglutination inhibition, enzyme inhibition, and wound repair has been discussed. The sulfated chitosan and its derivatives, especially self-assembly forming, have a role in drug delivery. The high sorption capacities of modified sulfated chitosan are of relevance too. The action of adsorption of metal ions by sulfated chitosan (not discussed here) can be of great advantage for the recovery of valuable metals. The rapid progress in the applicability of these derivatives is anticipated.

REFERENCES

Amiji, M.M. 1998. Platelet adhesion and activation on an amphoteric chitosan derivative bearing sulfonate group. *Coll. Surf. B: Biointerfaces* 10: 263–271.

Archibald, P.J., M.D. Fenn, and A.B. Roy. 1981. ^{13}C NMR studies of D-glucose and D-galactose monosulphates. *Carbohydr. Res.* 93: 177–190.

Artan, M., F. Karadeniz, M.Z. Karagozlu, M.M. Kim, S.K. Kim. 2010. Anti-HIV-1 activity of low molecular weight sulfated chitooligosaccharides. *Carbohydr. Res.* 345: 656–662.

Baumann, H. and V. Faust. 2001. Concepts for improved regioselective placement of O-sulfo, N-sulfo, N-acetyl, and N-carboxymethyl groups in chitosan derivatives. *Carbohydr. Res.* 331: 43–57.

Berth, G., A. Voigt, H. Dautzenberg, E. Donath, and H. Mohwald. 2002. Polyelectrolyte complexes and layer-by-layer capsules from chitosan/chitosan sulfate. *Biomacromolecules* 3: 579–590.

Brugnerotto, J., J. Lizardi, F.M. Goycoolea, W. Arguelles-Monal, J. Desbrieres, and M. Rinaudo. 2001. An infrared investigation in relation with chitin and chitosan characterization. *Polymer* 42: 3569–3580.

Cao, L., J. Wang, J. Hou, W. Xing, and C. Liu. 2014a. Vascularization and bone regeneration in critical sized defect using 2-N,6-O-sulfated chitosan nanoparticles incorporating BMP-2. *Biomaterials* 35: 684–698.

Cao, L.J., J. Werkmeister, W.V. Glattauer, K.M. Mc Lean, and C. Liu. 2014b. Bone regeneration using photocrosslinked hydrogel incorporating rhBMP-2 loaded 2-N, 6-O-sulfated chitosan nanoparticles. *Biomaterials* 35: 2730–2742.

Crini, G., G. Toni, M. Guerrini, B. Marte, M. Weltrowski, M. Morcellet, and C. Cosentino. 1997a. Synthesis, NMR study and preliminary sorption properties of two N-benzyl sulfonated chitosan derivatives. *J. Carbohydr.Chem.* 16: 681–689.

Cushing, I.B., R.V. Davis, E.J. Kratovil, and D.W. Mac Corquodale. 1954. The Sulfation of chitin in chlorosulfonic acid and dichloroethane. *J. Am. Chem. Soc.* 76: 4590–4591.

Drozd, N.N., A.I. Sher, V.A. Makarov, G.A. Vichoreva, I.N. Gorbachiova, and L.S. Galbraich. 2001. Comparison of antitrombin activity of the polysulphate chitosan derivatives in vitro and in vivo system. *Thromb. Res.* 102: 445–455.

Fan, L., P. Wu, J. Zhang, S. Gao, L. Wang, M. Li, M. Sha, W. Xie, and M. Nie. 2012. Synthesis and anticoagulant activity of the quaternaryammonium chitosan sulfates. *Int. J. Biol. Macromol.* 50: 31–37.

Gamzazade, A., A. Sklyar, S. Nasibov, I. Sushkov, A. Shashkov, and Y. Knirel. 1997a. Structural features of sulfated chitosans. *Carbohydr. Polym.* 34:113–116.

Gamzazade, A.I., S.M. Nasibovb, and S.V. Rogozhin. 1997b. Study of lipoprotein sorption by some sulfoderivatives of chitosan. *Carbohydr. Polym.* 34: 381–384.

Gilbert, E.E. 1962. The reactions of sulfur trioxide and its adducts with organic compounds. *Chem. Rev.* 62: 549–589.

Green, S., M. Roldo, D. Douroumis, N. Bouropoulos, D. Lamprou, and D.G. Fatouros. 2009. Chitosan derivatives alter release profiles of model compounds from calcium phosphate implants. *Carbohydr. Res.* 344: 901–907.

Hagiwara, K., Y. Kuribayashi, H. Iwai, I. Azuma, S. Tokura, K. Ikuta, and C. Ishihara. 1999. A sulfated chitin inhibits hemagglutination by Theileriasergentimerozoites. *Carbohydr. Polym.* 39: 245–248.

Hirano, S., M. Hasegawa, and J. Kinugawa. 1991. ^{13}C NMR analysis of some sulphate derivatives of chitosan. *Int. J. Biol. Macromol.* 13: 316–317.

Hirano, S. and J. Kinugawa. 1986. Effect of sulphated derivatives of chitosan on lipoprotein lipase activity of rabbit plasma after their intravenous injection. *Carbohydr. Res.* 150: 295–299.

Hirano, S., Y. Tanaka, M. Hasegawa, K. Tobetto, and A. Nishioka. 1985. Effect of sulfated derivatives of chitosan on some blood coagulant factors. *Carbohydr. Res.* 137: 205–215.

Holme, K.R., and A.S. Perlin. 1997. Chitosan N-sulfate. A water-soluble polyelectrolyte. *Carbohydr. Res.* 302: 7–12.

Horton, D. and E.K. Just. 1973. Preparation from chitin of (1→4)-2-amino-2-deoxy-β-D-glucopyranuronan and its 2-sulfoamino analog having blood-anticoagulant properties. *Carbohydr. Res.* 29: 173–179.

Huang, R., Y. Du, and J. Yang. 2003a. Preparation and anticoagulant activity of carboxybutyrylated hydroxyethyl chitosan sulfates. *Carbohydr. Polym.* 51: 431–438.

Huang, R., Y. Du, J. Yang, and L. Fan. 2003b. Influence of functional groups on the in vitro anticoagulant activity of chitosan sulfate. *Carbohydr. Res.* 338: 483–489.

Huang, R., Y. Du, L. Zheng, H. Liu, and L. Fan. 2004. A new approach to chemically modified chitosan sulfates and study of their influences on the inhibition of *Escherichia coli* and *Staphylococcus aureus* growth. *React. Funct. Polym.* 59: 41–51.

Huang, R., E. Mendis, and S.K. Kim. 2005. Factors affecting the free radical scavenging behavior of chitosan sulfate. *Int. J. Biol. Macromol.* 36:120–127.

Huynh, R., F. Chaubet, and J. Jozefonvicz. 2001. Anticoagulant properties of dextran methyl carboxylate benzylamide sulfate (DMCBSu): A new generation of bioactive functionalized dextran. *Carbohydr. Res.* 332: 75–83.

Illum, L. 1998. Chitosan and its use as a pharmaceutical excipient. *Pharm. Res.* 15: 1326–1331.

Ishihara, C., S. Shimakawa, M. Tsuji, J. Arikawa, and S. Tokura. 1995. A sulfated chitin, SCM-chitin III, inhibits the clearance of human erythrocytes from the blood circulation in erythrocyte-transfused SCID mice. *Immunopharmacol.* 29: 65–71.

Jayakumar, R., N. New, H. Nagagama, T. Furuike, and H. Tamura. 2008. Synthesis, characterization and biospecific degradation behavior of sulfated chitin. *Macromol. Symp.* 264: 163–167.

Je, J.Y., E.K. Kim, C.B. Ahn, S.H. Moon, B.T. Jeon, B. Kim, T.K. Park, and P.J. Park. 2007. Sulfated chitooligosaccharides as prolyl endopeptidase inhibitor. *Int J Biol Macromol.* 41: 529–533.

Je, J.Y., P.J. Park, and S.K. Kim. 2005. Prolyl, endopeptidase inhibitory activity of chitosan sulfates with different degree of deacetylation. *Carbohydr. Polym.* 60: 553–556.

Jeon, Y.J. and S.K. Kim. 2000. Production of chitooligosaccharides using an ultrafiltration membrane reactor and their antibacterial activity. *Carbohydr. Polym.* 41: 133–141.

Ji, X., Z. Zhong, X. Chen, R. Xing, S. Liu, L. Wang, and P. Li. 2007. Preparation of 1,3,5-thiadiazine-2-thione derivatives of chitosan and their potential antioxidant activity in vitro. *Bioorg. Med. Chem. Lett.* 17: 4275–4279.

Jiang, M., H. Ouyang, P. Ruan, H. Zhao, Z. Pi, S. Huang, P. Yi, and M. Crepin. 2011. Chitosan derivatives inhibit cell proliferation and induce apoptosis in breast cancer cells. *Anticancer Res.* 31: 1321–1328.

Jordan, J.L., S. Henderson, C.M. Elson, J. Zhou, A. Kydonieus, J. Downie, and D.T.D.G. Lee. 2007. Use of a sulfated chitosan derivative to reduce bladder inflammation in the rat. *Urology.* 70: 1014–1018.

Kim, J.H., Y.S. Kim, J.W. Hwang, Y.K. Han, J.S. Lee, S.K. Kim, Y.J. Jeon, S.H. Moon, B.T. Jeon, Y.Y. Bahk, and P.J. Park. 2014. Sulfated chitosan oligosaccharides suppress LPS-induced NOProduction via JNK and NF-κB Inactivation. *Molecules* 19: 18232–18247.

Kong, X., J. Wang, L. Cao, Y. Yu, and C. Liu. 2014. Enhanced osteogenesis of bone morphology protein-2 in2-N,6-O-sulfated chitosan immobilized PLGA scaffolds. *Coll. Surf B Biointerfaces.* 122: 359–367.

Kurita, K., K Sugita, N. Kodaira, M. Hirakawa, and J. Yang. 2005. *Biomacromolecules* 6: 1414–1418.

Lin, C.W. and J.C. Lin. 2001. Surface characterization and platelet compatibility evaluation of surface-sulfonated chitosan membrane. *J. Biomater. Sci. Polym. Edn.* 12: 543–557.

Liu, W., J. Zhang, N. Cheng, Z. Cao, and K. Yao. 2004. Anticoagulation activity of cross-linked N-sulfofurfuryl chitosan membranes. *J. Appl. Polym. Sci.* 94: 53–56.

Lu, X., H. Guo, L. Sun, L. Zhang, and Y. Zhang. 2013. Protective effects of sulfated chitooligosaccharides with different degrees of substitution in MIN6 cells. *Int. J. Biol. Macromol.* 52: 92–98.

Mariappan, M.R., J.G. Williams, and M.D. Pregaer. 1997. Chitosan and chitosan sulfate have opposing effects on collagen-fibroblast interactions. *Wound Rep. Reg.* 7: 400–406.

Mo, R., X. Jin, N. Li, C. Ju, M. Sun, C. Zhang, and Q. Ping. 2011. The mechanism of enhancement on oral absorption of paclitaxel by N-octyl-O-sulfate chitosan micelles. *Biomaterials* 32: 4609–4620.

Mourya, V.K. and N.N. Inamdar. 2008. Chitosan-modifications and applications: Opportunities galore. *React. Funct. Polym.* 68: 1013–1051.

Muhannad, J., H. Franz, B. Furkert, and W. Miiller. 2002. A new lipid emulsion formulation with high antimicrobial efficacy using chitosan. *Eur. J. Pharm. Biopharm.* 53: 115–123.

Murata, J., I. Saiki, K. Matsuno, S. Tokura, and I. Azuma. 1990. Inhibition of tumor cell arrest in lungs by antimetastatic chitin heparinoid. *Jpn. J. Cancer Res.* 81: 506–513.

Murata, J., I. Saiki, S. Nishimura, N. Nishi, S. Tokura, and I. Azuma. 1989. Inhibitory effects of chitin heparonoids. *Jpn. J. Cancer Res.* 80: 866–872.

Muzzarelli, R.A.A. 1992. Modified chitosans carrying sulfonic acid groups. *Carbohydr. Polym.* 19: 231–236.

Muzzarelli, R.A.A. and G. Giacomelli. 1987. The blood anticoagulant activity of N-carboxymethylchitosantrisulfate. *Carbohydr. Polym.* 7: 87–96.

Muzzarelli, R.A.A., F. Tanfani, and M. Emanuelli. 1984. Sulfated N-(carboxymethyl)chitosans: Novel blood anticoagulants. *Carbohydr. Res.* 126: 225–231.

Muzzarelli, R.A.A., F. Tanfani, M. Emanuelli, D.P. Pace, E. Chiurazzi, and M. Piani. 1986. Sulphated N-carboxymethylchitosans as blood anticoagulants. In: *Chitin in Nature and Technology*, R.A.A. Muzzarelli, C. Jeuniaux, G.W. Goodday (eds.). Plenum Press: New York, pp. 469–476.

Nagasawa, K., H. Harada, S. Hayashi, and T. Misawa. 1972. Sulfation of dextran with piperidine-N-sulfonic acid. *Carbohydr. Res.* 21: 420–426.

Nagasawa, K., Y. Tohira, Y. Inoue, and N. Tanoura. 1971. Reaction between carbohydrates and sulfuric acid: Part I. Depolymerization and sulfation of polysaccharides by sulfuric acid. *Carbohydr. Res.* 18: 95–102.

Naggi, A.M., G. Torri, T. Compagnoni, and B. Casu. 1986. Synthesis and physico-chemical properties of the polyampholyte chitosan 6-sulphate. In: *Chitin in Nature and Technology*, R.A.A. Muzzarelli, C. Jeuniaux, G.W. Gooday (eds.). Plenum Press: New York, pp. 371–377.

Nishimura, S., N. Nishi, and S. Tokura. 1986. Inhibition of the hydrolytic activity of thrombin by chitin heparinoids. *Carbohydr. Res.* 156: 286–292.

Nishimura, S.I., K. Hideaki, K. Shinada, T. Yoshida, S. Tokura, K. Kurita, H. Nakashima, N. Yamamoto, and T. Uryu. 1998. Regioselective syntheses of sulfated polysaccharides: Specific anti-HIV-1 activity of novel chitin sulfates. *Carbohydr. Res.* 306: 427–433.

Nishimura, S.I. and S. Tokura. 1987. Preparation and antithrombogenic activities of heparinoid from 6-O-(carboxymethyl) chitin. *Int. J. Biol. Macromol.* 9: 225–232.

Noreyka, R.M., V.S. Kolodzeykis, and G.E. Dugenas. 1985. Investigation of composition sulfated chitosan fractions. *Proceedings of the Conference 'Topical Questions of Developing Investigation and Production Medicinal Remedies'*. Kaunas, Lithuania, pp. 113–116.

Nudga, L.A., V.A. Petrova, A.D. Benkovich, and G.A. Petropavlovskii. 2001. Comparative study of reactivity of cellulose, chitosan, and chitin-glucan complex in sulfoethylation. *Russian J. Appl. Chem.* 74: 145–148.

Qu, G., Z. Yao, C. Zhang, X. Wu, and Q. Ping. 2009. PEG conjugated N-octyl-O-sulfate chitosan micelles for delivery of paclitaxel: In vitro characterization and in vivo evaluation. *Eur. J. Pharm. Sci.* 37: 98–105.

Ravi Kumar, M.N.V., R.A.A. Muzzarelli, C. Muzzarelli, H. Sashiwa, and A.J. Domb. 2004. Chitosan chemistry and pharmaceutical perspectives. *Chem. Rev.* 104: 6017–6084.

Roldo, M., K. Power, J.R. Smith, P.A. Cox, K. Papagelis, N. Bouropoulos, and D.F. Fatouros. 2009. N-Octyl-O-sulfate chitosan stabilizes single wall carbon nanotubes in aqueous media and bestows biocompatibility. *Nanoscale* 1: 366–373.

Ryu, B., S.W. Himaya, R.J. Napitupulu, T.K. Eom, and S.K. Kim. 2012. Sulfated chitooligosaccharide II (SCOS II) suppress collagen degradation in TNF-induced chondrosarcoma cells via NF-κB pathway. *Carbohydr. Polym.* 350: 255–261.

Ryu, B.H., S.T. Yang, and Y.H. Moon. 2001. Inhibition of chitin sulfate on human low density lipoprotein (LDL) oxidation by macrophages. *J. Fd. Hyg. Safety* 16: 342–348.

Saiki, I., J. Murata, J. Nakajima, S. Tokura, and I. Azuma. 1990. Inhibition by sulfated chitin derivatives of invasion through extracellular matrix and enzymatic degradation by metastatic melanoma cells. *Cancer Res.* 50: 3631–3637.

Schatz, C., A. Bionaz, J.M. Lucas, C. Pichot, C. Viton, A. Domard, and T. Delair. 2005. Formation of polyelectrolyte complex particles from self-complexation of N-sulfated chitosan. *Biomacromolecules* 6: 1642–1647.

Shelma, R. and C.P. Sharma. 2011. Development of lauroyl sulfated chitosan for enhancing hemocompatibility of Chitosan. *Coll. Surf. B: Biointerfaces* 84: 561–570.

Shigemasa, Y., H. Matsuura, H. Sashiwa, and H. Saimoto. 1996. Evaluation of different absorbance ratios from infrared spectroscopy for analyzing the degree of deacetylation in chitin. *Int. J. Biol. Macromol.* 18: 237–242.

Sosa, M., F. Fazely, J. Koch, S. Vercellotti, and R. Ruprecht. 1991. N-Carboxymethylchitosan-N,O-sulfate as an anti-HIV-1 agent. *Biochem. Biophys. Res. Commun.* 74: 489–496.

Tao, S., S. Gao, Y. Zhou, M. Cao, W. Xie, H. Zheng, and L. Fan. 2013. Preparation of carboxymethyl chitosan sulfate for improved cell proliferation of skin fibroblasts. *Int. J. Biol. Macromol.* 54: 160–165.

Terbojevich, M., C. Carraro, A. Cosani, B. Focher, A.M. Naggi, and G. Torri. 1989. Solution studies of chitosan 6-*O*-sulfate. *Makromolekular. Chemie* 190: 2847–2855.

Thanou, M., S. Henderson, A. Kydonieus, and C. Elson. 2007. N-sulfonato-N,O-carboxymethylchitosan: A novel polymeric absorption enhancer for the oral delivery of macromolecules. *J. Control. Rel.* 117: 171–178.

Tian, Q., X.H. Wang, W. Wang, C.N. Zhang, P. Wang, and Z. Yuan. 2012. Self-Assembly and liver targeting of sulfated chitosan nanoparticles functionalized with glycyrrhetinic acid. Nanomedicine: Nanotechnology, biology, and medicine 8: 870–879.

Vikhoreva, G., G. Bannikova, P. Stolbushkina, A. Panov, N. Drozd, V. Makarov, V. Varlamov, and L. Galbraikh. 2005. Preparation and anticoagulant activity of a low-molecular-weight sulfated chitosan. *Carbohydr. Polym.* 62: 327–332.

Vo, T.S. and S.K. Kim. 2010. Potential anti-HIV agents from marine resources: An overview. *Mar. Drugs* 8: 2871–2892.

Vongchan, P., W. Sajomsang, W. Kasinrerk, D. Subyen, and P. Kongtawelert. 2003. Anticoagulant activity of the chitosan polysulfate synthesized from marine crab shell by semi-heterogenous conditions. *Sci. Asia* 29: 115–120.

Vongchan, P., W. Sajomsang, D. Subyen, and P. Kongtawelert. 2002. Anticoagulant activity of a sulfated chitosan. *Carbohydr. Res.* 337: 1239–1242.

Warner, D.T. and L.L. Coleman. 1958. Selective Sulfonation of amino groups in amino alcohols. *J. Org. Chem.* 23: 1133–1135.

Whistler, R.J. and M. Kosik. 1971. Anticoagulant activity of oxidized and N- and O-sulfated chitosan. Arch. *Biochem. Biophys.* 142: 106–110.

Wolfrom, M.L. and T.M. Shienhan. 1959. The sulfonation of chitosan. *J. Am. Chem. Soc.* 81: 1764–1766.

Xing, R., S. Liu, H. Yu, Z. Guo, Z. Li, and P. Li. 2005b. Preparation of high-molecular weight and high-sulfate content chitosans and their potential antioxidant activity in vitro. *Carbohydr. Polym.* 61: 148–154.

Xing, R., S. Liu, H. Yu, Q. Zhang, Z. Li, and P. Li. 2004. Preparation of low-molecular-weight and high-sulfate-content chitosans under microwave radiation and their potential antioxidant activity in vitro. *Carbohydr. Res.* 339: 2515–2519.

Xing, R., H. Yu, S. Liu, W. Zhang, Q. Zhang, Z. Li, and P. Li. 2005a. Antioxidant activity of differently regioselective chitosan sulfates in vitro. *Bioorg. Med. Chem.* 13: 1387–1392.

Xu, J.C. and Y.L. Xiao. 1994. Preparation of hydrophilic chitosan. *Trans. Oceanol. Limnology* 1: 90–93.

Yang, J., K. Luo, D. Li, S. Yu, J. Cai, L. Chen, and Y. Du. 2013. Preparation, characterization and in vitro anticoagulant activity of highly sulfated chitosan. *Int. J. Biol. Macromol.* 52: 25–31.

Yao, Z., C. Zhang, Q. Ping, and L. Yu. 2007. A series of novel chitosan derivatives: Synthesis, characterization and micellar solubilization of paclitaxel. *Carbohyd. Polym.* 68: 78–792.

Yoshida, T., K. Hatanaka, T. Uryu, Y. Kaneko, E. Suzuki, H. Miyano, T. Mimura, O. Yoshida and N. Yamamoto. 1990. Synthesis and structural analysis of curdlan sulfate with a potent inhibitory effect in vitro of AIDS virus infection. *Macromolecules* 23: 3717–3722.

Yoshioka, H., S. Kazama, H. Tanizawa, S. Hirota, and M. Kamiya. 1993. Sulfated N-myristoyl chitosan as a surface modifier of liposomes. *Biosci. Biotech. Biochem.* 57: 1053–1057.

Yuan, L., Z. Yue, H. Chen, H. Huang, and T. Zhao. 2009. Interactions between lysozyme and regioselectively sulfated chitosan. *Coll. Surf. B: Biointerfaces* 73: 346–350.

Zhang, C., Q. Ping, H. Zhang, and J. Shen. 2003. Preparation of N-alkyl-O-sulfate chitosan derivatives and micellar solubilization of taxol. *Carbohydr. Polym.* 54: 137–141.

Zhang, C., P. Qineng, and H. Zhang. 2004. Self-assembly and characterization of paclitaxel-loaded N-octyl-O-sulfate chitosan micellar system. *Coll. Surf. B: Biointerfaces* 39: 69–75.

Zhang, C., G. Qu, Y. Sun, X. Wu, Z. Yao, Q. Guo, Q. Ding, S. Yuan, Z. Shen, Q. Ping, and H. Zhou. 2008. Pharmacokinetics, biodistribution, efficacy and safety of N-octyl-O-sulfate chitosan micelles loaded with paclitaxel. *Biomaterials* 29: 1233–1241.

Zhong, Z., X. Ji, R. Xing, S. Liu, Z. Guo, X. Chen, and P. Li. 2007. The preparation and antioxidant activity of the sulfanilamide derivatives of chitosan and chitosan sulfates. *Bioorg. Med. Chem.* 15: 3775–3782.

Zhong, Z., R. Xing, S. Liu, L. Wang, S. Cai, and P. Li. 2008. The antioxidant activity of the 2-(4(or2)-hydroxyl-5-chloride-1, 3-benzene-di-sulfanimide)-chitosan. *Eur. J. Med. Chem.* 43: 2171–2177.

Zhou, H., J. Qian, J. Wang, W. Yao, C. Liu, J. Chen, and X. Cao. 2009. Enhanced bioactivity of bone morphogenetic protein-2 with low dose of 2-N,6-O-sulfated chitosan in vitro and in vivo. *Biomaterials* 30: 1715–1724.

Zou, Y. and E. Khor. 2009. Preparation of sulfated-chitins under homogeneous conditions. *Carbohydr. Polym.* 77: 516–525.

8 Recent Advantages of Biopolymer Preparation and Applications in Bio-Industry

Bakrudeen Ali Ahmed Abdul, Mohaddeseh Adel,
Pegah Karimi, Masoud Abbaszadeh,
A. Kamaludeen, and A. Meera Moydeen

CONTENTS

8.1 INTRODUCTION

8.1.1 OUTLINE OF THE POLYMERS

Biopolymers are one of the main types of biomaterials family and they play an important role in human health. They are derived from natural sources and are mostly biodegradable; some are water soluble and not hazardous to the environment. Biopolymers are mostly produced by biological systems such as plants, animals, fungi, and microorganisms (Peralta et al. 2012), and are involved in plants, animals, and marines as natural building materials for their replication, transmission of foods, and energy transformation. Polymers are presented in various forms, such as fibers, papers, cloths, elastomers, plastics, enzymes, DNA, and major ingredients in soil and organisms (Carraher 2000). Biopolymers degrade by action of naturally occurring microorganisms, which has been dragging attention in recent years according to their role in various industrial and medical fields. They may be generated from microbial synthesized biopolymers, renewable resources, or petroleum-based chemicals (Khalil et al. 2013). A biopolymer is supposed to have specific properties, such as biocompatibility and biodegradable properties that enable them to be used in medicinal and other industrial usages. Biopolymers have various functions and characteristics due to their source they are originated from, and their chemical structure varies with extraction method, age, and type of algae (or) plants originated from the earth. Molecular weight (MW), degree of deacetylation (DDA), purity and crystallinity are the important characteristics of biopolymers (Schiffman and Schauer 2008).

8.1.2 TRADITIONAL APPLICATIONS OF BIOPOLYMERS

Polymers have a large number of applications in various industries, and listing them all is not possible. Initially, they were used in farming and packaging industries and also in other applications that required the minimum strength (Mohanty et al. 2005). In addition, the application of biopolymers, especially those originated from plants, in the food industry and food production was noticeable. One of the biopolymers that are originated from algae (brown seaweeds) is alginate, which has been used in the food industry since long time as a thickener and gelling agent. Thickening agents are helpful in adjusting the viscosity of products, making them more stable and easy to use. In 1992, Roller and Dea (1992) found that enzymes techniques may be suitable for increasing the opportunity to extract high-molecular-weight alginates which are considered to be a good gel former.

The other applications such as their usage in medical fields is one of the important; wound closure and products regarding healing the wounds, regenerative medicine, gene therapy, controlled drug delivery system, and medicinal implant devices in surgery (Nair and Laurencin 2007). In addition to simple staples, meshes, and clips, absorbable nonwoven materials to replace human tissue are used in wound healing. Moreover, drug delivery can be managed using biodegradable capsules (Penning et al. 1993). Other applications of polymers that are worth mentioning include soil retention sheeting, agriculture films, waste bags, packing materials, and food containers (Van de Velde and Kiekens 2002). The main reason of polymers applications is the high ability a property possesses in film forming. Most of the applications are due to fiber form of the biopolymers (Van de Velde and Kiekens 2002); nevertheless, the applications of biopolymers are infinite. Rubber is the best example of biopolymer that is not degradable. It is a commonly used elastomer in many human activities and derived from tropical trees (*Hevea brasiliensis*) whose commercial name is polyisoprene.

However, recent social concerns and environmental issues make the use of biopolymers and biodegradable materials an important issue. The rise of new emerging applications of biopolymers causes an increase in their production. The main issue of using biopolymers is that they should be stable while they are stored or used and their ability to degrade once disposed (Mohanty et al. 2005; Khalil et al. 2013). The innovation of biopolymers from renewable sources and in the development of materials from biopolymers brought the idea of preservation of fossil-based materials, reduction of the volume of waste, reduction of the amount of carbon dioxide released into the air, resulting in the reduction of air pollution and being a solution to the waste disposal problem (Mohanty et al. 2005).

8.1.3 CLASSIFICATION AND SYNTHESIS OF BIOPOLYMER

A polymer (or a macromolecule) is a molecule made from identical low molar mass units, called repeat units or monomers. As mentioned previously, proteins, polysaccharides, and rubber are polymers in which protein's repeat unit is categorized as amino acids and polysaccharide as sugar. Polymers are named after the number of repeat units they have possessed. For example, a polymer consisting of one type of monomers is called homo-polymer, and a polymer with two or more types of monomers is called a copolymer. A regular sequence of macromolecules having one repeated unit is the simplest polymer. When the two ends of a linear macromolecule are connected, a cyclic polymer molecule is formed. Furthermore, the combination of cyclic molecules and linear molecules creates a wide variety of macromolecules. Polyethylene and polypropylene belong to *polyolefins*, which include the major class of polymers (Sperling 2006).

Polymers are classified into two types: biopolymers and synthetic polymers. Different classifications are available for biopolymers based on the origin of the raw materials and their usage. Based on the degradability of biopolymers, they are classified into biodegradable and non-biodegradable. Based on their occurrence, they can be divided into natural biopolymers, such as proteins, polysaccharides, starch, cellulose, chitosan, agar, alginate, and carrageenan, and synthetic polymers, such as poly(glycolic acid) (PGA), poly(L-lactide) (PLA), poly(ε-caprolactone), polyesters, and polyphosphoester (Rhim et al. 2013; Tian et al. 2012). In the plant cell walls, after the production of polysaccharides such as cellulose and hemicelluloses, lignin fills the spaces between fibers and cement. Lignin is a phenolic compound that is resistant to microbial activity. The problem of science with lignin is that there is no exact method to isolate the lignin from its exact native structure (Figure 8.1). Consistency of fibers in industrial usage is an important factor (Mohanty et al. 2005).

In other classification forms, polymers are divided into few major groups such as elastomers, fibers, plastics, films, composites, and poly blends. Elastomers are a group of polymers that can be shaped when a force is applied and returned into their original shape when the force is removed, which is caused because of physical or chemical cross-links. In general, the cross-linked polymers are connected by many bonds and make a large molecule. A polymer is easily deformable and stretchable when the number of cross-links is low (Winnik 1999). The cross-links make a great diversity of structures according to the type of polymers, functionality, and amount of reactants (Carraher 2000).

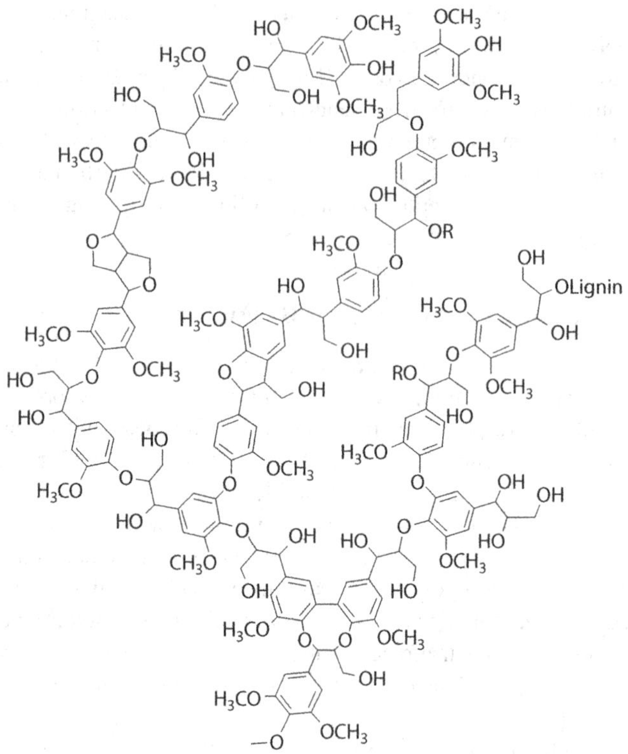

FIGURE 8.1 Lignin structure.

There are correlations, terms, and concepts for the synthesis of polymers. Polymers are synthesized by chain or stepwise polymerization. Although there are a few exceptions, including a correlation between vinyl polymers and the chain type of kinetics, and a correlation between condensation polymers and step-wise kinetics mentioned for the polymer synthesis. Condensation polymers are synthesized by three major techniques: the melt synthetic technique (high melt, bulk melt), solution polymerization, and interfacial polymerization. Free radical polymerization is the most important type of chain reaction polymerization. In free radical polymerization, initiation, propagation, and termination are the major steps. Initiation occurs when the free radicals attack the monomers and attach to them. Propagation occurs when monomers are added together rapidly, and termination occurs when two free radicals react together. In this method, the bulk solution, suspension, and emulsion polymerization are applied to produce polymers in chain reaction polymerization. Stepwise reactions require heating to begin the reaction, whereas chain processes start below the room temperature. Chain polymerization is usually faster than stepwise reaction due to the activation energy in controlling the step (Carraher 2000). Poly(ethylene terephthalate) and polyamides (known as nylon) are the polymers synthesized through stepwise polymerization reaction. Poly(ethylene terephthalate) is known as Dacron fiber with high crystallinity. In natural polymers, the organisms make the step polymerized polymers through an enzymatic polymer controlled reaction; a DNA (Sperling 2006).

8.1.4 BIOPOLYMERS MARKET VALUE AND DEMAND

Biopolymers market is growing rapidly and industries are having competitions in designing a biopolymer with superior functional attributes, abilities, and commercial value. These competitions are due to the eco-efficiency, green chemistry, renewable nature and industrial ecology of biopolymers, which lead the industries to the next generation of materials. The fibre reinforcement market value of biopolymers is derived from various sources that make it a very big business. Different sources of fiber reinforcement plastic composites such as marine sources are being used for various applications such as automotive, electronic component, miscellaneous, and aerospace. The demand for petrochemical-based polymers would reach up to 5% by 2020 according to the expectations of Toyota Company. The growth of market for biopolymers between 1999 to 2004 showed that the demand for biopolymers is increasing and the market is developing to a rich and mass production scale.

In 2007, the biopolymer production was 280M lb, which was increased to 740M lb/yr for PE/PP biopolymers during 2010–2012 in Brazil. Various factors control the market value of biopolymers. Factors such as high oil prices, depletion of oil reserves, the worldwide interest in renewable resources, waste management, concerns about greenhouse gas emission, legislative incentives, and commercial viability of production and processing affect the biopolymer market.

8.2 PREPARATION OF THE BIOPOLYMERS

8.2.1 PHYSICAL PROPERTIES

The physical properties of polymers depend on the factors such as interbonding, the presence of other polymer chains in their structure, chain size, MW, and nature of the backbone. The interbonding forces are divided into primary and secondary forces. The primary force is greater than 50 kcal/mole of interactions, whereas the secondary force is less than 10 kcal/mole of interactions. Polymers and small molecules join together by primary covalent bonds and secondary forces, respectively. The secondary forces and structural considerations determine the shape of polymer chains in the solid and mobile states. The combination of secondary and primary forces forms polymer structures in biopolymers (Carraher 2000).

While studying the physical properties of biopolymers, the density sounds a very important factor especially in designing parameters. The major part of a polymer structure is crystal which is caused the denser and higher melting point (Carraher 2000). Besides increasing the density values that imply a higher transportation cost, the implementation of materials becomes easier and less hazardous when lighter (Van de Velde and Kiekens 2002). Density is usually a useful factor in the calculation of specific properties; these properties imply a better understanding of the inner strength while building a new construct. For example, in case of flax amplification, poly-DL-lactide, poly-ε-caprolactone, and polyhydroxybutyrate are considerable choices due to lower density and lighter weight that they possess. Filler is another factor that enhances various physical properties such as heat deflection temperature, flexural modulus, flexural strength, and resistance of the composite. Fillers in the matrix composites affect the overall properties of the composite system (Khalil et al. 2013).

Several other factors of biopolymers are vapor transmission characteristics (mainly for film applications), crimp, impact properties, melt flow indices, coefficients of friction, hardness, compostabilities, water content or water uptake, contact angles with water, and surface energies (Van de Velde and Kiekens 2002). Water absorption is considered a negative factor in biopolymers due to making a disturbance in the fibre/polymer interface and cause to reduce the overall strength of the composite. Absorbing too much water can reduce the composite's strength (Van de Velde and Kiekens 2002). Degradation time of biopolymers is a factor that should be made as short as possible. When a polymer has a short degradation time, corrosion resistance should decrease. In high-performance composite, the polymers that have a longer degradation time are more likely to be used (Van de Velde and Kiekens 2002).

An issue in polymer science is to determine the form of polymer chains in space. The macromolecule dimensions can be obtained using scattering of X-rays, light, or neutrons. The polymer chain dimension can be obtained through indirect methods, such as the viscosity of the dilute solution and hydrodynamic property of chain molecules. Moreover, the size of a single macromolecule can be measured when it is dissolved in solution, but the molecular interactions, such as solvent and polymer interactions, cannot be ignored. The inherent structural factors such as the level of branching and the chemical structure of the base unit make the shape of polymers and may be different from the level of temperature, solvent, and flow (Winnik 1999).

8.2.2 Mechanical Properties

Polymer's persistency to deformation and their application for failure at static or dynamic loads make their mechanical properties. Various tests are available to determine the mechanical properties of biopolymers, of which the simplest one is tensile testing. There are two types of properties that are mostly correlated: tensile properties, such as ultimate tensile strain (ε, in %), elasticity modulus (E, in GPa), and tensile strength (s, in MPa), and flexural properties. When discussing a denser biopolymer, tensile properties are the best to study and lower density biopolymers tend to fail in this (Van de Velde and Kiekens 2002). In mechanical properties, the molecular mass is a very considerable factor for developing the biopolymer. For example, in poly-L-lactic acid, when the molecular mass is higher, a higher tensile strength is yielded (Fritz et al. 1994).

Filler content is one of the main important factors in the mechanical properties of biopolymers. It is added to polymer materials to enhance their nature, processing capabilities, and strength, and to reduce their cost production. By increasing the filler content, the tensile property decreases (Khalil et al. 2013). In unidirectional composites, most of the composite strength is provided by the reinforcement fiber (Van de Velde and Kiekens 2001). By using the rule of mixtures and typical polymer properties, the composite density can be obtained. When a composite is mixed with polyglycolide, a heavier composite with the same physical properties is obtained. However, the presence of polylactide and poly-ε-caprolactone in a composite makes it lighter with a high volume percentage (Van de Velde and Kiekens 2002). High volume percentage is a positive fact, as it results in less expensive polymers.

Furthermore, when choosing a matrix, any substance (even a weak substance such as polyhydroxyoctanoate) can be used, but the important fact is that the substance should have a high volume percentage. Decreasing the strength of the matrix results in a lighter composite and its mechanical properties are not affected (Van de Velde and Kiekens 2002). A lighter composite matrix is the best choice in preparing a polymer, whereas a heavier composite matrix has poor mechanical properties. The mechanical properties classified based on the density include specific tensile strength and tensile modulus. These equations show that tensile is an important factor and it is correlated with mechanical properties. Structural elements without reinforcements in biopolymers are considerable as specific properties settle the dimensions essential for a certain mechanical strength (Van de Velde and Kiekens 2002).

8.2.3 Thermal Properties

The thermal properties of polymers can be determined by different methods, but the most common one is differential scanning calorimetry (Jones and McClements 2010). When a polymer melts, it behaves like a liquid. By decreasing the temperature, the molten polymer's viscosity increases. As the temperature decreases enough, the individual chains start to solidify, and if it decreases further, the chains solidify outside of the domains of crystallinity. The degree of the crystallinity of the former causes the polymer materials to be flexible or rubbery. When a polymer is heated, it softens at a characteristic temperature range called glass transition temperature, which is a transition from a glass form to a rubber form and is measured under standard condition. This characteristic is very important as it can show the dramatic changes in the physical properties of the polymers, such as elasticity and stiffness. By measuring the physical, mechanical or thermodynamic properties as a function of temperature, the glass temperature of polymer can be observed (Winnik 1999). When the polymer temperature is reduced below the glass transition temperature, its flexibility decreases. Moreover, no segmental motion is available at the temperature below glass transition temperature, and if any dimensional changes occur, it is the result of the changes in primary valence bonds. However, the composite strength is mainly obtained from its fibers, and thus, the temperature does not have a major effect. Biopolymers with a lower glass transition melting point are more suitable to be used as matrix materials in producing composites with higher strength (Van de Velde and Kiekens 2002).

Another important parameter of biopolymers is their melting point. Biopolymers with a higher melting point have chain mobility and their mechanical properties are less. Besides the melting point, the process temperature is another parameter worth looking at, in which viscosity reduces when the process temperature increases (Van de Velde and Kiekens 2002). The process temperature of biopolymers is 20°C–100°C higher than their melting point (Van de Velde and Kiekens 2001). This higher temperature is mainly due to additives, which at reduced temperatures can impede thermal degradation. Moreover, lower melting point and process temperature are beneficial and energy cost saving because while producing a product, they prevent the degradation of the flax. This concludes that biopolymers with a high process temperature are not suitable to be used in flax combination as they lead to thermal degradation of the flax (Van de Velde and Kiekens 2002).

8.3   INDUSTRIAL APPLICATIONS OF POLYMER

8.3.1   INDUSTRIAL PURPOSE BIOPOLYMER PREPARATION

Recent advances in technologies in all areas from chemical synthesis or biosynthesis and benefits from sustainable, environmentally friendly products that decompose continuously, leaving behind no toxic trace and maintenance of physical health approaches companies to end manufacturing conventional nondegradable plastics and all products related.

Biopolymers are a specific type of polymers that break down into CO_2 and water by microorganisms. To provide general definition and clarify misconceptions, a biodegradable polymer can be degraded by naturally occurring microorganisms such as bacteria, fungi, and algae to yield water (H_2O), carbon dioxide (CO_2), methane (CH_4), biomass, and inorganic compounds, whereas a compostable plastic is biodegradable in a composting environment, result in the production of H_2O, CO_2, biomass, and inorganic compounds. The biodegradation during composting should be at a rate similar to other known compostable materials, and should not leave visual or toxic residue. In order to label a plastic as compostable one, it must meet scientific standards, such as the ASTM (American Society for Testing and Materials) specification. After discussing the different properties of a series of biodegradable polymers, it may be fulfilling to mention some current applications of biopolymers. Biomedical field has a large proportion of utilizing this technology and can be roughly divided into three categories: drug delivery systems, wound closure and healing products, and surgical implant devices. Drug delivery inside the human body can be quite easily controlled with the use of biodegradable capsules. In wound healing, sutures made of polyglycolic acid are absorbable and will be degraded by the body over time. Another related benefit of biopolymers is to use them as bio-restorable scaffolds for tissue engineering. Biopolymers are also applicable in food industry and feed additives, plastic industry, as packaging material for many purposes, agriculture, and environment pollution control.

8.3.2   BIOPOLYMERS RESOURCE FROM MARINE

Carrageenan (linear polysaccharide) obtained by extraction with water or alkaline water of a specific species of the class Rhodophycea (red seaweed), alginate (also linear polysaccharide) extracted from brown algae and chitosan are the examples of marine biopolymers. Chitosan is the second most abundant biopolymer after cellulose, and is unique and a typical marine polysaccharides. The wide variety of physicochemical and biological properties of polymers have found diverse applications in areas, ranging from medical to agrochemical, environmental, and different industrial uses. Chitosan and chitin (the primary structural component of of the outer skeleton of crustaceans) extracted from ciliates, amebae, cryophytes, some algae, yeasts, and fungi to the lower animals such as crustaceans, worms, insects, vertebrates, plants, and prokaryotes do not contain chitin. Chitosan is the N-deacetylated derivative of chitin (by treatment with hot alkali), with its structure composed of 2-amino-2-deoxy-β-D-glucose (GlcN) in a β(1,4) linkage and occasionally N-acetyl glucosamine (GlcNAc) residues. The structure of chitin and chitosan resembles that of cellulose except at position C-2, being replaced by acetamido and/or amino groups, respectively. The major procedure for obtaining chitosan is based on the alkaline deacetylation of chitin with strong alkaline solution (Srinivasa and Tharanathan 2007). According to chitin and chitosan's chemical structures and biological activities, their versatile uses in the biomedical, agricultural, environmental, and industrial have been discovered. Biocompatibility, renewable origin, nontoxicity, nonallergenicity, and biodegradability in the body are some features of these biopolymers, which make them biologically, economically, and medically eligible to be used in many purposes. These applications are summarized in Table 8.1.

8.3.3 PLASTIC INDUSTRY

Increased use of plastic packaging which is petroleum based and disposal of waste plastics are huge ecological problems, and the development of biodegradable plastics is an approach to protect and conserve ecology. Plastic wastes can

TABLE 8.1
Application of Chitin and Chitosan

Field	Form	Application	Reference
Medicine	Beads	Drug delivery	Cheba 2011
	Nanoparticles	Encapsulation of sensitive drugs	
	Microspheres	Enzyme immobilization	
	Fibers	Gene delivery vehicle	
	Films	Medical textiles	
		Wound care	
		Dialysis membrane	
		Antitumoral	
		Semipermeable film for wound dressing	
Genetic engineering	Vector	Gene carrier and DNA vaccine delivery, protects DNA from DNAase degradation	Cheba 2011
Food industry and food additives	Powder, gel, solution	Food preservative, antioxidant, emulsifier, thickener, stabilizer, clarifier, viscosifier, gelling agent, flavor, extender, livestock, and fish-feed additive	Cheba 2011
Water treatment	–	Chelation of metal ions, pesticides, phenols, dyes, dithiothreitol (DTT), polychlorinated biphenyl (PCBs), proteins, amino acids, detoxification of water from oil and greases, determination of lead in water samples, removal of dyes	Cheba 2011
Textile industry	–	Wool finishing, dying improvement, textile preservative and deodorant agent, textile printing and antimicrobial finishing flocculants, dye removal from textile waste water	Cheba 2011
Agriculture	–	Agriculture seed and fruit coating, fertilizer, biopesticide and fungicide growth enhancers, stimulator for the plant hormones responsible for root formation, stem growth, and fruit development	Cheba 2011
Other industry	–	Leather, plastics, cigarettes, and solid state batteries	Cheba 2011

TABLE 8.2

Biodegradation of Various Packaging Materials

Bioplastics (Plastic Packaging Films)	Duration of Bioplastics (Days)
Starch-based bioplastics	~40–60
Polymer-based films	~90–150
Chitosan-based films	~90–150
Cellulose-based films	>365
PLA-based films	150–240 (at 60°C)

be utilized as a renewable source of energy; nevertheless, burning the plastic in a conventional incinerator involves high-flame temperature, releasing a large amount of heat. Hence, the concept of biodegradability has both user-friendly and eco-friendly aspects, and the raw materials are essentially derived from either replicable agricultural feedstocks (cellulose, starch, and proteins) or marine resources (chitin/chitosan) (Srinivasa and Tharanathan 2007). Table 8.2 shows how long some common items will take to break down into their building locks and how it varies depending on the type, bacterial count, and moisture content; it is also possible that sewage sludge treatment impacts the duration of biodegradation (Srinivasa and Tharanathan 2007).

The name *chitin* is named after the Greek word *chiton*, meaning *coat of mail or envelop*. India has a coastline of 8129 km, and many varieties of fishes/shellfish resources are available. The commercial fishing of shrimp in India began in the 1960s when trawling was introduced and seafood export became a major growing industry. During crustacean processing, shell wastes accounting for up to 60% of the original materials are produced as waste by-products. One of the problems of the seafood industries is disposal of the solid wastes. In the 1970s, the Environmental Protection Agency-directed industries to stop dumping shell wastes of crab, lobster, and shrimp. As biodegradation of chitin in crustacean shell wastes is very slow, accumulation of large quantities of discards from the processing of crustaceans has become a major concern in the seafood industry in coastal areas. Globally, more than 100 million tons of chitin is produced, of which 2000 tons is produced in India. Hence, production of value-added products from such wastes and their application in different fields are of utmost interest. Using simple demineralization (treatment with hot dilute HCl) and deproteinization (treatment with hot dilute NaOH) steps, the amino polysaccharide chitin can be quantitatively recovered from crustacean wastes. Chitin is known to form a microfibrillar arrangement in living organisms. The fibrils having a diameter of 2.5–2.8 nm are usually embedded in the protein matrix; crustacean cuticles possess chitin microfibril with diameters as large as 25 nm (Srinivasa and Tharanathan 2007). Compared to plastic packaging films (~$2 per kg), chitosan is expensive (~$15.5 per kg), even though other biopolymers are much cheaper (e.g., corn starch and cellulose at $0.8–1.0 per kg). Nevertheless, for food coating and pharmaceutical applications, such high prices are tolerated, but such costs are too high for commodity packaging (Srinivasa and Tharanathan 2007) (Figure 8.2).

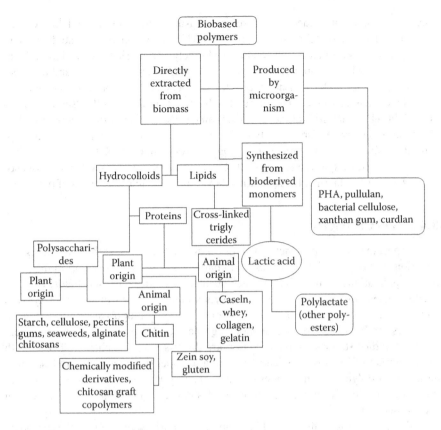

FIGURE 8.2 Biobased polymers.

8.3.4 AGRICULTURE POLYMER

Chitosan and its derivatives possess plant-protecting and antifungal properties, triggering a defense mechanism in plants against infection and parasitic attack, even at a very low concentration. It is used in the form of solution or as coating of the seed. It acts at several levels, by strengthening the root system and thickening the stem. It also behaves like fertilizer by accelerating the germination and growth of plants. Moreover, the activity of chitin and its derivatives on how it improves crop yield is detected. In addition to the direct effects on plant nutrition and plant growth stimulation, chitin-derived products have also been shown to be toxic to plant pests and pathogens, induce plant defenses, and stimulate the growth and activity of beneficial microbes (Sharp 2013).

8.3.5 CONDUCTING POLYMER

A research was conducted in 2008 (Khan 2008), and it reported that a chitosan–polyaniline (PANI) hybrid conducting biopolymer film was obtained on indium–tin-oxide (ITO) electrode using electrochemical polymerization process.

Electrochemical impedance spectroscopy measurements had showed low charge transfer resistance of PANI–chitosan and PANI. The aim of this study was to develop a process for metal-free conducting biopolymer matrices, which have advantages for technological applications, possess biodegradation property, and are cost-effective. Synthesis of metal nanoparticles is a very complex process and requires several chemical processes. Therefore, the chemicals used for synthesis and the non-degradable characteristics of metal oxides can have several environment issues when chemical wastes were disposed. Oxidative characteristics of nanomaterials can also limit the stability during storage and using electrodes in electrolytes. A process had been developed to synthesize a hybrid PANI–CS matrix as a metal-free biosensor with excellent conducting, biocompatible, and biodegradable properties of polymers.

8.4   CONCLUSION

The importance of biopolymers in many industrial and research fields drags the attention to study on their features and characteristics. The most important traditional applications of biopolymers include their uses in medicinal fields, packaging industries, and agricultural films. Polymers are classified in various ways and methods based on the origin of the raw materials into biopolymers and synthetic polymers, or biodegradable and nonbiodegradable. The syntheses of biopolymers by chain and/or stepwise polymerization are discussed in this chapter. The growth in the market of biopolymers leads to a great competition among the industries to design a biopolymer with a superior function. Physical, mechanical, and thermal properties of biopolymers are essential in designing a new biopolymer possessing such a function.

Chitin and chitosan, the second most abundant marine polymers, with their properties such as renewable resources, biocompatibility, and antimicrobial agents, have led to an increase in their applications in a wide spectrum in diverse fields of medicine, especially in drug delivery projects, waste management, food, agriculture, plastic industry, and a lot more that we still have not discovered about what biopolymers are capable to be used.

REFERENCES

Carraher, C.E. 2000. Introduction to polymer science and technology. In *Applied Polymer Science*, pp. 21–48. Elsevier: Oxford.
Cheba, B.A. 2011. Chitin and chitosan: Marine biopolymers with unique properties and versatile applications. *Global Journal of Biotechnology & Biochemistry* 6(3): 149–153.
Fritz, H.G., T. Seidenstücker, U. Bölz, M. Juza, J. Schroeter, and H-J. Endres. 1994. Use of whole cells and enzymes for the production of polyesters (Chapter 3) and Mimicking of natural substances (petroleum derived polymers) (Chapter 4). In study on *Production of Thermo-Bioplastics and Fibres Based Mainly on Biological Materials*, Agro-Industrial Research Division, Directorate-General XII Science, Research and Development, Brussels, Belgium, pp. 109–139.
Jones, O.G. and D.J. McClements. 2010. Functional biopolymer particles: Design, Fabrication, and Applications. *Comprehensive Reviews in Food Science and Food Safety* 9(4): 374–397.

Khalil, H.P.S.A., N.A.S. Aprilia, A.H. Bhat, M. Jawaid, M.T. Paridah, and D. Rudi. 2013. A Jatropha biomass as renewable materials for biocomposites and its applications. *Renewable and Sustainable Energy Reviews* 22: 667–685.

Khan, R. and M. Dhayal. 2008. Chitosan/polyaniline hybrid conducting biopolymer base impedimetric. *Biosensors and Bioelectronics* 24(6): 1700–1705.

Mohanty, A.K., M. Misra, L.T. Drzal, E. Susan, E. Selke, B.R. Harte, and G. Hinrichsen. 2005. *Natural Fibers, Biopolymers, and Biocomposites*: An Introduction, Natural Fibers, Biopolymers and Biocomposites, Taylor & Francis: Boca Raton, pp. 15–18.

Nair, L.S. and C.T. Laurencin. 2007. Biodegradable polymers as biomaterials. *Progress in Polymer Science* 32(8): 762–798.

Penning, J.P., H. Dijkstra, and A.J. Pennings. 1993. Preparation and properties of absorbable fibres from L-lactide copolymers. *Polymer* 34(5): 942–951.

Peralta, J., M.A. Raouf, S. Tang, and R.C. Williams. 2012. Bio-renewable asphalt modifiers and asphalt substitutes. In K. Gopalakrishnan, M. Zhou, T. Jin, Z. Wu, and M. Chi (Eds.) *Sustainable Bioenergy and Bioproducts*, pp. 89–115. Springer: London.

Rhim, J.-W., H.-M. Park, and C.-S. Ha. 2013. Bio-nanocomposites for food packaging applications. *Progress in Polymer Science* 38(10): 1629–1652.

Roller, S. and I.C.M. Dea. 1992. Biotechnology in the production and modification of biopolymers for foods. *Critical Reviews in Biotechnology* 12(3): 261–277.

Schiffman, J.D. and C.L. Schauer. 2008. A review: Electrospinning of biopolymer nanofibers and their applications. *Polymer Reviews* 48(2): 317–352.

Sharp, R.G. 2013. A review of the applications of chitin and its derivatives in agriculture to modify plant-microbial interactions and improve crop yields. *Argonomy* 3(4): 778–757.

Sperling, L.H. 2006. Chain structure and configuration. In *Introduction to Physical Polymer Science*, 4th edition, Hoboken, NJ, pp. 29–70. Wiley.

Srinivasa, P.C. and R.N. Tharanathan. 2007. Chitin/Chitosan—safe, ecofriendly packaging materials with multiple. *Food Reviews International* 23(1): 53–72.

Tian, H., Z. Tang, X. Zhuang, X. Chen, and X. Jing. 2012. Biodegradable synthetic polymers: Preparation, functionalization and biomedical application. *Progress in Polymer Science* 37(2): 237–280.

Van de Velde, K. and P. Kiekens. 2001. Thermoplastic polymers: Overview of several properties and their consequences in flax fibre reinforced composites. *Polymer Testing* 20(8): 885–893.

Van de Velde, K. and P. Kiekens. 2002. Biopolymers: Overview of several properties and consequences on their applications. *Polymer Testing* 21(4): 433–442.

Winnik, F.M. 1999. Elements of polymer science. *Cosmetic Science and Technology Series* 22: 1–50.

9 Biological Applications of Marine Biopolymers

T. Rajeshwari, M. Saranya,
Govindasamy Rajakumar, and Ill-Min Chung

CONTENTS

9.1   INTRODUCTION

Biopolymer is a polymer that is produced by living beings. It is a biodegradable chemical compound that is regarded as the most organic compound in the ecosphere. The name *biopolymer* indicates that it is a biodegradable polymer. The term *biopolymers* is used to describe a variety of materials. In general, however, biopolymers fall into two principal categories: polymers that are produced by biological systems such as microorganisms, plants, and animals, and polymers that are synthesized chemically but are derived from biological starting materials such as amino acids, sugars, natural fats, or oils (Cappello 1992). Some biopolymer examples are proteins, carbohydrates, DNA, RNA, lipids, nucleic acids, peptides, and polysaccharides (such as glycogen, starch, and cellulose).

9.2 STRUCTURE OF BIOPOLYMER

The structure of biopolymers has been a subject of investigation ever since they were discovered. So far, the most accurate methods for structure determination have been X-ray diffraction techniques. These techniques are, however, restricted to crystallizable molecules, and it has not been established if the molecular structure in a crystal is identical to that in solution. Many methods have been developed or adopted to probe biopolymer properties in solution. The most common are dynamic light scattering (Berne and Pecora 1976), transient electric birefringence (Eden and Elias 1983), and nuclear magnetic resonance and ultracentrifugation (Cantor and Schimmel 1980; Figure 9.1).

9.3 PHYSICOCHEMICAL PROPERTIES OF BIOPOLYMER

Biopolymers are polymers produced by living organisms. As they are polymers, they contain monomeric units that are covalently bonded to form larger structures. There are three main classes of biopolymers based on the differing monomeric units used and the structure of the biopolymer formed: Polynucleotides, which are long polymers composed of 13 or more nucleotide monomers; polypeptides, which are short polymers of amino acids; and polysaccharides, which are often linear bonded polymeric carbohydrate structures (Figure 9.2).

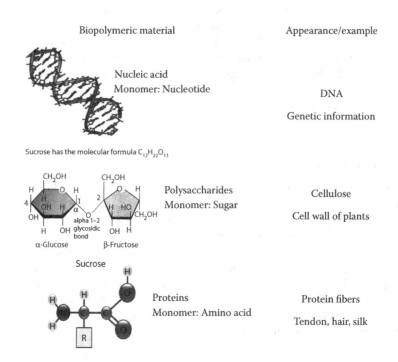

FIGURE 9.1 Biopolymer and its appearance.

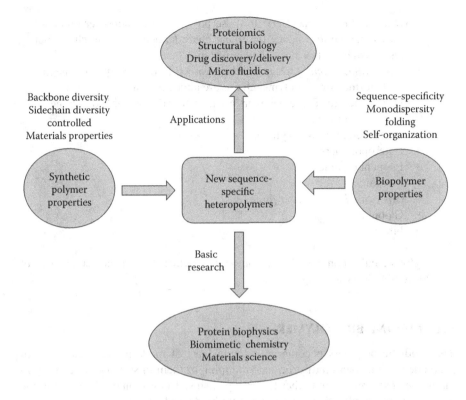

FIGURE 9.2   Biopolymers from polysaccharides and agroproteins.

Polymers are classified as follows:

1. Classification by source
2. Classification by structure
3. Classification by synthesis
4. Classification by molecular forces

- *Classification by source*
  - Natural (nucleic acids, polysaccharides, protein, natural rubber [polyisoprene])
  - Synthetic (polyethelene, teflon, polyvinilchloride, polystyrene)
- *Classification by structure*
  - *Linear polymers*: In these polymers, the monomers are joined together to form long straight chains of polymer molecules. They have high melting point, high densities, and high tensile (pulling) strength because of the close packing of polymer chains.

- • *Branched chain polymers*: In these polymers, the monomer units not only combine to produce the linear chain (called the main chain) but also form branches along the main chain.
- • *Three-dimensional (3D) network polymers*: In these polymers, the initially formed linear polymer chains are joined together to form a 3D network structure. These polymers are also called cross-linked polymers.
- • *Classification by synthesis*
  - • Carbon containing polymers
  - • Heteropolymers
  - • Element organic
  - • Inorganic
- • *Classification by molecular forces*
  - • Globular
  - • Fibril

The high-molecular compounds are compounds, which have a molecular mass of 10,000–10,000,000 Da.

9.4 MARINE BIOPOLYMER

The synthetic polymers become an essential part of modern life. Excess use of synthetic polymers and indiscriminate dumping of them in soil and water are polluting the environment and other living organisms. To overcome this problem, the production and applications of eco-friendly biodegradable products (such as biopolymer) from marine sources are becoming predictable from the last decade and also good alternatives of synthetic polymers. Keeping this point in mind, several studies aimed at isolating and identifying the biopolymers producing organisms from marine sources that can be effectively utilized for the synthesis of biopolymers (Muthezhilan et al. 2014) for treating diseases such as diabetes, inflammatory, and hypersensitivity.

Phycocolloids (production of biopolymers) are extracted from seaweeds and algal species, namely, hypnea, eucheuma, and gracilaria (red algae); and sargassum, turbinaria, and ulva (brown algae) (Jhurry et al. 2006). Poly-3-hydroxybutyrates (large-scale production of biopolymer) are extracted from marine bacteria of AMET 5111 *Pseudomonas* spp. (Muthezhilan et al. 2014). Fucoidans, carrageenans, and agar (polysaccharide) are extracted from red edible seaweeds, brown algae, and brown seaweeds (Jhurry et al. 2006).

9.5 APPLICATIONS

9.5.1 GENERAL APPLICATIONS OF MARINE BIOPOLYMER

Chitosan is a natural nontoxic biopolymer produced by the deacetylation of chitin, a major component of the shells of crustaceans such as crab, shrimp, and crawfish. Chitooligosaccharides (COSs) are the degraded products of chitosan or chitin prepared by enzymatic or chemical hydrolysis of chitosan. Chitosan and its derivatives have shown various functional properties that have made them possible to be used in many fields, including food (Shahidi et al. 1999), cosmetics (Kumar et al. 2000), biomedicine (Felt et al. 1998), agriculture (Yamada et al. 1993), environmental protection (Peniche-Covas et al. 1992), and wastewater management (Jeuniaux 1986).

Chitosan has three types of reactive functional groups: an amino group and both primary and secondary hydroxyl groups at the C-2, C-3, and C-6 positions, respectively. Chemical modifications of these groups have provided numerous useful materials in different fields of application. Currently, chitosan has received considerable attention for its commercial applications in the biomedical, food, and chemical industries (Knorr 1984; Kurita 1986; Razdan and Pettersson 1994; Furusaki et al. 1996; Muzzarelli 1977; Kurita 1998). Due to its unique biological characteristics, including biodegradability and nontoxicity, many applications have been found either alone or blended with other natural polymers (starch, gelatin, and alginates) in the food, pharmaceutical, textile, agriculture, water treatment, and cosmetics industries (Roberts 1992; Arvanitoyannis et al. 1998; Arvanitoyannis 1999; Haque et al. 2005; Kim et al. 2005; Yamada et al. 2005; Table 9.1).

In agriculture, chitosan has been described as a plant antivirus and an additive in liquid multicomponent fertilizers (Struszczyk et al. 1989), and it has also been investigated as a metal-recovering agent in agriculture and industry (Onsoyen and Skaugrud 1990). Chitosan has been noted for its application as a film-forming agent in cosmetics (Lang and Clausen 1989), a dye binder for textiles, a strengthening additive in paper (Ashford et al. 1977), and a hypolipidic material in diets (Fukada et al. 1991; Table 9.2).

The biopolymers from bacteria will help to produce biodegradable products in large quantities at a very low cost (Muthezhilan et al. 2014). Phycocolloids (marine biopolymer) from seaweeds are used for food, medicine, cosmetic

TABLE 9.1
Commercial Applications of Chitosan

S. No.	Commercial Sector	Applications
1	Agriculture	Defensive mechanism in plants, stimulation of plant growth, seed coating, frost protection, time release of fertilizers, and nutrients into the soil
2	Water and waste treatment	Flocculant to clarify water (drinking water, pools), removal of metal ions, ecological polymer (eliminate synthetic polymers), and reduce odors
3	Food and beverages	Not digestible by human (dietary fiber), bind lipids (reduce cholesterol), preservative, thickener and stabilizer for sauces, protective, fungistatic, antibacterial coating for fruit
4	Cosmetics and toiletries	Maintain skin moisture, treat acne, improve suppleness of hair, reduce static electricity in hair, tone skin, oral care (tooth paste, chewing gum)
5	Biopharmaceutics	Immunologic, antitumoral, hemostatic and anticoagulant, healing, and bacteriostatic

TABLE 9.2

Applications of Chitin and Chitosan

Area of Application	Examples
Antimicrobial agent	Bactericidal, fungicidal, and measure of mold contamination in agricultural commodities
Edible film industry	Controlled moisture transfer between food and the surrounding environment, controlled release of antimicrobial substances, controlled release of antimicrobial substances, controlled release of antioxidants, controlled release of nutrients, flavor and drugs, reduction of oxygen partial pressure, controlled rate of respiration, temperature control, controlled enzymatic browning in fruits, and reverse osmosis membranes
Additives	Clarification and deacidification of fruits and beverages, natural flavor extender, texture controlling agent, emulsifying agent, food mimetic, thickening and stabilizing agent, and color stabilization
Nutritional quality	Dietary fiber, hypocholesterolemic effect, livestock and fish feed additive, reduction of lipid absorption, production of single-cell protein, antigastritis agent, and infant feed ingredient
Recovery of solid materials from food processing wastes	Affinity flocculation and fractionation of agar
Purification of water	Recovery of metal ions, pesticides, phenols, and PCBs, and removal of dyes
Waste water treatment	Removal of metal ions, flocculant/coagulation of protein, dye, and aminoacids
Food industry	Removal of dye, suspended solids, as a preservative, color stabilization, food stabilizer, thickener and gelling agent, and animal feed additive
Agriculture	Seed coating, fertilizer, controlled agro chemical release, and prevention of decay of fruits and vegetables
Biotechnology	Enzyme immobilization, protein separation, cell recovery, and chromatography
Cosmetics	Moisturizer; face, hand and body creams; and bath lotion
Other applications	Enzyme immobilization, encapsulation of nutraceuticals, chromatography, and analytical reagents

products, pharmaceuticals, fertilizers, and animal feed production (Jhurry et al. 2006). Carrageenans are widely used in the food industry for their gelling, thickening, and stabilizing properties. Their main application is in dairy and meat products, due to their strong binding to food proteins. Fucoidan is used as an ingredient in some dietary supplement products. Agarose is frequently used in molecular biology for the separation of large molecules, especially DNA, by electrophoresis (FAO 2011).

The complex sulfated polysaccharide (SP) from ulvan can also be of potential interest for food, pharmaceutical, and agricultural applications (Lahaye and Axelos 1993; Costa et al. 2010; Wijesekara et al. 2011; Stengel et al. 2011; Alves et al. 2012).

Besides their use as food, the macroalgae of the genus *Ulva* can also have applications in the removal of nutrients from effluent waters of sewage, industry, and mariculture. Studies showed that some *Ulva* species have been tagged as a pollution indicator due to their biomass accumulation when they inhabited in highly polluted waters (Lahaye et al. 1998; Largo et al. 2004; Wolf et al. 2012). For instance, *Ulva lactuca* has proven to be a good seaweed biofilter in the treatment of fishpond effluents.

Regarding industrial applications of galactans extracts from algae, they are generally around the texture (gelling and thickening properties), but now they are also used as cosmetic and biomedical products.

9.5.2   MEDICAL APPLICATIONS OF MARINE BIOPOLYMER

Marine biopolymers have so many medical applications, for example, chitosan, a biopolymer of glucosamine derived from chitin used for tissue engineering applications: tissue and organ loss or damage is a major human health problem. Transplantation of tissue or organs is a standard therapy to treat the tissue- or organ-damaged patients. However, this therapy is severely limited due to the shortage of donors. Tissue engineering is one of the available therapies to treat the loss or damaged tissue and organ. Chitosan is a promising polymer for tissue engineering for its nontoxicity, biocompatibility, and biodegradability. Moreover, it has structural similarity to glucosaminoglycans, which are the major components of the extracellular matrix (Giri et al. 2012). Tissue engineering is a highly interdisciplinary field that combines the principles and methods of life sciences and engineering to utilize the structural and functional relationships in normal and pathological tissue to develop biological substitutes to restore, maintain, or improve biofunction. Chitosan and its derivatives are promising candidates as a supporting material for tissue engineering applications due to their porous structure, gel forming properties, ease of chemical modification, high affinity for *in vivo* macromolecules, and so on. In-Yong et al. (2008) focused on the various types of chitosan derivatives and their use in various tissue engineering applications, namely, the skin, bone, cartilage, liver, nerve, and blood vessel.

Exopolysaccharides (EPSs) are extracellular carbohydrate polymers produced and secreted by microorganisms, which are accumulated outside the cells. Some new EPSs produced by bacteria isolated from extreme marine environments showed the promising properties for tissue engineering in bone healing (Nichols et al. 2005). In tissue engineering, special interest is paid to stem cells and the design of bioactive nanopatterned scaffolds of different polymeric materials, including EPS, with specific ligands that direct and enhance cell function and differentiation of embryonic stem cells (Evans et al. 2006).

Chitosan in bone tissue engineering: A biodegradable scaffold in tissue engineering serves as a temporary skeleton to accommodate and stimulate new tissue growth. Zhensheng et al. (2005) reported thon the development of a biodegradable porous scaffold made from naturally derived chitosan and alginate polymers with significantly improved mechanical and biological properties compared to its chitosan counterpart. Enhanced mechanical properties were attributable to the formation of a complex structure of chitosan and alginate. Bone-forming osteoblasts readily attached to the chitosan–alginate scaffold, proliferated well, and deposited calcified matrix. The chitosan–alginate scaffold could be prepared from solutions of physiological pH, which might have provided a favorable environment for incorporating proteins with less risk of denaturation. Chitosan is also used as an adjuvant with bone cements to increase its injectability while keeping the chemicophysical properties suitable for surgical use with respect to setting time and mechanical properties. A new robotic desktop rapid prototyping (RP) system was designed by Ang et al. (2002) to fabricate the scaffolds for tissue engineering applications. Neutralization of the chitosan forms a gel-like precipitate, and the hydrostatic pressure in the sodium hydroxide (NaOH) solution keeps the cuboid scaffold in shape. Results of *in vitro* cell culture studies revealed the scaffold biocompatibility. The results of this preliminary study using the RP robotic dispensing system demonstrated its potential in fabricating 3D scaffolds with regular and reproducible macropore architecture.

Chitosan in cartilage tissue engineering: Silk fibroin/chitosan-blended scaffolds were fabricated and studied by Nandana et al. (2011) for cartilage tissue engineering. Silk fibroin served as a substrate for cell adhesion and proliferation, whereas chitosan has a structure similar to that of glycosaminoglycans and shows promise for cartilage repair. They compared the formation of cartilaginous tissue in silk fibroin/chitosan-blended scaffolds seeded with bovine chondrocytes and cultured *in vitro* for 2 weeks. The amount of glycosaminoglycan and collagen accumulated in all the scaffolds was the highest in the silk fibroin/chitosan (1:1) blended scaffolds. The results suggested that silk/chitosan scaffolds may be a useful alternative to synthetic cell scaffolds for cartilage tissue engineering. 3D scaffolds are especially important for fabricating articular cartilage. Chitosan was chosen by Francis Suh and Howard (2000) as a scaffolding material in articular cartilage engineering due to its structural similarity with various glycosaminoglycans (GAGs) found in articular cartilage. The *in vitro* tissue-engineered cartilage reconstructions were made by mixing sheep chondrocytes with a chitosan hydrogel.

Fucoidans, carrageenans, and agar (polysaccharide) are extracted from red edible seaweeds, brown algae, and brown seaweeds used as anticoagulant, antithrombotic, antiviral, antiproliferative, and antitumor agents. Some of the important marine biopolymers and their medical applications are briefly described in Sections 9.5.2.1 through 9.5.2.7.

9.5.2.1 Antidiabetic Activity

Diabetes mellitus is often simply referred to as diabetes. Diabetes is a group of metabolic diseases in which a person has high blood sugar, either because the body does not produce enough insulin or because cells do not respond to the insulin that is produced. This high blood sugar produces the classical symptoms of polyuria, polydipsia, and polyphagia. Diabetes mellitus is often called *the silent killer*, because it causes serious complications without serious symptoms and can affect many of the major organs in the body (Papaspyros 1964). It is a chronic disorder that affects the metabolism of carbohydrates, fats, proteins, and electrolytes in the body, leading to severe complications that are classified into acute, subacute, and chronic (Rang et al. 1991). The marine biopolymers used for the treatment of diabetes are *Ulva*, *Conus geographus*, and chitin.

9.5.2.1.1   Ulva

Diabetes mellitus is the most common endocrine disorder, with more than 150 million people suffering worldwide (World Health Organization 1985). Literature surveys indicate more than 400 plant species have antidiabetic activity, and most of the natural products used for diabetes treatments have been isolated from plants (Rai 1995). In contrast, the antidiabetic effects of compounds derived from marine bacteria and fungi remain poorly investigated, but may be of great promise in the search for novel drugs.

Diabetes mellitus is classified into two types: type1 (insulin dependent) and type 2 (non-insulin dependent). Type 2 diabetes mellitus is divided into two categories: obese type with hyperinsulinemia and nonobese type with hypoinsulinemia. It is established that obesity causes peripheral insulin resistance, which leads to hyperinsulinemia. Obesity-related type 2 diabetes mellitus is also characterized by hypertriglyceridemia and hyperinsulinemia. Improving the abnormality of lipid metabolism and glucose metabolism may be useful in preventing the development or progression of obesity-related type 2 diabetes mellitus. Miura et al. (1995) first showed that chitosan given as a 5% food mixture produces consistent blood glucose and lipid-lowering effects in normal mice and neonatal streptozotocin-induced diabetic mice.

In recent years, the significance of marine algae as a supply for new bioactive substances has been growing very rapidly (Smit 2004; Athukorala et al. 2006; Boopathy and Kathiresan 2010; Gamal 2010; Wijesekara et al. 2011; Mohamed et al. 2012) owing to their capacity to produce metabolites that exhibit various biological activities such as antidiabetic, antihypertensive, anticancer, antiobesity, antihyperlipidemic, antioxidant (Shalaby 2011), antibacterial, anti-inflammatory, antiproliferative, and antiviral (Xu et al. 2004; Cabrita et al. 2010). Although not many members of the genus *Ulva* have been extensively investigated, there are some interesting aspects of biological activities of the extracts and isolated metabolites. It is important to mention also that ulvan, a major SP found in the cell wall of green algae, is composed mainly of rhamnose, glucuronic acid, iduronic acid, xylose, glucose, sulfate with small amounts of iduronic acid, and traces of galactose, and represents 8%–9% of the algae dry weight (Ray and Lahaye 1995; Quemener et al. 1997; Lahaye 1998; Lahaye et al. 1999; Lahaye and Robic 2007; Robic et al. 2009; Boopathy and Kathiresan 2010; Stengel et al. 2011; Wijesekara et al. 2011).

The presence of the sulfate groups and the unusual chemical composition and structure of ulvan render it different biological properties (Lahaye and Robic 2007; Wijesekara et al. 2011; Alves et al. 2012). This complex SP can also be of potential interest for food, pharmaceutical, and agricultural applications. In recent years, ulvan has been extensively investigated for the development of novel drugs and functional foods (Lahaye and Robic 2007; Lahaye et al. 1999; Wijesekara et al. 2011). On account of its peculiar composition and structure (Robic et al. 2009), it represents a potential source of new functional biopolymer, and it is widely used as a biomaterial for tissue engineering in regenerative medicine.

Furthermore, studies showed that SPs can also exhibit beneficial biological activities such as anticoagulant, antiviral, antioxidant, anti-inflammatory (Costa et al. 2010), and antiproliferative (Mohamed et al. 2012). As attention has been focused on natural antioxidants in the past few years, because synthetic antioxidants such as butylated hydroxyanisole and butylated hydroxytoluene were found to implicate in liver damage and carcinogenesis, several natural SPs, including ulvan, were evaluated for their antioxidant activity. Interestingly, ulvan from *U. pertusa* and acetylated and benzoylated ulvans were found to have the antioxidant activity, including the scavenging activity against superoxide and hydroxyl radicals, reducing power and chelating ability (Qi et al. 2006).

9.5.2.1.2 Conus geographus

The venoms of predatory marine cone snails are remarkably potent and diverse. Most bioactive venom components are small disulfide-rich peptides, termed conotoxins (Olivera and Just 1996) that target specific receptors and ion channel subtypes located in the prey's nervous system (Terlau and Olivera 2004; Olivera and Teicher 2007). Here, evidence for specialized insulin in the venom of *Conus geographus* that is part of the chemical arsenal used by the snail for capturing prey. The venom gland of cone snails is highly specialized for conotoxin biosynthesis and secretion (Safavi-Hemami et al. 2014). Discovery of that insulin expressed in the venom gland of *C. geographus* at levels comparable to conotoxins was unexpected. When injected into fish, this insulin significantly lowers blood glucose levels, and direct application into the water column significantly reduces locomotor activity. This peptide has unusual features, including posttranslational modifications unprecedented in insulin but often found in conotoxins.

9.5.2.1.3 Chitin

Chitin (Figure 9.3), a mucopolysaccharide and the supporting material of crustaceans and insects, is the second most abundant polymer after cellulose found in nature; it is produced by many living organisms and is present usually in a complex with other polysaccharides and proteins. It was found as a major component in arthropods (insects, crustaceans, arachnids, and myriapods), nematodes, algae, and fungi (Rudall and Kenchington 1973; Muzzarelli 1977; Willis 1999; Synowiecki and Al-Khateeb 2003).

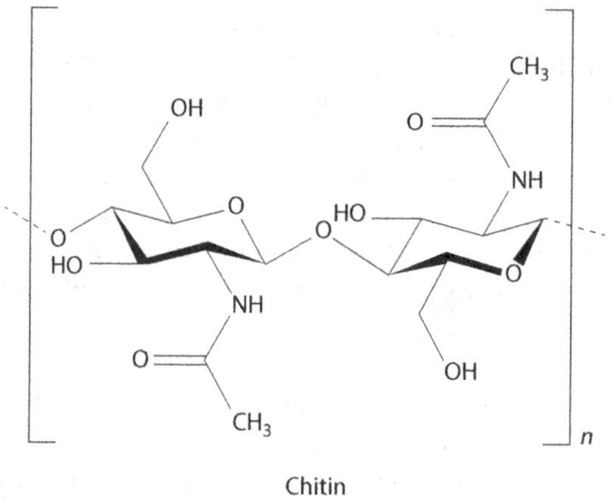

Chitin

FIGURE 9.3 Chitin.

Besides its application as a starting material for the synthesis of chitosan and chitooligosaccharides, chitin itself has been a center of many therapeutic applications and is thought to be a promising biomaterial for tissue engineering and stem cell technologies (Wan and Tai 2013).

9.5.2.1.4 Chitosan

Chitosan (Figure 9.4), a biopolymer of glucosamine derived from chitin that is chemically similar to that of cellulose, is not digestible by mammalian digestive enzymes and acts as a dietary fiber in the gastrointestinal tract (Gallaher et al. 2000). One of the recently reports demonstrated that chitosan has a hypoglycemic effect in streptozotocin (STZ)-induced diabetic animals (Yao et al. 2006). Other studies also found that low-molecular-weight chitosan (average molecular weight -2×10^4 Da) (Kondo et al. 2000; Hayashi and Ito 2002), and chitosan oligosaccharides (Lee et al. 2003), can reduce the plasma glucose level in diabetic animals (Table 9.3).

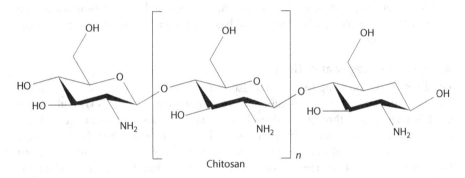

Chitosan

FIGURE 9.4   Chitosan.

TABLE 9.3

Biomedical Applications of Biopolymer

Potential Biomedical Applications	Principal Characteristics
Medical	Wound and bone healing, blood cholesterol control, skin burn, contact lens, surgical sutures, dental plaque inhibition, clotting agent, and antitumor
Surgical sutures	Biocompatible
Dental implants	Biodegradable
Artificial skin	Renewable
Rebuilding of bone	Film forming
Corneal contact lenses	Hydrating agent
Time release drugs for animals and humans	Nontoxic and biological tolerance
Encapsulating material	Hydrolyzed by lyzosyme, wound healing properties, efficient against bacteria, viruses, and fungi

Due to the presence of hydroxyl, amine, and acetylated amine groups, chitosan, low-molecular-weight chitosan, and COS interact readily with various cell receptors that trigger a cascade of interconnected reactions in living organisms resulting in antidiabetic effects (Ju et al. 2010).

9.5.2.1.5 Fucoxanthin

Fucoxanthin is the main pigment found in brown algae and possesses antidiabetic (Maeda et al. 2007) and antioxidant activities (Sachindra et al. 2007).

Marine algae are a natural resource representing many interests in the medical, therapeutic, and nutritional fields. In industrialized countries, a large number of research teams are investigating the ways of isolating polysaccharides, known to be very important in the medicinal and pharmaceutical fields such as anticoagulants (Ushakova et al. 2008), anti-inflammatory drugs (Cardozo et al. 2010), and antidiabetes induced by alloxan (Huang et al. 2006).

Fucoxanthin has been reported to have an antidiabetic effect (Maeda et al. 2009), which has an unique structure containing an allenic bond and a 5,6-monoepoxide (Holdt and Kraan 2011), whose structure has been linked to the anti-obesity effect (Miyashita 2009).

9.5.2.2 Anticoagulant Activity

Disorders in blood coagulation increase the risk of hemorrhage or thrombosis (Rivas et al. 2011). Anticoagulants prevent coagulation (Desai 2004) and can be used *in vivo* to treat thrombotic disorders. Heparin, an anticoagulant used widely in venous thromboembolic disorders, was discovered more than 50 years ago. However, it has several side effects, including thrombocytopenia, hemorrhage, and ineffectiveness due to congenital or acquired antithrombin deficiencies and inability to inhibit thrombin bound to fibrin (Pereira et al. 2002). Moreover, it is primarily extracted from pig intestines or bovine lungs, where it exists in low levels. Therefore, alternative anticoagulants are necessary for safer and more effective therapy.

9.5.2.2.1 Chitosan

The chemical modification of the amino and hydroxyl groups can generate products for pharmaceutical applications; for example, sulfated chitosan possesses a wide range of biological activities. Thus, chitosan sulfates, as the nearest structural analogs of the natural blood anticoagulant heparin, demonstrate the anticoagulant, antisclerotic, and antiviral activities (Hirano et al. 1985; Nishimura et al. 1998; Drozd et al. 2001; Vongchan et al. 2002; Desai 2004).

It has been used extensively as a biomaterial, due to its anticoagulant properties (Dutkiewicz and Kucharska 1992) and its action as a promoter of wound healing in the field of surgery (Muzzarelli et al. 1989).

9.5.2.2.2 Fucoidans

Fucoidans (Wang et al. 2012) are a group of sulfated heteropolysaccharides found in the cell wall of some members of Phaeophyceae. Drozd et al. (2006) elucidated the pharmacology of the fucoidans (Wang et al. 2012) from the marine algae

Fucus evanescens and *Laminaria cichorioides*, showing that these SPs inhibited both thrombin and factor Xa with a comparable potency to nonfractioned and low-molecular-weight heparin. In rats, intravenous injection of fucoidans dose-dependently increased the anticoagulant activity in the plasma. Interestingly, fucoidans can form complexes with protamine sulfate. Furthermore, the anticoagulation activity was increased with an increased fucoidan sulfate content (Shanthi et al. 2014).

Fucoidans (SPs) are involved extensively in the cell walls of brown macroalgae. They show various physiological and biological features, such as the anticoagulant, antioxidant, antiviral, and antithrombotic activities, in addition to the impact on the inflammatory and immune systems (Wijesekara et al. 2011).

9.5.2.2.3 Marine Proteins

Interest in marine proteins might be directly correlated not only to the intact protein but also to the possibility of generating bioactive peptides. In this sense, different peptides derived from marine proteins have been identified as having the antioxidant activity (Byun et al. 2009), and also the anticoagulant, antihypertensive, or antimicrobial activities (Ngo et al. 2011). These peptides have been isolated from diverse marine sources such as algae, crustaceans, and also different fish species.

Many marine organisms produce polysaccharides that have diverse applications, due to their biofunctional properties, and much research has been conducted to assess the possible use of these polysaccharides. Marine polysaccharides, including cellulose, fucan, glucosaminglycan, glucan, chitin, chitosan, laminaran, carrageenan, agar, and alginic acid, have anticoagulant, immunostimulatory, and antioxidative effects. Thus, these compounds could potentially be developed into therapeutics and nutraceuticals (Laurienzo 2010; Vo and Kim 2010; Gupta and Abu-Ghannam 2011; Wang et al. 2012; Thomas and Kim 2013).

Therapeutic interest of algal SPs as an anticoagulant agent has recently been the focus. In the future, algal (Rhodophyta, Phaeophyta, and Chlorophyta) SPs can be developed as anticoagulant/antithrombotic agents or could be used as a model for the same (Shanmugam and Mody 2000).

The first report on marine algal extracts possessing the blood anticoagulant properties was done by Chargaff et al. (1936), demonstrating the anticoagulant activity in an extract of a red alga *Iridae laminarioides*. This material, a *galactan sulfuric acid ester*, was shown to possess 30 U/mg of heparin equivalence. Subsequent studies described similar anticoagulant properties in agar and carrageenan. A group of 19 species belonging to red, brown, and green algae were screened by Elsener in 1938, but the anticoagulant activity was found only in *Delesseria sanguinea* (red alga).

Carrageenan of *Grateloupia turuturu* also showed the anticoagulant activity (Efimov et al. 1983). Sulfated galactan from *G. indica* of Indian waters exhibited the anticoagulant activity as potent as heparin. Carrageenan is derived from a number of seaweeds of the class Rhodophyceae. It is a generic name for a family of gel-forming and viscosifying polysaccharides. It is a sulfated polygalactan with 15%–40% of ester sulfate content. The principal basis of the anticoagulant activity of carrageenan appears to be an antithrombic property. The mechanism underlying the anticoagulant activity of carrageenan involves thrombin inhibition. There is either antithrombin potentiation via heparin cofactor II and/or a direct antithrombin effect (Buck et al. 2006).

Literature speaking about galactan from fungi is little but exists. The genus *Pleurotus* is known as a producer of this polysaccharide. Unconnected to their natural biological implication in animal, algae, and plants, galactans could act as a potential pharmacological product in mammalian systems. For example, sulfated galactan could modulate the anticoagulant activity (Pereira et al. 2002). Glycosaminoglycans were extracted from the dry tissue of marine clam Scapharca inaequivalvis, composed of dermatan sulfate and heparin sulfate.

9.5.2.3 Antiallergic Activity

Allergy is a common form of hypersensitivity with an incidence that has increased dramatically in the developed world during the past 50 years, and, at present, it affects >25% of the population in these countries (Larche et al. 2006). Atopic individuals show a dysregulated immune response to nonpathogenic proteins, called allergens, present either in the environment (i.e., dust, pollen) or in food (i.e., eggs, milk, nuts). This response starts, like any acquired immune response, with antigenic sensitization. Allergen is taken by dendritic cells and presented to specific Th cells by means of major histocompatibility complex class II and costimulatory molecules (CD80, CD86), thus performing the immunological synapse (Valenta et al. 2004).

Bae et al. (2013) demonstrated that oral administration of chitin (α and β) is beneficial in preventing food allergies. The oral administration of chitin was accomplished by milling it to a particle size less than 20 μm and mixing it with feed. Their results showed that α-form reduced the serum levels of peanut-specific immunoglobulin E (IgE) and both the forms decreased the levels of interleukins (ILs), IL-5 and IL-10, and increased the levels of IL-12. Dietary supplementation of chitin has shown to exert positive immunomodulatory effects (Harikrishnan et al. 2012a, 2012b).

Chitosan lacks irritant or allergic effects and is biocompatible with both healthy and infected human skin (Malette et al. 1986). When chitosan was administered orally in mice, the lethal dose, 50% (LD50) was found to be in excess of 16 g/kg, which is higher than that of sucrose (Arai et al. 1968). Chitosan is compatible with lots of biologically active components incorporated in cosmetic products composition. It may be noted that substances absorbing the harmful ultraviolet radiation or different dyes can be easily covalently linked to chitosan amino groups.

Compositions based on chitosan and other hydrocolloids containing antiallergic and anti-inflammatory substances of vegetable origin, new types of depilatory, and means for curling and doing the hair are being work out. According to Nawanopparatsakul et al. (2005), chitosan and its derivatives offer in three areas of cosmetics: hair care, skin care, and oral care. Facial mask prepared by using curcuminoids showed skin irritation, but incorporation of chitosan in this preparation reduced this untoward effect.

9.5.2.4 Anti-Inflammatory

Inflammation is a local response of living mammalian tissues to injury. It is a body defense reaction in order to eliminate or limit the spread of injurious agents. There are various components to an inflammatory reaction injury. Edema formation, leukocyte infiltration, and granuloma formation represent such components of inflammation (Mitchell and Cotron 2010). The inflammatory process can be elicited by numerous internal or external stimuli. Inflammatory diseases are usually treated with drugs that inhibit inflammatory processes. Anti-inflammatory refers to substances or treatments that reduce inflammation. Macrophages are key players in inflammation (Kazlowska et al. 2010). Due to the presence of hydroxyl, amine, and acetylated amine groups, chitosan, low-molecular-weight chitosan, and COS interact readily with various cell receptors that trigger a cascade of interconnected reactions in living organisms resulting in anti-inflammatory (Fernandes et al. 2010) and anticancerogenic (Huang et al. 2005) effects.

Fucoxanthin is the main pigment found in brown algae and possesses anti-inflammatory activity (Shiratori et al. 2005). Marine sources are widely regarded as possessing interesting lipid compositions, which make them attractive as a source for lipid extraction. The main polar lipids found in these substrates include monogalactosyl diacylglycerols, digalactosyl diacylglycerols, and phosphatidylglycerols. These polar lipids possess several functional activities, but are mainly referenced in the literature for their anti-inflammatory activities (Larsen et al. 2003; Bruno et al. 2005).

Sterols and some of their derivatives were found previously to play an important role in lowering LDL cholesterol levels *in vivo* (Francavilla et al. 2010). Other bioactivities are associated with sterols and include anti-inflammatory and antiatherogenic activity (Francavilla et al. 2010). In addition, phytosterols (C_{28} and C_{29} sterols) are the important precursors of compounds, including vitamins. For example, ergosterol is a precursor of vitamin D_2 and cortisone.

Macroalgae are regarded as a rich source of SPs. For example, the alga *Chondrus crispus* is traditionally employed for the extraction of carrageenan (also known as Irish moss), a highly SP. Among their associated bioactive properties, the anti-inflammatory, immunomodulating, anticancer, antiviral, or antioxidant activities have been pointed out (Li et al. 2008).

Phycobiliproteins are one of the most important groups of proteins from seaweed. These water-soluble proteins, mainly found in some blue-green and red algae, are characterized by possessing a tetrapirrolic ring covalently attached to their structure. This pigment can be either phycocyanobilin (blue-green algae) or phycoerythrobilin (red algae), and it is partially responsible for the functional properties associated with these proteins, mainly anti-inflammatory, hepatoprotective, and antioxidant activities (Bhat et al. 1998; Bhat and Madyastha 2000; Romay et al. 2003).

Fucoidan extracted from brown seaweeds, which have a higher sulfate content, was reported to have the anti-inflammatory activity in several cell lines (Lutay et al. 2011). Sulfated galactan could modulate the anti-inflammatory activity (Berteau and Mulloy 2003).

9.5.2.5 Immunoadjuvants

An adjuvant is an agent that stimulates the immune system, increasing the response to a vaccine, while not having any specific antigenic effect. Adjuvants perform one or more of the three main functions: (1) They provide a *depot* for the antigen for slow release, (2) they facilitate targeting of the antigen to immune cells and enhance phagocytosis, and (3) they modulate and enhance the type of immune response induced by the antigen alone (Trujillo-Vargas et al. 2005; Cox et al. 2006; Lutsiak et al. 2006; Petrovsky 2006). They may also provide the danger signal the immune system needs in order to respond to the antigen as it would to an active infection (Janeway et al. 2001). Thus, they play a significant role in every aspect of the immune response.

Clinically, immunomodulators can be classified into the following three categories:

1. *Immunoadjuvants*: They are used to enhance the efficacy of vaccines and therefore could be considered specific immune stimulants. They hold the promise of being the true modulators of the immune response. It has been proposed that they be exploited as selectors between cellular and humoral helper T1 (Th1) and helper T2 cells (Th2), immunoprotective, immunode-structive, and reagenic (IgE) versus IgG-type immune responses posing a real challenge to vaccine designers (Hofmeyr 2001).

2. *Immunostimulants*: They are inherently nonspecific as they are envisaged as an enhancement to a body's resistance to infection. They can act through innate and adaptive immune responses. In healthy individuals, they are expected to serve as prophylactic and promoter agents, that is, as immu-nopotentiators, by enhancing the basic level of immune response. In the individual with impairment of immune response, they are expected to act as immunotherapeutic agents (Alfons and Patrick 2001).

3. *Immunosuppressants*: They are a structurally and functionally heteroge-neous group of drugs, which are often concomitantly administered in com-bination of regimens to treat various types of organ transplant rejection and autoimmune diseases (El-Sheikh 2008).

It has been used extensively as a biomaterial (Shigemasa and Minami 1995) due to its immunostimulatory activities (Nishimura et al. 1987). Due to the presence of hydroxyl, amine, and acetylated amine groups, chitosan, low-molecular-weight chitosan, and COS interact readily with various cell receptors that trigger a cascade of interconnected reactions in living organisms resulting in immunostimulative effects (Moon et al. 2007).

Carrageenan (SPs) from marine algae can have diverse biological activities, including immunomodulatory effects (Necas and Bartosikova 2013).

The main properties of chitin and chitosan, applied for specific applications, such as biocompatibility, renewable origin, nontoxicity (Kumar et al. 2000), nonal-lergenicity, and biodegradability in the body (Patil et al. 2000). In addition, it has attractive biological activities (immunoadjuvant, antithrombogenic, antifungal, anti-bacterial, antitumor, and anticholesteremic agents) and bioadhesivity (especially of chitosan and its derivatives) (Venter et al. 2006).

The Th1 adjuvant effect of chitin microparticles in inducing viral-specific immu-nity has also been reported by Hamajima et al. (2003).

9.5.2.6 Antihypersensitivity

A hypersensitivity reaction refers to a state of altered reactivity in which the body mounts an amplified immune response to a substance. In 1963, Gell and Coombs (1963) classified hypersensitivity reactions into five different groups (types I, II, III, IV, and V), which depended upon the severity and latency of a reaction. A summary of the hypersensitivity reactions is presented in Table 9.4.

TABLE 9.4
Summary of the Hypersensitivity Reactions

	Antigens	Effectors	Tissue Damage
Type I Hypersensitivity			
Anaphylaxis	Insect venoms, drugs, food	IgE on basophils and mast cells	Edema, bronchoconstriction, vascular collapse, and death
Asthma and hay fever	House dust mites, cats, cockroaches, molds	IgE on mast cells and Th2 cells	Bronchoconstriction, edema, mucus production, inflammation, and epithelial cell damage
Food allergy	Peanuts, nuts, egg, milk, shellfish, and fish	IgE on mast cell and Th2 cells	Diarrhea, vomiting, urticaria, and eczema
Type II Hypersensitivity			
Good pasture syndrome	Basement membrane	Antibody and complement	Nephritis
Drug sensitivity	Quinidine bound to platelets	Antibody and complement	Purpura and thrombocytopenia
Hemolytic disease of the newborn	Rh antigen on the red blood cells	Opsonization of red blood cells	Anemia
Myasthenia gravis	Acetylcholine receptor	Antibody	Paralysis
Type III Hypersensitivity			
Arthus reaction	Soluble antigens	Immune complexes, complement, basophils, platelets, and neutrophils	Local inflammatory reaction
Extrinsic allergic alveolitis	Inhaled antigens, molds, mushroom spores, and bird proteins	Immune complexes, antibody, complement, and monocytes	Monocytic lung inflammation and edema
Serum sickness	Foreign serum proteins	Immune complexes, complement, basophils, platelets, and neutrophils	Joint inflammation and vasculitis
Systemic lupus erythematosus	Autoantigens, DNA, ribonuclear proteins, histones, and cytoplastic antigens	Immune complexes and complement	Nephritis, vasculitis, and pleuritis
Type IV Hypersensitivity			
Delayed hypersensitivity	Proteins, viruses, bacteria (tuberculin), autoantigens, and grafts	T cells and macrophages	Monocytic inflammation, islet destruction in diabetes, and chronic graft rejection

(Continued)

TABLE 9.4 (*Continued*)
Summary of the Hypersensitivity Reactions

	Antigens	Effectors	Tissue Damage
Contact hypersensitivity	Poison ivy, rubber chemicals, chromate, 2,4-Dinitrofluorobenzene (DNFB), 2,4-Dinitrochlorobenzene (DNCB), and topical antibiotics	T cells and macrophages	Monocytic skin inflammation
Th2 responses	House dust mites, and food and helminth parasites	T cells and eosinophils	Inflammation and cell destruction
Type V Hypersensitivity			
Graves disease	Thyroid-stimulating hormone receptor	Antireceptor and antibody	Goiter and thyrotoxicosis

9.5.2.7 Anticholesteremic Activity

Most of the naturally occurring polysaccharides, namely, cellulose, dextrin, pectin, alginic acid, agar, agarose, and carrageenan, are naturally acidic in nature, whereas chitin and chitosan are the examples of highly basic polysaccharides. They have several properties such as solubility in various media, solution, viscosity, metal chelation, and structural characteristics. The chemical properties of chitosan are due to the presence of linear polyamine and reactive amino groups, which can chelate many transitional metal ions. Chitin also has biological properties as follows: it is biocompatible, accelerates the formation of osteoblast that is responsible for bone formation, anticholesteremic, hemostatic, fungistatic, spermicidal, antitumor, and accelerates bone formation (Pal et al. 2014).

The main biological activities of chitin and chitosan applied for specific applications are as follows: anticholesteremic, immunoadjuvant, antithrombogenic, antifungal, antibacterial, and antitumor agents, and bioadhesivity (especially of chitosan and its derivatives (Venter et al. 2006).

The biological properties of chitosan are as follows: (1) It is anticholesteremic, (2) it has regenerative effect on connective gum tissue, (3) it is hemostatic and fungistatic, (4) it is antitumor, (5) it is biocompatible, (6) it accelerates bone formation, and (7) it is immunoadjuvant (Dutta et al. 2004).

9.6 CONCLUSIONS AND FUTURE PERSPECTIVES

In summary, marine biopolymer has been extensively utilized as a biomaterial for many biomedical applications, particularly in the areas of drug delivery, *in vitro* cell culture, wound and bone healing, blood cholesterol control, skin burn, contact lens, surgical sutures, dental plaque inhibition, clotting agent, antitumor, and tissue engineering. The most attractive features of marine biopolymers for these applications include biocompatible, biodegradable, renewable, nontoxic, biological tolerance, mild gelation conditions, and simple modifications to prepare biopolymer derivatives with new properties. Chitin and chitosan have emerged as the most extensively explored marine biomaterials due to very good cytocompatibility and biocompatibility, biodegradation, sol/gel transition properties, and chemical versatility, which make possible further modifications to tailor their properties. In the future, effort should be made on chemical derivatization of biopolymer to create next-generation marine biomaterials having enhanced or altogether new properties. A thorough understanding of the chemistry of marine biopolymer is vital to this goal. An important challenge that remains is the development of biopolymer particles, with a narrow size distribution, high mechanical and chemical stability, and feasibility to scale up to medical and industrial-scale production volumes.

REFERENCES

Ahmad, Z., R. Pandey, S. Sharma, and G.K. Khuller. 2006. Pharmacokinetic and pharmacodynamic behaviour of antitubercular drugs encapsulated in alginate nanoparticles at two doses. *International Journal of Antimicrobial Agents* 27: 420–427.

Alfons, B., and M. Patrick. 2001. Modes of action of Freund's adjuvants in experimental models of autoimmune diseases. *Journal of Leukocyte Biology* 70: 849–60.

Alves, A., R.A. Sousa, and R.L. Reis. 2012. *In vitro* cytotoxicity assessment of ulvan, a polysaccharide extracted from green algae. *Phytotherapy Research* 27(8): 1143–1148. doi:101002/ptr.4843.

Ang, T.H., F.S.A. Sultana, D.W. Hutmacher, Y.S. Wong, J.Y.H. Fuh, X.M. Mo, H.T. Loh, E. Burdet, and H.S. Teoh. 2002. Fabrication of 3D chitosan–hydroxyapatite scaffolds using a robotic dispensing system. *Materials Science and Engineering* 20: 35–42.

Arai, K., T. Kinumaki, and T. Fujita. 1968. Toxicity of chitosan. *Bulletin of Tokai Regional Fisheries Research Laboratory* 56: 89–94.

Arvanitoyannis, I.S. 1999. Totally and partially biodegradable polymer blends based on natural and synthetic macromolecules: Preparation, physical properties, and potential as food packaging materials. *Journal of Macromolecular Science* C 39: 205–271.

Arvanitoyannis I.S., A. Nakayama, and S.I. Aiba. 1998. Chitosan and gelatin based edible films: State diagrams, mechanical and permeation properties. *Carbohydrate Polymers* 37: 371–382.

Ashford, N.A., D.B. Hattis, and A.E. Murray. 1977. Industrial Prospects for chitin and protein from shellfish wastes. MIT Sea Grant Program, Massachusetts Institute of Technology. Report no. MITSG 77-3, Index no. 77-703-Zle.

Athukorala, Y., W.K. Jung, T. Vasanthan, and Y.J. Jeon. 2006. An anticoagulative polysaccharide from an enzymatic hydrolysate of *Ecklonia cava*. *Carbohydrate Polymers* 66: 184–191.

Bae, M. J., H.S. Shin, E.K. Kim, J. Kim and D.H. Shon. 2013. Oral administration of chitin and chitosan prevents peanut-induced anaphylaxis in a murine food allergy model. *International Journal of Biological Macromolecules* 61: 164–168.

Berne, B., and R. Pecora. 1976. *Dynamic Light Scattering*. John Wiley & Sons, New York.

Berteau, M., and B. Mulloy. 2003. Sulfated fucans, fresh perspectives: Structures, functions, and biological properties of sulfated fucans and an overview of enzymes active toward this class of polysaccharide. *Glycobiology* 13: 29–40.

Bhat, B.V., N.W. Gaikwad, and K.M. Madyastha. 1998. Hepatoprotective effect of C-phycocyanin:protection for carbon tetrachloride and R-(+)-pulegone-mediated hepatotoxicty in rats. *Biochemical and Biophysical Research Communications* 249: 428–431.

Bhat, B.V., and K.M. Madyastha. 2000. C-Phycocyanin: A potent peroxyl radical scavenger *in vivo* and *in vitro*. *Biochemical and Biophysical Research Communications* 275: 20–25.

Boopathy, N.S., and K. Kathiresan. 2010. Anticancer drugs from marine flora: An overview. *Journal of Oncology*. doi:10.1155/2010/214186.

Bruno, A., C. Rossi, G. Marcolongo, A. Di Lena, A. Venzo, C.P. Berrie, D. Corda. 2005. Selective *in vivo* anti-inflammatory action of the galactolipid monogalactosyldiacylglycerol. *European Journal of Pharmacology* 524: 159–168.

Buck, C.B., C.D. Thompson, J.N. Roberts, M. Muller, D.R. Lowy, and J.T. Schiller. 2006. Carrageenan is a potent inhibitor of papillomavirus infection. *PLoS Pathogens* 2: 0671–80.

Byun, H.G., J.K. Lee, H.G. Park, J.K. Jeon, and S.K. Kim. 2009. Antioxidant peptides isolated from the marine rotifer, *Brachionus rotundiformis*. *Process Biochemistry* 44: 842–846.

Cabrita, M.T., C. Vale, and A.P. Rauter. 2010. Halogenated compounds from marine algae. *Marine Drugs* 8: 2301–2317.

Cantor, P., and R. Schimmel. 1980. Biophysical chemistry, Vol. II. In C.J. Van Oss (Ed.), *Techniques for the Study of Biological Structure and Function*. W.H. Freeman and Company, New York.

Cappello, J. 1992. Genetic production of synthetic protein polymers. *Materials Research Bulletin* 17: 45–53.

Cardozo, M.L., C.A. Xavier, M.B. Bezerra, A.O. Paiva, and E.L. Leite. 2010. Assessment of zymozan-induced leukocyte influx in a rat model using sulfated polysaccharides. *Planta Medica* 76: 113–9.

Chargaff, E., F.W. Bancroft, and M.S. Brown. 1936. Studies on the chemistry of blood coagulation: II. On the inhibition of blood clotting by substances of high molecular weight. *Journal of Biological Chemistry* 115: 155–161.

Costa, L.S., G.P. Fidelis, S.L. Cordeiro, R.M. Oliveira, D.A. Sabry, R.B. Camara, L.T. Nobre, M.S. Costa, J. Almeida-Lima, E.H. Farias, E.L. Leite, and H.A. Rocha. 2010. Biological activities of sulfated polysaccharides from tropical seaweeds. *Biomedicine and Pharmacotherapy* 64: 21–28.

Cox, E., F. Verdonck, D. Vanrompay, and B. Goddeeris. 2006. Adjuvants modulating mucosal immune responses or directing systemic responses towards the mucosa. *Veterinary Research* 37: 511–539.

Desai, U.R. 2004. New antithrombin-based anticoagulants. *Medical Research Review* 24: 151–181.

Drozd, N.N., A.I. Sher, V.A. Makarov, G.A. Vichoreva, I.N. Gorbachiova, and L.S. Galbraich. 2001. Comparison of antitrombin activity of the polysulphate chitosan derivatives *in vitro* and *in vivo* system. *Thrombosis Research* 102: 445–455.

Drozd, N.N., A.S. Tolstenkov, V.A. Makarov, T.A. Kuznetsova, N.N. Besednova, N.M. Shevchenko, and T.N. Zvyagintseva. 2006. Pharmacodynamic parameters of anticoagulants based on sulfated polysaccharides from marine algae. *Bulletin of Experimental Biology and Medicine* 142: 591–593.

Dutkiewicz, J., and M. Kucharska. 1992. *Advances in Chitin and Chitosan*. Elsevier Science, London.

Dutta, P.K., J. Dutta, and V.S. Tripathi. 2004. Chitin and chitosan: Chemistry, properties and applications. *Journal of Scientific and Industrial Research* 63: 20–31.

Eden, D., and J.G. Elias. 1983. Measurements of Suspended Particles by Quasi-Elastic Light Scattering. In B. Dahneke (Ed.), *Measurement of Suspended Particles by Quasi-Elastic Light Scattering*, Wiley-Interscience, New York.

Efimov, V.S., A.I. Usov, T.S. Ol'skaya, A. Baliunis, A. Rozkin, and M. Ya. 1983. Carrageenan of Grateloupia turuturu also showed anticoagulant activity. *Farmakologiia i Toksikologiia* (Moscow) 46: 61–67 (in Russian).

El-Sheikh, A.L.K. 2008. *Renal Transport and Drug Interactions of Immuno Suppressants (thesis)*, p. 62, Radbound University, Nijmegen, the Netherlands.

Evans, N.D., E. Gentleman, and J.M. Polak. 2006. Scaffolds for stem cells. *MaterialsToday* 9: 26–33. doi:10.1016/S1369-7021(06)71740-0.

FAO. Agar and Carrageenan Manual. Fao.org (1965-01-01). Retrieved on 2011-12-10.

Felt, O., P. Buri, and R. Gurny. 1998. Chitosan: A unique polysaccharide for drug delivery. *Drug Development and Industrial Pharmacy* 24: 979–993.

Fernandes, J.C., H. Spindola, V. De Sousa, A. Santos-Silva, M.E. Pintado, F.X. Malcata, and J.E. Carvalho. 2010. Antiinflammatory activity of chitooligosaccharides *in vivo*. *Marine Drugs* 8: 1763–1768.

Francavilla, M., P. Trotta, and R. Luque. 2010. Phytosterols from *Dunaliella tertiolecta* and *Dunaliella salina*: A potentially novel industrial application. *Bioresource Technology* 101: 4144–4150.

Francis Suh, J.K., and W.T. Howard. 2000. Application of chitosan-based polysaccharide in cartilage tissue engineering: A review. *Biomaterials* 21: 2589–2598.

Fukada, Y., K. Kimura, and Y. Ayaki. 1991. Effect of chitosan feeding on intestinal bile acid metabolism in rats. *Lipids* 26: 395–399.

Furusaki, E., Y. Ueno, N. Sakairi, N. Nishi, and S. Tokura. 1996. Facile preparation and inclusion ability of a chitosan derivative bearing carboxymethyl-β-cyclodextrin. *Carbohydrate Polymers* 29: 29–34.

Gallaher, C.M., J. Munion, Jr. R Hesslink, J. Wise, and D.D. Gallaher. 2000. Cholesterol reduction by glucomannan and chitosan is mediated by changes in cholesterol absorption and bile acid and fat excretion in rats. *The Journal of Nutrition* 130: 2753–2759.

Gamal, A.A.E. 2010. Biological importance of marine algae. *Saudi Pharmaceutical Journal* 18: 1–25.

Gell, P.G.H., and R.R.A. Coombs. 1963. The classification of allergic reactions underlying disease. In R.R.A. Coombs, P.G.H. Gell (Eds.), *Clinical Aspects of Immunology*. Blackwell Science, Oxford.

Giri, T.K., T. Amrita, A. Amit, B. Ajazuddin, B. Hemant, and D.K. Tripathi. 2012. Modified chitosan hydrogels as drug delivery and tissue engineering systems: Present status and applications. *Acta Pharmaceutica Sinica B* 2: 439–449.

Gupta, S., and N. Abu-Ghannam. 2011. Bioactive potential and possible health effects of edible brown seaweeds. *Trends in Food Science and Technology* 22: 315–326.

Hamajima, K., Y. Kojima, K. Matsui, Y. Toda, N. Jounai, T. Ozaki, K.Q. Xin, P. Strong, and K. Okuda. 2003. Chitin micro-particles: A useful adjuvant for inducing viral specific immunity when delivered intranasally with an HIV-DNA vaccine. *Viral Immunology* 16: 541–547.

Haque, T., H. Chen, W. Ouyang, C. Martoni, B. Lawuyi, A.M. Urbanska, and S. Prakash. 2005. Superior cell delivery features of poly(ethylene glycol) incorporated alginate, chitosan, and poly-L-lysine microcapsules. *Molecular Pharmaceutics* 2: 29–36.

Harikrishnan, R., J.S. Kim, C. Balasundaram, and M.S. Heo. 2012a. Dietary supplementation with chitin and chitosan on haematology and innate immune response in *Epinephelus bruneus* against *Philasterides dicentrarchi*. *Experimental Parasitology* 131: 116–124.

Harikrishnan, R., J.S. Kim, C. Balasundaram, and M.S. Heo. 2012b. Immunomodulatory effects of chitin and chitosan enriched diets in *Epinephelus bruneus* against *Vibrio alginolyticus* infection. *Aquaculture* 326–329: 46–52.

Hayashi, K., and M. Ito. 2002. Antidiabetic action of low molecular weight chitosan in genetically obese diabetic KK-Ay mice. *Biological and Pharmaceutical Bulletin* 25: 188–192.

Hirano, S., Y. Tanaka, M. Hasegawa, K. Tobetto, and A. Nishioka. 1985. Effect of sulfated derivatives of chitosan on some blood coagulant factors. *Carbohydrate Research* 137: 205–215.

Hofmeyr, S.A. 2001. An interpretative introduction to the immune system. In I. Cohen, L. Segel (Eds.), *Design Principles for the Immune System and Other Distributed Autonomous Systems*, p. 3e24, Oxford University Press, New York.

Holdt, S.L., and S. Kraan. 2011. Bioactive compounds in seaweed: Functional food applications and legislation. *Journal of Applied Phycology* 23: 543–97.

Huang, R., E. Mendis, N. Rajapakse, and S.K. Kim. 2006. Strong electronic charge as an important factor for anticancer activity of chitooligosaccharides (COS). *Life Sciences* 78: 2399–2408.

Huang, Z.X., X.T. Mei, D.H. Xu, S.B. Xu, and J.Y. Lv. 2005. Protective effects of polysaccharide of *Spirulina platensis* and *Sargassum thunbeergii* on vascular of alloxan induce diabetic rats. *Zhongguo Zhong Yao Za Zhi.* 30: 211–215.

In-Yong, K., S.-J. Seo, H.-S. Moon, M.-K. Yoo, I.-Y. Park, B.-C. Kim, and C.-S. Cho. 2008. Chitosan and its derivatives for tissue engineering applications. *Biotechnology Advances* 26: 1–21.

Jag, P., H.O. Verma, V.K. Munka, S.K. Maurya, D. Roy, and J. Kumar. 2014. Biological method of chitin extraction from shrimp waste an eco-friendly low cost technology and its advanced application. *International Journal of Fisheries and Aquatic Studies* 1: 104–107.

Janeway, C.A., P. Travers, M. Walport, M.J. Shlomchik. 2001. Immunobiology 5th ed. In *The Immune System in Health and Disease*. Garland Science publishing, New York.

Jeuniaux, C. 1986. Chitosan as a tool for the purification of waters. In R.A.A. Muzzarelli, C. Jeuniaux, G.W. Gooday (Eds.), *Chitin in Nature and Technology*, pp. 551–570. Plenum Press, New York.

Jhurry, D., A. Bhaw-Luximon, T. Mardamootoo, and A. Ramanjooloo. 2006. Biopolymers from the mauritian marine environment. *Macromolecular Symposia* 231: 16–27.

Ju, C., W. Yue, Z. Yang, Q. Zhang, X. Yang, Z. Liu, and F. Zhang. 2010. Antidiabetic effect and mechanism of chitooligosaccharides. *Biological and Pharmaceutical Bulletin* 33: 1511–1516.

Kazlowska, K., T. Hsu, C.C. Hou, W.C. Yang, and G.J. Tsai. 2010. Anti-inflammatory properties of phenolic compounds and crude extract from *Porphyra dentata*. *Journal of Ethanopharmacology* 128: 123–130.

Kim, H.J., F. Chen, X. Wang, and N.C. Rajapakse. 2005. Effect of chitosan on the biological properties of sweet basil (*Ocimum basilicum* L.). *Journal of Agricultural and Food Chemistry* 53: 3696–3701.

Knorr, D. 1984. Use of chitinous polymers in food: A challenge for food research and development. *Food Technology* 38: 85–97.

Kondo, Y., A. Nakatani, K. Hayash, and M. Ito. 2000. Low molecular weight chitosan prevents the progression of low dose streptozotocin induced slowly progressive diabetes mellitus in mice. *Biological and Pharmaceutical Bulletin* 23: 1458–1464.

Kumar, M.N.V.R., R.A.A. Muzzarelli, C. Muzzarelli, H. Sashiwa, and A.J. Domb. 2000. Chitosan chemistry and pharmaceutical perspectives. *Reactive and Functional Polymers* 46: 1–27.

Kurita, K. 1986. Chemical modifications of chitin and chitosan, In R. Muzzarelli (Ed.), *Chitin in Nature and Technology*, pp. 287–293. Plenum Press, New York.

Kurita, K. 1998. Chemistry and application of chitin and chitosan. *Polymer Degradation and Stability* 59: 117–120.

Lahaye, M. 1998. NMR spectroscopic characterisation of oligosaccharides from two *Ulva rigida* ulvan samples (Ulvales, Chlorophyta) degraded by a lyase. *Carbohydrate Research* 314: 1–12.

Lahaye, M., and M.A.V. Axelos. 1993. Gelling properties of water-soluble polysaccharides from proliferating marine green seaweeds (*Ulva* spp.). *Carbohydrate Polymers* 22: 261–265.

Lahaye, M., E.A.C. Cimadevilla, R. Kuhlenkamp, B. Quemener, V. Lognoné, and P. Dion. 1999. Chemical composition and 13C NMR spectroscopic characterisation of ulvans from *Ulva* (Ulvales, Chlorophyta). *Journal of Applied Phycology* 11: 1–7.

Lahaye, M., F. Inizan, and J. Vigouroux. 1998. NMR analysis of the chemical structure of ulvan and of ulvan-boron complex formation. *Carbohydrate Polymers* 36: 239–249.

Lahaye, M., and A. Robic. 2007. Structure and functional properties of ulvan, a polysaccharide from green seaweeds. *Biomacromolecules* 8: 1765–1774.

Lang, G. and T. Clausen. 1989. The use of chitos an in cosmetics, In G. Skjoak-Brok, T. Anthonsen, P. Sandford (Eds.), *Chitin and Chitosan*, pp. 139–147. Elsevier Science, London.

Larche, M., C.A. Akdis, and R. Valenta. 2006. Immunological mechanisms of allergen-specific immunotherapy. *Nature Review Immunology* 6: 761–71.

Largo, D.B., J. Sembrano, M. Hiraoka, and M. Ohno. 2004. Taxonomic and ecological profile of "green tide" species of *Ulva* (Ulvales Chlorophyta) in central Philippines. *Hydrobiol* 512: 247–253.

Larsen, E., A. Kharazmi, L.P. Christensen, and S.B. Christensen. 2003. An anti-inflammatory galactolipid from rose hip (*Rosa canina*) that inhibits chemotaxis of human peripheral blood neutrophils in vitro. *Journal of Natural Products* 66: 994–995.

Laurienzo, P. 2010. Marine polysaccharides in pharmaceutical applications: An overview. *Marine Drugs* 8: 2435–2465.

Lee, H.W., Y.S. Park, J.W. Choi, S.Y. Yi, and W.S. Shin. 2003. Antidiabetic effects of chitosan oligosaccharides in neonatal streptozotocin induced noninsulin-dependent diabetes mellitus in rats. *Biological and Pharmaceutical Bulletin* 26: 1100–1103.

Li, B., F. Lu, X. Wei and R. Zhao. 2008. Fucoidan: Structure and bioactivity. *Molecules* 13:1671–1695.

Lutay, N., I. Nilsson, T. Wadstrom, and A. Ljungh. 2011. Effect of heparin, fucoidan and other polysaccharides on adhesion of enterohepatic helicobacter species to murine macrophages. *Applied Biochemistry and Biotechnology* 164: 1–9.

Lutsiak, M.E., G.S. Kwon, and J. Samuel. 2006. Biodegradable nanoparticle delivery of a Th2-biasedpeptide for induction of Th1 immune responses. *Journal of Pharmacy Pharmacology* 58: 739–747.

Maeda, H., M. Hosokawa, T. Sashima, and K. Miyashita. 2007. Dietary combination of fucoxanthin and fish oil attenuates the weight gain of white adipose tissue and decreases blood glucose in obese/diabetic KK-Ay mice. *Journal of Agricultural and Food Chemistry* 55: 7701–7706.

Maeda, H., M. Hosokawa, T. Sashima, K. Murakami-Funayama, and K. Miyashita. 2009. Anti-obesity and anti-diabetic effects of fucoxanthin on diet-induced obesity conditions in a murine model. *Molecular Medicine Reports* 2: 897–902.

Malette, W., H. Quigley, and E. Adickes. 1986. *Chitin in Nature and Technology*. Plenum Press, New York.

Mitchell, R.N., and R.S. Cotron. 2010. Robinsons Basic Pathology. In *Robinsons Basic Pathology*, edn. 7, pp. 34–42. Harcourt Pvt. Ltd, New Delhi, India.

Miura, T., M. Usami, Y. Tsuura, H. Ishida, and Y. Seino. 1995. Hypoglycemic and hypolipidemic effect of chitosan in normal and neonatal streptozotocin-induced diabetic mice. *Biological and Pharmaceutical Bulletin* 18: 1623–1625.

Miyashita, K. 2009. The carotenoid fucoxanthin from brown seaweed affects obesity. *Lipid Technology* 21: 186–90.

Mohamed, S., S.N. Hashim, and A.H. Rahman. 2012. Seaweeds: A sustainable functional food for complementary and alternative therapy. *Trends in Food Science and Technology.* 23: 83–96.

Moon, J.S., H.K. Kim, H.C. Koo, Y.S. Joo, H.M. Nam, Y.H. Park, and M.I. Kang. 2007. The antibacterial and immunostimulative effect of chitosan-oligosaccharides against infection by *Staphylococcus aureus* isolated from bovine mastitis. *Applied Microbiology and Biotechnology* 75: 989–998.

Muzzarelli, R., G. Biagini, A. Pugnaloni, O. Filippini, V. Baldassarre, C. Castaldini, and C. Rizzoli. 1989. Reconstruction of parodontal tissue with chitosan. *Biomaterials* 10: 598–603.

Muthezhilan, R., C.P. Kaarthikeyan, M. Jayaprakashvell, and A. Jaffar Hussain. 2014. Isolation, optimization and production of biopolymer (poly 3-hydroxy butyrate) from marine bacteria. *PakistanJournal of Biotechnology* 11: 59–66.

Muzzarelli, R.A.A. 1977. *Chitin.* Pergamon Press, New York.

Nandana, B., T. Quynhho. C. Albert, L. David, L. Robert, C. Subhas. 2011. Potential of 3-D tissue constructs engineered from bovine chondrocytes/silk fibroin-chitosan for in vitro cartilage tissue engineering. *Biomater.* 32: 5773–5781.

Nawanopparatsakul, S., J. Euasathien, C. Eamtawecharum, P. Benjasirimingokol, S. Soiputtan, P. Toprasri. 2005. Skin irritation test of curcuminoids facial mask containing chitosan as a binder. *Silpakorn University Journal of Social Sciences, Humanities and Arts* 5(1–2): 140–147.

Necas, J., and L. Bartosikova. 2013. Carrageenan: A review. *Review Article Veterinarni Medicina* 58: 187–205.

Ngo, D.H., I. Wijesekara, T.S. Vo, Q.V. Ta, and S.V. Kim. 2011. Marine food-derived functional ingredients as potential antioxidants in the food industry: An overview. *Food Research International* 44: 523–529.

Nichols, C.A.M., J. Guezennec, and J.P. Bowman. 2005. Bacterial polysaccharides from extreme marine environments with special considerations of the southern ocean, sea ice and deep-sea hydrothermal vents: A review. *Marine Biotechnology* 7: 253–271. doi:10.1007/s10126-004-5118-2.

Nishimura, K., S.I. Nishimura, and H. Seo. 1987. Effect of multiporous microspheres derived from chitin and partially deacetylated chitin on the activation of mouse peritoneal macrophages. *Vaccine* 5: 136–140.

Nishimura, S., H. Kai, K. Shinada, T. Yoshida, S. Tokura, K. Kurita, H. Nakashima, N. Yamamoto, and T. Uryu. 1998. Regioselective syntheses of sulfated polysaccharides: Specific anti-HIV-1 activity of novel chitin sulfates. *Carbohydrate Research* 306: 427–433.

Olivera, B.M., and E.E. Just. 1996. Conus venom peptides, receptor and ion channel targets, and drug design: 50 million years of neuropharmacology. *Molecular Biology of the Cell* 8: 2101–2109.

Olivera, B.M., and R.W. Teicher. 2007. Diversity of the neurotoxic Conus peptides: A model for concerted pharmacological discovery. *Molecular Interventions* 7: 251–260.

Onsoyen, E., and O. Skaugrud. 1990. Metal recovery using chitosan. *Journal of Chemical Technology and Biotechnology* 49: 395–404.

Papaspyros, N.S. 1964. The history of diabetes. In G.T. Verlag (Ed.), *The History of Diabetes Mellitus*, pp. 4–5. Thieme, Stuttgart, Germany.

Patil, R.S., V. Ghormade, and M.V. Deshpande. 2000. Chitinolytic enzymes: An exploration. *Enzyme and Microbial Technology* 26: 473–483.

Peniche-Covas, C., L.W. Alvarez, and W. Arguelles-Monal. 1992. Adsorption of mercuric ions by chitosan. *Journal of Applied Polymer Science* 46: 1147–1150.

Pereira, M.S., F.R. Melo, and P.A. Mourao. 2002. Is there a correlation between structure and anticoagulant action of sulfated galactans and sulfated fucans? *Glycobiology.* 12: 573–580.

Petrovsky, N. 2006. Novel human polysaccharide adjuvants with dual Th1 and Th2 potentiating activity. *Vaccine* 24: 26–29.

Qi, H., Q. Zhang, T. Zhao, R. Hu, K. Zhang, and Z. Li. 2006. *In vitro* antioxidant activity of acetylated and benzoylated derivatives of polysaccharide extracted from *Ulva pertusa* (Chlorophyta). *Bioorganic and Medicinal Chemistry Letters* 16: 2441–2445.

Quemener, B., M. Lahaye, and C. Bobin-Dubigeon. 1997. Sugar determination in ulvans by a chemical-enzymatic method coupled to high performance anion exchange chromatography. *Journal of Applied Phycology* 9: 179–188.

Rai, M.K. 1995. A review on some antidiabetic plants of India. *Ancient Science of Life* 14: 42–54.

Rang, H.P., M.M. Dale, and J.M. Ritters. 1991. The endocrine pancreas and the control of blood glucose. In B. Simmons, S. Beasley (Eds.), *Pharmacology*, Vol. 3, pp. 403–410, Longman Group, UK.

Ray, B., and M. Lahaye. 1995. Cell-wall polysaccharides from the marine green alga *Ulva "rigida"* (Ulvales, Chlorophyta), chemical structure of ulvan. *Carbohydrate Research* 274: 313–318.

Razdan, A., and D. Pettersson. 1994. Effect of chitin and chitosan on nutrient digestibility and plasma lipid concentrations in broiler chickens. *British Journal of Nutrition* 72: 277–288.

Rivas, G.G., C.M.G. Gutierrez, G.A. Arteaga, I.E.S. Mercado, and N.E.A. Sanchez. 2011. Screening for anticoagulant activity in marine algae from the Northwest Mexican Pacific coast. *Journal of Applied Phycology* 23: 495–503.

Roberts, G.A.F. 1992. *Chitin Chemistry*. MacMillan Press, London.

Robic, A., D. Bertrand, J.F. Sassi, and Y. Lerat. 2009. Determination of the chemical composition of ulvan, a cell wall polysaccharide from *Ulva* spp. (Ulvales, Chlorophyta) by FT-IR and chemometrics. *Journal of Applied Phycology* 21: 451–456.

Romay, C.H., R. Gonzalez, N. Ledón, D. Remirez, and V. Rimbau. 2003. C-Phycocyanin: Abiliprotein with antioxidante, anti-inflammatory and neuroprotective effects. *Current Protein and Peptide Science* 4: 207–216.

Rudall, K.M., and W. Kenchington. 1973. The chitin system. *Biological Reviews of the Cambridge Philosophical Society* 48: 597–636.

Sachindra, N.M., E. Sato, H. Maeda, M. Hosokawa, Y. Niwano, M. Kohno, and K. Miyashita. 2007. Radical scavenging and singlet oxygen quenching activity of marine carotenoid fucoxanthin and its metabolites. *Journal of Agricultural and Food Chemistry* 55: 8516–8522.

Safavi-Hemami, H., H. Hu, D.G. Gorasia, P.K. Bandyopadhyay, P.D. Veith, N.D. Young, E.C. Reynolds, M. Yandell, B.M. Olivera, and A.W. Purcell. 2014. Combined proteomic and transcriptomic interrogation of the venom gland of *Conus geographus* uncovers novel components and functional compartmentalization. *Molecular and Cellular Proteomics* 13: 938–953.

Shahidi, F., J.K.V. Arachchi, and Y.J. Jeon. 1999. Food applications of chitin and chitosans. *Trends in Food Science and Technology* 10: 37–51.

Shalaby, E.A. 2011. Algae as promising organisms for environment and health. *Plant Signaling and Behavior* 6: 1338–1350.

Shanmugam, M., and K.H. Mody. 2000. Heparinoid-active sulphated polysaccharides from marine algae as potential blood anticoagulant agents. *Current Science* 79: 25.

Shanthi, N., T. Eluvakkal, and K. Arunkumar. 2014. Characterization of galactose rich fucoidan with anticoagulation potential isolated from *Turbinaria decurrens* Bory de Saint-Vincent occurring along the coast of Gulf of Mannar (Pamban), India. *Journal of Pharmacognosy Phytochemistry* 3: 132–137.

Shigemasa, Y., and S. Minami. 1995. *Biotechnology & Genetic Engineering Reviews*. Intercept, Andover, MA.

Shiratori, K., K. Ohgami, I. Ilieva, X.H. Jin, Y. Koyama, K. Miyashita, K. Yoshida, S. Kase, and S. Ohno. 2005. Effects of fucoxanthin on lipopolysaccaride-induced inflammation in vitro and in vivo. *Experimental Eye Research* 81: 422–428.

Smit, A.J. 2004. Medicinal and pharmaceutical uses of seaweed natural products: A review. *Journal of Applied Phycology* 16: 245–262.

Stengel, D.B., S. Connan, and Z.A. Popper. 2011. Algal chemodiversity and bioactivity: Sources of natural variability and implications for commercial application. *Biotechnological Advances* 29: 483–501.

Struszczyk, H., H. Pospieszny, and S. Kotlinski. 1989. Some new application of chitosan. In G. SkjoakBrok, T. Anthonsen, P. Sandford (Eds.), *Chitin and Chitosan*, pp. 733–742. Elsevier Science, London.

Synowiecki, J., and N.A. Al-Khateeb. 2003. Production, properties, and some new applications of chitin and its derivatives. *Critical Reviews in Food Science and Nutrition* 43: 145–171.

Terlau, H., and B.M. Olivera. 2004. Conus venoms: A rich source of novel ion channel-targeted peptides. *Physiological Reviews* 84: 41–68.

Thomas, N.V., and S.K. Kim. 2013. Beneficial effects of marine algal compounds in cosmeticals. *Marine Drugs* 11: 146–164.

Trujillo-Vargas, C.M., K.D. Mayer, T. Bickert, A. Palmetshofer, S. Grunewald, J.R. Ramirez-Pineda, T. Polte, G. Hansen, G. Wohlleben, and K.J. Erb. 2005. Vaccinations with T-helper type 1 directing adjuvants have different suppressive effects on the development of allergen-induced T-helper type 2 responses. *Clinical and Experimental Allergy* 35: 1003–1013.

Ushakova, N.A., G.E. Morozevich, N.E. Ustiuzhanina, M.I. Bilan, and A.L. Usov. 2008. Anticoagulant activity of fucoidans from brown algae. *Biomed Khim* 54: 597–606.

Valenta, R., T. Ball, M. Focke, B. Linhart, N. Mothes, V. Niederberger, S. Spitzauer, I. Swoboda, S. Vrtala, K. Westritschnig, and D. Kraft. 2004. Immunotherapy of allergic disease. *Advances in Immunology* 82: 105–153.

Venter, J.P., A.F. Kotze, R. Auzely-Velty, and M. Rinaudo. 2006. Synthesis and evaluation of the mucoadhesivity of a CD-chitosan derivative. *International Journal of Pharmaceutics*. 313: 36–42.

Vo, T.S., and S.K. Kim. 2010. Potential anti-HIV agents from marine resources: An overview. *Marine Drugs*. 8: 2871–2892.

Vongchan, P., W. Sajomsang, D. Subyen, and P. Kongtawelert. 2002. Anticoagulant activity of sulfated chitosan. *Carbohydrate Research*. 337: 1233–1236.

Wan, A.C.A., and B.C.U. Tai. 2013. Chitin-a promising biomaterial for tissue engineering and stem cell technologies. *Biotechnology Advances* 31: 1776–1785.

Wang, W., S.X. Wang, and H.S. Guan. 2012. The antiviral activities and mechanisms of marine polysaccharides: An overview. *Marine Drugs*. 10: 2795–2816.

Wijesekara, I., R. Pangestuti, and S.K. Kim. 2011. Biological activities and potential health benefits of sulfated polysaccharides derived from marine algae. *Carbohydrate Polymers* 84: 14–21.

Willis, J.H. 1999. Cuticular proteins in insects and crustaceans. *American Zoologist*. 39: 600–609.

Wolf, M.A., K. Sciuto, C. Andreoli, and I. Moro. 2012. *Ulva* (Chlorophyta, Ulvales) biodiversity in the North Adriatic Sea (Mediterranean Italy): Cryptic species and new introductions. *Journal of Phycology* 48: 1510–1521.

World Health Organization. 1985. Diabetes Mellitus: Report of a WHO Study Group, WHO Technical Report Series, p. 727, World Health Organization, Geneva, Switzerland.

Xu, N., X. Fan, X. Yan, and C.K. Tseng. 2004. Screening marine algae from China for their antitumor activities. *Journal of Applied Phycology* 16: 451–456.

Yamada, A., N. Shibbuya, O. Komada, and T. Akatsuka. 1993. Induction of phytoalexin formation in suspension-cultured rice cells by N-acetylchitooligosaccharides. *Bioscience, Biotechnology and Biochemistry* 57: 405–409.

Yamada, K., Y. Akiba, T. Shibuya, A. Kashiwada, K. Matsuda and M. Hirata. 2005. Water purification through bioconversion of phenol compounds by tyrosinase and chemical adsorption by chitosan beads. *Biotechnology Progress* 21: 823–829.

Yao, H.T., S.Y. Hwang, and M.T. Chiang. 2006. Effect of chitosan on plasma cholesterol and glucose concentration in streptozotocin induced diabetic rats. *Taiwan Journal of Agriculturaland Chemistry and Food Science* 44: 122–132.

Zhensheng, L., R.R. Hassna, D.H. Kip, X. Demin, and Z. Miqin. 2005. Chitosan–alginate hybrid scaffolds for bone tissue engineering. *Biomaterials* 26: 3919–3928.

10 Role of Chitosan in Enhancing Crop Production

Apiradee Uthairatanakij and Pongphen Jitareerat

CONTENTS

10.1 INTRODUCTION

Chitosan, a polycationic β-1,4-linked-D-glucosamine polymer, is a polysaccharide polymer and a derivative of chitin, which is present in the shell of crustaceans such as the shells of crab and shrimp, an abundant by-product of seafood processing, via a deacetylation reaction (removal of acetyl groups $COCH_3$ from the chitin original structure) with alkali (Kurita et al. 1979). It has a rigid and specific crystalline structure that exists in nature in different polymorphic forms having various properties (Prashanth and Tharanathan 2007). Chitosan has been widely used to stimulate plant growth and seed germination, and enhances the yields of numerous crops (Vander 1998; Kowalski et al. 2006; Nge et al. 2006). It is reported to influence the production of substances related to stress response such as phytoalexins (Walker-Simmons et al. 1983) and acts as a biocontrol agent (El-Ghaouth et al. 1994). In addition, chitosan is also reported to be involved in plant resistance to pathogen infection (Rabea et al. 2003; Pichyangkura and Chadchawan 2015). Chitosan and its derivatives, such as glycol chitosan and carboxymethyl chitosan, are known to form a semipermeable film around plant tissues; they are inhibitory to a number of pathogenic fungi, and they also induce host defense responses (El-Ghaouth et al. 1994). In addition, the systemic disease protection elicited by chitosan has been reported (Corsi et al. 2015).

The aim of this chapter is to reveal the application of chitosan in agricultural field. Chitosan enhances plant growth, plant elicitor, and secondary metabolite production in plants, which provide them resistance against biotic and abiotic stresses.

This chapter delineates the potential application of chitosan coatings for enhancing the crop production.

10.2   THE POTENTIAL OF BIOSTIMULANTS TO IMPROVE PLANT GROWTH

Chitosan is a nontoxic and environmentally friendly biopolymer, and considered as a plant growth promoter in some plant species. Pichyangkura and Chadchawan (2015) reviewed that chitosan induces several defense genes in plants, such as pathogenesis-related (PR) genes (glucanase and chitinase) and also induces many enzymes in the reactive oxygen species scavenging system, including superoxide dismutase, catalase, and peroxidase; therefore, chitosan has been used as a biostimulant to stimulate plant growth and stress tolerance, and to induce pathogen resistance. Biostimulants are obtained from different organic materials and include humic substances, complex organic materials, beneficial chemical elements, peptides and amino acids, inorganic salts, seaweed extracts, antitranspirants, amino acids, other N-containing substances, and chitin and chitosan derivatives (Nardi et al. 2016).

Foliar spraying with chitosan at 0.1% (w/v) increased the growth parameters (shoot height, leaf number/plant, plant fresh weight) and also induced the activity levels of defense enzymes such as protease inhibitors, β-1,3-glucanases, peroxidases, and polyphenol oxidases (PPOs) in the leaves and rhizomes of turmeric plants, resulting in high yield and curcumin content (Anusuya and Sathiyabama 2016). Chitosan with low and high molecular weights at different dilutions, that is, standard, 1:1, 1:2, 1:3, 1:4, 1:5, and 1:10, markedly enhanced the tomato (*Lycopersicon esculentum*) growth parameters, that is, root and shoot length and weights. Similarly, foliar applications of chitosan resulted in yield increases of nearly 20% in tomatoes (Walker et al. 2004). Mondal et al. (2012) also reported the effect of foliar application of chitosan on growth and yield in okra. Chitosan works as a positive factor in enhancing the shoot and root lengths, fresh and dry weights of shoots and roots, and leaf area of bean plants (Sheikha and Al-Malki 2011). Tamala et al. (2007) revealed that the application of chitosan concentration at 80 mg L^{-1} had higher plant height, number of leaves per plant, inflorescences length, diameter of rachis, diameter of peduncle than untreated plants with no significant differences. Foliar spraying fertilizer (20-20-20) combined with 20 mg/L chitosan also significantly increased the weight of inflorescences and leaf area. Similarly, foliar application of chitosan at early growth stages in maize improved the morphological (plant height, leaf number per plant, leaf length and breadth, leaf area per plant) and physiological (total dry mass/plant, absolute growth rate, and harvest index) parameters and yield components, with the highest seed yield recorded in 100 and 125 ppm of chitosan (Mondal et al. 2013). Shehata et al. (2012) observed that foliar application of chitosan at 4 mL/L obtained the highest vegetative growth, yield, and quality of cucumber plants. Wang et al. (2016) revealed that chitosan oligosaccharides (COSs) could affect the production quality of wheat (*Triticum aestivum* L.) and impacted the grain yield significantly in all irrigated cultivars, but did not have a significant effect of COS on rain-fed cultivar.

The influence of 0.5% chitosan solutions with low molecular weight (2 kDa), medium molecular weight (50 kDa), and high molecular weight (970 kDa) on the growth and yield of flowers and corms of potted *Gompey* freesia showed that regardless of the molecular weight of the compound, the chitosan-treated plants had more leaves and shoots, flowered earlier, and formed more flowers and corms. The application of medium- and high-molecular-weight chitosan resulted in higher plants with a higher relative chlorophyll content (Salachna and Zawadzińska 2015). Chamnanmanoontham et al. (2014) reported that the application of oligomeric chitosan with an 80% degree of deacetylation (DDA) at 40 mg/L significantly enhanced the vegetative growth, in terms of the leaf and root fresh weights and dry weights of rice seedlings compared to the control, suggesting that chitosan enhanced the seedling growth via multiple and complex networks between the nucleus and the chloroplast.

Ziani et al. (2010) found that chitosan coating significantly differed on the increasing artichoke seed germination, decreased the number of type of fungi, and increased plant growth. In addition, chitosan with lower molecular weight gave better results from both microbial and germination point of view. Goñi et al. (2013) found that the contact of lettuce seeds with a 10 g/L chitosan solution for 10 minutes maintained the highest germination percentage. Li et al. (2013) observed that fresh and dry weights of watermelon seedlings planted in soil were increased by chitosan-treated seed, but not by chitosan leaf spraying. In addition, Saharan et al. (2015) observed that Cu-chitosan nanoparticles showed a substantial growth-promoting effect on tomato seed germination, seedling length, and fresh and dry weights at 0.08%, 0.10%, and 0.12% level.

It has been reported that the addition of chitosan to a liquid culture medium also enhances the shoot growth of *Lippia dulcis* Trev. (Sauerwein et al. 1991). Chitosan enhances the *in vitro* micropropagation of *Dendrobium Eiskul*. Using 80% *N*-deacetylated oligomeric (O-80) forms of crab (*Portunus pelagicus*), chitosan applied during shoot induction of protocorm-like bodies (PLBs) at 10 or 20 mg/L was the most appropriate chitosan and also induced further PLB formation. The addition of 10 mg/L of O-80 or polymeric (P-80) form gave the best quantity and quality, respectively, of plantlets, whereas 20 mg/L of P-70 chitosan as a supplement during exflasking enhanced both the survival rate and the growth of the plantlets at 1 month after exflasking (Pornpienpakdee et al. 2010). Samarfard et al. (2013) showed that PLBs of *Phalaenopsis gigantea* inoculated in liquid New Dogashima Medium and Vacin and Went (VW) supplemented with 10 mg/L chitosan observed the highest PLB multiplication and stimulated the formation of juvenile leaves. *Dendrobium Queen Pink* protocorms cultured in modified VW medium supplemented with chitosan at 60 mg/L for a year had the highest plant height, root length, and leaf area compared to other treatments, but no statistical difference on the number of leaves, roots, and new shoots. Moreover, all concentrations of chitosan increased the number of stomata compared with the control, but there was no difference in the number and size of the chloroplasts (Obsuwan et al. 2013). Teixeira Da Silva et al. (2013) reported that using 0.1–1.0 mg/L chitosan produced more PLBs/PLB and a greater fresh weight than Teixeira Cymbidium basal medium without plant growth regulator (PGRs).

El-Tanahy et al. (2012) showed that the use of chitosan at the concentration of 5% combined with the inorganic fertilizer (NPK) had the best effect on plant vegetative growth (number, plant height, fresh and dry weights of leaves and shoots), yield (pod weight, length and diameter and number of seeds, seed yield), and also seed quality (total protein, total carbohydrates N, P, and K). Chitosan has also been used in various forms. It can be more effective as a plant growth enhancer and as an antifungal agent when applied in the form of submicron dispersions compared to applying chitosan in the conventional form. The highest number of shoots (19), maximum stem diameter (0.23 m), and maximum stem length (2.80 m) and chlorophyll content were observed in plants treated with submicron chitosan dispersions (SCD) of 600 nm droplet size of 1.0% chitosan (Zahid et al. 2013). In addition, chitosan application can be used to enhance waxy corn yield and also to reduce chemical fertilizer uses in waxy corn growth (Boonlertnirun et al. 2011). López-Mondéjar et al. (2012) reported that the incorporation of the chitin-rich residues obtained from several industries into the growing media enhanced the growth (first leaf length, stem length, and shoot dry weight) of muskmelon seedlings. In addition, the use of these residues with *Trichoderma harzianum* as amendments of growing media enhanced the growth of muskmelon seedlings and decreased the weight loss due to the pathogen infection. Tomato treated with chitosan in combination of *Pseudomonas* spp. had higher plant height, biomass and chlorophyll content, number of fruits per plant, fruit yield, and shelf life of fruits than the diseased control treatment (Mishra et al. 2014). It has been reported that chitosan increased the growth rates of roots and shoots of daikon radish (*Raphanus sativus* L.) (Tsugita et al. 1993). Utsunomiya and Kinai (1994) applied COSs to soil used for cultivating passion fruit (*Passiflora edulis* Sims). They showed that COSs advanced flowering time and increased flower numbers (Utsunomiya and Kinai 1994). The effect of chitosan on the growth of gerbera plants has been studied. The results showed that chitosan significantly enhanced growth factors in terms of the average values of flower-stem length, the number of growing leaves, (including leaf width and length), and the number of flowers per bush (Wanichpongpan et al. 2000). Chitosan also promoted the growth of various crops such as cabbage (*Brassica oleracea* L. var. Capitata) (Hirano 1988), soybean sprouts (Lee et al. 2005), and sweet basil (Kim 2005). Chitogel, a derivative of chitosan, was found to improve vegetative growth of grapevine plantlets (AitBarka et al. 2004). This study showed that the average O_2 production of plantlets cultured on medium supplemented with 1.75% chitogel increased 2-fold, whereas the CO_2 fixation increased only 1.5-fold, indicating that chitogel had a beneficial effect on net photosynthesis in plantlets and confirmed its positive effects on grapevine physiology (AitBarka et al. 2004). It has also been shown that chitosan promotes vegetative growth and enhances various processes in developing flower buds, including induction of flowering of Lisianthus (*Eustoma grandiflorum*) (Ohta et al. 1999; Uddin et al. 2004). Spraying with chitosan at 600 mg/L increased the width of the sepals of *Dendrobium* Red Sonia ##17 at harvest (Uthairatanakij et al. 2006). Several experiments on the effects of concentration and frequency of chitosan application were conducted in various crops such as chili, Chinese cabbage, celery, bitter cucumber, and rice (Chandrkrachang et al. 2003). The data showed that chitosan concentration and frequency of application significantly increased the growth rates of chili and the harvest yield of Chinese cabbage (Chandrkrachang et al. 2003). Lee et al. (1999) found that chitosan treatment increased the yield and marketability of soybean sprouts. In contrast, *Phaseolus vulgaris* grown in hydroponic culture and treated with COSs at high dose had shorter shoots and roots, but COS did not affect chlorophyll *a*, *b*, and carotenoid concentrations (Chatelain et al. 2014). However, the mechanism of action of chitosan on plant growth remains still unclear.

10.3 CHITOSAN INFLUENCING STRESSES

Chitosan was used as an elicitor molecule to enhance plant resistance to the stress. It clearly induced resistance to osmotic stress (a surrogate for drought stress) in the "Leung Pratew 123" ("LPT123") rice (*Oryza sativa* L. "Leung Pratew123") by enhancing plant growth and maintenance of the photosynthetic pigments during osmotic stress, but not in the derived mutated line, LPT123-TC171. H_2O_2 is proposed to be one of the key components for plant growth stimulation during osmotic (drought) stress by chitosan (Pongprayoon et al. 2013). Moreno et al. (2008) demonstrated that foliar spray of chitosan reduced abiotic stress in winter for broccoli grown under hydroponic conditions in the greenhouse. Also, chitosan sprayed at head induction and during development enhanced its nutritional quality to deliver a health-promoting food. Jabeen and Ahmad (2013) indicated that the low concentrations of chitosan exhibited positive effects on salt stress alleviation through the decrease of CAT and POX activities in safflower and sunflower crops, and also increased the percentage of germination. Under the increasing water-deficit stress, the percentage of germination was increased by low concentrations of chitosan (0.05%–0.4%), but malondialdehyde (MDA) and proline contents and CAT and POX activities were decreased in safflower (*Carthamus tinctorius* L.) (Mahdavi et al. 2011).

10.4 CHITOSAN AS PLANT ELICITOR

Chitosan is an exogenous elicitor of response mechanisms and has been demonstrated to induce plant defenses in chili seeds (Photchanachai et al. 2006); fresh cut broccoli, raspberry, and many other fruits and vegetables (Moreira et al. 2011); avocado (Bill et al. 2014); tomato (Sathiyabama et al. 2014); and dragon fruit (Ali et al. 2014). Application of chitosan and chitin oligomers increased the activities of phenylalanine ammonia lyase (PAL) and tyrosine ammonia lyase (TAL), the key enzymes of the phenyl propanoid pathway, in soybean leaves (Khan et al. 2003) and sweet basil (*Ocimum basilicum* L.) (Kim et al. 2005). The products of PAL and TAL are modified via the phenyl propanoid pathways to produce precursors of secondary metabolites, including lignin, flavonoid pigments, and phytoalexins, which play an important role in plant–pathogen interactions (Morrison and Buxton 1993). It has been shown that chitosan can induce chitinase and chitosanase, which are the members of a group of plant PR proteins (Collinge et al. 1993; Loon et al. 1994). These PR proteins can degrade the cell walls of some phytopathogens and consequently may play a role in host plant defense systems (Dixon et al. 1994; Graham and Sticklen 1994). Oxidation of phenolic compounds associated with enhanced resistance to pathogens may involve PPO, which could generate reactive oxygen species (Mayer 2006). It was found that 0.01 mg/mL of chitosan applied as a foliar spray increased the enzymatic (peroxidase, catalase, and phenylalanine ammoniumlyase) and nonenzymatic (total phenolics, flavonoids, and proteins) defensive metabolites and the total antioxidant activity of the spinach leaves (Singh 2016). Chitosan can also induce plant immune systems (systemic acquired resistance or SAR), which is long lasting and often confers broadbased resistance to different pathogens. SAR develops in uninfected parts of the plant. As a result, the entire plant is more resistant to the secondary infection. Representative proteins of SAR include antifungal chitinases, β-1,3-glucanases, and PR-1 and PR-5 (Sathiyabama and Balasubramaman 1998). The effectiveness in eliciting SAR was tested on kiwi micropropagated plants using 15 and 50 mg/L of chitosan. It was found that chitosan enhanced the activity of enzymes involved in detoxification processes (guaiacol peroxidase and ascorbate peroxidase) and in increasing plant defense barriers (PAL and PPO) (Corsi et al. 2015). The increase in the total phenolic content, lignin synthesis, and the activities of PAL, peroxidase, PPO, and cinnamyl alcohol dehydrogenase was triggered by the chitosan elicitor; thus, chitosan could induce effective defense responses in tomato plants against *Ralstonia solanacearum* (Mandal et al. 2013). Chitosan at the concentration of 1.0 mg/mL also significantly reduced Cercospora leaf spot severity when applied at 1 and 3 days prior to inoculation, and chitosan-treated plants showed higher peroxidase activity at the time of inoculation. In addition, chitosans in the form of microparticles (CS) or nanoparticles (CSNPs) were investigated through minimum bactericidal concentration against *Pseudomonas fluorescens*, *Erwinia carotovora*, and *Escherichia coli*. The results showed that the antibacterial activity was significantly enhanced in the CSNPs compared to CS microparticles, especially for chitosan nanoparticles from crab shells (Mohammadi et al. 2016). Zahid et al. (2013) demonstrated that low-molecular-weight chitosan in the form of nanoemulsions (droplet size 600 nm) at 1.0% concentration showed the best results in terms of inhibiting conidial germination and reducing the dry weight of mycelia and sporulation compared to untreated control; thus, nano-emulsions could be used to control anthracnose disease of dragon fruit plants. In addition, mycelial growth and disease incidence/severity were significantly suppressed by 600 nm submicron chitosan dispersion at 1% chitosan concentration, and host resistance was stimulated in dragon fruit plants; therefore chitosan dispersions significantly enhanced the production of plant defense-related enzymes such as PO, PPO, and PAL (Zahid et al. 2013). Moreover, at 0.12% concentration, Cu-chitosan nanoparticles caused 70.5% and 73.5% inhibition of mycelial growth and 61.5% and 83.0% inhibition of spore germination in inhibited *Alternaria solani* and *Fusarium oxysporum* (Saharan et al. 2015). All the concentrations of chitosan (0, 5, 50, 100, and 500 µg.a.i./mL) significantly reduced the radial growth of *Verticillium dahlia in vitro* after 120 hours; chitosan (100 µg.a.i./plant) applied by foliar spray on potato seedlings at 15, 25, and 40 days after sowing significantly decreased disease severity and increased the fresh weights of tubers (Amini 2015). Chitosan significantly reduced the disease incidence of early blight caused by *A. solani* in potato plants due to an increase of chitinase activity and new isoforms of chitinase (Abd-El-Kareem and Haggag 2014; Sathiyabama et al. 2014). Similarly, disease severity of bacterial spot caused by *Xanthomonas gardneri* was greatly reduced by chitosan (3.0 mg/mL) up to 85% compared to the control, and the application of chitosan at 5 days before inoculation showed larger reduction in disease severity and a high level of peroxidase activity. However, the in vitro growth of *X. gardneri* was not affected by chitosan treatment (De Jail et al. 2014). Application of *Pseudomonas* spp. combined with chitosan could reduce the severity of tomato leaf curl virus by 48% at 45 days after inoculation (DAI), resulting in the highest phenol content, peroxidase, PPO, chitinase, and PALase activities (Mishra et al. 2014). Chitosan conferred a high protection of grapevine leaves against gray mold caused by *Botrytis cinerea*. Treatment of grapevine leaves by chitosan led to a marked induction of lipoxygenase, PAL, and chitinase activities, three markers of plant defense responses. Strong reduction of *B. cinerea* infection was achieved with 75–150 mg/L chitosan (Trotel-Aziz et al. 2006). Cobos et al. (2015) showed that the infection rate in pruning wounds of grapevine trunk inoculated with *Diplodia seriata* and *Phaeomoniella chlamydospora* was significantly reduced in plants treated with COS. Rahman et al. (2014) indicated that COSs could inhibit fungal germination and growth (*B. cinerea* Pers. Ex Fr. and *Mucor piriformis* Fischer) and that the effect depended highly on the level of polymerization of the oligomers. In some studies, it was observed that COSs at 50 μg m/L reduced the disease symptoms caused by *Sclerotinia sclerotiorum* in *Brassica napus* L. *in vivo* compared to the control plants due to the induced bursts of cytosolic Ca^{2+}, nitric oxide, and hydrogen peroxide (Yin et al. 2013). Chitosan A at 0.40 mg m/L significantly repressed the growth of *Acidovorax citrulli* in watermelon seedling and reduced the disease index of watermelon seedlings planted in soil and the death rate of seedlings planted in perlite; thus, the efficacy of chitosan as an antibacterial agent may be attributed to membrane lysis (Li et al. 2013). Wang et al. (2012) demonstrated that chitosan significantly inhibited the germination of the resting spores of the clubroot pathogen and reduced the disease index of clubroot of Chinese cabbage and the number of the resting spores in soil compared to the control regardless of the chitosan type and concentration as well as the application method. The mechanism of chitosan in protection of rice from *Rhizoctonia solani* pathogen was attributed to direct destruction of the mycelium, evidenced by scanning and transmission electron microscopic observations and pathogenicity testing; indirect induced resistance was evidenced by the changes in the activities of the defense-related PAL, peroxidise, and PPO in rice seedling (Liu et al. 2012). Also, de Oliveira Junior et al. (2012) reported that chitosan had a direct effect on hyphal morphology changes, for example, mycelial aggregation and structural changes such as excessive branching, swelling of the cell wall, and hyphae size reduction.

10.5 ELICITOR FOR THE PRODUCTION OF SECONDARY METABOLITES

The use of biotic or abiotic elicitors is one of the ways to increase the yields of secondary metabolites in *in vitro* cultures (Bohlmann and Eilert 1994). Hairy root cultures of *Brugmansia candida* supplemented with chitosan at certain concentrations were found to increase the content of root scopolamine and hyoscyamine, which are valuable anticholinergic drugs employed as antispasmodics and in the treatment of motion sickness. Both are the members of the tropane group of alkaloids (Hashimoto et al. 1993). Hairy root cultures of *Hyoscyamus muticus* treated with chitosan produced fivefold more hyoscyamine than the control (Sevón et al. 1992). Chitosan added to suspension cell cultures of parsley (*Petroselinum crispum*) elicited a rapid deposition of the β-1,3-glucan and callose in the cell walls and a slower formation of coumarins (Conrath et al. 1989). The application of chitosan to the culture media has been shown to enhance the production of hernandulcin, a minor constituent (0.004% dry weight) of the essential oil obtained from the aerial parts of *L. dulcis* Trev (Sauerwein et al. 1991). Treating hairy root cultures of *Trigonella foenum-graecum* L. with 40 mg/L chitosan induced a threefold increase in diosgenin, a spirostanol important for the synthesis of steroid hormones (Merkli et al. 1997). Adventitious root culture elicitor treated with various combinations of chitosan and pectin or chitosan alone resulted in enhanced biosynthesis of secondary metabolites, but inhibited root growth. The optimum concentration of elicitor for enhancing metabolite biosynthesis was found at the concentration of 0.2 mg/mL chitosan, in which 103.16, 48.57, and 75.32 mg/g dry weight of anthraquinones, phenolics, and flavonoids, respectively, were achieved (Baque et al. 2012). In addition, chitosan-oil coating exhibited significantly higher levels of total phenolics, flavonoids, and individual phenolic compounds than the control, resulting in the reduction of microbial count in shiitake mushroom (Jiang et al. 2012). Moreover, chitosan induces the accumulation of phytoalexins resulting in antifungal responses and enhances protection from further infections (Hadwiger and Beckman 1980; Vasyukova et al. 2001). Chitosan also enhances phytoalexin production in germinating peanut (Cuero et al. 1991) and also induces the formation of phytoalexins in legumes and solanaceous plants (Cote and Hahn 1994). Thus, chitosan may be involved in the signaling pathway for the biosynthesis of phenolics (Figure 10.1).

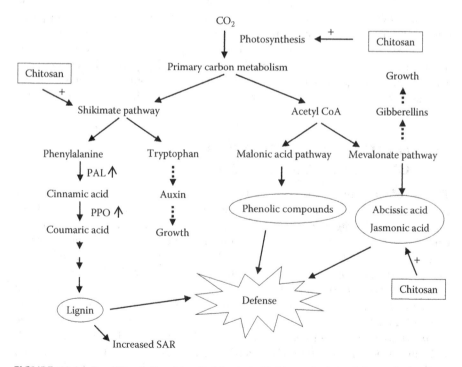

FIGURE 10.1 Possible relationship of chitosan with biosynthetic pathways of phytohormones and secondary metabolites involved in plant growth and disease resistance.

10.6 POSTHARVEST APPLICATION

Due to certain harmful effects of synthetic fungicides on human health and environment, there is a need to look for some safe alternatives. Chitosan is a natural substance obtained from various species, particularly from the exoskeletons of crustaceans. It is biodegradable, has low potential toxicity, is common in the environment, and is not harmful to people, pets, wildlife, or the natural environment; also it was found to be nontoxic when fed to mice, rats, and rabbits (EPA 1995). It has been used in postharvest treatment to maintain postharvest quality and control diseases in mango (Muangdech 2016), navel orange fruit (Youssef et al. 2015), guava, (Hong et al. 2012), and banana (Gol and Rao 2011). Pomegranate fruits coated with chitosan delayed the decrease in total soluble solids (TSS) and titratable acidity (TA) percent, a* value of arils, anthocyanins, flavonoids, total phenolics content, and antioxidant activity, but less than application of carnauba wax (Meighani et al. 2014). Hong et al. (2012) demonstrated that application of 2.0% chitosan significantly reduced firmness and weight loss, delayed changes in chlorophyll and MDA contents and TSS, and retarded the loss of titratable acidity and vitamin C in guava fruits during 12 days of storage. Abbasi et al. (2009) indicated that irradiated Crab chitosan (200 kGy) treated fruits maintained the eating quality up to 4 weeks of storage at 15°C ± 1°C and 85% relative humidity. Chitosan has been used to prevent microbial deterioration of refrigerated fresh produces. Moreira et al. (2011) reported that chitosan coating significantly reduced all microbiological population counts, except lactic acid bacteria. In addition, dos Santos et al. (2012) demonstrated the potential of the combination of chitosan and *Origanum vulgare* L. essential oil at subinhibitory concentrations to control postharvest pathogenic fungi in grape fruits, in particular, *Rhizopus stolonifer* and *Aspergillus niger*. Jiang et al. (2012) found that shiitake (*Lentinus edodes*) mushrooms treated with chitosan-oil coating maintained tissue firmness, inhibited the increase of respiration rate, reduced microorganism counts (yeasts and molds and pseudomonad), and maintained the overall quality of shiitake mushroom during the storage at 4°C. Moreover, chitosan in postharvest treatment may be used in combination with other techniques. Djioua et al. (2010) observed that hot water dipping 50°C for 30 minutes and chitosan coating, either alone or in combination, did not affect the taste and the flavor of mango slices, but could not inhibit the microbial growth for 9 days at 6°C.

10.7 CONCLUSION

Chitosan is a nontoxic, biocompatible, and biodegradable biopolymer. The applicability of chitosan is directly related with its physicochemical properties such as the degree of deacetylation and molecular weight. From this review, it is clear that chitosan and its derivatives are excellent in promoting plant growth, have high antibacterial activity, increase disease resistance, reduce stress and also induce the production of secondary metabolites. In addition, chitosan can be applied after harvest to maintain and extend the storage life and shelf life of produces. Therefore, chitosan can be an alternative substance for improving crop production.

REFERENCES

Abbasi, N.A., Z. Iqbal, M. Maqbool, and I.A. Hafiz. 2009. Postharvest quality of mango (*Mangifera indica* L.) fruit as affected by chitosan coating. *Pakistan Journal of Botany* 41: 343–357.

Abd-El-Kareem, F. and W.M. Haggag. 2014. Chitosan and citral alone or in combination for controlling early blight disease of potato plants under field conditions. *Research Journal of Pharmaceutical, Biological and Chemical Sciences* 5: 941–949.

AitBarka, E., P. Eullaffroy, C. Clément, and G. Vernet. 2004. Chitosan improves development, and protects *Vitis vinifera* L. against *Botrytis cinerea*. *Plant Cell Report* 22: 608–614.

Ali, A., N. Zahid, S. Manickam, Y. Siddiqui, P.G. Alderson, and M. Maqbool. 2014. Induction of lignin and pathogenesis related proteins in dragon fruit plants in response to submicron chitosan dispersions. *Crop Protection* 63: 83–88.

Amini, J. 2015. Induced resistance in potato plants against verticillium wilt invoked by chitosan and Acibenzolar-S-methyl. *Australian Journal of Crop Science* 9(6): 570–576.

Anusuya, S. and M. Sathiyabama. 2016. Effect of chitosan on growth, yield and curcumin content in turmeric under field condition. *Biocatalysis and Agricultural Biotechnology* 6: 102–106.

Baque, M.A., S.H. Moh, E.J. Lee, J.J. Zhong, and K.Y. Paek. 2012. Production of biomass and useful compounds from adventitious roots of high-value added medicinal plants using bioreactor. *Biotechnology Advances* 30: 1255–1267.

Bill, M., D. Sivakumar, L. Korsten, and A.K. Thompson. 2014. The efficacy of combined application of edible coatings and thyme oil in inducing resistance components in avocado (*Persea americana Mill.*) against anthracnose during post-harvest storage. *Crop Protection* 64: 159–167.

Bohlmann, J. and U. Eilert. 1994. Elicitor induced secondary metabolism in *Ruta graveolens* L. Role of chorismate utilizing enzymes. *Plant Cell Tissue and Organ Culture* 38: 189–198.

Boonlertnirun, S., R. Suvannasara, P. Promsomboon, and K. Boonlertnirun. 2011. Application of chitosan for reducing chemical fertilizer uses in waxy corn growing. *Thai Journal of Agricultural Science* 44: 22–28.

Chamnanmanoontham, N., W. Pongprayoon, R. Pichayangkura, S. Roytrakul, and S. Chadchawan. 2014. Chitosan enhances rice seedling growth via gene expression network between nucleus and chloroplast. *Plant Growth Regulation* 75: 101–114.

Chandrkrachang, S., P. Sompongchaikul, and S. Teuntai. 2003. Effect of chitosan applying in multicuture crop plantation. *The National Chitin-Chitosan Conference,* July 17–18, 2003, Chulalongkorn University, Bangkok, Thailand, pp. 158–160.

Chatelain, P.G., M.E. Pintado, and M.W. Vasconcelos. 2014. Evaluation of chitooligosaccharide application on mineral accumulation and plant growth in *Phaseolus vulgaris*. *Plant Science* 215–216: 134–140.

Cobos, R., R.M. Mateos, J.M. Álvarez- Pérez, M.A. Olego, S. Sevillano, S. González-García, E. Garzón, and J.J.R. Coque. 2015. Effectiveness of natural antifungal compounds to control infection through 3 pruning wounds by grapevine trunk disease pathogens. *Applied and Environmental Microbiology*. doi:10.1128/AEM.01818-15.

Collinge, D.B., K.M. Kragh, J.D. Mikkelsen, K.K. Nielsen, U. Rasmussen, and K. Vad. 1993. Plant chitinase. *Plant Journal* 3: 31–40.

Conrath, U., A. Domard, and H. Kauss. 1989. Chitosan-elicited synthesis of callose and of coumarin derivates in parsley cell suspension cultures. *Plant Cell Reports* 8: 152–155.

Corsi, B., C. Forni, and L. Riccioni. 2015. In vitro cultures of *Actinidia deliciosa* (A. Chev) C.F. Liang & A.R. Ferguson: A tool to study the SAR induction of chitosan treatment. *Organic Agriculture* 5: 189–198.

Cote, F. and M.G. Hahn. 1994. Oligosaccharin: Structures and signal transduction. *Plant Molecular Biology* 26: 1379–1411.

Cuero, R.G., G. Osugi, and A. Washington. 1991. N-carboxymethyl chitosan inhibition of flatoxin production: Role of zinc. *Biotechnology Letters* 13: 41–44.

De Jail, N.G., C. Luiz, A.C.D.R. Neto, and R.M. Di Piero. 2014. High-density chitosan reduces the severity of bacterial spot and activates the defense mechanisms of tomato plants. *Tropical Plant Pathology* 39: 434–441.

de Oliveira Junior, E.N., T.T. Franco, and I.S. de Melo. 2012. Changes in hyphal morphology due to chitosan treatment in some fungal species. *Brazilian Archives of Biology and Technology* 55: 637–646.

Dixon, R.A., M.J. Harrison, and C.J. Lamb. 1994. Early events in the activation of plant defenses. *Annual Review of Phytopatholgy* 32: 479–510.

Djioua, T., F. Charles, J.R.M. Freire, H. Filgueiras, M.N. Ducamp-Collin, and H. Sallanon. 2010. Combined effects of postharvest heat treatment and chitosan coating on quality of fresh-cut mangoes (*Mangifera indica* L.). *International Journal of Food Science and Technology* 45: 849–855.

dos Santos, N.S.T., A.J.A. Athayde Aguiar, C.E.V. de Oliveira, C. Veríssimo de Sales, S. de Meloe Silva, R. Sousa da Silva, T.C.M. Stamford, and E.L. de Souza. 2012. Efficacy of the application of a coating composed of chitosan and *Origanum vulgare* L. Essential oil to control *Rhizopus stolonifer* and *Aspergillus niger* in grapes (*Vitislabrusca* L.). *Food Microbiology* 32: 345–353.

El-Ghaouth, A. 1994. Effect of chitosan on cucumber plants: Suppression of *Pythium aphanidermatum* and induction of defense reactions. *Phytopathology* 84: 313–320.

El-Tanahy, A.M.M., A.R. Mahmoud, M.M. Abde-Mouty, and A.H. Ali. 2012. Effect of chitosan doses and nitrogen sources on the growth, yield and seed quality of cowpea. *Australian Journal of Basic and Applied Sciences* 6: 115–121.

EPA. 1995. Poly-D-Glucosamine (chitosan); Exemption from the requirement of a tolerance U.S. Environmental Protection Agency, Final Rule. *Federal Register* 60(75): 19523–19524.

Gol, N.B. and T.V.R. Rao. 2011. Banana fruit ripening as influenced by edible coatings. *International Journal of Fruit Science* 11: 119–135.

Goñi, M.G., M.R. Moreira, G.E. Viacava, and S.I. Roura. 2013. Optimization of chitosan treatments for managing microflora in lettuce seeds without affecting germination. *Carbohydrate Polymers* 92: 817–823.

Graham, L.S. and M.B. Sticklen. 1994. Plant chitinases. *Canadian Journal of Botany* 72: 1057–1083.

Hadwiger, L.A. and J.M. Beckmann. 1980. Chitosan as a component of pea-*Fusarium solani* interactions. *Plant Physiology* 66(2): 205–211.

Hashimoto, T., D.J. Yun, and Y. Yamada. 1993. Production of tropane alkaloids in genetically engineered root cultures. *Phytochemistry* 32: 713–718.

Hirano, S. 1988. The activation of plant cells and their self-defence function against pathogens in connection with chitosan (in Japanese with English summary). *Nippon Nogeikagaku Kaishi* 62: 293–295.

Hong, K., J. Xie, L. Zhang, D. Sun, and D. Gong. 2012. Effects of chitosan coating on postharvest life and quality of guava (*Psidium guajava* L.) fruit during cold storage. *Scientia Horticulturae* 144: 172–178.

Jabeen, N. and R. Ahmad. 2013. The activity of antioxidant enzymes in response to salt stress in safflower (*Carthamus tinctorius* L.) and sunflower (*Helianthus annuus* L.) seedlings raised from seed treated with chitosan. *Journal of the Science of Food and Agriculture* 93: 1699–1705.

Jiang, T., L. Feng, and X Zheng. 2012. Effect of chitosan coating enriched with thyme oil on postharvest quality and shelf life of shiitake mushroom (Lentinusedodes). *Journal of Agricultural and Food Chemistry* 60: 188–196.

Khan, W., B. Prithiviraj, and D.L. Smith. 2003. Chitosan and chitin oligomers increase phenylalanine ammonia-lyase and tyrosine ammonia-lyase activities in soybean leaves. *Journal of Plant Physiology*, 160: 859–863.

Kim, H.J. 2005. Characterization of bioactive compounds in essential oils, fermented anchovy sauce, and edible plants, and, induction of phytochemicals from edible plants using methyl jasmonate (MeJA) and chitosan. Dissertation of Clemson University, p. 178.

Kim, H.J., F. Chen, X. Wang, and N.C. Rajapakse. 2005. Effect of chitosan on the biological properties of sweet basil (*Ocimum basilicum* L.). *Journal of Agricultural Food Chemistry* 53: 3696–3701.

Kowalski, B., F.J. Terry, L. Herrera, and D.A. Peñalver. 2006. Application of soluble chitosan in vitro and in the greenhouse to increase yield and seed quality of potato minitubers. *Potato Research* 49: 167–176.

Kurita, K.K., T.T. Sannan, and Y.Y. Iwakura. 1979. Studies on chitin. VI. Binding on metal cations. *Journal of Applied Polymer Science* 23: 511–515.

Lee, Y.S., C.S. Kang, and Y.S. Lee. 1999. Effects of chitosan on production and rot control of soybean sprouts. *Korean Journal of Crop Science* 44: 368–372.

Lee, Y.S., Y.H. Kim, and S.B. Kim. 2005. Changes in the respiration, growth, and vitamin C content of soybean sprouts in response to chitosan of different molecular weights. *HortScience* 40: 1333–1335.

Li, B., Y. Shi, C. Shan, Q. Zhou, M. Ibrahim, Y. Wang, G. Wu, H. Li, G. Xie, and G. Sun. 2013. Effect of chitosan solution on the inhibition of *Acidovorax citrulli* causing bacterial fruit blotch of water melon. *Journal of the Science of Food and Agriculture* 93: 1010–1015.

Liu, H., W. Tian, B. Li, G. Wu, M. Ibrahim, Z. Tao, Y. Wang, G. Xie, H. Li, and G. Sun. 2012. Antifungal effect and mechanism of chitosan against the rice sheath blight pathogen, *Rhizoctoniasolani*. *Biotechnology Letters* 34: 2291–2298.

Loon, L.C.V., W.S. Pierpoint, T. Boller, and V. Conejero. 1994. Recommendations for naming plant pathogenesis-related proteins. *Plant Molecular Biology Reporter* 12: 245–264.

López-Mondéjar, R., J. Blaya, M. Obiol, M. Ros, and J.A. Pascual. 2012. Evaluation of the effect of chitin-rich residues on the chitinolytic activity of *Trichoderma harzianum*: In vitro and greenhouse nursery experiments. *Pesticide Biochemistry and Physiology* 103: 1–8.

Mahdavi, B., S.A.M.M. Sanavy, M. Aghaalikhani, M. Sharifi, and A. Dolatabadian. 2011. Chitosan improves osmotic potential tolerance in safflower (*Carthamus tinctorius* L.) seedlings. *Journal of Crop Improvement* 25: 728–741.

Mandal, S., I. Kar, A.K. Mukherjee, and P. Acharya. 2013. Elicitor-induced defense responses in *Solanum lycopersicum* against *Ralstonia solanacearum*. *The Scientific World Journal*. doi:10.1155/2013/561056.

Mayer, A.F. 2006. Polyphenol oxidases in plants and fungi: Going places? A review. *Phytochemistry* 67: 2318–2331.

Meighani, H., M. Ghasemnezhad, and D. Bakhshi. 2014. Effect of different coatings on postharvest quality and bioactive compounds of pomegranate (*Punicagranatum* L.) fruits. *Journal of Food Science and Technology* 52: 4507–4514.

Merkli, A., P. Christen, and I. Kapetanidis. 1997. Production of diosgenin by hairy root cultures of *Trigonella foenum-graecum* L. *Plant Cell Reports* 16: 632–636.

Mishra, S., K.S. Jagadeesh, P.U. Krishnaraj, A.S. Byadagi, and A.S. Vastrad. 2014. Field evaluation of chitosan and *Pseudomonas* sp. on the biological control of tomato leaf curl virus (Tolcv) in tomato. *Journal of Pure and Applied Microbiology* 8: 681–688.

Mohammadi, A., M. Hashemi, and S.M. Hosseini. 2016. Effect of chitosan molecular weight as micro and nanoparticles on antibacterial activity against some soft rot pathogenic bacteria. *LWT – Food Science and Technology*. 71: 347–355.

Mondal, M.M.A., A.B. Puteh, N.C. Dafader, M.Y. Rafii, and M.A. Malek. 2013. Foliar application of chitosan improves growth and yield in maize. *Journal of Food, Agriculture and Environment* 11: 520–523.

Mondal, M.M.A., A.B. Puteh, M.A. Malek, M.R. Ismail, and M. Ashrafuzzaman. 2012. Effect of foliar application of chitosan on growth and yield in okra. *Australian Journal of Crop Science* 6: 918–921.

Moreira, M.D.R., A. Ponce, R. Ansorena, and S.I. Roura. 2011. Effectiveness of edible coatings combined with mild heat shocks on microbial spoilage and sensory quality of fresh cut broccoli (*Brassica oleracea* L.). *Journal of Food Science* 76: M367–M374.

Moreno, D.A., C. Lopez-Berenguer, M.C. Martinez-Ballesta, M. Carvajal, and C. Garcia-Viguera. 2008. Basis for the new challenges of growing broccoli for health in hydroponics. *Journal of the Science of Food and Agriculture* 88: 1472–1481.

Morrison, T.A. and D.R. Buxton. 1993. Activity of phenylalanine ammonialyase, tyrosine ammonia-lyase, and cinnamyl alcohol dehydrogenase in the maize stalks. *Crop Science.* 33: 1264–1268.

Muangdech, A. 2016. Research on using natural coating materials on the storage life of mango fruit cv. Nam Dok Mai and technology dissemination. *Walailak Journal of Science and Technology* 13: 205–220.

Nardi, S., D. Pizzeghello, M. Schiavon, and A. Ertani. 2016. Plant biostimulants: Physiological responses induced by protein hydrolyzed-based products and humic substances in plant metabolism. *Scientia Agricola (Piracicaba, Braz.)* 73(1). doi:10.1590/0103-9016-2015-0006.

Nge, K.L., N. Nwe, S. Chandrkrachang, and W.F. Stevens. 2006. Chitosan as a growth stimulator in orchid tissue culture. *Plant Science* 170: 1185–1190.

Obsuwan, K., K. Sawangsri, A. Thongpukdee, and C. Thepsithar. 2013. The response of growth and development from in vitro seed propagation of dendrobium orchid to chitosan. *Acta Horticulturae* 970: 173–176.

Ohta, K., A. Tanguchi, N. Konishi, and T. Hosoki. 1999. Chitosan treatment affects plant growth and flower quality in *Eustoma grandiflorum*. *HortScience* 34: 233–234.

Photchanachai, S., J. Singkaew, and J. Thamtong. 2006. Effects of chitosan seed treatment on *Collectotrichum* sp. and seedling growth of chilli cv. Jinda. *Acta Horticulture* 712: 585–590.

Pichyangkura, R. and S. Chadchawan. 2015. Biostimulant activity of chitosan in horticulture. *Scientia Horticulturae* 196: 49–65.

Pongprayoon, W., S. Roytrakul, R. Pichayangkura, and S. Chadchawan. 2013. The role of hydrogen peroxide in chitosan-induced resistance to osmotic stress in rice (*Oryza sativa.* L.). *Plant Growth Regulation.* doi:10.1007/s10725-013-9789-4.

Pornpienpakdee, P., R. Singhasurasak, P. Chaiyasap, R. Pichyangkura, R. Bunjongrat, S. Chadchawan, and P. Limpanavech. 2010. Improving the micropropagation efficiency of hybrid Dendrobium orchids with chitosan. *Scientia Horticulturae* 124: 490–499.

Prashanth, K.V.H. and R.N. Tharanathan. 2007. Chitin/chitosan: Modifications and their unlimited application potential. *Trends in Food Science and Technology* 18: 117–131.

Rabea, E.I., M.E.-T. Badawy, C.V. Stevens, G. Smagghe, and W. Steurbaut. 2003. Chitosan as antimicrobial agent: Applications and mode of action. *Biomacromolecules* 4(6): 1457–1465.

Rahman, M.H., L.G. Hjeljord, B.B. Aam, M. Sørlie, and A. Tronsmo. 2014. Antifungal effect of chito-oligosaccharides with different degrees of polymerization. *European Journal of Plant Pathology* 141: 147–158.

Saharan, V., G. Sharma, M. Yadav, M.K. Chowdhary, S.S. Sharma, A. Pal, R. Raliya, and P. Biswas. 2015. Synthesis and *in vitro* antifungal efficacy of Cu–chitosan nanoparticles against pathogenic fungi of tomato. *International Journal of Biological Macromolecules* 75: 346–353.

Salachna, P. and A. Zawadzińska. 2015. Comparison of morphological traits and mineral content in *Eucomis autumnalis (Mill.)* Chitt. plants obtained from bulbs treated with fungicides and coated with natural polysaccharides. *Journal of Ecological Engineering* 16(2): 136–142.

Samarfard, S., M.A. Kadir, S.B. Kadzimin, S. Ravanfar, and H.M. Saud. 2013. Genetic stability of in vitro multiplied *Phalaenopsis gigantea* protocorm-like bodies as affected by chitosan. *Notulae Botanicae Horti Agrobotanici Cluj-Napoca* 41: 177–183.

Sathiyabama, M., G. Akila, and R.E. Charles. 2014. Chitosan-induced defence responses in tomato plants against early blight disease caused by *Alternaria solani* (Ellis and Martin) Sorauer. *Archives of Phytopathology and Plant Protection* 47: 1777–1787.

Sathiyabama, M. and R. Balasubramanian. 1998. Chitosan induces resistance component in arachishipogaea against leaf rust caused by *Puccinia arachidis* Speg. *Crop Protection* 17: 307–313.

Sauerwein, M., H.M. Flores, T. Yamazaki, and K. Shimomura. 1991. *Lippia dulcis* shoot cultures as a source of the sweet sesquiterpene hernandulcin. *Plant Cell Reports* 9: 663–666.

Sevón, N., R. Hiltunen, and K.M. Oksman-Caldentey. 1992. Chitosan increases hyoscyamine content in hairy root cultures of *Hyoscyamus muticus. Pharmaceutical and Pharmacological Letters* 2: 96–99.

Shehata, S.A., Z.F. Fawzy, and H.R. El-Ramady. 2012. Response of cucumber plants to foliar application of chitosan and yeast under greenhouse conditions. *Australian Journal of Basic and Applied Sciences* 6: 63–71.

Sheikha, S.A. and F.M. Al-Malki. 2011. Growth and chlorophyll responses of bean plants to the chitosan applications. *European Journal of Scientific Research* 50(1): 124–134.

Singh, S. 2016. Enhancing phytochemical levels, enzymatic and antioxidant activity of spinach leaves by chitosan treatment and an insight into the metabolic pathway using DART-MS technique. *Food Chemistry* 199:176–84.

Tamala, W., P. Jitareerat, A. Uthairatanakij, and K. Obsuwan. 2007. Effect of preharvest chitosan sprays on growth of Curcuma "Laddawan" (*Curcuma alismatifolia* × *Curcuma cordata*). *Acta Horticulture* 755:387–394.

Teixeira, D.S.J.A., A. Uthairatanakij, K. Obsuwan, K. Shimasaki, M. Tanaka. 2013. Elicitors (chitosan and hyaluronic acid) affect protocorm-like body formation in hybrid cymbidium. *The Asian and Australian Journal of Plant Science and Biotechnology* 7(1): 77–81.

Trotel-Aziz, P., M. Couderchet, G. Vernet, and A. Aziz. 2006. Chitosan stimulate defense reaction in grapevine leaves and inhibits development of *Botrytis cinerea. European Journal of Plant Pathology* 114: 405–413.

Tsugita, T., K. Takahashi, T. Muraoka, and H. Fukui. 1993. The application of chitin/chitosan for agriculture (in Japanese). In *7th Symposium on Chitin and Chitosan*. Fukui, Japan: Japanese Society for Chitin and Chitosan, pp. 21–22.

Uddin, A.F.M.J., F. Hashimoto, K. Shimiza, and Y. Sakata. 2004. Monosaccharides and chitosan sensing in bud growth and petal pigmentation in *Eustomagrandiflorum* (Raf.) Shinn. *Scientia Horticulturae* 100: 127–138.

Uthairatanakij, A., P. Jitareerat, S. Kanlayanarat, C. Piluek, and K. Obsuwan. 2006. *Efficacy of Chitosan Spraying on Quality of Dendrobium Sonia # 17 Inflorescence.* Korea: World Horticultural Congress.

Utsunomiya, N. and H. Kinai. 1994. Effect of chitosan-oligosaccharides soil conditioner on the growth of passion fruit. *Journal of the Japanese Society for Horticultural Science* 64: 176–177.

Vander, P. 1998. Comparison of the ability of partially N-acetylated chitosans and chitooligosaccharides to elicit resistance reactions in wheat leaves. *Plant Physiology* 118: 1353–1359.

Vasyukova, N.I., L.I. Zinoveva, E.A. Iĺinskaya, G.I. Perekhod, N.G. Chalenko, A.V. Iĺina, V.P. Varlamov, and O.L. Ozeretskovskaya. 2001. Modulation of plant resistance to diseases by water-soluble chitosan. *Applied Biochemistry and Microbiology* 37: 103–109.

Walker, R., S. Morris, P. Brown, and A. Gracie. 2004. Evaluation of potential for chitosan to enhance plant defense. A Report for the Rural Industries Research and Development Corporation, Australia, RIRDC Publication No. 04.

Walker-Simmons, M., L. Hadwiger, and C.A. Ryan. 1983. Chitosans and pectic polysaccharides both induce the accumulation of the antifungal phytoalexin pisatin in pea pods and antinutrient proteinase inhibitors in tomato leaves. *Biochemical and Biophysical Research Communications* 110: 194–199.

Wang, M., Y. Wang, H. Wu, J. Xu, T. Li, D. Hegebarth, R. Jetter, L. Chen, and Z. Wang. 2016. Three TaFAR genes function in the biosynthesis of primary alcohols and the response to abiotic stresses in *Triticum aestivum*. *Scientific Reports* 6: 25008.

Wang, Y.L., B. Li, X. Chen, Y. Shi, Q. Zhou, H. Qiu, M. Ibrahim, G.L. Xie, and G.C. Sun. 2012. Effect of chitosan on seed germination, seedling growth and the club root control in Chinese cabbage. *Journal of Food Agriculture and Environment* 10: 673–675.

Wanichpongpan, P., K. Suriyachan, and S. Chandrkrachang. 2000. Effect of chitosan on the growth of Gerbera flower plant (*Gerbera jamesonii*). In Uragami, T., K. Kurita, T. Fukamizo, (Eds.), *Proceedings of the Eighth International Chitin and Chitosan Conference and Fourth Asia Pacific Chitin and Chitosan Symposium*, September 21–23, 2000, pp. 198–201. Yamaguchi, Japan.

Yin, H., Y. Li, H.Y. Zhang, W.X. Wang, H. Lu, K. Grevsen, Z. Xa, and Y. Du. 2013. Chitosan oligosaccharides-triggered innate immunity contributes to oilseed rape resistance against *Sclerotinia sclerotiorum*. *International Journal of Plant Sciences* 174: 722–732.

Youssef, A.R.M., E.A.M. Ali, and H.E. Emam. 2015. Influence of postharvest applications of some edible coating on storage life and quality attributes of navel orange fruit during cold storage. *International Journal of ChemTech Research* 8: 2189–2200.

Zahid, N., P.G. Alderson, A. Ali, M. Maqbool, and S. Manickam. 2013. In vitro control of *Colletotrichum gloeosporioides* by using chitosan loaded nano emulsions. *Acta Horticulturae* 1012: 769–774.

Ziani, K., B. Ursúa, and J.I. Maté. 2010. Application of bioactive coatings based on chitosan for artichoke seed protection. *Crop Protection* 29(8): 853–859.

Section III

**Biomedical Applications
of the Marine Biopolymers**

11 Marine Biopolymers for Anticancer Drugs

T. Gomathi, P.N. Sudha, Jayachandran Venkatesan, and Sukumaran Anil

CONTENTS

11.1 INTRODUCTION

A large number of polymers, differing widely in structure and function, are synthesized in living organisms. It is a fairly ubiquitous compound produced by many organisms: cell walls of fungi and algae, exoskeletons of insects, mollusks (endoskeleton of cephalopods), and shells of crustaceans. Annually, polymers has been estimated that on the order of 10^{10}–10^{11} tons are produced by living organisms (Revathi et al. 2012). Biopolymers are the waste extracts of marine organisms, produced each year by the shellfish processing industries (approximately 75% of the total weight of crustaceans [shrimp, crabs, prawns, lobster, and krill]) ending up as by-products (Kuddus and Ahmad 2013). Usually, seafood wastes are thrown away at sea, burned, landfilled, or simply left out to spoil (Xu et al. 2013). Therefore, the extraction and its use as is or after further processing may be a way to minimize the waste and to produce valuable compounds with remarkable biological properties and crucial application in various fields. The properties of the polymers mainly depend on the physicochemical nature. This chapter describes the various marine biopolymers, and their properties and applications in drug delivery.

11.1.1 Objectives

Cancer is one of the leading diseases in which uncontrolled manipulation and spread of abnormal forms of the body's own cells takes place through invasion or by implantation into distinct sites by metastasis. Homeostasis within a cell is regulated by the balance between proliferation, growth arrest, and apoptosis. Imbalance between cell growth and death may result in cancer. There are many types of cancer such as lung, ovarian, skin, breast, prostate, colorectal, and bladder. Despite huge advances in prevention and treatment, experts' opinion is that cancer is poised to become the leading cause of death worldwide as people refuse to ditch bad habits and the population ages. Cancer is one of the disastrous diseases to mankind for centuries even after a lot of research work has been carried out in this field.

The main approaches in cancer treatment are surgical excision, radiation therapy, and chemotherapy. The choice of therapy depends on the cancer type and its development stage.

Chemotherapy, which is used alone or in combination with other forms of treatment, is the treatment of cancer with one or more cytotoxic anticancer drugs, aiming at curing cancer, prolonging life, or palliating symptoms. Conventional chemotherapeutic drugs are distributed nonspecifically in the body where they affect both cancerous and normal cells, resulting in dose-related side effects and inadequate drug concentrations in the cancerous tissues. Nonspecific drug delivery leads to significant complications that represent a serious obstacle to effective anticancer therapy. The ideal delivery carrier for anticancer drug should be able to transport the drug specifically to the cancerous tissues and release the drug molecules inside the tissues. Delivering therapeutics to the entire region of tumor in an appropriate concentration is an intricate task and is not easily achievable with conventional cancer therapy techniques. An anticancer drug used in chemotherapy often requires modification to increase solubility, circulation time, and alteration to reduce adverse side effects and nonspecific activity (Liang et al. 2006).

11.2 MARINE BIOPOLYMERS

11.2.1 Alginate

Alginate is a linear, naturally occurring anionic polysaccharide, extracted from brown sea algae, containing D-mannuronic (M) and L-guluronic (G) acids. Its distinctive properties, for example, hydrophilicity, biocompatibility, mucoadhesiveness, nontoxicity, and inexpensiveness, make it a suitable drug delivery carrier. Also its capability to form gel in the presence of divalent cations has been exploited to incorporate numerous drugs, proteins, or enzymes (Tønnesen and Karlsen 2002).

The mechanism of gelation has been intensively investigated by circular dichroism and nuclear magnetic resonance studies. The gelation and cross-linking are due to the stacking of the guluronic acid (G) blocks of alginate chains with the formation of the egg-box junction (Katchalsky et al. 1961; Boyce et al. 1974).

11.2.2 CARRAGEEN

Carrageenan is an anionic, sulfated polysaccharide and is commonly isolated from red seaweed. It is mainly composed of D-galactose and 3,6-anhydro-D-galactose with glyosidic units. It has been widely used for functional food applications and cancer treatments (Holdt and Kraan 2011; Lordan et al. 2011). Recently, it has also been used for several biomedical applications (Mihaila et al. 2013), which were intensively reviewed by Li et al. (2014). The extraction procedure, structure, and subsequent product applications have also been discussed by Prajapati et al. (2014) in detail (Melo-Silveira et al. 2013). Three different types of carrageenan are available, depending on the extraction procedure: kappa (κ), iota (ι), and lamda (λ) carrageenan (Kadajji and Betageri 2011).

These biocompatible and biodegradable biomacromolecules are extensively used in food and pharmaceutical industries. In pharmaceutical industry, these play a significant role as gelling agents in controlled drug release and prolonged retention. Their anticancer, antioxidant, anticoagulant, antihyperlipid, antiviral, and immunomodulatory activities have gained several pharmacological applications (Li et al. 2014; Prajapati et al. 2014).

11.2.3 CHITIN/CHITOSAN

Chitosan is a natural polysaccharide and is considered the largest biomaterial after cellulose in terms of utilization and distribution (Mincea et al. 2012). Chitin is the primary component of arthropod exoskeletons (e.g., insects and crustaceans), cephalopod beaks and shells (e.g., squid), fungi cell walls, and mollusk radulae (chitinous feeding ribbons). Marine crustacean shells (crab and shrimp) are the major commercial sources of chitosan, the partially deacetylated derivative of chitin. Chitin, chitosan, and their derivatives have gained increasing application in biological and biomedical applications.

Chitin and its derivatives are renewable, biocompatible, biodegradable, and nontoxic compounds that have many biological properties such as anticancer (Salah et al. 2013), antioxidant (Yen et al. 2008), antimicrobial (Goy et al. 2009), and anticoagulant (Vongchan et al. 2003) properties. In addition, they are used as biomaterials in a wide range of applications: for biomedical purposes such as for artificial skin, bones, and cartilage regeneration (Dash et al. 2011; Parvez et al. 2012); for food preservation such as for edible films (Muzzarelli and Muzzarelli 2005); and for pharmaceutical purposes such as for drug delivery (Riva et al. 2011).

Chitosan is approved as a nontoxic, biocompatible polymer by the U.S. Food and Drug Administration for wound dressing. The LD50 (Lethal Dose, 50%) of chitosan in mice after oral administration is 16 g/kg body weight, which is almost equal to household sugar or salt. No side effects were reported in human up to 4.5 g/day oral administration of chitosan. However, when taken regularly for 12 weeks, it showed mild nausea and constipation in humans (Baldrick 2010). Although chitosan alone is considered to be safe for oral administration, its properties may change completely upon chemical modification. Moreover, it is well known that the pharmacokinetic properties of a drug or excipient change considerably when included in a nanoparticulate system (Kean and Thanou 2010). Thus, their *in vivo* fate is decided by the size, charge, and surface modifications of the nanoparticles (NPs).

11.3 ANTICANCER DRUGS—OVERVIEW

11.3.1 5-Fluorouracil

5-Fluorouracil (5-FU) is a pyrimidine analog with the chemical name 2,4-dihydroxy-5-fluoropyrimidine. It is one of the most widely used antineoplastic drugs for the treatment of breast cancer (Longley et al. 2003), gastric cancer (Dickson and Cunningham 2004), pancreatic cancer (Pasetto et al. 2004), brain tumor (Lesniak and Brem 2004), liver cancer (Elias et al. 2003), and colorectal cancer (Dodov et al. 2009; Dev et al. 2010). It is a cytotoxic agent that interferes with inhibiting the biosynthesis of deoxyribonucleotides for DNA replication by the inhibition of thymidylate synthase activity, leading to thymidine depletion, incorporation of deoxyuridine triphosphate into DNA, and cell death. An additional mechanism of cytotoxicity of 5-FU is the incorporation of uridine triphosphate into RNA, which disrupts RNA synthesis and processing. However, it metabolizes so fast that the biological half-life is only 10–20 minutes (Sanoj Rejinold et al. 2011; Kevadiya et al. 2012). Therefore, to obtain an effective clinical blood drug concentration, people often choose to increase drug mass or to administer the drug to patients continually or repeatedly, which enhances the toxic side effects of 5-FU.

11.3.2 Curcumin

Curcumin is a yellow spice derived from the roots of the plant *Curcuma longa*. It exhibits a wide range of pharmacological effects such as anti-inflammatory, anticancer, and antiangiogenic properties (Maheshwari et al. 2006; Aggarwal et al. 2007; Zhang et al. 2007). Its therapeutic activity against hepatocarcinoma cells has been studied and proved to be promising (Kunnumakkara et al. 2008; Darvesh et al. 2012; Ahmed et al. 2014). Despite its therapeutic efficacy and safety, curcumin has not been widely utilized for treatment. Poor absorption, rapid metabolism, and fast elimination attenuate the bioavailability of curcumin. Compared to other synthetic and natural anticancer drugs, curcumin has drawn special attention because it can suppress cell proliferation by inducing cell cycle arrest and can cause apoptosis in various cancer cells (Choudhuri et al. 2005).

11.3.3 Methotrexate

Methotrexate (MTX) is a hydrophilic small-molecule anticancer agent (log *P*, −1.8 and molecular weight, 454.5 Da) widely used in the central nervous system malignancies (Abrey et al. 2000). It was originally developed and continues to be used for chemotherapy, either alone or in combination with other agents. It is effective for the treatment of a number of cancers, including breast, head and neck, leukemia, lymphoma, lung, osteosarcoma, bladder, and trophoblastic neoplasms. MTX-based chemotherapy has improved the survival rates for this patient population. However, a major defect in this context is poor drug permeability through the blood–brain barrier (Gao and Jiang 2006).

11.3.4 DOXORUBICIN

Chemically, doxorubicin (DOX) hydrochloride is (8*S*,10*S*)-10-[(3-amino-2,3,6-trideoxy-L-lyxo-hexopyranosyl)oxy]-8-glycolyl-7,8,9,10-tetrahydro-6,8,11-trihydroxy-1-methoxy5,12-naphthacenedione. DOX is a cytotoxic anthracycline antibiotic isolated from the cultures of *Streptomyces peucetius* var. caesius. It consists of a naphthacenequinone nucleus linked through a glycosidic bond at a ring atom 7 to an amino sugar, daunosamine. The anthracycline ring is lipophilic, but the saturated end of the ring system contains abundant hydroxyl groups adjacent to the amino sugar, producing a hydrophilic center. Thus, the molecule is amphoteric that contains acidic functions in the ring phenolic groups and a basic function in the sugar amino group. It binds to the cell membrane and plasma protein. Usually, it is supplied in the hydrochloride form as a sterile red-orange lyophilized powder containing lactose and as a sterile parenteral, isotonic solution with sodium chloride for intravenous use only. Several mechanisms have been proposed to explain the DOX antitumor activity. There are two major mechanisms: the intercalation into DNA, leading to inhibition of the DNA synthesis or poisoning of topoisomerase II, and generation of free radicals, leading to DNA and cell membrane damage (Qin Tian et al. 2010).

11.3.5 LENALIDOMIDE

Lenalidomide, a thalidomide analog, is an immunomodulatory compound used for the treatment of myelodysplastic syndromes, with pleiotropic activities including induction of apoptosis, inhibition of angiogenesis, and broad immunomodulatory effects. The introduction of lenalidomide and other new anticancer agents, such as thalidomide and bortezomib, has a major impact on the outcomes in patients with multiple myeloma (MM), significantly improving 5–10 years of survival rates. Lenalidomide has a dual mode of action including tumoricidal and immunomodulatory effects. Kumar and Rajkumar (2006) gave a detailed clinical response of thalidomide and lenalidomide in the treatment of MM.

Lenalidomide is off-white to pale-yellow solid powder. As lenalidomide is an effective derivative of thalidomide in medical oncology therapeutics, lower solubility may limit its effectiveness. In general, the formulation of a drug in soluble form is much essential and more challenging. Many researchers extended their research to increase drug solubility, where the solubility renders the stability of the compound.

11.4 NEED FOR DRUG CARRIER

Cancer therapy remains challenging, even with the development of a large number of anticancer drugs. Delivery of drugs to the receptors at a particular site has the potential to reduce side effects and to increase pharmacological response. Among the different routes of targeting a drug, the oral route remains to be the choice of administration (Krishnaiah et al. 2002).

Nanotechnology, a newly evolved discipline, includes the formation, management, and application of structures in the nanometer size range (Athar and Das 2013). The unique properties of nanomaterials can be applied to solve different problems, including new ways of drug delivery. According to the guidelines of the National Institutes of Health, an NP is any material that is used in the formulation of a drug resulting in a final product smaller than 1 micron in size (Babu et al. 2013). From the scientific evidence accumulated to date, it has been already demonstrated that NPs hold an incredible potential in various biomedical applications, including effective drug delivery systems (Li et al. 2014a, 2014b; Safari and Zarnegar 2014).

In the past few decades, nanomedicine, the exploitation of the unique properties of nanoscale and nanostructured materials in medical applications, has been explored extensively as a promising strategy in the advancement of anticancer therapies with the ability to overcome many of the limitations common to chemotherapeutic agents (Lammers et al. 2008, 2012; Farrell et al. 2011). NPs ranging in size from 1 to 1000 nm have been designed as drug delivery vehicles from a wide variety of materials, including lipid-based amphiphiles (liposomes, hexasomes, cubosomes) (Drummond and Fong 2000; Sagnella et al. 2010, 2011), metallic (iron oxide, gold) (Cho et al. 2008; Boyer et al. 2010; Huang et al. 2012), carbon nanotubes (Cho et al. 2008), mesoporous silicates (Slowing et al. 2008), or polymers (Markovsky et al. 2012).

Biomaterials made from proteins, polysaccharides, and synthetic biopolymers are preferred, but lack the mechanical properties and stability in aqueous environments necessary for medical applications. Cross-linking improves the properties of the biomaterials, but most cross-linkers either cause undesirable changes to the functionality of the biopolymers or result in cytotoxicity. Compared with water-insoluble polymers, water-soluble polymers have a wide range of industrial applications such as food, pharmaceuticals, paint, textiles, paper, constructions, adhesives, coatings, and water treatment.

11.5 DRUG DELIVERY APPLICATIONS

Drug delivery is becoming an increasingly important aspect for medicine field, as more potent and specific drugs are being developed. No longer depending on small-molecule drugs, this field now not only encompasses the prolonging duration of drug release but also focuses on customized systems that are designed to achieve specific spatial and temporal control.

11.5.1 ALGINATE

Alginate beads have the following advantages: (1) Alginate is known to be nontoxic when taken orally, and also to have a protective effect on the mucous membranes of the upper gastrointestinal tract (Koji et al. 1982); (2) as dried alginate beads have the property of reswelling, they can act as a controlled-release system; (3) as their property of reswelling is susceptible to environmental pH, acid-sensitive drugs incorporated into the beads would be protected from gastric juice (Haug et al. 1967; Yotsuyanagi et al. 1987). The physical characteristics of calcium alginate gel beads are also influenced by the alginate concentration and molecular size, the calcium concentration, and the gelling time.

Oral administration of anticancer drug is a viable alternative to intravenous injection, because it can maintain an optimum blood drug concentration and improves convenience and compliance of patients (Guo et al. 2014). Also the porosity gives alginate beads not only a fast release pattern of incorporated drugs but also a very low efficiency of incorporation of low-molecular-weight drugs, except for sparingly soluble drugs (Pfister et al. 1986). Therefore, it appears that alginate beads can be used for a controlled release system of macromolecular drugs or low-molecular-weight drugs bound to macromolecules through covalent or noncovalent bonds.

Dodov et al. (2009) prepared lectin-conjugated chitosan–Ca–alginate microparticles (MPs) loaded with acid-resistant particles of 5-FU for efficient local treatment of colon cancer. MPs were prepared by a novel one-step spray-drying technique and after wheat germ agglutinin (WGA) conjugation, and characterized for size, swelling behavior, surface charge, entrapment efficiency, and *in vitro* drug release. The prepared MPs were spherical, with 6.73 g/mg of WGA conjugated onto their surface. The size and zeta potential increased after conjugation, from 6.6 to 14.7 m and from 9.6 to 15.3 mV, whereas drug encapsulation was 75.6% and 72.8%, respectively, after conjugation. Functionalized MPs showed excessive mucoadhesiveness *in vitro*, due to the positive surface charge, pH-dependent swelling of the matrix, and lectin–sugar recognition.

Dey and Sreenivasan (2014), have developed alginate–curcumin conjugate for enhancing solubility and stability of curcumin. The conjugate is found to be cytotoxic toward L-929 cells. The aim of this work is to check the suitability of the alginate–curcumin conjugate for the enhanced delivery of curcumin to hepatocytes by attaching a galactose moiety on alginate.

Sarika et al. (2016) synthesized galactosylated alginate–curcumin conjugate (LANH$_2$-ALG Ald-Cur) is synthesized for targeted delivery of curcumin to hepatocytes exploiting asialoglycoprotein receptor on hepatocytes (Sarika et al. 2016). The synthetic procedure includes the oxidation of alginate (ALG), the modification of lactobionic acid, the grafting of targeting group (modified lactobinic acid, LANH$_2$), and the conjugation of curcumin to alginate. Alginate–curcumin conjugate (ALG–Cur) without the targeting group is also prepared for the comparison of properties. LANH$_2$–ALG Ald–Cur self-assembles to micelle with a diameter of 235 ± 5 nm and a zeta potential of −29 mV in water. Cytotoxicity analysis demonstrates the enhanced toxicity of LANH$_2$–ALG Ald–Cur over ALG–Cur on HepG2 cells. Cellular uptake studies confirm that LANH$_2$–ALG Ald–Cur can selectively recognize HepG2 cells and shows higher internalization than ALG–Cur conjugate. Results indicate that LANH$_2$–ALG Ald–Cur conjugate micelles are the suitable candidates for targeted delivery of curcumin to HepG2 cells.

Arıca et al. (2002) formulated 5-FU using alginate beads by the gelation of alginate with calcium cations. The effect of polymer concentration and the drug loading (1.0%, 5.0%, and 10%) on the release profile of 5-FU was investigated. As the drug load increased, larger beads were obtained in which the resultant beads contained higher 5-FU content. The encapsulation efficiencies obtained for 5-FU loads of 1.0%, 5.0%, and 10% (w/v) were 3.5%, 7.4%, and 10%, respectively. Scanning electron microscopy and particle size analysis revealed differences between the formulations as to their appearance and size distribution. The amount of 5-FU released from the alginate beads increased with decreasing alginate concentrations.

DOX-loaded glycyrrhetinic acid (GA)-modified alginate (ALG) NPs (DOX/GA-ALG NPs) were prepared by Zhang et al. (2012) for targeting therapy of liver cancer. The biodistribution of DOX/GA-ALG NPs in Kunming mice and their antitumor activity against liver tumors *in situ* and its side effects were investigated. The biodistribution data showed that the concentration of DOX in the liver reached 67.8 ± 4.9 mg/g after intravenous administration of DOX/GA-ALG NPs, which was 2.8-fold and 4.7-fold higher compared to non-GA-modified NPs (DOX/CHO-ALG NPs) and DOX-HCl, respectively. Histological examination showed tumor necrosis in both experimental groups. Most importantly, the heart cells and the liver cells surrounding the tumor were not affected by administration of DOX/GA-ALG NPs, whereas myocardial necrosis and apparent liver cell swelling were observed after DOX-HCl administration.

Self-assembled core/shell NPs were synthesized by Wang et al. (2015) from water-soluble alginate substituted by hydrophobic phytosterols. Folate, a cancer cell-specific ligand, was conjugated to the phytosterol–alginate (PA) NPs for targeting folate receptor-overexpressing cancer cells. The physicochemical properties of folate-phytosterol-alginate (FPA) NPs were characterized by nuclear magnetic resonance, transmission electron microscopy, dynamic light scattering, electrophoretic light scattering, and fluorescence spectroscopy. DOX, an anticancer drug, was entrapped inside the prepared NPs by dialysis method. The identification of the prepared FPA NPs to folate receptor-overexpressing cancer cells (KB cells) was confirmed by cytotoxicity and folate competition assays. Compared to the pure DOX and DOX/PA NPs, the DOX/FPA NPs had lower half maximal inhibitory concentration (IC50) value to KB cells because of folate receptor-mediated endocytosis process, and the cytotoxicity of DOX/FPA NPs to KB cells could be competitively inhibited by free folate.

Alginate–calcium carbonate–DOX-p53 NPs were prepared by a coprecipitation technique. *p53* is a tumor suppressor gene that plays a pivotal role in DNA repair, apoptosis, and cell cycle regulation. Zhao et al. (2012a, 2012b) stated that "inhibiting p53 mutations, the reintroduction of wild type (wt) p53 into tumor cells harboring p53 mutations, may also enhance the sensitivity of tumor cells to chemotherapeutic agents through the inhibition of the P-gp expression related to drug resistance. On the other hand, wt p53 protein is positive in response to a variety of stress signals including DNA damage caused by antitumor drugs." Thus, the combination of p53 and DOX may increase the efficacy of the cancer treatment. The developed particle size, ~100–400 nm, depended on the polymer content. The NPs showed a high drug encapsulation efficiency and completely inhibited the growth of the HeLa cells. These NPs were used for both gene and drug delivery purposes (Zhao et al. 2012a, 2012b).

11.5.2 CARRAGEENAN

Long-term NP stability is a major challenge of polysaccharide-based NPs used for drug delivery system (DDS). Rodrigues et al. (2015) reported chitosan–carrageenan NPs that were developed using a simple polyelectrolyte complexation method. The developed NPs were stored at 4°C in an aqueous solution, and their size and zeta potential were measured. No statistically significant changes were observed in the size and zeta potential. This indicated that the stability of the NPs was not dependent on the mass ratio of polymers (Rodrigues et al. 2015). In the work from the same group, the addition of sodium tripolyphosphate (TPP) to the chitosan–carrageenan mixture was observed to increase the stability of the NPs for more than 250 days (Rodrigues et al. 2012), suggesting that TPP can act as an effective stabilizer. Carneiro et al. (2013) reported that γ-Fe_2O_3 NP-coated citrate and rhodium (II) citrate enhanced the cytotoxicity on breast carcinoma. Degraded ι-carrageenan (ι-car) was also reported to have the antitumor activity toward human osteosarcoma cell line both *in vitro* and *in vivo* (Jin et al. 2013). Hence, the synergic effect of the NPs and polysaccharides could be a new area of research, which could confer beneficial functionalities and multiple bioapplications to the product developed.

11.5.3 CHITOSAN

The increased interest in chitosan, particularly its use in the pharmaceutical field, is attributed to its favorable properties such as biocompatibility, ability to bind some organic compounds, susceptibility to enzymatic hydrolysis, and intrinsic physiological activity combined with nontoxicity and heavy metal ions (Ravi Kumar 2000; Wang et al. 2003). These properties are particularly amenable to a wide variety of biomedical applications in drug delivery and targeting, wound healing, and tissue engineering, and in the area of nanobiotechnology.

Cationic polymers are widely used as carriers for nonviral genetic material delivery (Kiang et al. 2004; Gao et al. 2009; Liang et al. 2012). They can condense with genetic materials through electrostatic interaction to form polyplexes and facilitate the cellular uptake by cells (Gao et al. 2009; Kiang et al. 2004). In addition, the amine group of polyplexes is quick on the uptake of the cell-absorbing protons, facilitating the escape of the polyplexes from endosome or lysosome through a triggered osmotic swelling effect (Suh et al. 1994; Boussif et al. 1995).

Chitosan has attracted attention as a material for drug delivery anticancer drugs. In this regard, chitosan-based delivery systems range from MPs to NP composites and films. Laxmi et al. (2007) showed the preparation of niosomal MTX in chitosan gel, tested the same for irritation and sensitization on healthy human volunteers, and also compared its efficacy with a marketed MTX gel in the treatment of localized psoriasis. Results showed that no significant irritation and sensitization is produced from niosomal MTX gel and is more efficacious than marketed MTX gel. In 2008, Xu et al. (2008) prepared DOX–chitosan polymeric micelles. These micelles had excellent drug-loading properties and were found suitable for targeting the liver and spleen, and considerably reduced drug toxicity to the heart and kidney. Chourasia et al. (2004) prepared a similar multiparticulate system by coating cross-linked chitosan microspheres with Eudragit® L-100 and S-100 (Rohm Pharmaceuticals, Darmstadt, Germany) as pH-sensitive polymers for targeted delivery of metronidazole, a broad-spectrum antibacterial agent. *In vitro* drug release studies were performed in conditions simulating a stomach-to-colon transit in the presence and absence of rat cecal contents. The results showed a pH-dependent release of the drug attributable to the presence of the Eudragit coating. Moreover, the release of drug was found to be higher in the presence of rat cecal contents, indicating the susceptibility of the chitosan matrix to colonic enzymes. Similar nanoparticular systems for colon-specific delivery of metronidazole were reported by Elzatahry and Eldin (2008).

Jain et al. (2007) developed chitosan hydrogel beads, exhibiting pH-sensitive properties and specific biodegradability for colon-targeted delivery of satranidazole. Azadi et al. (2013) prepared MTX-loaded hydrogel NPs and, after *in vitro* characterization, investigated their transport across the blood–brain barrier *in vivo* in intact animals. The *in vitro* drug release study indicated non-Fickian diffusion kinetic, apparently governed by both diffusion of the drug out of the NPs and swelling/ disintegration of the polymeric network as characterized by a Weibull model for both surface-treated and untreated nanogels. After intravenous administration of surface-modified and unmodified nanogels compared to the free drug, all with the same dose of 25 mg/kg, remarkably higher brain concentrations of MTX were achieved with the nanogel formulations in comparison with the free drug (in some cases, more than tenfold); but there were no significant differences between the surface-modified and unmodified nanogels in all the time points tested. Hyaluronic acid-coupled chitosan NPs bearing 5-FU were also prepared by an ionotropic gelation method for the effective delivery of the drug to the colon tumors (Jain and Jain, 2008). Chitosan-based delivery systems have been widely studied for colonic drug targeting because this system can protect therapeutic agents from the hostile conditions of the upper gastrointestinal tract and release the entrapped agents specifically at the colon through degradation of the glycosidic linkages of chitosan by colonic microflora (Hejazi and Amiji, 2003). Tozaki et al. (1997) investigated the use of chitosan capsules for colon-specific delivery of 5-aminosalicylic acid.

Xing et al. (2010) developed chitosan–alginate NPs by an emulsion method to incorporate 5-FU. 5-FU is a pyrimidine analog drug that has been used to treat cancer for several decades. The resulting particle size was found to be ~200 nm. A drug release of 50% was observed at 12 hours *in vitro* (Xing et al. 2010). Using the same 5-FU drug, sodium alginate–chitosan NPs were prepared by an ionic gelation technique. The developed NPs showed a size ranging from ~329–505 nm. The encapsulation efficiency of 5-FU mainly depended on the molar ratios of sodium alginate and chitosan (6%–26%) (Nagarwal et al. 2012). Das et al. (2010) developed alginate–chitosan–pluronic F127 NPs for curcumin drug delivery. The encapsulation efficiency of the NPs was improved by the addition of pluronic F127. The size of the NPs was found to be ~100 nm.

Shim et al. (2009) prepared chitosan-modified poly(lactic-*co*-glycolic acid) NPs containing paclitaxel (C-NPs-paclitaxel) with a mean diameter of 200–300 nm by a solvent evaporation method. The study demonstrated that the *in vitro* uptake of the NPs by a lung cancer cell line (A549) was significantly increased by chitosan modification. In particular, a lung-specific increase in the distribution index of paclitaxel (i.e., area under the curve (AUC) [lung]/AUC [plasma]) was observed for C-NPs-paclitaxel, when administered to lung-metastasized mice via the tail vein at a paclitaxel dose of 10 mg/kg. Transient formation of nanoparticle aggregates in the bloodstream, followed by enhanced trapping in the lung capillaries, was proposed as the mechanism of lung tumor-specific distribution of C-NPs-paclitaxel. Also, the authors showed that under acidic tumor conditions, C-NPs became more positive and interacted strongly with the negatively charged tumor cells (Yang et al. 2009). The enhanced interaction between C-NPs and tumor cells in the acidic microenvironment might be the underlying mechanism of lung tumor-specific accumulation of paclitaxel from C-NPs-paclitaxel.

Chitosan was also used in the preparation of films for drug delivery systems (Shu et al. 2002; Perugini et al. 2003). Films prepared using chitosan have been utilized for oral delivery of many drugs such as chlorhexidine digluconate (Senel et al. 2000), 5-FU (Ouchi et al. 1989), mitoxantrone (Jameela and Jayakrisnan 1995), cytarabine (Blanco et al. 2000), and paclitaxel (Miwa et al. 1998). The characteristics of chitosan including the drug delivery behavior of nanocomposite films prepared from the mixture of chitosan and organic rectorite, which is a type of layered silicate, were investigated (Wang et al. 2007).

11.6   CONCLUSION

In summary, biopolymers have been extensively utilized for many biomedical applications, particularly in drug delivery. The most attractive features of these applications include good cytocompatibility and biocompatibility, biodegradation, sol/gel transition properties, chemical versatility, and simple modifications to prepare new derivatives with new properties. In the future, an effort should be made on chemical derivatization to create next-generation biomaterials having enhanced or altogether new properties. A thorough understanding of the chemistry of biopolymers is vital to this goal and feasibility to scale up to industrial-scale production volumes.

REFERENCES

Abrey, L.E., J. Yahalom, and L.M. De Angelis. 2000. AL primary central nervous system lymphoma: A curable brain tumor. *J. Clin. Oncol.* 18:3144–3150.
Aggarwal, B.B., Y.J. Surh, and S. Shishodia. 2007. *The Molecular Targets and Therapeutic Uses of Curcumin in Health and Disease.* New York: Springer.
Ahmed, H.H., W.G. Shousha, A.B. Shalby, H.A. El-Mezayen, N.S. Ismaiel, and N.S. Mahmoud. 2014. Curcumin: A unique antioxidant offers a multimechanistic approach for management of heptacellular carcinoma in rat model. *Tumor Biol.* 36:1667–1678.
Arıca, B., S.C. alış, H.S. Kas, M.F. Sargon, and A.A. Hıncal. 2002. 5-Fluorouracil encapsulated alginate beads for the treatment of breast cancer. *Inter. J. Pharm.* 242:267–269.
Athar, M. and A.J. Das. 2013. Therapeutic nanoparticles: State-of-the-art of nanomedicine. *Adv. Mater. Lett.* doi:10.5185/amlett.5475.

Azadi, A., M. Hamidi, and M.-R. Rouini. 2013. Methotrexate-loaded chitosan nanogels as 'trojan horses' for drug delivery to brain: preparation and in vitro/in vivo characterization, *Int. J. Biol. Macromol.* 9(62):523–30.

Babu, A., A.K. Templeton, A. Munshi, and R. Ramesh. 2013. Nanoparticle-based drug delivery for therapy of lung cancer: Progress and challenges. *J. Nanomater.* 1–11. doi:10.1155/2013/863951.

Baldrick. P. 2010. The safety of chitosan as a pharmaceutical excipient. *Regul. Toxicol. Pharmacol.* 56:290–299.

Blanco, M.D., C. Gomez, R. Olmo, E. Muñiz, and J.M. Teijon. 2000. Chitosan microspheres in PLG films as devices for cytarabine release. *Int. J. Pharm.* 202:29–39.

Boussif, O. et al. 1995. A versatile vector for gene and oligonucleotide transfer into cells in culture and in vivo: polyethylenimine. *Proc. Natl. Acad. Sci.* 92:7297.

Boyce, T.A., A.A. McKinnon, E.R. Morris, D.A. Rees, and D. Thorn. 1974. Chain conformations in the sol-gel transitions for polysaccharide systems, and their characterization by spectroscopic methods. *Faraday Disc. Chem. Sot.* 57:221–229.

Boyer, C. et al. 2010. Anti-fouling magnetic nanoparticles for siRNA delivery. *J. Mater. Chem.* 20:255–65.

Carneiro, M.L. et al. 2013. Antitumor effect and toxicity of free rhodium (II) citrate and rhodium (II) citrate-loaded maghemite nanoparticles in mice bearing breast cancer. *J. Nanobiotechnol.* 11:4.

Cho, K.J., X. Wang, S.M. Nie, Z. Chen, and D.M. Shin. 2008. Therapeutic nanoparticles for drug delivery in cancer. *Clin. Cancer. Res.* 14:1310–6.

Choudhui, T., S. Pal, T. Das, and G. Sa. 2005. Curcumin selectively induces apoptosis in deregulated cyclin D1-expressed cells at G2 phase of cell cycle in a p53-dependent manner. *J. Biol. Chem.* 280:20059–20068.

Chourasia, M.K. and S.K. Jain. 2004. Design and development of multiparticulate system for targeted drug delivery to colon. *Drug Deliv.* 11:201–207.

Darvesh, A.S., B.B. Aggarwa, and A. Bishayee. 2012. Curcumin and liver cancer: A review. *Curr. Pharm. Biotechnol.* 13:218–228.

Das, R.K., N. Kasoju, and U. Bora. 2010. Encapsulation of curcumin in alginate-chitosan-pluronic composite nanoparticles for delivery to cancer cells. *Nanomed. Nanotechnol. Biol. Med.* 6:153–160.

Dash, M., F. Chiellini, R.M. Ottenbrite, and E. Chiellini. 2011. Chitosan—A versatile semi-synthetic polymer in biomedical applications. *Progr. Polym. Sci.* 36:981–1014.

Dev, A. et al. 2010. Novel carboxymethyl chitin nanoparticles for cancer drug delivery applications. *Carbohydr. Polym.* 79:1073–1079.

Dey, S. and K. Sreenivasan. 2014. Conjugation of curcumin onto alginate enhances aqueous solubility and stability of curcumin. *Carbohydrate Polymers* 99:499–507.

Dickson, J.L. and D. Cunningham. 2004. Systemic treatment of gastric cancer. *Eur. J. Gastroenterol. Hepatol.* 16:255–263.

Dodov, M.G., S. Calis, M.S. Crcarevska, N. Geskovski, V. Petrovska, and K. Goracinova. 2009. Wheat germ agglutinin-conjugated chitosan–Ca–alginate microparticles for local colon delivery of 5-FU: Development and in vitro characterization *Inter. J. Pharm.* 381:166–175.

Drummond, C.J. and C. Fong. 2000. Surfactant self-assembly objects as novel drug delivery vehicles. *Curr. Opin. Coll. Interf. Sci.* 4:449–56.

Elias, D., J.F. Ouellet, N. Bellon, J.P. Pignon, M. Pocard, and P. Lasser. 2003. Extrahepatic disease does not contraindicate hepatectomy for colorectal liver metastases. *Br. J. Surg.* 90:567–74.

Elzatahry, A.A. and M.S.M. Eldin. 2008. Preparation and characterization of metronidazole loaded chitosan nanoparticles for drug delivery application. *Polym. Adv. Technol.* 19:1787–1791.

Farrell, D., K. Ptak, N.J. Panaro, and P. Grodzinski. 2011. Nanotechnology-based cancer therapeutics—promise and challenge—Lessons learned through the NCI alliance for nanotechnology in cancer. *Pharm. Res.* 28:273–8.

Gao, K. and X. Jiang. 2006. NPDDS for cancer treatment: Targeting nanoparticles, a novel approach. *Int. J. Pharm.* 310:213–219.

Gao, X., R. Kuruba, K. Damodaran, B.W. Day, D. Liu, and S. Li. 2009. *J. Control. Release* 137:38.

Goy, R.C., D. de Britto, and O.B.G. Assis. 2009. A review of the antimicrobial activity of chitosan. *Polimeros.* 19:241–247.

Guo, H., F. Zhao, W. Wang, Y. Zhou, Y. Zhang, and G. Wets. 2014. Modeling the Perceptions and Preferences of Pedestrians on Crossing Facilities. *Discrete Dynamics in Nature and Society* 2014:8.

Haug, A., B. Larsen, and O. Smidsrod. 1967. Alkaline degradation of alginate. *Acta Chem. Stand.* 21:2859–2870.

Hejazi, R. and M. Amiji. 2003. Chitosan-based gastrointestinal delivery systems. *J. Control. Release* 89:151–165.

Holdt, S.L. and S. Kraan. 2011. Bioactive compounds in seaweed: Functional food applications and legislation. *J. Appl. Phycol.* 23:543–597.

Huang, K.Y. et al. 2012. Size dependent localization and penetration of ultrasmall gold nanoparticles in cancer cells, multicellular spheroids, and tumors in vivo. *ACS Nano.* 6:4483–93.

Jain, A. and S.K. Jain. 2008. In vitro and cell uptake studies for targeting of ligand anchored nanoparticles for colon tumors. *Eur. J. Pharm. Sci.* 35:404–416.

Jain, S.K., A. Jain, Y. Gupta, and M. Ahirwar. 2007. Design and development of hydrogel beads for targeted drug delivery to the colon. *AAPS Pharm. Sci. Tech.* 8:56.

Jameela, S.R. and A. Jayakrisnan. 1995. Glutaraldehyde cross-linked chitosan microspheres as a long acting biodegradable drug delivery vehicle: Studies on the in vitro release of mitoxantrone and in vivo degradation of microspheres in rat muscle. *Biomaterials* 16:769–75.

Jin, J., L. Cai, Z.M. Liu, and X.S. Zhou. 2013. MiRNA-218 inhibits OS cell migration and invasion by downregulating of TIAM1, MMP2 and MMP9. *Asian Pac. J. Cancer Prev.* 14:3681–3684.

Kadajji, V.G. and G.V. Betageri. 2011. Water soluble polymers for pharmaceutical applications. *Polymers* 3:1972–2009.

Katchalsky, A., R.E. Cooper, J. Upadhyay, and A. Wassermann. 1961. Counterion fixation in alginates. *J. Chem. Sot.* 5198–5204.

Kean, T. and M. Thanou. 2010. Biodegradation, biodistribution and toxicity of chitosan. *Adv. Drug Deliv. Rev.* 62:3–11.

Kevadiya, B.D., T.A. Patel, D.D. Jhala, R.P. Thumbar, H. Brahmbhatt, M.P. Pandya, S. Rajkumar, G.V. Joshi, P.K. Gadhia, C.B. Tripathi, and H.C. Bajaj. 2012. Layered inorganic nanocomposites: a promising carrier for 5-fluorouracil (5-FU). *Eur. J. Pharm. Biopharm.* 81:91.

Kiang, T., J. Wen, H.W. Lim, and K.W. Leong. 2004. *Biomaterials* 25: 5293.

Koji, D., Y. Chiaki, Y. Mamabu, O. Masayuki, M. Takashi, and K. Hisanao. 1982. Pharmacological studies of sodium alginate. IV. Erythrocyte aggregation by sodium alginate. *Yakugaku Zasshi* 102:573–578.

Krishnaiah, Y.S., V. Satyanarayana, and P. Bhaskar. 2002. Influence of Limonene on the bioavailability of nicardipine hydrochloride from membrane-moderated transdermal therapeutic systems in human volunteers. *Int. J. Pharm.* 247:91–102.

Kuddus, S.M. and R.I.Z. Ahmad. 2013. Isolation of novel chitinolytic bacteria and production optimization of extracellular chitinase. *J. Genet. Eng. Biotech.* 11:39–46.

Kumar, S., and S.V. Rajkumar. 2006. Thalidomide and lenalidomide in the treatment of multiple myeloma. *Euro. J. Cancer* 42(11):1612–1622.

Kunnumakkara, A.B., P. Anand, and B.B. Aggarwal. 2008. Curcumin inhibits proliferation, invasion, angiogenesis and metastasis of different cancers through interaction with multiple cell signaling proteins. *Cancer Lett.* 269:199–225.

Lammers, T., W.E. Hennink, and G. Storm. 2008. Tumour-targeted nanomedicines: Principles and practice. *Br. J. Cancer* 99:392–397.

Lammers, T., F. Kiessling, W.E. Hennink, and G. Storm. 2012. Drug targeting to tumors: Principles, pitfalls and (pre-) clinical progress. *J. Control. Release* 161:175–187.

Laxmi, P.K., S.D. Gayathri, B. Shyamala, and S. Sachidanand. 2007. Niosomal methotrexate gel in the treatment of localized psoriasis: Phase I and Phase II studies. *Ind. J. Dermatol. Venereol Leprol.* 73:157–161.

Lesniak, M.S. and H. Brem. 2004. Targeted therapy for brain tumors. *Nat. Rev. Drug Discov.* 3:499–508.

Li, L., R. Ni, Y. Shao, and S. Mao. 2014. Carrageenan and its applications in drug delivery. *Carbohydr. Polym.* 103:1–11.

Li, N., Y. Chen, Y.M. Zhang, Y. Yang, Y. Su, J.T. Chen, and Y. Liu. 2014a. Polysaccharide-gold nanocluster supramolecular conjugates as a versatile platform for the targeted delivery of anticancer drugs. *Sci. Rep.* 4:4164. doi:10.1038/srep04164.

Li, Y., Y. Yang, W. Zhang, and X. Chen. 2014b. Nanotechnology: Advanced materials and nanotechnology for drug delivery. *Adv. Mater.* 26(31):5576. doi:10.1002/adma.201470215.

Liang, H.F., C.T. Chen, S.C. Chen, A.R. Kulkarni, Y.L. Chiu, M.C.S. Chen, and H.W. Sung. 2006. Paclitaxel-loaded Poly (-glutamic acid) -poly(lactide) nanoparticles as a targeted drug delivery system for the treatment of liver cancer. *Biomaterials* 27:2051–2059.

Liang, Y., Z. Liu, X. Shuai, W. Wang, J. Liu, W. Bi, C. Wang, X. Jing, Y. Liu, and E. Tao. 2012. *Biochem. Biophys. Res. Commun.* 421:690.

Longley, D.B., D.B. Harkin, and P.G. Johnston. 2003. 5-Fluorouracil: Mechanisms of action and clinical strategies. *Nat. Rev. Cancer* 3:330–338.

Lordan, S., R.P. Ross, and C. Stanton. 2011. Marine bioactives as functional food ingredients: Potential to reduce the incidence of chronic diseases. *Mar. Drugs* 9:1056–1100.

Maheshwari, R.K., A.K. Singh, J. Gaddipati, and R.C. Srimal. 2006. Multiple biological activites of curcumin. *Life Sci.* 78:2081–2087.

Markovsky, E. et al. 2012. Administration, distribution, metabolism and elimination of polymer therapeutics. *J. Control. Release* 161:446–60.

Melo-Silveira, R.F., J. Almeida-Lima, and H.A.O. Rocha. 2013. Application of marine polysaccharides in nanotechnology. In *Marine Medicinal Glycomics,* G. Santulli ed., New York: Nova Science Publishers, pp. 95–114.

Mihaila, S.M., A.K. Gaharwar, R.L. Reis, A.P. Marques, M.E. Gomes, and A. Khademhosseini. 2013. Photocrosslinkable κ-carrageenan hydrogels for tissue engineering applications. *Adv. Healthc. Mater.* 2:895–907.

Mincea, M., A. Negrulescu, and V. Ostafe. 2012. Preparation, modification, and applications of chitin nanowhiskers: A review. *Rev. Adv. Mater. Sci.* 30:225–42.

Miwa, A., A. Ishibe, M. Nakano, T. Yamahira, S. Itai, S. Jinno, and H. Kawahara. 1998. Development of novel chitosan derivatives as micellar carriers of taxol. *Pharm. Res.* 15:1844–50.

Muzzarelli, R.A.A. and C. Muzzarelli. 2005. Chitosan chemistry: Relevance to the biomedical sciences. *Adv. Polym. Sci.* 186:151–209.

Nagarwal, R.C., R. Kumar, and J. Pandit. 2012. Chitosan coated sodium alginate–chitosan nanoparticles loaded with 5-FU for ocular delivery: In vitro characterization and in vivo study in rabbit eye. *Eur. J. Pharm. Sci.* 47:678–685.

Ouchi, T., T. Banba, M. Fujimoto, and S. Hamamoto. 1989. Synthesis and antitumor activity of chitosan carrying 5-fluorouracil. *Makromol. Chem. Phys.* 190:1817–25.

Parvez, S. et al. 2012. Preparation and characterization of artificial skin using chitosan and gelatin composites for potential biomedical application. *Polym. Bull.* 69:715–731.

Pasetto, L.M., A. Jirillo, M.Stefani, S. Monfardini. 2004. Old and new drugs in systemic therapy of pancreatic cancer. *Crit. Rev. Oncol. Hematol.* 49:135–151.

Perugini, P., I. Genta, B. Conti, T. Modena, and F. Pavanetto. 2003. Periodontal delivery of ipriflavone: New chitosan/PLGA film delivery system for a lipophilic drug. *Int. J. Pharm.* 252:1–9.

Pfister, G., M. Bahadir, and F. Korte. 1986. Release characteristics of herbicides from calcium alginate gel formulations. *J. Control. Release* 3:229–233.

Prajapati, V.D., P.M. Maheriya, G.K. Jani, and H.K. Solanki. 2014. Carrageenan: A natural seaweed polysaccharide and its applications. *Carbohydr. Polym.* 105:97–112.

Ravi Kumar, M.N.V. 2000. A review of chitin and chitosan applications. *React. Func. Polym.* 46:1–27.

Rejinold, N.S. et al. 2011. Biodegradable and thermo-sensitive chitosan-g-poly(N-vinyl caprolactam) nanoparticles as a 5-fluorouracil carrier. *Carbohydr. Polym.* 83:776–786.

Revathi, M., R. Saravanan, and A. Shanmugam. 2012. Production and characterization of chitinase from *Vibrio* speices, a head waste of shrimp *Metapenaeus dobsonii* (Miers, 1878) and chitin of *Sepiella inermis* Orbigny, 1848. *Adv. Biosci. Biotech.* 3:392–397.

Riva, R., H. Ragelle, A. des Rieux, N. Duhem, C. Jerome, and V. Preat. 2011. Chitosan and Chitosan Derivatives in Drug Delivery and Tissue Engineering, *Adv. Polym.* Sci. 244: 19–44.

Rodrigues, S., L. Cardoso, A.M.R. da Costa, and A. Grenha. 2015. Biocompatibility and stability of polysaccharide polyelectrolyte complexes aimed at respiratory delivery. *Materials* 8:5647–5670.

Rodrigues, S., A.M.R.D. Costa, and A. Grenha. 2012. Chitosan/carrageenan nanoparticles: Effect of cross-linking with tripolyphosphate and charge ratios. *Carbohydr. Polym.* 89:282–289.

Safari, J. and Z. Zarnegar. 2014. Advanced drug delivery systems: Nanotechnology of health design—A review. *J. Saudi Chem. Soc.* 18:85–99.

Sagnella, S.M., C.E. Conn, I. Krodkiewska, M. Moghaddam, J.M. Seddon, and C.J. Drummond. 2010. Ordered nanostructured amphiphile self-assembly materials from endogenous nonionic unsaturated monoethanolamide lipids in water. *Langmuir* 26:3084–94.

Sagnella, S.M. et al. 2011. Nanostructured nanoparticles of self-assembled lipid pro-drugs as a route to improved chemotherapeutic agents. *Nanoscale* 3:919–24.

Salah, R. et al. 2013. Anticancer activity of chemically prepared shrimp low molecular weight chitin evaluation with the human monocyte leukaemia cell line, THP-1. *Int. J. Bio. Macromol.* 52:333–339.

Sarika, P.R., N.R. Jamesa, P.R. Anil Kumar, K. Deepa, and D.K. Raj. 2016. Galactosylated alginate-curcumin micelles for enhanced delivery of curcumin to hepatocytes. *Int. J. Bio. Macromol.* 86:1–9.

Senel, S., G. Ikinci, S. Kas, A. Yousefi-Rad, M.F. Sargon, and A.A. Hincal. 2000. Chitosan films and hydrogels of chlorhexidine gluconate for oral mucosal delivery. *Int. J. Pharm.* 193:197–203.

Shu, X.Z. and K.J. Zhu. 2002. The influence of multivalent phosphate structure on the properties of ionically cross-linked chitosan films for controlled drug release. *Eur. J. Pharm. Biopharm.* 54:235–43.

Slowing, I.I., J.L. Vivero-Escoto, C.W. Wu, and V.S.Y. Lin. 2008. Mesoporous silica nanoparticles as controlled release drug delivery and gene transfection carriers. *Adv. Drug Deliv. Rev.* 60:1278–88.

Suh, J., H.J. Paik, and B.J. Hwang. 1994. Ionization of poly(ethylenimine) and poly(allylamine) at various pHs. *Bioorg. Chem.* 22:318.

Tian, Q. et al. 2010. Glycyrrhetinic acid modified chitosan/poly(ethylene glycol) nanoparticles for liver-targeted delivery. *Biomaterials* 31:4748–4756.

Tønnesen, H.H. and J. Karlsen. 2002. Alginate in drug delivery systems. *Drug Develop. Indus. Phar.* 28(6):621–630.

Tozaki, H., J. Komoike, C. Tada, T. Maruyama, A. Terabe, T. Suzuki, A. Yamamoto, and S. Muranishi. 1997. Chitosan capsules for colon-specific drug delivery: Improvement of insulin absorption from the rat colon. *J. Pharm. Sci.* 86:1016–1021.

Vongchan, P., W. Sajomsang, W. Kasinrerk, D. Subyen, and P. Kongtawelert. 2003. Anticoagulant activities of the chitosan polysulfate synthesized from marine crab shell by semi-heterogeneous conditions. *Sci. Asia* 29:115–120.

Wang, H., Y. Wang, E. Rayburn, D.L. Hill, J.J. Rinehart, and R. Zhang. 2007. Dexamethasone as a chemosensitizer for breast cancer chemotherapy: Potentiation of the antitumor activity of adriamycin, modulation of cytokine expression, and pharmacokinetics. *Int. J. Oncol.* 30:947–953.

Wang, J. et al. 2015. Folate mediated self-assembled phytosterol-alginate nanoparticles for targeted intracellular anticancer drug delivery. *Coll. Surf. B: Biointerfaces* 129:63–70.

Wang, X.H., F.Z. Cui, and Y.H. Zhang. 2003. Preparation and characterization of collagen/chitosan matrices as potential biomaterials. *J. Bioact. Comp. Polym.* 18:453–467.

Xing, J., L. Deng, and A. Dong. 2010. Chitosan/alginate nanoparticles stabilized by poloxamer for the controlled release of 5-fluorouracil. *J. Appl. Polym. Sci.* 117:2354–2359.

Xu, Y. et al. 2013. Transformation of the matrix structure of shrimp shells during bacterial deproteination and demineralization. *Microb. Cell Factories* 12:90.

Xu, X.Y., J.P. Zhou, and L. Li. 2008. Preparation of doxorubicin-loaded chitosan polymeric micelle and study on its tissue biodistribution in mice. *Acta. Pharm. Sin.* 43:743–748.

Yang, R., W.S. Shim, F.D. Cui, G. Cheng, X. Han, Q.R. Jin, D.D. Kim, S.J. Chung, and C.K. Shim. 2009. Enhanced electrostatic interaction between chitosan-modified PLGA nanoparticle and tumor. *Int. J. Pharm.* 371:142–147.

Yen, M.T., J.H. Yang, and J.L. Mau. 2008. Antioxidant properties of chitosan from crab shells. *Carbohydr. Polym.* 74:840–844.

Yotsuyanagi, T., T. Ohkubo, T. Ohhashi, and K. Ikeda. 1987. Calcium-induced gelation of alginic acid and pH-sensitive reswelling of dried gels. *Gem. Pharm. Bull.* 35:1555–1563.

Zhang, C., W. Wang, T. Liu, Y. Wu, H. Guo, P. Wang, Q. Tian, Y. Wang, and Z. Yuan. 2012. Doxorubicin-loaded glycyrrhetinic acid-modified alginate nanoparticles for liver tumor chemotherapy. *Biomaterials* 33:2187–2196.

Zhang, H.G., H. Kim, C. Liu, S. Yu, J. Wang, W.E. Grizzle, R.P. Kimberly, and S. Barnes. 2007. Curcumin reverses breast tumor exosomes mediated immune suppression of NK cell tumor cytotoxicity. *Biochim. Biophys. Acta* 1773:1116–1123.

Zhao, D., C.J. Liu, R.X. Zhuo, and S.X. Cheng. 2012a. Alginate/CaCO3 hybrid nanoparticles for efficient codelivery of antitumor gene and drug. *Mol. Pharm.* 9:2887–2893.

Zhao, D., R.X. Zhuo, and S.X. Cheng. 2012b. Alginate modified nanostructured calcium carbonate with enhanced delivery efficiency for gene and drug delivery. *Mol. Biosyst.* 8:753–759.

12 Drug Delivery Applications of Chitosan

*Sougata Jana, Kalyan Kumar Sen, Arijit Gandhi,
Subrata Jana, and Chandrani Roy*

CONTENTS

12.1   INTRODUCTION

Many therapeutically promising drugs and biomolecules are characterized by a marked instability due to inherent physicochemical and biopharmaceutical features that make their administration extremely challenging. Therefore, finding adequate alternatives has become a major challenge among scientists, and researchers have given their efforts toward the design of suitable targeted drug delivery systems that release the drugs or bioactive agents at the desired site of action. This could increase patient compliance and therapeutic efficacy of pharmaceutical agents through improved pharmacokinetics and biodistribution. These drug delivery carriers should be able to enhance physicochemical stability and protection of encapsulated drugs (Chiellini et al. 2008; Luppi et al. 2010). The choice of the carrier molecule is of high importance because it significantly affects the pharmacokinetics and pharmacodynamics of the drugs. A wide range of natural or synthetic polymers have been employed as drug carriers. Among them, natural polysaccharides have received increasing attention because of their outstanding physical and biological properties (Liu et al. 2008). Chitosan, a cationic, nontoxic, biocompatible natural polymer produced by the deacetylation of chitin, has received considerable attention due to its biological activities and properties in commercial applications. Chitin was first isolated and characterized from mushrooms, by French chemist Henri Braconnot in 1811. Now it is manufactured by chemically treating the shells of crustaceans, such as shrimps and crabs. Chitosan was obtained from partial deacetylation of chitin and composed of copolymers of glucosamine and *N*-acetylglucosamine (Jana et al. 2013). Within the past 20 years, a considerable amount of work has been done on chitosan and its potential use in drug delivery systems. Chitosan exhibited properties such as controlled drug release, mucoadhesion, *in situ* gellation, transfection, permeation enhancement, and efflux pump inhibitory properties (Grabovac et al. 2005; Sun et al. 2010; Bernkop-Schnürch and Dünnhaupt 2012). As the only natural positive polysaccharide, chitosan is especially advantageous in forming stable complex with negative compounds, which makes chitosan a good candidate for the drug encapsulation and controlled release (Illum et al. 2001). Due to chemical modifications, most of these properties can even be further improved. On account of these advantages, chitosan and its derivatives are used to deliver a wide variety of drugs, protein peptides, genes, and vaccines through different delivery systems such as microparticles, nanoparticles, hydrogels, was films.

12.2 CHEMICAL STRUCTURE

Chitin is a linear polysaccharide consisting of (1–4)-linked 2-acetamido-2-deoxy-β-D-glucopyranose. It is the second most plentiful natural polymer, after cellulose, with which it bears a structural resemblance. Chitosan is made by alkaline N-deacetylation of chitin. It is a linear polysaccharide consisting of (1–4)-linked 2-amino-2-deoxy-β-D-glucopyranose (Figure 12.1).

A sharp nomenclature with respect to the degree of N-deacetylation has not been defined between chitin and chitosan. The commercially available chitosan

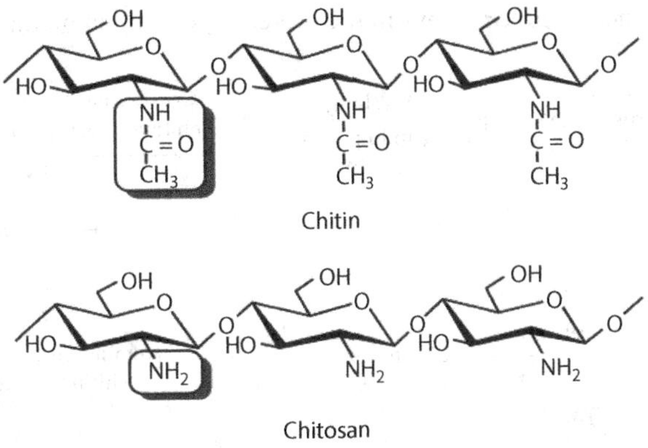

FIGURE 12.1   Chemical structures of chitin and chitosan.

is normally a polymer with less than 20%–25% acetyl content. Chitosan has three types of reactive functional groups: an amino group and both primary and secondary hydroxyl groups at the C-2, C-3, and C-6 positions, respectively. Its advantage over other polysaccharides is that its chemical structure allows specific modifications, especially $-NH_2$ group in the C-2 position (Domard and Cartier 1992; Majeti and Kumar 2000; Jana et al. 2013).

12.3 METHOD OF PREPARATION OF CHITOSAN

The different local resources used to extract chitosan are shrimp shell and crab shell. The shells of these species were scraped free of loose tissue, washed, dried, and grounded to pass through sieve. Then they were subjected to demineralization, deproteinization, and deacetylation (Figure 12.2).

Demineralization was carried out by dilute HCl solution. The treatments with hydrochloric acid and their durations (24–72 hours) depend on the nature of species. It was observed that the emission of CO_2 gas depends upon the mineral content of different species and penetration in the shell's mass (Trung et al. 2006).

Deproteinization of chitin was carried out by using NaOH at 60°C. The treatment was repeated several times. The absence of proteins was indicated by the absence of color of the medium at the last treatment, which was left overnight. Then the resulting solution was washed with water to neutrality and with ethanol. The purified chitin was dried at 50°C to constant weight. Sometimes, decolorization was done to remove natural pigment. The deacetylation process was carried out by adding 50% NaOH and then boiled at 100°C for 2 hours on a hot plate. The samples were then placed under the hood and cooled for 30 minutes at room temperature. Afterward, the samples were washed continuously with the 50% NaOH and filtered in order to retain the solid matter, which is the chitosan. The samples were then left uncovered and oven dried at 110°C for 6 hours. The chitosan obtained was in a creamy-white form (Muzzarelli and Rochetti 1985).

Deacetylation of chitin was also bone by biological method. In this method, chitosan was produced from chitin by using the enzyme chitin deacetylase. The deproteinized sample was prepared by *Serratia marcescens* culture, which was inoculated and incubated for 7 days in the protease production medium. Then it was

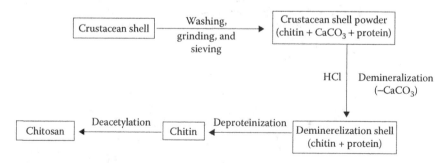

FIGURE 12.2 Synthetic pathway of chitosan.

decontaminated and the collected particles were dried under sunlight and powdered. The prepared chitin and 1 mL of chitin deacetylase producing culture in Lactobacilli MRS broth 7406 were inoculated in the 50 ml of nutrient broth and incubated for 5 days. Then the medium was collected and centrifuged. The pellet was dried under sunlight, and chitosan was prepared in powder form (Babu et al. 2012).

The obtained chitosan has to be purified to make it suitable for pharmaceutical use. The purification process was designed in three steps:

1. Removal of insolubles with filteration in which chitosan was dissolved in acetic acid and the insolubles were removed by filteration
2. Reprecipitation of chitosan with 1 N NaOH
3. Demetallization of retrieved chitosan by adding 10% aqueous solution of sodium dodecyl sulfate and stirring for 30 minutes for dissolving the protein left over finally. After that, 5% w/v ethylenediaminetetraacetic acid was added and stirred at room temperature for 2 hours for precipitation of heavy metals

The water-insoluble chitosan precipitate was collected by centrifugation and washed several times with distilled water by resuspension and recentrifugation for 30 minutes. The residue obtained was dried in hot air oven at 60°C gently to prevent physical damage in the chain structure (Puvvada et al. 2012).

12.4 PROPERTIES OF CHITOSAN

The physical, chemical, and biological properties of chitosan are discussed in Sections 12.4.1 and 12.4.2 (RaviKumar 2000; Singala and Chawla 2001; Dutta et al. 2004; Shaji et al. 2010; Gaikwad and Pande 2013).

12.4.1 PHYSICAL AND CHEMICAL PROPERTIES

12.4.1.1 Molecular Weight and Degree of Deacetylation
The molecular weight (MW) of chitosan ranges from 1×10^5 to 3×10^5. The degree of acetylation of chitosan ranges from 66% to 99.8%. The process of deacetylation involves the removal of acetyl groups from the molecular chain of chitin, leaving behind a compound (chitosan) with a high-degree chemical reactive amino group ($-NH_2$).

12.4.1.2 Solubility
Chitosan is sparingly soluble in water and practically insoluble in ethanol (95%), other organic solvents, and neutral and alkaline solutions at pH > 6.5. It dissolves readily in dilute and concentrated solutions of most organic acids and to some extent in mineral inorganic acids. Upon dissolution, the group of the polymer becomes protonated, resulting in a positively charged polysaccharide ($-NH^{3+}$) and chitosan salts (chloride, glutamate, etc.) that are soluble in water.

12.4.1.3 Viscosity

It acts as a pseudoplastic material exhibiting a decrease in viscosity with an increasing rate of shear. Generally, the viscosity of chitosan is <5 cps; it increases with increasing chitosan concentration, decreasing temperature, and increasing degree of deacetylation.

12.4.1.4 Cationic Polyamine

Chitosan has high charge density at pH 6.5. It forms gel with a number of multivalent anions at low pH range and chelates certain heavy transition metal ions by residual amino groups.

12.4.1.5 Water-Holding Property

Water uptake of chitin, microcrystalline chitin, and chitosan ranges from 325% to 440% (w/w), and the difference is possibly due to differences in the amount of salt-forming groups and differences in the protein contents of the materials.

12.4.1.6 Permeation-Enhancing Property

The mechanism being responsible for the permeation-enhancing effect of chitosan is also based on the positive charges of the polymer, which seems to interact with the cell membrane resulting in a structural reorganization of tight junction-associated proteins.

12.4.1.7 Gelation Property

Aldehydes or carboxylic anhydrides react with chitosan in aqueous organic acid solution to give various forms of gels. The ionotropic gelation of chitosan with different anionic counterions results in gels with a good mechanical stability.

12.4.2 Biological Properties of Chitosan

The biological properties of chitosan are as follows:

1. Biocompatible
2. Safe and nontoxicity
3. Biodegradable to normal body constituents
4. Binds to mammalian and microbial cells aggressively
5. Nonimmunogenic
6. Anticholesteremic
7. Anti-inflammatory
8. Antitumor
9. Antiviral
10. Antibacterial
11. Antifungal
12. Hemostatic
13. Wound healing accelerator activity
14. No effects on serum electrolyte levels or fat-soluble vitamin levels

15. No information about allergic reactions related to these products has been available. β-(1,4)-Glycosidic bond of chitosan will only be degraded by microfloral β-glycosidases in the lower part of the colon and result in nontoxic degradation products.

12.5   DIFFERENT DERIVATIVES OF CHITOSAN

Chitosan may be readily derivatized by utilizing the reactivity of the primary amino group and the primary and secondary hydroxyl groups.

12.5.1   N-CARBOXYMETHYL CHITOSAN

Carboxymethyl chitosan was synthesized by reaction of chitosan with sodium monochloracetate in the presence of NaOH. N-Carboxymethyl chitosan can also produced by reaction of chitosan with glyoxylic acid in the presence of a reducing agent (Rinaudo 2006). Carboxymethyl chitosan acts as permeation eanhancer by enhancing paracellular transport by reversible opening of intestinal tight junctions. This derivative is water soluble in a wide range of pH.

12.5.2   N-SULFONATED CHITOSAN

It is amphoteric in nature. It can be prepared under heterogeneous reaction condition using 2-sulfobenzoic acid anhydride (Chen et al. 1998). It is a novel polymeric absorption enhancer for the oral delivery of macromolecules.

12.5.3   N-TRIMETHYL CHITOSAN

N-trimethyl chitosan (TMC) can be synthesized by dissolving chitosan and sodium iodide in aqueous solution of 1-methyl-2-pyrrolidinone followed by addition of sodium hydroxide and methyl iodide (Amidi et al. 2006). This cationic derivative is found to be water soluble over all the practical pH range. The degree of quarternization depends on the MW of chitosan.

12.5.4   N-SUCCINYL CHITOSAN

It can be synthesized by the introduction of succinyl groups at the N-position of the glucosamine units of chitosan. It is water soluble and low toxic. It has a reactive amino group, a carboxyl group, and both primary and secondary hydroxyl groups at the C-3 and C-6 positions, respectively. This feature makes it possible to exhibit chelation with various metal ions. It can also be synthesized by using chitosan with succinic anhydride (Jayakumar et al. 2010).

12.5.5   CHITOSAN ESTERS

Chitosan esters, such as chitosan succinate and chitosan phthalate, have been used successfully as potential matrices for the colon-specific oral delivery. By converting the polymer from an amine to a succinate form, the solubility profile is changed significantly. The modified polymers are insoluble under acidic conditions and act as sustained release for the encapsulated agent under basic conditions and also for colon-targeted system (Aiedeh and Taha 2001).

12.5.6 THIOLATED CHITOSAN

Various properties of chitosan can be improved by the incorporation of thiol groups. Due to the formation of disulfide bonds with mucus glycoproteins, mucoadhesiveness is augmented. The permeation through mucosa can be enhanced by utilizing thiolated instead of unmodified chitosan. Moreover, thiolated chitosans display *in situ* gelling features due to the pH-dependent formation of inter- and intramolecular disulfide bonds. Thiolated chitosan was synthesized by the reaction of 1% v/v acetic acid solution of chitosan with 2-iminothiolane HCl (Bernkop-Schnurch et al. 2003). The formation of disulfide bonds by air oxidation during synthesis is avoided by performing the process at a pH below 5. At this pH range, the concentration of thiolate anions, representing the reactive form for oxidation of thiol groups, is low, and the formation of disulfide bonds can be almost excluded.

12.5.7 N-METHYLENE PHOSPHONIC CHITOSAN

These anionic derivatives, with some amphoteric character, were synthesized under various conditions and proved to have good complexing efficiency for cations such as Ca^{2+} and those of transition metals (Cu(II), Cd(II), Zn(II), etc.) (Ramos et al. 2003).

12.5.8 PHOSPHORYLATED CHITOSAN

It is synthesized by graft copolymerization technique by reacting 2-carboxethylphosphonic acid and chitosan in the presence of 1-ethyl-3-(3-dimethylaminopropyl) carbodiimide catalyst (Jayakumar et al. 2006). The phosphorylated chitosan has zwitterionic in nature and has improved antimicrobial property.

12.6 CHITOSAN-BASED DELIVERY SYSTEMS

12.6.1 MICROPARTICLES AND NANOPARTICLES

Many methods used in the development of polymeric micro- and nanoparticulate drug delivery devices using chitosan and its derivatives. Selection of any of the methods depends upon the factors such as particle size requirement, thermal and chemical stability of the active agent, release kinetic profiles, and stability of the final product.

12.6.1.1 Ionic Gelation

The use of complexation between positively chargerd chitosan and oppositely charged macromolecules to prepare chitosan particles is very simple and mild process. In this method, chitosan is dissolved in aqueous acidic solution. This solution is

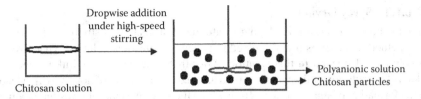

FIGURE 12.3 Schematic representation of preparation of chitosan particulate systems by ionic gelation method.

then added dropwise to polyanionic tripolyphosphate (TPP) solution under constant stirring. Due to the complex formation between oppositely charged species, chitosan undergoes ionic gelation and precipitates to form spherical particles (Figure 12.3) (Shu et al. 2000).

Insulin-loaded chitosan nanoparticles have been prepared by mixing insulin with TPP solution and then adding this to chitosan solution under constant stirring (Fernandez-Urrusuno et al. 1999). Ko et al. (2002) prepared chitosan microparticles with TPP by the ionic cross-linking method. Particle sizes of TPP-chitosan microparticles varied from 500 to 710 µm with drug encapsulation efficiencies >90% (Ko et al. 2002).

12.6.1.2 Emulsion Cross-Linking

In this method, the chitosan aqueous solution is emulsified in the oil phase. Therefore, water-in-oil (w/o) emulsion is prepared and stabilized using a surfactant. The stable emulsion is cross-linked by using an appropriate cross-linking agent to harden the droplets. Particles are filtered and washed properly and then dried (Figure 12.4).

For example, Jameela et al. (1998) prepared chitosan microspheres in the size range of 45–300 µm for the controlled release of progesterone. An aqueous acetic acid dispersion of chitosan containing progesterone was emulsified in the oil phase consisting of liquid paraffin and petroleum ether stabilized by using sorbitan sesquioleate, and droplets were hardened by glutaraldehyde cross-linking (Jameela et al. 1998).

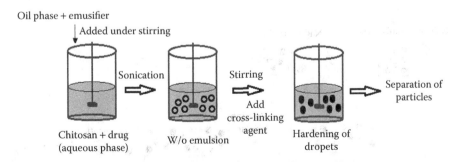

FIGURE 12.4 Schematic representation of preparation of chitosan particulate systems by emulsion cross-linking method.

12.6.1.3 Spray Drying

This method is based on the drying of atomized droplets in a stream of hot air. In this method, chitosan is first dissolved in aqueous acetic acid solution. Then drug is dissolved or dispersed in this solution. After that, a suitable cross-linking agent is added. This solution or dispersion is then atomized in a stream of hot air, which leads to the formation of small droplets, from which the solvent evaporates instantaneously leading to the formation of free-flowing particles. For example, vitamin D_2 (VD2), also called as ergocalciferol, was efficiently encapsulated into chitosan microspheres prepared by spray-drying method. The microencapsulated product was coated with ethyl cellulose. The sustained release property of VD2 microspheres was used for the treatment of prostatic disease (Shi and Tan 2002).

12.6.1.4 Emulsion Droplet Coalescence

This method is a derivation of the emulsification cross-linking method and was first reported for microparticle preparation (Tokumitsu et al. 1999a). The same authors later adapted the method to prepare chitosan nanoparticles loaded with gadopentetic acid (Tokumitsu et al. 1999b).

In this method, chitosan is dissolved in the aqueous solution of drug, and this chitosan–drug solution is added in an oil phase containing stabilizer. The mixture is stirred with a high-speed homogenizer, thus forming w/o emulsion. In parallel, another w/o emulsion is prepared by adding NaOH to a similar outer phase. Both emulsions are then mixed using a high-speed homogenizer, leading to droplet coalescence. This results in the solidification of chitosan particles by action of NaOH, which acts as a precipitating agent.

Afterward, a further set of washing and centrifugation steps is applied using toluene, ethanol, and water (Figure 12.5).

12.6.1.5 Emulsion Solvent Diffusion

This method is generally used to prepare chitosan nanoparticles. It involves the addition of an organic phase (e.g., methylene chloride and acetone) containing the hydrophobic drug to an aqueous solution containing chitosan and a stabilizer (e.g., poloxamer, lecithin) under stirring. This leads to the formation of a w/o emulsion,

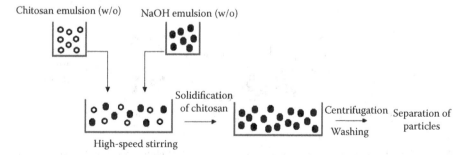

FIGURE 12.5 Schematic representation of preparation of chitosan particulate systems by emulsion droplet coalescence method.

which is then subjected to high-pressure homogenization. Methylene chloride is subsequently removed under reduced pressure at room temperature. At this stage, acetone diffuses to the aqueous phase, decreasing chitosan solubility, and, thus, nanoparticles are formed upon polymer precipitation. An additional amount of water is usually added in order to permit the complete diffusion of acetone. Finally, nanoparticles are isolated by centrifugation (El-Shabouri 2002).

12.6.1.6 Coacervation/Precipitation

In this process, the polymer is solubilized to form a solution. This is followed by the addition of a solute, which forms insoluble polymer derivative and precipitates the polymer. This process avoids the use of toxic organic solvents and glutaraldehyde used in the other methods of preparation of chitosan particles. For example, chitosan microspheres loaded with recombinant human interleukin-2 (rIL-2) have been prepared by dropping of rIL-2 with sodium sulfate solution in acidic chitosan solution. Protein and sodium sulfate solutions were added to chitosan solution, and during the precipitation of chitosan, the protein was incorporated into microspheres (Ozbas-Turan et al. 2002). Chitosan–DNA nanoparticles have been prepared using the complex coacervation technique. The particle size was optimized to 100–250 nm with a narrow distribution. The surface charge of these particles was slightly positive. The chitosan–DNA nanoparticles could partially protect the encapsulated plasmid DNA from nuclease degradation (Mao et al. 2001).

12.6.1.7 Reverse Micellar Method

In this method, a w/o microemulsion is prepared using a lipophilic surfactant that is dissolved in an appropriate organic solvent, such as n-hexane. Surfactants such as sodium bis(ethyl hexyl) sulfosuccinate or cetyl trimethylammonium bromide are used. An aqueous phase comprising chitosan, the drug, and glutaraldehyde, is then added over the organic phase under continuous stirring. Reverse micelles are produced at this stage. Thereafter, particles are extracted following solvent evaporation. It is seen that an increase in the cross-linking rate results in the production of larger particles (Figure 12.6) (Banerjee et al. 2002).

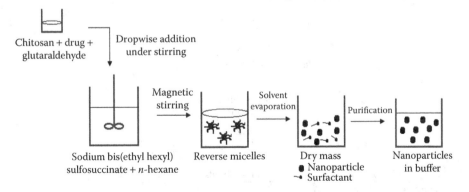

FIGURE 12.6 Schematic representation of preparation of chitosan particulate systems by reverse micellar method.

Compared to other emulsion-based methods, the reverse micellar method has the advantage of producing ultrafine nanoparticles of ~100 nm or even less (Tang et al. 2007).

12.6.2 HYDROGELS

Hydrogels are composed of cross-linked polymer networks that have a high number of hydrophilic groups or domains. These networks have a high affinity for water. Water penetrates these networks causing swelling. The schematic representation of the general method of preparation of chitosan hydrogels is given in Figure 12.7.

12.6.2.1 Physical Association Networks

12.6.2.1.1 Ionic Complexes

Due to the presence of cationic amino groups of chitosan, ionic interactions can occur between chitosan and negatively charged molecules and anions. Ionic complexation can be accompanied by other secondary interchain interactions, including hydrogen bonding between chitosan's hydroxyl groups and the ionic molecules, or interactions between deacetylated chitosan chains after neutralization of their cationic charge (Dambies et al. 2001, Shu et al. 2001).

12.6.2.1.2 Polyelectrolyte Complexes

The associations between the chitosan polymer and polyelectrolytes are stronger than other secondary binding interactions such as hydrogen bonding or van der Waals interactions. Chitosan-based polyelectrolyte complex (PEC) networks have been produced by water-soluble anionic macromolecules such as DNA, anionic polysaccharides (e.g., alginate, carboxymethyl cellulose, pectin), and proteins (e.g., gelatin, albumin).

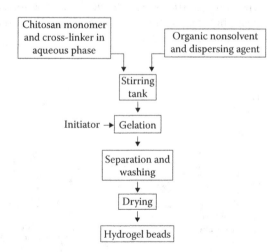

FIGURE 12.7 Schematic representation of general method of preparation of chitosan hydrogels.

12.6.2.1.3 Physical Mixtures and Secondary Bonding

Hydrogels can be formed by polymer blends between chitosan and other water-soluble nonionic polymers. The chain–chain interactions act as cross-linking sites of the hydrogel.

For example, hydrogel consisting of a polymer blend of chitosan and polyethylenimine was prepared. By mixing the polymer with chitosan, a three-dimensional (3D) hydrogel was formed within 5 minutes that was stable under cell culture conditions and could support the growth of primary human skeletal cells (Khan et al. 2009).

12.6.2.1.4 Thermoreversible Hydrogels

These hydrogel systems form transient gels or liquid states depending on the environmental temperature. Bhattarai et al. (2005) developed an injectable, thermoreversible gel that utilized chitosan chain interactions for gelation. The gel was formed by a chitosan-g-PEG copolymer that was produced by chemically grafting monohydroxy PEG onto the chitosan backbone using Schiff base and sodium cyanoborohydride chemistry (Bhattarai et al. 2005). Recently, researchers have developed other hydrogels using chitosan copolymers in combination with poly(N-isopropyl acrylamide) and poloxamers whose hydrophobic group interactions dominate at elevated temperatures. These polymers have been recognized as good candidates for *in situ*, reversible hydrogel formation (Hoffman 2002).

12.6.2.2 Cross-Linked Networks

12.6.2.2.1 Chemical Cross-Linking by Cross-Linkers

Many molecules have been used to cross-link chitosan polymers, including glutaraldehyde, diglycidyl ether, diisocyanate, and diacrylate. These hydrogels have improved mechanical properties compared to physical hydrogels. Cross-linked chitosan networks can be prepared using the available $-NH_2$ and $-OH$ groups (Hennink and van Nostrum 2002).

12.6.2.2.2 Polymer–Polymer Cross-Linking

This process avoids the use of chemical cross-linkers. This approach can be used to form covalently bonded hydrogels *in situ*. For example, a biodegradable hydrogel composed of chitosan and hyaluronic acid polymers was produced by *in situ* polymer–polymer bonding. Schiff bases were formed between the polymers when N-succinylated chitosan and aldehyde-terminated hyaluronic acid were mixed together at physiological pH for 1–4 minutes. The hydrogel was stable for at least 4 weeks (Tan et al. 2009). Chitosan hydrogels have also used Michael addition reactions to form polymer–polymer linkages (Metters and Hubbell 2005).

12.6.2.2.3 Interpenetrating Polymer Networks

Interpenetrating polymer network (IPN) is a combination of at least two polymer chains each in network form, of which at least one is synthesized and/or cross-linked in the immediate presence of the other without any covalent bond between them. When two separate polymer systems that are cross-linked to form a single polymer network, it is called semi-IPN. If the two separate polymers are independently cross-linked, it is called full-IPN. Here, a cross-linked chitosan network is allowed to swell in an aqueous solution of polymer monomers. These monomers are then polymerized, forming a physically entangled polymer mesh called an interpenetrating network (Lee et al. 2000; Myung et al. 2008).

12.6.2.2.4   Photo-Cross-Linking

In this method, polymer mixtures formed hydrogels *in situ* using photo-sensitive functional groups. By adding these reactive groups to chitosan, the polymer can form cross-linkages upon irradiation with ultraviolet (UV) light. This technique has several advantages such as ease of formation, speed, safety, and low cost. For example, a thermo-sensitive, chitosan-pluronic hydrogel was also produced by UV photo-cross-linking (Yoo 2007). The chitosan and pluronic groups were functionalized with photosensitive acrylate groups that were cross-linked by UV exposure. The resultant polymers could then form a physical network at temperatures above the lower critical solution temperature. The hydrogel showed the sustained release of encapsulated human growth hormone and plasmid DNA (Yoo 2007; Lee et al. 2009).

Chitosan-based drug delivery systems prepared by different methods are summarized in Table 12.1.

TABLE 12.1
Chitosan-Based Drug Delivery Systems Prepared by Different Methods

Type of System	Method of Preparation	Drugs or Biomolecules
Microparticles	Ionic gelation	Felodipine
	Emulsion cross-linking	Cisplatin, pentazocine, phenobarbitone, theophylline, diclofenac sodium, griseofulvin, aspirin
	Coacervation/precipitation	Propranolol
	Spray drying	Ketoprofen, bovine serum albumin, ampicillin, oxytetracycline
Nanoparticles	Emulsification and cross-linking	5-FU
	Emulsion droplet coalescence	5- flurouracil, gadopentetic acid
	Emulsion solvent diffusion	Cyclosporine-A
	Reverse micellar	Oligonucleotides, doxorubicin
	Ionic gelation	Insulin, bovine serum albumin, polypeptidic mixtures, ovalbumin, tetanus toxoid, estradiol, carvacrol, heparin, cyclosporin A, saponin, epidermal growth factor receptor
	Modified ionic gelation with radical polymerization	Insulin, BSA, silk peptide
	Desolvation	DNA
Hydrogels	Cross-linking	Aspirin, theophylline, lidocaine
	Physical association	DNA, chondroitin sulfate, hyaluronic acid, heparin
Films	Solution casting	Acyclovir,progesterone, beta-oestradiol
Tablets	Matrix coating	Salicylic acid, theophylline propranolol

12.7   APPLICATIONS OF CHITOSAN AND ITS DERIVATIVES

12.7.1   APPLICATIONS BASED ON INHERENT PROPERTIES OF CHITOSAN

12.7.1.1   Antioxidant Activity

Chitins and chitosans have shown an important biological antioxidant effect that has potentials for a wide variety of applications. However, they are insoluble in water, which is the limiting factor for its utilization in living systems. Therefore, it is important to produce soluble chitin or chitosan derivatives by hydrolysis. To overcome this fact, N-acetyl chitooligosaccharides (NA-COSs) with different MWs produced from crab chitin hydrolysis were evaluated in live cells (Chen et al. 2003). Two kinds of NA-COSs with MWs of 1–3 and <1 kDa exhibited an inhibitory effect against DNA and protein oxidation. Also intracellular glutathione level and intracellular radical scavenging effect were increased in their presence in mouse macrophages (RAW 264.7) and exerted an inhibitory effect against cellular oxidative stress. It was also described that COS is able to protect hydrogen peroxide-induced oxidative stress on human embryonic hepatocytes (L02 cells) (Xu et al. 2010). Administration of chitosans with low MW was reported to inhibit neutrophil activation and oxidation of serum albumin commonly observed in patients undergoing hemodialysis, resulting in the reduction of oxidative stress associated with uremia (Anraku et al. 2008). However, the cellular antioxidant effects of carboxylated COSs, a chemically modified derivative of COS, were evaluated by the ability to inhibit lipid and protein oxidation.

12.7.1.2   Anti-Inflammatory Effects

The anti-inflammatory effects of chitin, chitosan, and their derivatives were reported by a number of researchers. The most important factor in chronic inflammation has been known to be the nuclear factor-kappa B (NF-κB) transcription factor that plays a critical role in regulating genes that encoding pro-inflammatory cytokines, adhesion molecules, cyclooxygenase-2 (COX-2), and inducible nitric oxide synthase (Albert and Baldwin 2001). In particular, current approaches to the treatment of inflammation rely on the selective inhibition of COX-2 activity. Chitosan was able to partially inhibit the secretion of both interleukin (IL)-8 and tumor necrosis factor (TNF)-α from mast cells, demonstrating that water-soluble chitosan has the potential to reduce the allergic inflammatory response (Kim et al. 2004a). As mast cells are necessary for allergic reactions and have been involved in a number of neuroinflammatory diseases, chitosan may help to prevent or alleviate some of these complications. In another study, it was demonstrated that COSs enhanced the migration of the mouse peritoneal macrophages into inflammatory areas (Moon et al. 2007). TNF-α and IL-6 secretion was found to be inhibited in the presence of chitosan oligosaccharide (COS) in RAW 264.7 cells, suggesting that COS may possess an anti-inflammatory effect via the inhibition of TNF-α in inflammation (Yoon et al. 2007). Matrix metalloproteases are a family of secreted or transmembrane endopeptidases that degrade extracellular matrix components (Gorzelanny et al. 2007).

12.7.1.3 Antimicrobial Effects

For the past 15 years, the antimicrobial activity of chitin, chitosan, and their derivatives against bacteria, yeast, and fungi has received attention. In particular, water-
soluble chitosan derivatives were investigated for their antimicrobial activity (Qin
et al. 2004). The mechanism of the antimicrobial activity of chitosan and its derivatives involves cell lysis, breakdown of the cytoplasmic membrane barrier, and chelation of trace metal cations by the chitosan. In the killing of gram-negative bacteria,
a cationic chitosan must interact with bacterial cell membranes. The antibacterial
effect of chitosan is higher than that of chitin because chitosan possesses a number
of polycationic amines, which can interact with the negatively charged residues of
carbohydrates, lipids, and proteins located on the cell surface of bacteria, which subsequently inhibit the growth of bacteria. This interaction between positively charged
chitosan molecules and negatively charged microbial cell membranes results in the
leakage of intracellular constituents. In addition, it can be suggested that chitosan
and its derivatives not only bind to bacterial genes but also chelate metals such as
calcium, magnesium, and zinc ions, leading to the inhibition of transcription and
translation. The antibacterial effects are dependent on their degree of polymerization
or MW (Chung et al. 2004; Je and Kim 2006).

12.7.1.4 Immuno-Stimulating and Anticancer Effects

The mechanism of the antitumor activity of chitosan is enhanced by acquired immunity via accelerating T-cell differentiation to increase cytotoxicity and maintain
T-cell activity. Maeda and Kimura (2004) studied the antitumor effects of various
low-molecular-weight chitosans, such as water-soluble 21- or 46-kDa molecules with
low viscosity, produced by enzymatic hydrolysis of >650-kDa chitosan. The results
indicated there was a decrease in tumor growth and final tumor weight in sarcoma
180-bearing mice due to an increase of natural killer (NK) cell activity (Maeda and
Kimura 2004). Chitosan was also found to significantly inhibit human hepatocellular (HepG2) carcinoma cell proliferation, downregulation of cell cycle-related gene
expressions with decreased DNA content, and upregulation of p21 *in vitro* (Shen
et al. 2009). Amino derivatives of chitosan, such as aminoethyl, dimethylamino-
ethyl, and diethylaminoethyl chitosan, not only significantly induce cell death but
also inhibit proliferation of human gastric adenocarcinoma cells (Karagozlu et al.
2010). Generally, it was observed that the low-molecular-weight water-soluble chitosans might be useful in preventing tumor growth, partly through enhancing the cytotoxic activity against tumors as an immunomodulator (Kimura and Okuda 1999).

12.7.1.5 Anticoagulant Activity

A study of the anticoagulant activity showed that chitosan sulfates with lower MW
demonstrated a regular increase of anti-Xa activity like heparins. Vikhoreva et al.
(2005) demonstrated that sulfated chitosan derivatives and nonfractionated heparin
accelerate thrombin inactivation by forming an equimolar complex with antithrombin III. The anticoagulant activity of chitosan sulfates was determined according
to their ability to inhibit IIa and Xa factors. Xa factor is an important ingredient of
prothrombinase complex, from which thrombin is formed; the latter further directly
affects the thrombin formation process (Vikhoreva et al. 2005).

12.7.1.6 Hypocholesterolemic Effect

There are also studies concerning the role of chitosan in reducing the total cholesterol level. The influence of the MW on hypocholesterolemic effect was also evaluated. Xu et al. (2007) investigated the correlation between feeding chitosan (MW: 120 kDa) and lipid metabolism in hyperlipidemic rats. The cholesterol-lowering effect of chitosan was noted. The same results were achieved by Osman et al., (2010), although they used high-molecular-weight chitosan. The hypocholesterolemic effect of chitosan samples on human patients has also been recorded. Jaffer and Sampalis (2007) observed a lowering of serum cholesterol concentration after patients were treated with low-molecular-weight chitosan (40 kDa). It can be concluded that chitosans with different MWs are capable of lowering cholesterol levels, although the mechanisms of this effect are still not clear.

12.7.2 DELIVERY OF DIFFERENT CATEGORIES OF DRUGS AND BIOACTIVES

12.7.2.1 Delivery of Anti-Inflammatory Drugs

Shiraishi et al. (1993) prepared indomethacin-loaded chitosan microspheres by polyelectrolyte complexation of sodium TPP and chitosan. Kumbar et al. (2002) prepared chitosan microspheres of diclofenac sodium with three different cross-linking methods. Chitosan microspheres of ketoprofen have also been prepared by a multiple emulsion (o/w/o), which produced satisfactory yields of microspheres (Pavanetto et al. 1996). Yamada et al. (2001) prepared ketoprofen microspheres by the *dry-in-oil* method using ethylcellulose as a matrix polymer. Bead formulations containing acetaminophen were prepared using the combination of carboxymethyl cellulose sodium, cellulose microcrystalline (Avicel RC-591), and chitosan (Goskonda and Upadrashta 1993).

12.7.2.2 Delivery of Antibiotics

Hejazi and Amiji (2003) examined the gastric residence time of tetracycline-loaded chitosan microspheres (prepared by ionic cross-linking and precipitation method) following their oral administration in gerbils. Chandy and Sharma (1993) monitored the *in vitro* release profile of ampicillin from chitosan beads and microgranules. Amoxicillin- and metronidazole-loaded chitosan microspheres for stomach specific drug delivery were prepared for the treatment of *Helicobacter pylori* infection (Shah et al. 1999). Wong et al. (2002) studied the influence of microwave irradiation on the sulfathiazole release properties of alginate–chitosan and chitosan beads prepared by extrusion.

12.7.2.3 Delivery of Anticancer Drugs

Chandy et al. (2000) investigated the potential of chitosan-coated polylactic acid (PLA)/polylactic-*co*-glycolic acid (PLGA) microspheres for the targeted delivery of 5-fluorouracil (5-FU) to treat cerebral tumors. They demonstrated the possibility of entrapping an antiproliferative agent, cisplatin, in a series of surface-coated biodegradable microspheres composed of PLA–poly(caprolactone) blends coated with chitosan (Chandy et al. 2002). Chitosan microspheres loaded with cytarabine were embedded in a PLGA film to constitute a co-matrix system (Blanco et al. 2000). The possibility of encapsulating taxol-loaded PLA microspheres within heparin–chitosan spheres to develop a prolonged release co-matrix form was also investigated (Chandy et al. 2001). Sustained plasma levels of methotrexate were obtained when drug-loaded chitosan and chitin microspheres were administered to mice bearing Ehrlich ascites tumors (Singh and Udupa 1998).

12.7.2.4 Delivery of Anti-Infective Agents

Giunchedi et al. investigated the development of buccal tablets based on chitosan microspheres containing chlorhexidine diacetate (Giunchedi et al. 2002). Microspheres containing the mucoadhesive polymer chitosan hydrochloride, with matrix polymer Eudragit RS were prepared using pipemidic acid as a model drug (Bogataj et al. 2000). Hari et al. prepared microcapsules by adding dropwise a solution of sodium alginate containing nitrofurantoin into a chitosan–$CaCl_2$ system (Hari et al. 1996).

12.7.2.5 Delivery of Cardiac Agents

Casein–chitosan microspheres containing diltiazem hydrochloride were also prepared using aqueous coacervation technique (al-Suwayeh et al. 2003). Lim and Wan (1998) reported that propranolol-loaded chitosan microspheres prepared by emulsification coacervation technique. The formulation and *in vitro* release profile of the isosorbide-5-mononitrate-loaded chitosan microspheres was investigated by Farivar et al. (1993). The release of the drug from chitosan microspheres was compared with marketed formulations (Farivar et al. 1993).

12.7.2.6 Protein and Peptide Delivery

Generally, administration of proteins and peptides via nonparenteral routes has been considered a challenging task due to the poor absorption and severe enzymatic degradation. Owing to their unique mucoadhesive and/or absorption-enhancing properties, chitosans and their derivatives have been extensively investigated for the delivery of therapeutic proteins and peptides via mucosal (oral, buccal, nasal, pulmonary, and vaginal) and transdermal routes (Amidi et al. 2010).

Yang et al. (2007) prepared an inhalable chitosan-based powder formulation of salmon calcitonin-containing mannitol (as a cryoprotecting agent) using a spray-drying process. The effect of chitosan on the physicochemical stability of the protein was investigated with chromatographic and spectrometric techniques. The dissolution rate of the protein decreased when formulated with chitosan, which might be due to an irreversible complex formation between the (aggregated) protein and chitosan during the drying process (Yang et al. 2007). In another study, the potential of chitosan oligomers for delivery of proteins was studied. The absorption of interferon (INF)-α in rats was improved after pulmonary administration of aqueous solutions of the oligomers and INF. Among various oligomers, glucosamine hexamers at a concentration of 0.5% (w/v) showed the highest efficacy (Yamada et al. 2005).

Exogenous insulin has been widely used to combat diabetes mellitus. Oral delivery of insulin is quite challenging. There are several barriers preventing insulin from reaching the bloodstream, such as enzymatic degradation, inactivation by the acidic environment in the stomach, and poor absorption at the intestinal mucosa. Many studies have reported that chitosan significantly improved the delivery of therapeutic insulin. Insulin-loaded nanoparticles were obtained by ionic gelation of a chitosan solution with TPP solution also containing insulin. The insulin-loaded chitosan nanoparticles had a good loading capacity (65%–80%) and were fully recovered from the powder formulations after contact with an aqueous medium, and showed a fast release of insulin (Grenha et al. 2005).

Mao et al. (2006) utilized chitosan derivatives to synthesize insulin–polyelectrolyte nanocomplexes by self-assembly methods. On account of the electrostatic interactions between the negatively charged insulin and the positively charged chitosan, the insulin was safely encapsulated in chitosan nanoparticles for oral delivery.

Poly(ethylene glycol)-grafted-chitosan copolymers have been synthesized to increase chitosan's solubility and to improve its the biocompatibility. PEGylated chitosan nanoparticles, prepared by reacting PEG-aldehyde with amine groups of chitosan, were studied by Zhang et al. (2008c). Furthermore, insulin-loaded PEG–chitosan nanoparticles were prepared by ionic gelation of PEG–chitosan with TPP. The MW of chitosan and PEG affected the release kinetics of insulin. Formulations made of higher MW chitosan showed a faster and higher burst release than those made of lower MW chitosan, which has higher chain flexibility to yield a tighter network (Zhang et al. 2008c)

Chitosan-coated gold nanoparticles have been investigated for mucosal protein delivery. Chitosan was used as a reducing agent in the synthesis of gold nanoparticles and also as a mucoadhesive and penetration enhancer. Insulin was efficiently adsorbed through electrostatic interaction onto the surface of the coated nanoparticles, and they were colloidally stable for 6 months. Intranasal (i.n.) administration of these nanoparticles in diabetic rats showed an improved pharmacodynamic effect as evidenced by higher reduction in blood glucose levels (Bhumkar et al. 2007).

Ye et al. (2006) prepared a multilayer chitosan/alginate self-assembled coating on melamine formaldehyde (MF) microparticles, of which after deposition of the multilayer the MP template was removed by dissolving the core at low pH. Insulin was post-loaded into the hollow chitosan/alginate microparticles. To slow down the release kinetics, cross-linked particles were prepared by adding a calcium chloride solution to the insulin-loaded particles. The chitosan/alginate particles showed a sustained release of insulin of 80% in 15 hours, which was decreased to 50% for the cross-linked particles (Ye et al. 2006).

Moreover, chitosan-coated nanoparticles fabricated via self-assembly processes have been investigated in the delivery of proteins. Haidar et al. (2008) prepared cationic liposomes where the surface of the nanoparticles gradually adsorbed alginate and chitosan via the self-assembly technique. The resulting chitosan-coated nanoparticles exhibited slow release of the bovine serum albumin (BSA) over ~30 days (Haidar et al. 2008).

12.7.2.7   Gene Delivery

Chitosan has the ability to interact ionically with negatively charged DNA to form polyelectrolyte complexes, which results in better DNA protection against nuclease degradation. Several interesting studies describing the potential use of chemically modified chitosan in gene delivery have been reported. Self-aggregated nanoparticles were prepared by hydrophobic modification of chitosan with deoxycholic acid in aqueous media. Self-aggregates have a small size (mean diameter of 160 nm) with a unimodal size distribution. They can form charge complexes when mixed with plasmid DNA. The usefulness of self-aggregates/DNA complex for transfer of genes into mammalian cells *in vitro* has been suggested (Lee et al. 1998).

Numerous studies have been reported on the prophylactic and therapeutic use of genetic vaccines for combating a variety of infectious diseases in animal models. Cui and Mumper (2001) investigated the topical application of chitosan-based nanoparticles containing plasmid DNA as a potential approach to genetic immunization. Recently, Sajomsang et al. (2009) examined a methylated chitosan derivative/DNA complex containing different aromatic moieties. Of all the derivatives tested, *N*-(4-pyridinylmethyl) chitosan exhibited the highest transfection efficiency in human hepatoma cells (Huh 7 cells) (Sajomsang et al. 2009). Zhang et al. (2007) modified chitosan with alpha-methoxy-omega-succinimidyl-PEG to prolong gene transfer for improved gene expression compared to nonmodified chitosan/DNA complex both *in vitro* and *in vivo* (Zhang et al. 2007). Water-soluble chitosan was coupled with lactobionic acid-bearing galactose group as the specific ligand to asialoglycoprotein (ASGP) receptor of hepatocytes. This targeted DNA delivery system exhibited much enhanced gene delivery on human hepatoblastoma HepG2 cells than unmodified chitosan (Kim et al. 2004b).

12.7.2.8 Vaccine Delivery

Chitosan-based carriers have been extensively studied for parenteral and mucosal delivery of antigens. The intravenous (i.v.) administration of phagocytosable chitin microparticles resulted in activation of alveolar macrophages, which showed upregulation of the expression of IL-12, TNF-α, and IL-18, leading to the production of INF-γ by NK cells (Bourbouze et al. 1991). Zaharoff et al. (2007) showed that chitosan when dissolved in buffer pH 6.2, there was enhancement of immunoadjuvant properties of cytokines such as granulocyte-macrophage colony-stimulating factor (GM-CSF), when coadministered subcutaneously. Chitosan also prolonged dissemination of GM-CSF at the site of injection resulting in prolonged exposure of immune cells to this cytokine and enhancing the immunoadjuvant properties of GM-CSF (Zaharoff et al. 2007). Another research work showed that intramuscular administration of soluble chitosan with monovalent and trivalent split inactivated influenza vaccine resulted in strong humoral and cell-immunity responses against A- and B-type human influenza viruses (Ghendon et al. 2009). In another study, i.n. immunization with diphtheria toxoid (DT)-loaded TMC microparticles induced the formation of both immunoglobulin G (IgG) and immunoglobulin A (IgA) (van der Lubben et al. 2002).

The potential of TMC as an adjuvant for mucosal vaccination was shown in guinea pigs after pulmonary administration of DT-loaded TMC microparticles. The animals that received TMC–DT microparticle powders showed comparable or superior systemic and local immune responses compared to the animals that received a subcutaneously administered alum-adsorbed DT vaccine (Amidi et al. 2007).

PECs made by electrostatic interaction of positively charged chitosan and negatively charged dextran sulfate were investigated by Drogoz et al. (2008) for the delivery of the capsid protein of HIV-1 virus (p24).

Chitosan and its derivatives were also used as a coating material for negatively charged particles loaded with an antigen. Nagamoto et al. (2004) prepared chitosan-coated emulsions. A model antigen, albumin, and cholera toxin, as an adjuvant, were loaded into the particles. After administration, the chitosan-coated formulations induced high-serum IgG and mucosal IgA antibody titers in rats (Nagamoto et al. 2004).

It was seen that chitosan particles have been formulated with other polymers, for example, alginate to increase both the mucoadhesion properties of the vaccine and the colloidal stability of the particles, as well as to improve the release characteristics of a loaded antigen. In a study, mucoadhesive chitosan-coated PLGA microparticles loaded with hepatitis B surface antigen (HBsAg) were designed. Intranasally administered chitosan-coated PLGA particles exhibited stronger local and cell-mediated immune responses against HBsAg (Zhao et al. 2006). In another study, Pluronic® F127 was used as a mucosal adjuvant in chitosan particles loaded with *Bordetella bronchiseptica* antigens. The adjuvanted formulations remarkably improved systemic IgG and IgA antibodies compared to control free antigen after i.n. administration (Kang et al. 2007). Zhu et al. (2007) prepared chitosan microparticles loaded with a tuberculosis subunit antigen for subcutaneous immunization. Upon subcutaneous immunization, the chitosan formulations elicited higher serum IgG, IgG1, and IgG2a antibodies, and INF-γ levels than free antigen in phosphate-buffered saline (Zhu et al. 2007). Generally, it was found that the type and immunogenicity of antigens as well as the type and adjuvant activity of chitosan also play an important role in type of immune responses and adjuvant activity of chitosan formulations.

12.7.3 Targeted Drug Delivery to Different Organs/Cells

12.7.3.1 Ocular Drug Delivery

Chitosan-based systems are nowadays widely utilized for improving the retention and biodistribution of drugs applied topically onto the eye. Besides its low toxicity and good ocular tolerance, chitosan exhibits favorable biological behavior, such as bioadhesion- and permeability-enhancing properties, and also interesting physicochemical characteristics, which make it a unique material for the design of ocular drug delivery vehicles. Chitosan gels, chitosan-coated colloidal systems, and chitosan nanoparticles are able to enhance and prolong the retention of drugs on the eye surface. Chitosan was found to facilitate the transport of drugs to the inner eye or able to facilitate the accumulation of drug into the corneal/conjunctival epithelia (Alonso and Sánchez 2003).

Chitosan enhances the cornea contact time through its mucoadhesion mediated by electrostatic interaction between its positively charged chitosan and negatively charged mucin. Its ability to transient opening tight junction is believed to improve drug bioavailability.

Cao et al. (2007) investigated a novel thermosensitive copolymer poly(*N*-isopropylacrylamide)–chitosan for its thermosensitive *in situ* gel-forming properties and potential utilization for ocular drug delivery for timolol maleate over a period of 12 hours (Cao et al. 2007).

Effort was done to design a submicron-sized liposomal nonsteroidal anti-inflammatory drug (NSAID) preparation that targets the retina via topical instillation of eyedrops. Bromfenac (BRF)-loaded liposomes were prepared using the calcium acetate gradient method. Surface modification with chitosan was achieved using electrostatic interactions of negatively charged liposomes. Release of BRF from liposomes was sustained for several hours depending on the lipid concentration, inner water phase, initial drug amounts, and surface properties. BRF release was significantly prolonged by liposome encapsulation, and further by chitosan modification. Importantly, modification of liposomes with chitosan did not alter drug release profiles. However, polymer modification of liposomes reduced the initial rate of drug release (Tsukamoto et al. 2013).

Diebold et al. (2007) evaluated chitosan-based colloidal nanosystem with the potential to deliver drugs to the ocular surface. This nanosystem, liposome–chitosan nanoparticle (LCS–NP) complexes, was created as a complex between liposomes and chitosan nanoparticles. The conjunctival epithelial cell line instituto de oftalmobiologia aplicada (IOBA)-normal human conjunctiva (NHC) was exposed to several concentrations of three different LCS–NP complexes to determine the cytotoxicity. The uptake of LCS–NP by the IOBA-NHC conjunctival cell line and by primary cultured conjunctival epithelial cells was examined by confocal microscopy. Eyeball and lid tissues from LCS–NP-treated rabbits were evaluated for the *in vivo* uptake and acute tolerance of the nanosystems. The *in vitro* toxicity of LCS–NP in the IOBA-NHC cells was very low. LCS–NPs were identified inside IOBA-NHC cells after 15 minutes and inside primary cultures of conjunctival epithelial cells after 30 minutes. These data demonstrate that LCS–NPs are potentially used as drug carriers for the ocular surface (Diebold et al. 2007). In another study, the feasibility of *in situ* thermosensitive hydrogel based on chitosan in combination with disodium α-D-glucose 1-phosphate (DGP) was studied for the ocular drug delivery system (Chen et al. 2012). Aqueous solution of chitosan/DGP underwent sol–gel transition as temperature increased, which was flowing sol at room temperature and then turned into nonflowing hydrogel at physiological temperature. The properties of gels were characterized regarding gelation time, gelation temperature, and morphology. The sol–gel phase transition behaviors were affected by the concentrations of chitosan, DGP, and the model drug levocetirizine dihydrochloride (LD). The developed hydrogel presented a characteristic of a rapid release at the initial period followed by a sustained release and remarkably enhanced the cornea penetration of LD. The results of ocular irritation demonstrated the excellent ocular tolerance of the hydrogel. The ocular residence time for the hydrogel was significantly prolonged compared with eyedrops. The drug-loaded hydrogel produced more effective antiallergic conjunctivitis effects compared with LD aqueous solution. De Campos et al. (2004) prepared chitosan-based fluorescent (CS-fl) nanoparticles by ionotropic gelation. CS-fl nanoparticles were stable upon incubation with lysozyme and did not affect the viscosity of a mucin dispersion. *In vivo* studies showed that the amounts of CS-fl in the cornea and conjunctiva were significantly higher for CS-fl nanoparticles than for control CS-fl solution; these amounts were fairly constant for up to 24 hours (De Campos et al. 2004).

12.7.3.2 Transdermal Drug Delivery

Transdermal drug delivery system has been used for the drug administration via the skin for both local therapeutic effects and systemic delivery. As a substitute for the oral route, transdermal drug delivery has a number of significant advantages, including the ability to avoid problems of gastric irritation, pH, and emptying rate effects; avoid hepatic first-pass metabolism, thereby increasing the bioavailability of drug; reduce the risk of systemic side effects; rapid termination of therapy by removal of the device or formulation; and the reduction of fluctuations in plasma levels of drugs. Due to good bioadhesive property, film-forming property, and the ability to sustain the release of the active constituents, chitosan has been used in topical delivery systems.

Varshosaz et al. (2006b) prepared the gel-containing lidocaine (LC) as a local anesthetic agent with three different MWs and concentrations of chitosan for prolonging anesthetic effect of this drug for transdermal delivery. Lecithin was used as a permeation enhancer. Viscosity, bioadhesion, drug release from synthetic membranes, and drug permeation through biological barrier (rat skin) was studied. It was found that by increasing the concentration and MW of chitosan, there was an increase in both the rate and the extent of drug release and was probably because of the increase in repulsive forces between LC and chitosan cations. In another study, matrix-type transdermal patches were prepared using alprazolam as a model drug and employing the combinations of chitosan-polyvinyl alcohol cross-linked with maleic anhydride (Maji et al. 2013). The skin irritation study indicated that neither the polymer nor the drug caused any noticeable irritation or inflammation on or around the patch area, either during the period of study or after removal of the patch. Hemant and Shivakumar (2010) evaluated chitosan acetate films designed for transdermal delivery of propranolol hydrochloride. The permeability coefficient was 6.12×10^{-4} and 0.97×10^{-4} g.cm^2/day for chitosan acetate and chitosan, respectively. fourier transform infrared spectroscopy (FTIR) and differential scanning calorimetry (DSC) results indicated that there was no chemical interaction between the drug and the polymers used (Hemant and Shivakumar 2010). Madhulatha and Ravikiran (2013) prepared a sustained release transdermal therapeutic system containing ibuprofen with different ratios of chitosan, hydroxylpropyl methylcellulose (HPMC), and combination of chitosan–HPMC by solvent evaporation technique (Madhulatha and Ravikiran 2013).

In a study, a novel transdermal film of ondansetron HCl was developed with high MW chitosan as matrix polymer and 2-(2-ethoxy-ethoxy) ethanol (Transcutol®) as plasticizer. In vitro permeation study on *stratum corneum* intercellular lipids upto 24 hours showed that the chitosan gels consisting of Transcutol® as plasticizer and terpenes as penetration enhancer may be used to prepare transdermal films of ondansetron due to the good mechanical properties and bioadhesiveness of the transdermal films (Can et al. 2013).

Development of transdermal drug delivery system of ketoprofen drug with chitosan was also carried out for the treatment of arthritis (Ramchandani and Balakrishnan 2012).

Thein-Han and Stevens (2004) analyzed the release of a drug from a transdermal delivery system with a rate-controlling chitosan membrane *in vitro* and *in vivo*. LC hydrochloride, a local anesthetic, was used as the model drug. The *in vitro* permeability of various chitosan membranes for the drug was investigated using a Franz diffusion cell. Drug release was slower through chitosan membranes with a higher degree of deacetylation and a larger thickness (Thein-Han and Stevens 2004).

Allena et al. (2012) observed that chitosan:HPMC in the ratio of 5:1 along with dibutyl phthalate as a plasticizer was very promising in controlling the release of metformin via a transdermal drug delivery system.

To improve the physiochemical properties of biopatch materials, silver compounds of various concentrations were synthesized in chitosan solution and formed to silver hybridized porous chitosan structures. With this aim, Kim et al. (2013) ascertained that it was optimal to combine silver nitrate of 3%, chitosan of 1% (MW <1000 kDa), and sodium borohydride of 0.003% for achieving high mechanical strength and drug delivery efficiency. Drug release rate and hydrophilic ratio were increased due to an increase in silver concentration. Further, the initial drug release of the silver-hybridized porous chitosan patch was approximately 1.5 times faster than that of the chitosan patch as control. These results indicate that silver-hybridized porous chitosan patch can be widely used as a sterilizing transdermal drug delivery system in various fields (Kim et al. 2013).

12.7.3.3   Nasal Drug Delivery

The nasal mucosa provides a potentially good route for systemic drug delivery. One of the most important features of the nasal route is that it avoids first-pass hepatic metabolism, thereby reducing metabolism. The application of mucoadhesive polymers in nasal drug delivery systems has gained to promote dosage form residence time in the nasal cavity and improve the intimacy of contact with absorptive membranes of the biological system (Lisbeth 2003; Wang et al. 2008b).

Among the polymers widely used as nasal drug particulate carriers, the positively charged polymer, chitosan, is the most attractive because of its hydrogel nature, which leads to the opening of the tight junctions and its intimate contact with the negatively charged mucosa membrane. With regard to nasal administration, chitosans have been used for the preparation of gels, solid inserts, powders, and nanoparticles in which a 3D network can be recognized. *In vivo* evaluation in rabbits has proved that chitosan nanoparticles were able to improve the nasal absorption to a great extent compared with chitosan solution due to the intensified contact of the nanoparticle with the nasal mucosa (Calvo et al. 1999).

Chavan and Doijad (2010) employed a technique of spray drying for developing a microparticulate nasal drug delivery system for rizatriptan benzoate using chitosan as base. The loading of rizatriptan benzoate into chitosan microparticles led to an improvement of its dissolution rate. The rate of dissolution increased with an increase in the proportion of chitosan. With the increase in the proportion of chitosan in formulation, it has been observed that the mucoadhesive strength of microparticles was increased due to decreasing mucocilliary clearance, which increased the residence time of drug in nasal cavity, thus increasing absorption (Chavan and Doijad 2010). A new thermosensitive hydrogel was designed and prepared by simply mixing N-[(2-hydroxy-3-trimethylammonium)propyl] chitosan chloride and PEG with a small amount of α-β-glycerophosphate (Wu et al. 2007). It can be dropped or sprayed easily into the nasal cavity and spread on the nasal mucosa in solution state. After being administered into the nasal cavity, the solution transformed into viscous hydrogel at body temperature, which the decreased nasal mucociliary clearance rate and released drug slowly. Therefore, in this study, insulin as a model drug was entrapped in this formulation, and its release behavior *in vitro* was also investigated. The cytoxicity and the change of the blood glucose concentration after nasal administration of this hydrogel were also investigated. The hydrogel formulation decreased the blood glucose concentration apparently (40%–50% of the initial blood glucose concentration) for at least 4–5 hours after administration, and no apparent cytoxicity was found after application.

Dyer et al. (2002) prepared insulin-chitosan nanoparticles by the ionotropic gelation of chitosan glutamate and TPP pentasodium and by simple complexation of insulin and chitosan. The nasal absorption of insulin after administration in chitosan nanoparticle formulations and in chitosan solution and powder formulations was evaluated in anesthetised rats and/or in conscious sheep (Dyer et al. 2002). In another study, i.n. administration was investigated as a potential route to enhance systemic and brain delivery of didanosine (ddI) using chitosan nanoparticles. ddI-loaded chitosan nanoparticles were prepared through ionotropic gelation of chitosan with tripolyphosphonate anions. The nanoparticles were administered i.n. to rats, compared to i.n. and i.v. administration of ddI in solution. The concentrations of ddI in the blood, cerebrospinal fluid (CSF), and brain tissues were analyzed by ultra performance liquid chromatography. The brain/plasma, olfactory bulb/plasma, and CSF/plasma concentration ratios were significantly higher ($P < .05$) after i.n. administration of ddI nanoparticles or solution than those after i.v. administration of ddI aqueous solution (Al-Ghananeem et al. 2009). Pentazocine-loaded chitosan microspheres for intranasal systemic delivery significantly improved the bioavailability with sustained and controlled blood-level profiles compared to i.v. and oral administration (Kean et al. 2005). (Wang et al. 2009) showed that insulin-loaded thiolated chitosan nanoparticles substantially improved absorption of insulin across nasal mucosa compared to non-thiolated chitosan nanoparticles and soluble chitosan. Likely, thiolated chitosan nanoparticles have higher mucoadhesion properties and thus a longer residence time in nasal cavity. Moreover, thiolated chitosan nanoparticles showed a faster swelling and release compared to chitosan nanoparticles, which might facilitate the diffusion of the encapsulated drug. *In vivo* evaluations showed that after intranasal administration of the insulin-loaded thiolated nanoparticles to rats, the blood glucose levels of the animals rapidly decreased (Wang et al. 2009).

12.7.3.4 Colon-Targeted Drug Delivery

Colonic drug delivery has gained an increased importance not just for the delivery of the drugs for the treatment of local diseases associated with the colon such as Crohn's disease, ulcerative colitis, and irritable bowel syndrome but also for the potential it holds for the systemic delivery of proteins and therapeutic peptides. To achieve successful colon-targeted drug delivery, a drug needs to be protected from degradation, release, and/or absorption in the upper portion of the gastrointenstinal tract and then ensures abrupt or controlled release in the proximal colon. The use of biodegradable polymers holds great importance to achieve targeted drug release into the colon. Among them, chitosan is a well-accepted and a promising polymer for drug delivery in the colonic part, because it can biodegraded by the microflora present in the colon.

Pandey et al. (2013) prepared a PEC between chitosan (polycation) and pectin (polyanion) and developed enteric coated tablets for colon delivery using the PEC. Drug-loaded enteric coated tablets were prepared by wet granulation method using PEC to sustain the release at the colon, and coating was done with Eudragit S100 (Evonik Laboratory, Mumbai, India) to prevent the early release of the drug in the stomach and intestine. The optimized formulation containing 1.1% of PEC and 3% of coating showed highest swelling and release in alkaline pH mechanism of which was found to be microbial enzyme-dependent degradation established by *ex-vivo* study using rat caecal content (Pandey et al. 2013). Kawadkar and Ram (2007) prepared the chitosan-coated microsphere matrix system for the treatment of ulcerative colitis. In this study, the microspheres of chitosan HCl was directly compressed with the 5-aminosalicylic acid (5-ASA) into matrices. These matrices were compressed into tablets or capsules and coated. The release of 5-ASA from these compressed matrices by the polymer-degrading action of the cecal microflora was evaluated *in vitro* using rat cecal microflora in virtue of the similarity with human intestinal microflora, and it provided a better release of 5-ASA in the colon having ulcerative colitis (Kawadkar and Ram 2007). Lorenzo-Lamosa et al. (1998) proposed the design of microencapsulated chitosan microspheres for colonic drug delivery. They prepared the pH-sensitive multicore microparticulate system containing chitosan microcores entrapped into enteric acrylic microspheres. Sodium diclofenac was efficiently entrapped within these chitosan microcores and then microencapsulated into Eudragit L-100 and Eudragit S-100 to form a multireservoir system. *In vitro* release study revealed no release of the drug in gastric pH for 3 hours, and after the lag time, a continuous release for 8–12 hours was observed in the basic pH (Lorenzo-Lamosa et al. 1998). Chourasia et al. (2004) prepared a similar multiparticulate system by coating cross-linked chitosan microspheres with Eudragit L-100 and S-100 as pH-sensitive polymers for targeted delivery of the broad-spectrum antibacterial agent metronidazole. The results showed a pH-dependent release of the drug that was attributable to the presence of Eudragit coating. Moreover, the release of drug was found to be higher in the presence of rat cecal contents, indicating the susceptibility of the chitosan matrix to colonic enzymes.

In another study, a pH-dependent colon-targeted drug delivery system containing ornidazole-loaded chitosan beads was prepared for the management of amebiasis. The beads were prepared using different ornidazole and chitosan ratios by ionic gelation technique. Acrycoat S100 (Coral Pharma Chem, Ahmedabad) was used as a pH-dependent polymer for coating of chitosan beads exploiting oil-in-oil solvent evaporation method. The release profile of ornidazole was found to be pH dependent. In the acidic medium, the release rate was much slower; however, the drug was released quickly at pH 7 (Kumar et al. 2013). A colon-specific, pulsatile device for trimetazidine HCl using chitosan as a carrier was developed to achieve the time- or site-specific release of trimetazidine, based on chronopharmaceutical considerations. The basic design consists of an insoluble hard gelatine capsule body, filled with chitosan microsphere of trimetazidine and sealed with a hydrogel plug. The entire device was enteric coated, so that the variability in gastric emptying time can be overcome and a colon-specific release can be achieved. *In vitro* release studies of pulsatile device revealed that increasing the hydrophilic polymer content resulted in delayed release of trimetazidine from microspheres (Kumar et al. 2011). Orally administrable hydrogel was prepared by cross-linking chitosan with γ-poly(glutamic acid) for an excellent pH-responsive colon-targeted drug delivery system (Park et al. 2013). The surfaces of cross-linked hydrogel have a homogeneous pore array with a pore size corresponding to the varied blending ratio. The swelling ratio was dramatically changed by increasing the pH from 3 to 6, and the responsiveness of swelling ratio to the reversible pH changes between 3 and 10 was reliable for 72 hours. The drug diffusion rate was mainly dependent on the pH, and a water-soluble tetrazolium assay indicated that cytocompatibility of the hydrogel was in an acceptable range. Behin et al. (2013) evaluated Eudragit-coated chitosan microspheres of metronidazole for colon targeting. Chitosan microspheres were prepared by emulsion dehydration method using different ratios of drug and polymer. Eudragit-coated chitosan microspheres were performed by solvent evaporation method. The *in vitro* release of optimized formulation was found to be only 13.03% in 5 hours, but it showed a high and fast increase in drug release from the sixth hour in pH 6.8 phosphate buffer. It showed 90.52% drug release after 12 hours. The results clearly demonstrated that the Eudragit S100-coated metronidazole chitosan microspheres is a potential system for colon-specific drug delivery (Behin et al. 2013). Varshosaz et al. (2006a) prepared and evaluated chitosan microspheres coated with cellulose acetate butyrate. These microspheres were prepared by emulsion solvent evaporation technique for the delivery of 5-ASA into the colon (Varshosaz et al. 2006a).

Although chitosan is able to target drugs into the colon, the application has often been limited in colonic targeting of drugs because of its high solubility in gastric fluids, sometimes resulting in the burst release of the drug in the stomach (Park et al. 2010).

12.7.3.5 Buccal Drug Delivery

The buccal region of the oral cavity is an attractive target for administration of the drug of choice, particularly in overcoming problems such as high first-pass metabolism and drug degradation in the gastrointestinal environment Moreover, a rapid onset of action can be achieved relative to the oral route, and the formulation can be removed if therapy is required to be discontinued. Chitosan, being a mucoadhesive polymer, is used to improve drug delivery by enhancing the dosage form's contact time and residence time with the mucous membranes, and it can act as an absorption enhancer. The mucoadhesive property of Chitosan is either due to its ability to form secondary chemical bonds such as hydrogen bonds or ionic interactions between the positively charged amino groups of chitosan and the negatively charged mucin.

Sarath chandran et al. (2013) investigated the formulation of bisoprolol fumarate buccal patches for controlled release medication in order to treat blood pressure and cardiac diseases. The buccal patches were prepared by solvent casting method using chitosan. *In vitro* diffusion profile of bisoprolol fumerate from chitosan was showing good initial burst release along with an excellent controlled release profile for a duration of 12 hours. Based on the investigation results, the authors suggested that 2% is the optimum concentration to develop a good buccal patch containing bisoprolol fumerate. Design and development of such buccal patches may be highly beneficial, which can deliver drug up to a period of 12 hours. Hence, application of buccal patches may ensure the sufficient level of bisoprolol fumarate in the body to avoid the possible angina attack for hypertensive patients (Sarath chandran et al. 2013).

In another research, bioadhesive buccal tablets of repaglinide was prepared using HPMC K15M as a sustained release polymer, chitosan as a bioadhesive polymer, and ethyl cellulose as an impermeable backing layer. Tablets containing HPMC K15M and chitosan in the ratio of 1:1 and lactose as a filler had the maximum percentage of *in vitro* drug release. The swelling index, friability, and *in vitro* drug release were affected by the type of filler as dicalcium phosphate had good binding ability compared to lactose. The surface pH of all tablets was found to be satisfactory (between 6.26 and 7.01), close to neutral pH; hence, buccal cavity irritation should not occur with these tablets, and these tablets also showed adequate mucoadhesive strength. Thus, buccal adhesive tablet of repaglinide could be an alternative route to bypass hepatic first-pass metabolism and to improve the bioavailability of repaglinide (Patel et al. 2012).

A buccal drug delivery system using a novel catechol-functionalized chitosan (Cat-CS) hydrogel was also developed where catechol functional groups were covalently bonded to the backbone of chitosan and cross-linked the polymer with a nontoxic cross-linker genipin. The gelation time and the mechanical properties of Cat-CS hydrogels were similar to those of chitosan-only hydrogels. Catechol groups significantly enhanced mucoadhesion *in vitro*. The new hydrogel systems sustained the release of LC for about 3 hours. *In vivo* study to rabbit buccal mucosa indicated that no inflammation was observed on the buccal tissue (Xu et al. 2015).

Kshirasagar et al. (2012) prepared mucoadhesive buccal patches with chitosan dissolved in glacial acetic acid and glycerol as a plasticizer. Mucoadhessive patch containing 20 mg of fluxotine HCl was evaluated with respect to its *in vitro* drug permeation through goat buccal mucosa in 3 hours by using Franz diffusion cell (Kshirasagar et al. 2012).

In another study, an attempt was made to develop bilayered chitosan containing mucoadhesive buccal patches to ensure satisfactory unidirectional release of metoprolol tartarate. Mucoadhesive bilayered buccal patches of metoprolol tartarate were formulated using chitosan as the mucoadhesive polymer and the base matrix for the drug. The impermeable backing layer was of ethyl cellulose to ensure a unidirectional drug release. Patches containing lower drug concentration had higher bioadhesive strength with extended drug release. Stability studies were conducted in simulated saliva, and it was found that both drug and the patches were stable. The bilayered buccal patches of metoprolol tartarate can be formulated using chitosan as the mucoadhesive polymer to obtain satisfactory unidirectional drug release with adequate mucoadhesion (Furtado et al. 2010).

Recently, it has been shown that chitosan with thiol groups provide much higher adhesive properties. To date, three different thiolated chitosan derivatives have been synthesized: chitosan–thioglycolic acid conjugates, chitosan–cysteine conjugates, and chitosan–4-thio-butyl-amidine conjugates. The improved mucoadhesive properties of thiolated chitosans are explained by the formation of covalent bonds between thiol groups of the polymer and cysteine-rich subdomains of glycoproteins in the mucus layer. These covalent bonds are supposedly stronger than the noncovalent bonds such as ionic interactions of chitosan with anionic substructures of the mucus layer. This theory was supported by the results of tensile studies with tablets of thiolated chitosans, which demonstrated the correlation between the degree of modification with thiol bearing moieties and the adhesive properties of the polymer (Andreas and Hopf 2001; Hornof et al. 2003; Leitner et al. 2003).

12.7.3.6 Liver-Targeted Drug Delivery

Liver is a vital organ responsible for functions, including detoxification, protein synthesis, and the production of biochemicals necessary for the sustenance of life. Therefore, patients with chronic liver diseases such as viral hepatitis, liver cirrhosis, and hepatocellular carcinoma need attention to sustain life and as a result are often exposed to the prolonged treatment with drugs/herbal medications. Lack of site-specific delivery of these medications to the hepatocytes/nonparenchymal cells and adverse effects associated with their off-target interactions limits their continuous use. To overcome this, it is necessary for the development and fabrication of targeted delivery systems, which can deliver the drug at the desired site of action for a defined period of time.

A liver-targeted drug delivery carrier, composed of chitosan/PEG-glycyrrhetinic acid (CTS/PEG-GA) nanoparticles, was prepared by an ionic gelation process, in which GA acted as the targeting ligand. The cellular uptake was evaluated using human hepatic carcinoma cells (QGY-7703 cells). The anti-neoplastic effect of the doxorubicin HCl-loaded nanoparticles (DOX-loaded nanoparticles) was also investigated in $vitro$ and in $vivo$. The results showed that the CTS/PEG-GA nanoparticles were remarkably targeted to the liver and kept at a high level during the experiment. The DOX-loaded nanoparticles were greatly cytotoxic to QGY-7703 cells, and the IC_{50} (50% inhibitory concentration) for the free doxorubicin HCl and the DOX-loaded CTS/PEG-GA nanoparticles were 47 and 79 ng/mL, respectively. Moreover, the DOX-loaded CTS/PEG-GA nanoparticles could effectively inhibit tumor growth in H22 cell-bearing mice (Tian et al. 2010). In another study, (Yang et al. 2009) prepared polyion complex micelles (PIC micelles) based on methoxy PEG-$graft$-chitosan and lactose-conjugated PEG-$graft$-chitosan for liver-targeted delivery of diammonium glycyrrhizinate (DG). DG has been used in the treatment of chronic hepatitis and immunodeficiency virus infection. Pharmacokinetic experiments carried out using rats showed that the area under the curve values of DG for PIC micelles was higher than that for DG injection (Yang et al. 2009). Nanoparticles composed of galactosylated COS (Gal-CSO) and adenosine triphosphate (ATP) were prepared for hepatocellular carcinoma cell-specific uptake, and the characteristics of Gal-CSO/ATP nanoparticles were evaluated. The cytotoxicity of Gal-CSO/ATP nanoparticles was examined by the methyl tetrazolium assay, and the IC_{50} values were calculated with HepG2 cells. It was also found that the Gal-CSO/ATP nanoparticles could be uptaken by HepG2 cells, due to the expression of the ASGP receptor on their surfaces (Zhu et al. 2013).

It had also been reported that ASGP receptors were overexpressed on the surface of hepatoma cells, and targeting could be done through the introduction of galactose residues, which can specifically bind to the ASGP receptors on hepatoma cells, into drug carriers. Kim et al. (2006a) prepared 99mTc hydrazine nicotinamide-galactosylated chitosan and showed that 16% of the injected dose could accumulate in the liver within 120 minutes of injection. Wang et al. (2006) also prepared galactosylated liposomes and showed a relatively high liver-targeting efficiency (64.6%). The density and the activity of the ASGP receptors, however, are lower in patients suffering from liver disease, because of the presence in serum of inhibitors that reduce the binding capacity of primary hepatocellular carcinomas by 95%. Thus, ASGP receptor-mediated targeting to the liver may not be so effective under pathological conditions (Stockert and Morell 1983).

Liver cirrhosis complications are difficult to treat by active drug delivery, because of drug-metabolizing enzymes secreted by liver. The difficulties are solved by a specific liver targeting by galactosylated chitosan nanoparticles loaded with Silymarin. Targeted delivery of drug to hepatic cells can be successfully achieved by binding to ASGP receptor that is present in liver cells. Pharmacokinetic parameters showed evidence to confirm that galactosylated chitosan nanoparticles might be the best carrier for targeting liver cells (Venugopal et al. 2014).

Sahu et al. (2012) developed piperine-loaded chitosan microspheres to evaluate the enhanced hepatoprotective activity in paracetamol-induced hepatotoxic mice model. Piperine was extracted from *Piper longum* (*Pippali*). Solvent evaporation method was employed to fabricate the microspheres. In paracetamol-induced hepatotoxic mice model, serum glutamic oxaloacetic transaminase (SGOT) and serum glutamic pyruvic transaminase (SGPT) levels demonstrated no significant elevation in the blood by the microsphere formulation. The histopathology and enzyme-level results suggested that microsphere formulation can passively target hepatoprotective drug to the liver (Sahu et al. 2012). Kato et al. (2001) evaluated the potential of lactosaminated *N*-succinyl-chitosan (Lac-Suc), synthesized by reductive amination between *N*-succinyl-chitosan and lactose in the presence of sodium cyanoborohydride, as a liver-pecific drug carrier [44]. When Lac-Suc labeled with fluorescein isothiocyanate (FITC) was intravenously injected into mice, it initially undergoes fast hepatic clearance and showed maximum liver localization at 8 hours. The specific binding study of Lac-Suc to the ASGP receptors was examined, and the results revealed that the liver uptake of Lac-Suc was inhibited by asialofetuin, and it was suggested that the liver distribution of Lac-Suc should be concerned with the ASGP receptor (Kato et al. 2001).

12.7.3.7 Kidney- and Lung-Targeted Drug Delivery

For some drugs such as NSAIDS, kidney-targeted drug delivery is critical. To reduce the extra-renal toxicity of the drug and to improve its therapeutic efficiency for diseases occurring at the kidney, several strategies have been proposed for drug targeting to the kidney in the form of drug carrier conjugates. The mesangial cells of the glomerulus, the proximaltubular cells, and the interstitial fibroblasts are the principal targets for renal drug delivery because they play a pivotal role in many disease processes in the kidney.

Chitosan oligomers are water soluble and can be a potential drug carrier for renal targeting delivery. Zidovudine (AZT), an antiretroviral drug, has a very short half-life and is eliminated very quickly in human plasma and kidney after administration. To overcome this, AZT–chitosan oligomer conjugates were prepared and evaluated in terms of renal targeting. The *in vitro* release of AZT from AZT–chitosan oligomer conjugates was confirmed in mice plasma and renal homogenate. The pharmacokinetics study indicated longer mean retention time of AZT–chitosan oligomer conjugates. The AZT–chitosan oligomer conjugates were found accumulated in the kidney other than the heart, liver, spleen, lung, and brain after i.v. administration, in line with the evidence of the fluorescence imaging of FITC-labeled chitosan oligomer in 12 hours. Therefore, AZT–chitosan oligomer conjugates have the potential to be developed into a renal-targeted drug delivery system (Liang et al. 2012).

Renal fibrosis is a common progressive kidney disease, and there is a lack of efficient treatment for the condition. In this study, Qiao et al. (2014) designed a kidney-specific nanocomplex by forming a coordination-driven assembly from catechol-derived low-MW chitosan (HCA-Chi), metal ions (Cu), and active drug molecules. Autofluorescent DOX was selected to fabricate HCA-Chi–Cu–DOX ternary nanocomplex for investigating the cellular uptake behavior, transmembrane, and targeting properties. Uptake of HCA-Chi–Cu–DOX by HK-2 cells was dependent on the exposure time, concentration, and temperature, and was inhibited by blockers of megalin receptor. Tissue distribution showed that HCA-Chi–Cu–DOX nanocomplex was specifically accumulated in the kidney with a renal relative uptake rate of 25.6. It was concluded that HCA-Chi coordination-driven nanocomplex showed special renal targeting capacity and could be utilized to develop drug delivery systems for treating renal fibrosis (Qiao et al. 2014).

In order to evaluate the potential renal targeting profile of low-MW hydroxyethyl chitosan (LMWHC), prednisolone (Pre) was conjugated with LMWHC. To study the fate of LMWHC–Pre conjugate after i.v. administration, FITC was coupled to the conjugate to explore the renal targeting efficacy. The in *vivo* results showed that a significant amount of the conjugate was accumulated into the kidneys The preliminary pharmacodynamics study of LMWHC–Pre showed that the conjugate could effectively alleviate the nephrotic syndrome of rats induced by minimal change nephrosis model. Toxicity study also revealed that there was little glucocorticoid-induced osteoporosis by LMWHC–Pre upon 20 days of treatment. From this study, LMWHC–Pre may be employed as an effective potential drug candidate for the treatment of chronic renal disease (He et al. 2012).

Recently, the chitosan delivery system has been shown to target siRNA specifically to the kidneys in mice when administered intravenously. Two-dimensional and 3D bioimaging confirmed that chitosan-formulated siRNA is retained in the kidney for more than 48 hours where it accumulates in proximal tubule epithelial cells. Chitosan/siRNA nanoparticles, administered to chimeric mice with conditional knockout of the megalin gene, were distributed almost exclusively in cells that expressed megalin, implying that the chitosan/siRNA particle uptake was mediated by a megalin-dependent endocytotic pathway (Gao et al. 2014).

Delivering drugs to the lungs has many advantages because lungs have a large alveolar surface area, thin epithelial barrier, extensive vascularization, and relatively low enzymatic metabolic activity. i.v. injection of microspheres and inhalation are the possible routes for targeting drugs to the lungs. However, in some cases, it was found that microspheres with a particle diameter greater than 5 μm could block blood capillaries and induce chronic obstructive pulmonary emphysema. However, frequent inhalation may induce lung fibrosis. Therefore, designing a proper carrier system is essential for successful delivery of the drug to the lung. Wang et al. (2014) prepared docetaxel-loaded chitosan microspheres using a w/o emulsification method. *In vitro* release indicated that the drug-loaded microspheres had a well-sustained release efficacy, and *in vivo* studies showed that the microspheres were found to release the drug to a maximum extent in the target tissue (lung). The sustained release of DTX from microspheres revealed its applicability as a drug delivery system to minimize the exposure of healthy tissues while increasing the accumulation of therapeutic drug in target sites (Wang et al. 2014). Yang et al. (2009) prepared chitosan-modified PLGA nanoparticles containing paclitaxel with a mean diameter of 200–300 nm by a solvent evaporation method. The study demonstrated that the *in vitro* uptake of the nanoparticles by a lung cancer cell line (A549) was significantly increased by chitosan modification (Yang et al. 2009b).

12.7.3.8   Cancer-Targeted Drug Delivery

Anticancer drugs often suffer from poor solubility in water and thus need to use organic solvents for clinical applications, resulting in undesirable side effects such as venous irritation and respiratory distress (Torchilin 2004). Therefore, chitosan is used nowdays as a carrier system that encapsulates a large quantity of drugs and specifically targets tumor cells for successful cancer therapy. In recent years, chitosan–anticancer drug conjugates have been investigated. For example, DOX-conjugated glycol chitosan (GC) with a *cis*-aconityl spacer was synthesized by chemical attachment of *N-cis*-aconityl DOX to GC using carbodiimide chemistry. The hydrophobic nature of DOX within the conjugate allowed for its physical entrapment inside the nanoparticles. The release rate of DOX from the nanoparticles was significantly dependent on the pH. *In vivo* systemic administration of nanoparticles in mice indicated a significant accumulation into the tumor tissue (Son et al. 2003). *N*-Succinyl-chitosan was conjugated with mitomycin C (MMC) using carbodiimide chemistry. Due to the hydrophilic nature of *N*-succinyl-chitosan, the conjugate is water soluble when the MMC content in the conjugate is less than 12%. These conjugates exhibited good antitumor activities against various tumors such as murine leukemias (L1210 and P388), B16 melanoma, Sarcoma 180 solid tumor, and a murine liver metastatic tumor (M5076) (Kato et al. 2004).

TPP-cross-linked chitosan nanoparticles have been widely used to deliver various antitumor drugs. For example, Janes et al. (2001) effectively entrapped DOX into the TPP-cross-linked chitosan nanoparticles. DOX-loaded nanoparticles in human melanoma A375 cells and C26 murine colorectal carcinoma cells indicated that formulations containing dextran sulfate were able to maintain the cytostatic activity relative to free DOX.

Chitosan was also investigated as a carrier of hydrophilic drug such as, 5-FU by forming PEC nanoparticles with polyaspartic acid sodium salt. Both *in vitro* and *in vivo* study indicated sustained release of 5-FU from nanoparticles. From the *in vivo* animal test, it was found that the tumor inhibition rate of PEC nanoparticles is much higher than that of 5-FU alone (Zhang et al. 2008b).

Hydrophobically modified glycol chitosans (HGCs) were prepared by covalent conjugation of bile acid (deoxycholic acid) to the backbone of glycol chitosan using carbodiimide chemistry (Kwon et al. 2003). Animal experiments showed that HGCs prolonged blood circulation and exhibited high-tumor specificity for delivery of diverse anticancer drugs such as paclitaxel (Kim et al. 2006b), docetaxel (Hwang et al. 2008), camptothecin (Min et al. 2008), and cisplatin (Kim et al. 2008).

Recently, carboxymethyl chitosan has been modified with linoleic acid and used as a carrier for adriamycin. These self-assembled nanoparticles released adriamycin in a sustained manner, and the drug release rate was dependent on the linoleic acid degree of substitution on hydrophilic carboxymethyl chitosan. The *in vitro* antitumor activity of the drug-loaded nanoparticles against HeLa cells was also investicated (Tan et al. 2009). You et al. (2007) synthesized stearate-grafted COS (CSSA) by the reaction of carboxyl group of stearic acid with the amine group of chitosan. CSSA facilitated the effective internalization of the nanoparticles within the A549 cancer cells (You et al. 2007).

In another study, the effect of PEG conjugation on paclitaxel loaded *N*-octyl-sulfate chitosan nanoparticles was investigated by Qu et al. (2009). They found that PEG-conjugated particles were phagocytized less than unconjugated nanoparticles by the reticuloendothelial system (Qu et al. 2009).

Lin et al. (2008) prepared galactosylated chitosan-coated BSA nanoparticles containing 5-FU for the treatment of liver cancer. In this study, 5-FU was physically encapsulated into BSA nanoparticles, followed by surface coating with N-galactosylated chitosan by electrostatic interactions. Compared to the uncoated nanoparticles, coated nanoparticles showed a sustained release of 5-FU without the significant initial burst *in vitro* (Zhang et al. 2008a).

The decrease in extracellular pH values in the tumor tissue is primarily due to poor organization of the vasculature. This difference in pH between tumors and normal tissue has stimulated many investigators to design novel pH-sensitive carriers. For example, a camptothecin-loaded poly(*N*-isopropylacrylamide)/chitosan nanoparticle was prepared and its potential as a pH-sensitive carrier in tumor targeting was evaluated. The *in vitro* cytotoxicity of the drug-loaded nanoparticles was compared with free camptothecin against SW480 cells at pH values of 6.8 and 7.4. The drug-loaded nanoparticles significantly enhanced cytotoxicity at pH 6.8 but displayed minimal cytotoxicity at pH 7.4 (Fan et al. 2008). Zhang et al. (2006) prepared pH-responsive chitosan-based microgels by ionically cross-linking *N*-([2-hydroxy-3-trimethylammonium]propyl) chitosan chloride in the presence of TPP. These microgels were loaded with methotrexate and conjugated to apo-transferrin. The conjugated microgels exhibited a significant increase in cell mortality of HeLa cells, compared to nonconjugated microgels. This was due to pH-mediated release of methotrexate from the microgels by their swelling at the intracellular level.

Drug-loaded magnetic particles represent a promising alternative strategy in overcoming the blood–brain barrier. Hassan and Gallo (1993) developed magnetic chitosan microspheres containing oxantrazole, an anticancer drug, for the treatment of brain tumors. Zhu et al. (2009) developed chitosan-coated magnetic nanoparticles containing 5-FU through a reverse microemulsion method and showed that the drug release was occurred in a sustained manner into the SPCA-1 cancer cells. After accumulation of such type of magnetic carrier at the target tumor site *in vivo*, drugs were released from the magnetic carrier and effectively taken up by the tumor cells. The efficiency of the accumulation of carrier system depends on various parameters that include the intensity of the magnetic field, rate of blood flow, and surface characteristics of carriers.

Sahu et al. (2011) have prepared nanoparticles based on *O*-carboxymethyl chitosan modified with stearic acid and folic acid to achieve tumor cell-targeting properties. These nanoparticles showed an excellent cytotoxic property in comparison with the native drug (Sahu et al. 2011).

TABLE 12.2

Application Summery of Chitosan in Combination with Other Polymer(s)

Combination of Chitosan and Other Polymer(s)	Formulation	Drug/ Biomolecules	Reference
Chitosan + poly(*N*-isopropylacrylamide)	Hydrogel	Timolol	Cao et al. (2007)
Chitosan + disodium α-D-glucose 1-phosphate	Hydrogel	Levocetirizine dihydrochloride	De Campos et al. (2004)
Chitosan + (*N*-isopropylacrylamide)	Nanoparticle	Camptothecin	Fan et al. (2008)
N-Octyl-sulfate chitosan + PEG	Nanoparticles	Paclitaxel	Qu et al. (2009)
Chitosan + PEG + glycyrrhetinic acid	Nanoparticles	Doxorubicin HCl	Tian et al. (2010)
Chitosan + HPMC K15M + ethyl cellulose	Tablets	Repaglinide	Patel et al. (2012)
Chitosan + Eudragit S100	Microspheres	Metronidazole	Behin et al. (2013)
Chitosan + cellulose acetate butyrate	Microspheres	5-ASA	Varshosaz et al. (2006b)
Chitosan + Acrycoat S100	Beads	Ornidazole	Kumar et al. (2013)
Chitosan + Eudragit	Microspheres	Metronidazole	
Chitosan + Eudragit	Microparticles	Sodium diclofenac	Lorenzo-Lamosa et al. (1998)
N-[(2-Hydroxy-3-trimethylammonium) propyl] chitosan chloride + PEG	Thermosensitive hydrogel	Insulin	Wu et al. (2007)
Chitosan + HPMC	Transdermal patch	Metformin	Allena et al. (2012)
Chitosan + HPMC	Transdermal patch	Ibuprofen	Madhulatha and Ravikiran (2013)
Chitosan + polyvinyl alcohol	Transdermal patch	Alprazolam	Maji et al. (2013)
Chitosan + polylactate-*co*-glycolate	Microparticles	Hepatitis B surface antigen	Zhao et al. (2006)
Chitosan + alginate	Nanoparticles	Bovine serum albumin	Haidar et al. (2008)
Chitosan + PEG	Nanoparticles	Insulin	Zhang et al. (2008c)
Chitosan hydrochloride + Eudragit RS	Microspheres	Pipemidic acid	Bogataj et al. (2000)

In recent years, large numbers of single-walled carbon nanotube-based drug delivery systems have been designed and prepared. It has been shown that the single-walled carbon nanotubes combined with polysaccharides could greatly improve the therapeutic efficiency of the drug while reducing their toxicity. Ji et al. (2012) reported a drug delivery system based on folic acid-conjugated chitosan modified with single-walled carbon nanotubes for controllable release of DOX. It was observed that these formulations could effectively kill the HCC SMMC-7721 cell lines and depress the growth of liver cancer in mice (Ji et al. 2012).

Arya et al. (2011) prepared a targeted system based on herceptin-conjugated gemcitabine-loaded chitosan nanoparticles for pancreatic cancer therapy. A specific molecular targeting by anti-HER2 and higher uptake of these nanoparticless by malignant Mia Paca 2 and PANC 1 cells resulted in an enhanced cytotoxicity effect of the encapsulated drug, leading to more apoptosis in the pancreatic cancer cell lines (Arya et al. 2011).

The applications of chitosan in combination with other poymer(s) are summarized in Table 12.2.

12.8 CONCLUSION

Chitin and chitosan possess unique structures, multidimensional properties, highly sophisticated functions, and a wide range of applications, especially in the biomedical and pharmaceutical fields. Moreover, the chemical modification of chitosan enhances biological activities and raises the number of potential biomedical applications. *In vivo* residence time of the dosage form in the gastrointestinal tract and the bioavailability of various drugs can be increased by mucoadhesive and absorption enhancement properties of chitosan. Targeted ophthalmic, nasal, sublingual, buccal, gastrointestinal, colon-specific, and transdermal drug delivery is achieved by chitosan and its derivatives. Recently, chitosan has been also extensively explored in gene delivery. However, studies toward optimization of process parameters and scaleup from the laboratory to the production level are yet to be undertaken. Most of studies carried out are only in *in vitro* conditions. Therefore, more *in vivo* studies need to be carried out. In order to achieve an efficient drug delivery, special preparation techniques need to be developed by taking care of certain parameters such as crosslinker concentration, chitosan MW, and processing conditions.

REFERENCES

Aiedeh, K. and M.O. Taha. 2001. Synthesis of iron-cross-linked chitosan succinate and iron-cross-linked hy droxamated chitosan succinate and their in-vitro evaluation as potential matrix materials for oral theophylline sustained-release beads. *Eur. J. Pharm. Sci.* 13:159–168.

Albert, S. and J. Baldwin. 2001. Series introduction: The transcription factor NF-kB and human disease. *J. Clin. Investig.* 107:3–6.

Al-Ghananeem, A.A., H. Saeed, R.L. Florence, R.A. Yokel, and H. Malkawi. 2009. Intranasal drug delivery of didanosine-loaded chitosan nanoparticles for brain targeting; an attractive route against infections caused by AIDS viruses. *J. Drug Target.* 18:381–388.

Allena, R.T., H.K.S. Yadav, S. Sandina, and S.C.M. Prasad. 2012. Preparation and evaluation of transdermal patches of metformin hydrochloride using natural polymer for sustained release. *Int. J. Pharm. Pharm. Sci.* 4:297–302.

Alonso, M.J. and A. Sánchez. 2003. The potential of chitosan in ocular drug delivery. *J. Pharm. Pharmacol.* 55:1451–63.

al-Suwayeh, S.A., A.R. el-Helw, A.F. al-Mesned, M.A. Bayomi, and A.S. el-Gorashi. 2003. In vitro–in vivo evaluation of tableted caseinchitosan microspheres containing diltiazem hydrochloride. *Boll. Chim. Farm.* 142:14–20.

Amidi, M., E. Mastrobattista, W. Jiskoot, and W.E. Hennink. 2010. Chitosan-based delivery systems for protein therapeutics and antigens. *Adv. Drug. Deliv. Rev.* 62:59–82.

Amidi, M., H.C. Pellikaan, H. Hirschberg, A.H. de Boer, D.J. Crommelin, W.E. Hennink, G. Kersten, and W. Jiskoot. 2007. Diphtheria toxoid-containing microparticulate powder formulations for pulmonary vaccination: Preparation, characterization and evaluation in guinea pigs. *Vaccine* 25:6818–6829.

Amidi, M., S.G. Romeijn, G. Borchard, H.E. Junginger, W.E. Hennink, and W. Jiskoot. 2006. Preparation and characterization of protein-loaded N-trimethyl chitosan nanoparticles as nasal delivery system. *J. Control. Rel.* 111: 107–116.

Andreas, B.S. and T.E. Hopf. 2001. Synthesis and in vitro evaluation of chitosan-thioglycolic acid conjugates. *Sci. Pharm.* 69:109–118.

Anraku, M., M. Kabashima, H. Namura, T. Maruyama, M. Otagiri, J.M. Gebicki, N. Furutani, and H. Tomida. 2008. Antioxidant protection of human serum albumin by chitosan. *Int. J. Biol. Macromol.* 43:159–164.

Arya, G., M. Vandana, S. Acharya, and S.K. Sahoo. 2011. Enhanced antiproliferative activity of Herceptin (HER2)-conjugated gemcitabine-loaded chitosan nanoparticle in pancreatic cancer therapy. *Nanomedicine* 7:859–870.

Babu, N., D. Amirtham, and R. Ramachandran. 2012. Comparative analysis of anti microbial and chromium removal properties of chemically and biologically produced chitosan from shrimp shell waste. *Int. J. Res. Environ. Sci. Tech.* 2:119–123.

Banerjee, T., S. Mitra, A.K. Singh, R.K. Sharma, and A. Maitra. 2002. Preparation, characterization and biodistribution of ultrafine chitosan nanoparticles. *Int. J. Pharm.* 243:93–105.

Behin, S.R., I.S. Punitha, P. Prabhakaran, and J. Kundaria. 2013. Design and evaluation of coated microspheres of antiprotozoal drug for colon specific delivery. *Am. J. PharmTech. Res.* 3:555–569.

Bernkop-Schnürch, A. and S. Dünnhaupt. 2012. Chitosan-based drug delivery systems. *Euro. J. Pharm. Biopharm.* 81:463–469.

Bernkop-Schnurch, A., M. Hornof, and T. Zoidl. 2003. Thiolated polymers-thiomers: Synthesis and in vitro evaluation of chitosan-2-iminothiolane conjugates. *Int. J. Pharm.* 260:229–237.

Bhattarai, N., H.R. Ramay, J. Gunn, F.A. Matsen, and M.Q. Zhang. 2005. PEG-grafted chitosan as an injectable thermosensitive hydrogel for sustained protein release. *J. Control. Rel.* 103:609–624.

Bhumkar, D.R., H.M. Joshi, M. Sastry, and V.B. Pokharkar. 2007. Chitosan reduced gold nanoparticles as novel carriers for transmucosal delivery of insulin. *Pharm. Res.* 24:1415–1426.

Blanco, M.D., C. Gomez, R. Olmo, E. Muniz, and J.M. Teijon, J.M. 2000. Chitosan microspheres in PLG films as devices for cytarabine release. *Int. J. Pharm.* 202:29–39.

Bogataj, M., A. Mrhar, I. Grabnar, Z. Rajtman, P. Bukovec, S. Srcic, and U. Urleb. 2000. The influence of magnesium stearate on the characteristics of mucoadhesive microspheres. *J. Microencapsul.* 17:499–508.

Bourbouze, R., F. Raffi, G. Dameron, H. Hali-Miraftab, F. Loko, and J.L. Vilde. 1991. N-acetylbeta-D-glucosaminidase (NAG) isoenzymes release from human monocyt-ederived macrophages in response to zymosan and human recombinant interferon-gamma. *Clin. Chim. Acta* 199:185–194.

Calvo, P., C. Remunan-Lopez, and M.J. Alonso. 1999. Enhancement of nasal absorption of insulin using chitosan nanoparticles. *Pharm. Res.* 16:1576–81.

Cao, Y., C. Zhang, W. Shen, Z. Cheng, L. Yu, and Q. Ping. 2007. Poly (N-isopropyl acryl-amide) chitosan as thermosensitive in situ gel forming system for ocular drug delivery. *J. Control. Rel.* 120:186–194.

Can, A.S., M.S. Erdal, S. Güngör, and Y. Özsoy. 2013. Optimization and character-ization of chitosan films for transdermal delivery of ondansetron. *Molecules* 18:5455–5471.

Chandy, T., G.S. Das, and G.H. Rao. 2000. 5-Fluorouracil-loaded chitosan coated poly-lactic acid microspheres as biodegradable drug carriers for cerebral tumours. *J. Microencapsul.* 17:625–638.

Chandy, T., G.H. Rao, R.F. Wilson, and G.S. Das. 2001. Development of poly(lactic acid)/chitosan co-matrix microspheres: Controlled release of taxol–heparin for preventing restenosis. *Drug Deliv.* 8:77–86.

Chandy, T. and C.P. Sharma. 1993. Chitosan matrix for oral sustained delivery of ampicillin. *Biomaterials* 14:939–944.

Chandy, T., R.F. Wilson, G.H. Rao, and G.S. Das. 2002. Changes in cisplatin delivery due to surface-coated poly(lactic acid)-poly(epsilon-caprolactone) microspheres. *J. Biomater. Appl.* 16:275–291.

Chavan, J.D. and R.C. Doijad. 2010. Formulation and evaluation of chitosan based microparticulate nasal drug delivery system of rizatriptan benzoate. *Int. J. Pharm. Tech. Res.* 2:2391–2402.

Chen, A., T. Taguchi, K. Sakai, K. Kikuchi, M. Wang, and I. Miwa. 2003. Antioxidant activi-ties of chitobiose and chitotriose. *Biol. Pharm. Bull.* 26:1326–1330.

Chen, C.S., J.C. Su, and G.J. Tsai. 1998. Antimicrobial effect and physical properties of sul-fonated chitosan. In *Advances in Chitin Science*, Vol. III. R.H. Chen, H.C. Chen (eds.). Taiwan: Rita Advertising Co, pp. 278–282.

Chen, X., X. Li, Y. Zhou, X. Wang, Y. Zhang, Y. Fan, Y. Huang, and Y. Liu. 2012. Chitosan-based thermosensitive hydrogel as a promising ocular drug delivery system: Preparation, characterization, and in vivo evaluation. *J. Biomater. Appl.* 27:391–402.

Chiellini, F., A.M. Piras, C. Errico, and E. Chiellini. 2008. Micro/nanostructured polymeric systems for biomedical and pharmaceutical applications. *Nanomedicine* 3:367–393.

Chung, Y.C., Y.P. Su, C.C. Chen, G. Jia, H.L. Wang, J.C. Wu, and J.G. Lin. 2004. Relationship between antibacterial activity of chitosan and surface characteristics of cell wall. *Acta Pharmacol. Sinica* 25:932–936.

Cui, Z. and R.J. Mumper. 2001. Chitosan-based nanoparticles for topical genetic immuniza-tion. *J. Control. Rel.* 75:409–419.

Dambies, L., T. Vincent, A. Domard, and E. Guibal. 2001. Preparation of chitosan gel beads by ionotropic molybdate gelation. *Biomacromolecules* 2:1198–1205.

de Campos, A.M., Y. Diebold, E.L.S. Carvalho, A. Sánchez, and M.J. Alonso. 2004. Chitosan nanoparticles as new ocular drug delivery systems: In vitro stability, in vivo fate, and cellular toxicity. *Pharma. Res.* 21:803–810.

Diebold, Y., M. Jarrín, V. Sáez Carvalho, E.L. Orea, M. Calonge, B. Seijo, and M.J. Alonso. 2007. Ocular drug delivery by liposome–chitosan nanoparticle complexes (LCS-NP). *Biomaterials* 28:1553–1564.

Domard, A. and N. Cartier. 1992. Glucosamine oligomers: Solid-state crystallization and sustained dissolution. *Int. J. Biol. Macromol.* 14:100–106.

Drogoz, A., S. Munier, B. Verrier, L. David, A. Dornard, and T. Delair. 2008. Towards bio-compatible vaccine delivery systems: Interactions of colloidal PECs based on polysac-charides with HIV-1 p24 antigen. *Biomacromolecules* 9:583–591.

Dutta, P.K., J. Dutta, and V.S. Tripathi. 2004. Chitin and chitosan: Chemistry, properties and applications. *J. Sci. Indus. Res.* 63:20–31.

Dyer, A.M., M. Hinchcliffe, P. Watts, J. Castile, I. Jabbal-Gill, R. Nankervis, A. Smith, and L. Illum. 2002. Nasal delivery of insulin using novel chitosan based formulations: A comparative study in two animal models between simple chitosan formulations and chitosan nanoparticles. *Pharm. Res.* 19:998–1008.

El-Shabouri, M.H. 2002. Positively charged nanoparticles for improving the oral bioavail-ability of cyclosporin-A. *Int. J. Pharm.* 249:101–108.

Fan, L., H. Wu, H. Zhang, F. Li, T. Yang, C. Gu, and Q. Yang. 2008. Novel super pH-sensitive nanoparticles responsive to tumor extracellular pH. *Carbohyd. Polym.* 73:390–400.

Farivar, M., H.S. Kas, L. Oner, and A.A. Hincal. 1993. Isosorbide-5-mononitrate micro-spheres: Formulation and evaluation of in vitro release profiles by application of facto-rial design. *HU Ecz. Der.* 13:25–37.

Fernandez-Urrusuno, R., P. Cavlo, C. Remunan-Lopez, J.L. Vila-Jato, and M.J. Alonso. 1999. Enhancement of nasal absorption of insulin using chitosan nanoparticles. *Pharm. Res.* 16:1576–1581.

Furtado, S., S. Bharath, B.V. Basavaraj, S. Abraham, R. Deveswaran, and V. Madhavan. 2010. Development of chitosan based bioadhesive bilayered patches of metoprolol tartarate. *Int. J. Pharm. Sci. Rev. Res.* 4:198–202.

Gaikwad, U.V. and A.S. Pande. 2013. A review of biopolymer chitosan blends in polymer system. *Int. Res. J. Sci. Eng.* 1:13–16.

Gao, S., S. Hein, F. Dagnæs-Hansen, K. Weyer, C. Yang, R. Nielsen, E.I. Christensen, R.A. Fentonl, and J. Kjems. 2014. Megalin-Mediated specific uptake of chitosan/siRNA nanoparticles in mouse kidney proximal tubule epithelial cells enables AQP1 gene silencing. *Theranostics* 4:1039–1051.

Ghendon, Y., S. Markushin, Y. Vasiliev, I. Akopova, I. Koptiaeva, and G. Krivtsov. 2009. Evaluation of properties of chitosan as an adjuvant for inactivated influenza vaccines administered parenterally. *J. Med. Virol.* 81:494–506.

Giunchedi, P., C. Juliano, E. Gavini, M. Cossu, and M. Sorrenti. 2002. Formulation and in vivo evaluation of chlorhexidine buccal tablets prepared using drug-loaded chitosan microspheres. *Eur. J. Pharm. Biopharm.* 53:233–239.

Gorzelanny, C., B. Poppelmann, E. Strozyk, B. Moerschbacher, and S. Schneider. 2007. Specific interaction between chitosan and matrix metalloprotease 2 decreases the inva-sive activity of human melanoma cells. *Biomacromolecules* 8:3035–3040.

Goskonda, S.R. and S.M. Upadrashta. 1993. Avicel RC-591/chitosan beads by extrusion sphe-ronization technology. *Drug Dev. Ind. Pharm.* 19:915–927.

Grabovac, V., D. Guggi, and A. Bernkop-Schnürch. 2005. Comparison of the mucoadhesive properties of various polymers. *Adv. Drug Deliv. Rev.* 57:1713–1723.

Grenha, A., B. Seijo, and C. Remunan-Lopez. 2005. Microencapsulated chitosan nanopar-ticles for lung protein delivery. *Eur. J. Pharm. Sci.* 25:427–437.

Haidar, Z.S., R.C. Hamdy, and M. Tabrizian. 2008. Protein release kinetics for core–shell hybrid nanoparticles based on the layer-by-layer assembly of alginate and chitosan on liposomes. *Biomaterials* 29:1207–1215.

Hari, P.R., T. Chandy, and C.P. Sharma. 1996. Chitosan/calcium alginate microcapsules for intestinal delivery of nitrofurantoin. *J. Microencapsul.* 13:319–329.

Hassan, E.E. and J.M. Gallo. 1993. Targeting anticancer drugs to the brain. I: Enhanced brain delivery of oxantrazole following administration in magnetic cationic microspheres. *J. Drug Target.* 1:7–14.

He, X.K., Z.X. Yuan, X.I. Wu, C.Q. Xu, and W.Y. Li. 2012. Low molecular weight hydroxy-ethyl chitosan-prednisolone conjugate for renal targeting therapy: Synthesis, character-ization and in vivo studies. *Theranostics* 2:1054–1063.

Hejazi, R. and M. Amiji. 2003. Stomach-specific anti-H. pylori therapy. II. Gastric residence studies of tetracycline-loaded chitosan microspheres in gerbils. *Pharm. Dev. Technol.* 8:253–262.

Hemant, K.S.Y. and H.G. Shivakumar. 2010. Development of chitosan acetate films for trans-dermal delivery of propranolol hydrochloride. *Trop. J. Pharm. Res.* 9:197–203.

Hennink, W.E. and C.F. van Nostrum. 2002. Novel crosslinking methods to design hydrogels. *Adv. Drug Deliv. Rev.* 54:13–36.

Hoffman, A.S. 2002. Hydrogels for biomedical applications. *Adv. Drug Deliv. Rev.* 54:3–12.

Hornof, M.D., C.E. Kast, and B.S. Andreas. 2003. In vitro evaluation of the viscoelastic behav-ior of chitosan—thioglycolic acid conjugates. *Eur. J. Pharm. Biopharm.* 55:185–190.

Hwang, H.Y., I.S. Kim, I.C. Kwon, and Y.H. Kim. 2008. Tumor targetability and antitumor effect of docetaxel-loaded hydrophobically modified glycol chitosan nanoparticles. *J. Control. Rel.* 128:23–31.

Illum, L., I. Jabbal-Gill, M. Hinchcliffe, A. Fisher, and S. Davis. 2001. Chitosan as a novel nasal delivery system for vaccines. *Adv. Drug Deliv. Rev.* 51:81–96.

Jaffer, S. and J.S. Sampalis. 2007. Efficacy and safety of chitosan HEP-40™ in the man-agement of hypercholesterolemia: A randomized, multicenter, placebocontrolled trial. *Altern. Med. Rev.* 12:265–273.

Jameela, S.R., T.V. Kumary, A.V. Lal, and A. Jayakrishnan. 1998. Progesterone-loaded chito-san microspheres: A long acting biodegradable controlled delivery system. *J. Control. Rel.* 52:17–24.

Jana, S., A. Gandhi, K.K. Sen, and S.K. Basu. 2013. Biomedical applications of chitin and chitosan derivatives. In *Chitin and Chitosan Derivatives: Advances in Drug Discovery and Developments*, 1st editon, Chapter 18, Se-Kwon Kim (ed.). Boca Raton, FL: Taylor & Francis Group, LLC, pp. 337–360.

Janes, K.A., M.P. Fresneau, A. Marazuela, A. Fabra, and M.J. Alonso. 2001. Chitosan nanoparticles as delivery systems for doxorubicin. *J. Control. Rel.* 73:255–267.

Jayakumar, R., M. Prabaharan, S.V. Nair, S. Tokura, H. Tamura, and N. Selvamurugan. 2010. Novel carboxymethyl derivatives of chitin and chitosan materials and their biomedical applications. *Prog. Mater. Sci.* 55:675–709.

Jayakumar, R., R.L. Reis, and J.F. Mano. 2006. Phosphorous containing chitosan beads for controlled oral drug delivery. *J. Bioact. Compat. Polym.* 21:327–340.

Je, J. and S. Kim. 2006. Chitosan derivatives killed bacteria by disrupting the outer and inner membrane. *J. Agric. Food Chem.* 54:6629–6633.

Ji, Z., G. Lin, and Q. Lu. 2012. Targeted therapy of SMMC-7721 liver cancer in vitro and in vivo with carbon nanotubes based drug delivery system. *J. Colloid. Int. Sci.* 365:143–149.

Kang, M.L., H.L. Jiang, S.G. Kang, D.D. Guo, D.Y. Lee, C.S. Cho, and H.S. Yoo. 2007. Pluronic® F127 enhances the effect as an adjuvant of chitosan microspheres in the intranasal delivery of Bordetella bronchiseptica antigens containing dermonecrotoxin. *Vaccine* 25:4602–4610.

Karagozlu, M., J. Kim, F. Karadeniz, C. Kong, and S. Kim. 2010. Antiproliferative effect of aminoderivatized chitooligosaccharides on AGS human gastric cancer cells. *Process Biochem.* 45:1523–1528.

Kato, Y., H. Onishi, and Y. Machida. 2001. Biological characteristics of lactosaminated N-succinyl-chitosan as a liver-specific drug carrier in mice. *J. Control. Rel.* 70:295–307.

Kato, Y., H. Onishi, and Y. Machida. 2004. N-succinyl-chitosan as a drug carrier: Water insoluble and water-soluble conjugates. *Biomaterials* 25:907–915.

Kawadkar, J. and A. Ram. 2007. Colon targeted chitosan microsphere compressed matrices for the treatment of ulcerative colitis. *Pharma. Rev.* 5(4).

Kean, T., S. Roth, and T. Thanou. 2005. Trimethylated chitosans as non-viral gene delivery vectors: Cytotoxicity and transfection efficiency. *J. Control. Rel.* 103: 643–653.

Khan, F., R.S. Tare, R.O.C. Oreffo, and M. Bradley. 2009. Versatile biocompatible polymer hydrogels: Scaffolds for cell growth. *Angew. Chem. Int. Ed.* 48:978–982.

Kim, E.M., H.J. Jeong, S.L. Kim, M.H. Sohn, and J.W. Nah. 2006a. Asialoglycoprotein-receptor-targeted hepatocyte imaging using 99mTc galactosylated chitosan. *Nuc. Med. Biol.* 33:529–534.

Kim, J.H., S.I. Kim, I.B. Kwon, M.H. Kim, and J.I. Lim. 2013. Simple fabrication of silver hybridized porous chitosan-based patch for transdermal drug-delivery system. *Mate. Lett.* 95:48–51.

Kim, J.H., Y.S. Kim, S. Kim, K. Choi, H. Chung, S.Y. Jeong, R.W. Park, I.S. Kim, I.C. Kwon. 2006b. Hydrophobically modified glycol chitosan nanoparticles as carriers for pacli-taxel. *J. Control. Rel.* 111:228–234.

Kim, J.H., Y.S. Kim, K. Park et al. 2008. Antitumor efficacy of cisplatin-loaded glycol chito-san nanoparticles in tumor-bearing mice. *J. Control. Rel.* 127:41–49.

Kim, M., H. You, M. You, N. Kim, B. Shim, and H. Kim. 2004a. Inhibitory effect of water soluble chitosan on TNF α and IL 8 secretion from HMC 1. *Cells* 26:401–409.

Kim, T.H., I.K. Park, J.W. Nah, Y.J. Choi, and C.S. Cho. 2004b. Galactosylated chitosan/DNA nanoparticles prepared using water-soluble chitosan as a gene carrier. *Biomaterials* 25:3783–3792.

Kimura, Y. and H. Okuda. 1999. Prevention by chitosan of myelotoxicity, gastrointestinal toxicity and immunocompetent organic toxicity induced by 5-fluorouracil without loss of antitumor activity in mice. *Cancer Sci.* 90:765–774.

Ko, J.A., H.J. Park, S.J. Hwang, J.B. Park, and J.S. Lee. 2002. Preparation and characteriza-tion of chitosan microparticles intended for controlled drug delivery. *Int. J. Pharm.* 249:165–174.

Kumar, A.S.N., C. Pavanveena, and K. Kavitha. 2011. Colonic drug delivery system of trimetazidine hydrochloride for angina pectoris. *Int. J. Pharm. Pharm. Sci.* 3:22–26.

Kumar, D.V., A. Mishra, and T.S. Easwari. 2013. Formulation and development of acrycoat-coated chitosan beads of ornidazole for colon targeting. *Eur. J. App. Sci.* 5:47–52.

Kumbar, S.G., A.R. Kulkarni, and M. Aminabhavi. 2002. Crosslinked chitosan microspheres for encapsulation of diclofenac sodium: Effect of crosslinking agent. *J. Microencapsul.* 19:173–180.

Kshirasagar, N., N. Thamada, V.N.B.K. Naik, and M.S. Gopal. 2012. Design and evaluation of chitosan containing mucoadhesive buccal patch of Fluxotine Hcl. *Int. J. Sci. Res. Pub.* 2:1–5.

Kwon, S., J.H. Park, H. Chung, I.C. Kwon, and S.Y. Jeong. 2003. Physicochemical charac-teristics of self-assembled nanoparticles based on glycol chitosan bearing 5-β-cholanic acid. *Langmuir* 19:10188–10193.

Lee, J.I., H.S. Kim, and H.S. Yoo. 2009. DNA nanogels composed of chitosan and Pluronic with thermo-sensitive and photo-crosslinking properties. *Int. J. Pharm.* 373:93–99.

Lee, K.Y., I.C. Kwon, Y.H. Kim, W.H. Jo, and S.Y. Jeong. 1998. Preparation of chitosan self-aggregates as a gene delivery system. *J. Control. Rel.* 51:213–220.

Lee, S.J., S.S. Kim, and Y.M. Lee. 2000. Interpenetrating polymer network hydrogels based on poly(ethylene glycol) macromer and chitosan. *Carbohydr. Polym.* 41:197–205.

Leitner, V.M., G.F. Walker, and B.S. Andreas. 2003. Thiolated polymers: Evidence for the formation of disulphide bonds with mucus glycoproteins. *Eur. J. Pharm. Biopharm.* 56:207–214.

Liang, Z., T. Gong, X. Sun, J.Z. Tang, and Z. Zhang. 2012. Chitosan oligomers as drug carri-ers for renal delivery of zidovudine. *Carbohydr. Polym.* 87:2284–2290.

Lin. A., Y. Liu, Y. Huang, J. Sun, Z. Wu. et al. 2008. Glycyrrhizin surface-Modified chitosan nanoparticles for hepatocyte-targeted delivery. *Int. J. Pharm.* 359: 247–53.

Lim, L.Y. and L.S. Wan. 1998. Effect of magnesium stearate on chitosan microspheres prepared by an emulsification–coacervation technique. *J. Microencapsul.* 15:319–333.

Lisbeth, I. 2003. Nasal drug delivery—possibilities problems and solutions. *J. Control. Rel.* 87:187–98.

Liu, Z., Y. Jiao, Y. Wang, C. Zhou, and Z. Zhang. 2008. Polysaccharides-based nanoparticles as drug delivery systems. *Adv. Drug Deliv. Rev.* 60:1650–1662.

Lorenzo-Lamosa, M.L., C. Remunan-Lopez, J.L. Vila-Jato, and M.J. Alonso. 1998. Design of microencapsulated chitosan microspheres for colonic drug delivery. *J. Control. Rel.* 52: 109–118.

Luppi, B., F. Bigucci, T. Cerchiara, and V. Zecchi. 2010. Chitosan-based hydrogels for nasal drug delivery: From inserts to nanoparticles. *Expert. Opin. Drug Deliv.* 7:811–828.

Madhulatha, A. and N. Ravikiran. 2013. Formulation and evaluation of ibuporfen transdermal patches. *Int. J. Res. Pharm. Bio. Sci.* 4:351–362.

Maeda, Y. and Y. Kimura. 2004. Antitumor effects of various low-molecular-weight chitosans are due to increased natural killer activity of intestinal intraepithelial lymphocytes in sarcoma 180-bearing mice. *J. Nutr.* 134:945–950.

Majeti, N.V. and R. Kumar. 2000. A review of chitin and chitosan applications. *React. Func. Polym.* 46:1–27.

Maji, P., A. Gandhi, S. Jana, and N. Maji. 2013. Preparation and characterization of maleic anhydride cross-linked chitosan-polyvinyl alcohol hydrogel matrix transdermal patch. *J. Pharma. Sci. Tech.* 2:62–67.

Mao, H.Q., K. Roy, V.L. Troung-Le, K.A. Janes, K.Y. Lin, Y. Wang, J.T. August, and K.W. Leong. 2001. Chitosan DNA nanoparticles as gene delivery carriers: Synthesis, characterization and transfection efficiency. *J. Control. Rel.* 70:399–421.

Mao, S., U. Bakowsky, A. Jintapattanakit, and T. Kissel. 2006. Self-assembled polyelectrolyte nanocomplexes between chitosan derivatives and insulin. *J. Pharm. Sci.* 95:1035–1048.

Metters, A. and J. Hubbell. 2005. Network formation and degradation behavior of hydrogels formed by Michael-type addition reactions. *Biomacromolecules* 6:290–301.

Min, K.H., K. Park, Y.S. Kim, S.M. Bae, S. Lee, H.G. Jo, R.W. Park, and I.S. Kim. 2008. Hydrophobically modified glycol chitosan nanoparticles encapsulated camptothecin enhance the drug stability and tumor targeting in cancer therapy. *J. Control. Rel.* 127: 208–218.

Moon, J., H. Kim, H. Koo, Y.S. Joo, H.M. Nam, Y.H. Park, and M.I. Kang. 2007. The antibacterial and immunostimulative effect of chitosan-oligosaccharides against infection by Staphylococcus aureus isolated from bovine mastitis. *Appl. Microbiol. Biotechnol.* 75:989–998.

Muzzarelli, R.A.A. and R. Rochetti. 1985. Determination of the degree of deacetylation of chitosan by first derivative ultraviolet spectrophotometry. *J. Carbohydr. Polym.* 5:461–472.

Myung, D., D. Waters, M. Wiseman, P.E. Duhamel, J. Noolandi, C.N. Ta, and C.W. Frank. 2008. Progress in the development of interpenetrating polymer network hydrogels. *Polym. Adv. Technol.* 19:647–653.

Nagamoto, T., Y. Hattori, K. Takayama, and Y. Maitani. 2004. Novel chitosan particles and chitosan-coated emulsions inducing immune response via intranasal vaccine delivery. *Pharm. Res.* 21:671–674.

Osman, M., S.A. Fayed, I.M. Ghada, and R.M. Romeilah. 2010. Protective effects of chitosan, ascorbic acid and gymnema sylvestre against hypercholesterolemia in male rats. *Aust. J. Basic Appl. Sci.* 4:89–98.

Ozbas-Turan, S., J. Akbuga, and C. Aral. 2002. Controlled release of interleukin-2 from chitosan microspheres. *J. Pharm. Sci.* 91:124–125.

Pandey, S., A. Mishra, P. Raval, H. Patel, A. Gupta, and D. Shah. 2013. Chitosan–pectin polyelectrolyte complex as a carrier for colon targeted drug delivery. *J. Young Pharm.* 5:160–166.

Patel, D.M., P.M. Shah, and C.N. Patel. 2012. Formulation and evaluation of bioadhesive buccal drug delivery of repaglinide tablets. *Asian J. Pharm.* 6:171–179.

Park, B.G., H.S. Kang, W. Lee, J.S. Kim, and T.I. Son. 2013. Reinforcement of pH-responsive γ-poly(glutamic acid)/chitosan hydrogel for orally administrable colon-targeted drug delivery. *J. Appl. Polym. Sci.* 127:832–836.

Park, J.H., G. Saravanakumar, K. Kim, and I.C. Kwon. 2010. Targeted delivery of low molecular drugs using chitosan and its derivatives. *Adv. Drug Del .Rev.* 62:28–41.

Pavanetto, F., P. Perugini, B. Conti, T. Modena, and I. Genta. 1996. Evaluation of process parameters involved in chitosan microsphere preparation by the o/w/o multiple emulsion method. *J. Microencapsul.* 13:679–688.

Puvvada, Y.S., S. Vankayalapati, and S. Sukhavasi. 2012. Extraction of chitin from chitosan from exoskeleton of shrimp for application in the pharmaceutical industry. *Int. Curr. Pharm. J.* 1:258–263.

Qiao, H., M. Sun, and Z. Su. 2014. Kidney-specific drug delivery system for renal fibrosis based on coordination-driven assembly of catechol-derived chitosan. *Biomaterials* 35:7157–7171.

Qin, C., Q. Xiao, H. Li, M. Fang, Y. Liu, X. Chen, and Q. Li. 2004. Calorimetric studies of the action of chitosan-N-2-hydroxypropyl trimethyl ammonium chloride on the growth of microorganisms. *Int. J. Biol. Macromol.* 34:121–126.

Qu, G., Z. Yao, C. Zhang, X. Wu, and Q. Ping. 2009. PEG conjugated N-octyl-O-sulfate chitosan micelles for delivery of paclitaxel: In vitro characterization and in vivo evaluation. *Eur. J. Pharm. Sci.* 37:98–105.

Ramchandani, U. and S. Balakrishnan. 2012. Development and evaluation of transdermal drug delivery system of ketoprofen drug with chitosan for treatment of arthritis. *Eur. J. Appl. Sci.* 4:72–77.

Ramos, V.M., N.M. Rodriguez, M.F. Diaz, M.S. Rodriguez, A. Heras, and E. Agullo. 2003. N-methylene phosphonic chitosan: Effect of preparation methods on its properties. *Carbohydr. Polym.* 52:39–46.

RaviKumar, M.N.V. 2000. A review of chitin and chitosan applications. *React. Funct. Polym.* 46:1–27.

Rinaudo, M. 2006. Chitin and chitosan: Properties and applications. *Prog. Polym. Sci.* 31:603–632.

Sahu, P., A. Bhatt, A. Chaurasia, and V. Gajbhiye. 2012. Enhanced hepatoprotective activity of piperine loaded chitosan microspheres. *Int. J. Drug Dev. Res* 4:229–233.

Sahu, S.K., S. Maiti, T.K. Maiti, S.K. Ghosh, and P. Pramanik. 2011. Hydrophobically modified carboxymethyl chitosan nanoparticles targeted delivery of paclitaxel. *J. Drug Target.* 19:104–113.

Sajomsang, W., U. Ruktanonchai, P. Gonil, V. Mayen, and P. Opanasopit. 2009. Methylated N-aryl chitosan derivative/DNA complex nanoparticles for gene delivery: Synthesis and structure–activity relationships. *Carbohydr. Polym.* 78:743–752.

Sarath chandran, C., K.V. Shijith, K.V. Vipin, and A.R. Augusthy. 2013. Chitosan based mucoadhesive buccal patches containing bisoprolol fumarate. *Int. J. Adv. Pharm. Bio. Chem.* 2:465–469.

Shah, S., R. Qaqish, V. Patel, and M. Amiji. 1999. Evaluation of the factors influencing stomach-specific delivery of antibacterial agents for *Helicobacter pylori* infection. *J. Pharm. Pharmacol.* 51:667–672.

Shaji, J., V. Jain, and S. Lodha. 2010. Chitosan: A novel pharmaceutical excipient. *Int. J. Pharm. Appl. Sci.* 1:11–28.

Shen, K., M. Chen, H. Chan, J. Jeng, and Y. Wang. 2009. Inhibitory effects of chitooligosaccharides on tumor growth and metastasis. *Food Chem. Toxicol.* 47:1864–1871.

Shiraishi, S., T. Imai, and M. Otagiri. 1993. Controlled release of indomethacin by chitosan–polyelectrolyte complex: Optimization and in vivo/in vitro evaluation. *J. Control. Rel.* 25:217–225.

Singla, A.K. and M. Chawla. 2001. Chitosan. Some pharmaceutical and biological aspects-an update. *J. Pharm. Pharmacol.* 53:1047–1067.

Singh, U.V. and N. Udupa. 1998. Methotrexate loaded chitosan and chitin microspheres—in vitro characterization and pharmacokinetics in mice bearing Ehrlich ascites carcinoma. *J. Microencapsul.* 15:581–594.

Shi, X.Y. and T.W. Tan. 2002. Preparation of chitosan/ethylcellulose complex microcapsule and its application in controlled release of vitamin D-2. *Biomaterials* 23:4469–4473.

Shu, X.Z. and K.J. Zhu. 2000. A novel approach to prepare tripolyphosphate/chitosan complex beads for controlled release drug delivery. *Int. J. Pharm.* 201:51–58.

Shu, X.Z., K.J. Zhu, and W. Song. 2001. Novel pH-sensitive citrate cross-linked chitosan film for drug controlled release. *Int. J. Pharm.* 212:19–28.

Son, Y.J., J.S. Jang, Y.W. Cho, H. Chung, R.W. Park, I.C. Kwon, I.S. Kim, J.Y. Park, and S.B. Seo. 2003. Biodistribution and anti-tumor efficacy of doxorubicin loaded glycol-chitosan nanoaggregates by EPR effect. *J. Control. Rel.* 91:135–145.

Stockert, R.J. and A.G. Morell. 1983. Hepatic binding protein: The galactose-sepcific receptor of mammalian hepatocytes. *Hepatology* 3:750–757.

Sun, W., S. Mao, Y. Wang, V.B. Junyaprasert, T. Zhang, L. Na, and J. Wang. 2010. Bioadhesion and oral absorption of enoxaparin nanocomplexes. *Int. J. Pharm.* 386:275–281.

Tan, H., C.R. Chu, K.A. Payne, and K.G. Marra. 2009. Injectable in situ forming biodegradable chitosan-hyaluronic acid based hydrogels for cartilage tissue engineering. *Biomaterials* 30:2499–2506.

Tang, Z.X., J.Q. Qian, and L.E. Xi. 2007. Preparation of chitosan nanoparticles as carrier for immobilized enzyme. *Appl. Biochem. Biotechnol.* 136:77–96.

Thein-Han, W.W. and W.F. Stevens. 2004. Transdermal delivery controlled by a chitosan membrane. *Drug Develop. Indus. Pharm.* 30:397–404.

Tian, Q., C.N. Zhang, X.H. Wang, W. Huang, R.T. Cha, C.H. Wang, Z. Yuan, M. Liu, H.Y. Wan, and H. Tang. 2010. Glycyrrhetinic acid-modified chitosan/poly(ethylene glycol) nanoparticles for liver-targeted delivery. *Biomaterials* 31:4748–4756.

Tokumitsu, H., H. Ichikawa, and Y. Fukumori. 1999a. Chitosan-gadopentetic acid complex nanoparticles for gadolinium neutron capture therapy of cancer: Preparation by novel emulsion droplet coalescence technique and characterization. *Pharm. Res.* 16:1830–1835.

Tokumitsu, H., H. Ichikawa, Y. Fukumori, and L.H. Block. 1999b. Preparation of gadopentetic acid loaded chitosan microparticles for gadolinium neutron-capture therapy of cancer by a novel emulsion-droplet coalescence technique. *Chem. Pharm. Bull.* 47:838–842.

Torchilin, V.P. 2004. Targeted polymeric micelles for delivery of poorly soluble drugs. *Cell. Mol. Life Sci.* 61:2549–2559.

Trung, T.S., W.W. Thein-Han, N.T. Qui, C.H. Ng, and W.F. Stevens. 2006. Functional characteristics of shrimp chitosan and its membranes as affected by the degree of deacetylation. *Bioresour. Technol.* 97:659–663.

Tsukamoto, T., K. Hironaka, T. Fujisawa, D. Yamaguchi, K. Tahara, Y. Tozuka, H. Takeuchi. 2013. Preparation of bromfenac loaded liposomes modified with chitosan for ophthalmic drug delivery and evaluation of physicochemical properties and drug release profile. *Asian J. Pharm. Sci.* 8:104–109.

van der Lubben, I.M., J.C. Verhoef, M.M. Fretz, O. Van, I. Mesu, and G. Kersten. 2002. Trimethyl chitosan chloride (TMC) as a novel excipient for oral and nasal immunisation against diphtheria. *STP Pharm. Sci.* 12:235–242.

Varshosaz, J., A.J. Dehkordi, and S. Golafshan. 2006a. Colon-specific delivery of mesalazine chitosan microspheres. *J. Microencapsul.* 23:329–339.

Varshosaz, J., F. Jaffari, and S. Karimzadeh. 2006b. Development of bioadhesive chitosan gels for topicaldelivery of lidocaine. *Scientia Pharmaceutica Sci. Pharm.* 74:209–223.

Venugopal, V., J. Kumar, and S. Muralidharan. 2014. Targeted delivery of silymarin to liver cells by galactosylated na-noparticles: In-vitro & in-vivo evaluation studies. *Albanian J. Pharm. Sci.* 2:4–8.

Vikhoreva, G., G. Bannikova, P. Stolbushkina, A. Panov, and N. Drozd. 2005. Preparation and anticoagulant activity of a low-molecular weight sulfated Chitosan. *Carbohydr. Polym.* 62:327–332.

Wang, H., Y. Xu, and X. Zhou. 2014. Docetaxel-Loaded chitosan microspheres as a lung targeted drug delivery system: In vitro and in vivo evaluation. *Int. J. Mol. Sci.* 15:3519–3532.

Wang, S.N., Y.H. Deng, H. Xu, H.B. Wu, Y.K. Qiu, and D.W. Chen. 2006. Synthesis of a novel galactosylated lipid and its application to the hepatocyte-selective targeting of liposomal doxorubicin. *Eur. J. Pharm. Biopharm.* 62:32–38.

Wang, X., N. Chi, and X. Tang. 2008b. Preparation of estradiol chitosan nanoparticles for improving nasal absorption and brain targeting. *Eur. J. Pharm. Biopharm.* 70:735–740.

Wang, X., C. Zheng, Z.M. Wu, D.G. Teng, X. Zhang, Z. Wang, and C.X. Li. 2009. Chitosan-AC nanoparticles as a vehicle for nasal absorption enhancement of insulin. *J. Biomed. Mater. Res. B. Appl. Biomater.* 88B:150–161.

Wong, T.W., L.W. Chan, S.B. Kho, and P.W. Sia Heng. 2002. Design of controlled-release solid dosage forms of alginate and chitosan using microwave. *J. Control.Rel.* 84:99–114.

Wu, J., W. Wei, L.Y. Wang, Z.G. Su, and G.H. Ma. 2007. A thermosensitive hydrogel based on quaternized chitosan and poly(ethylene glycol) for nasal drug delivery system. *Biomaterials* 28:2220–2232.

Xu, G., X. Huang, L. Qiu, J. Wu, and Y. Hu. 2007. Mechanism study of chitosan on lipid metabolism in hyperlipidemic rats. *Asia Pac. J. Clin. Nutr.* 16:313–317.

Xu, J., S. Strandman, J.X.X. Zhu, J. Barralet, and M. Cerruti. 2015. Genipin-crosslinked catechol-chitosan mucoadhesive hydrogels for buccal drug delivery. *Biomaterials* 37:395–404.

Xu, Q., P. Ma, W. Yu, C. Tan, H. Liu, C. Xiong, Y. Qiao, and Y. Du. 2010. Chitooligosaccharides protect human embryonic hepatocytes against oxidative stress induced by hydrogen peroxide. *Mar. Biotechnol.* 12:292–298.

Yamada, K., M. Odomi, N. Okada, T. Fujita, and A. Yamamoto. 2005. Chitosan oligomers as potential and safe absorption enhancers for improving the pulmonary absorption of interferon-alpha in rats. *J. Pharm. Sci.* 94:2432–2440.

Yamada, T., H. Onishi, and Y. Machida. 2001. In vitro and in vivo evaluation of sustained release chitosan-coated ketoprofen microparticles. *Yakugaku Zasshi* 121:239–245.

Yang, M., S. Velaga, H. Yamamoto, H. Takeuchi, Y. Kawashima, L. Hovgaard, M. van de Weert, and S. Frokjaer. 2007. Characterisation of salmon calcitonin in spray-dried powder for inhalation. Effect of chitosan. *Int. J. Pharm.* 331:176–181.

Yang, R., W.S. Shim, F.D. Cui, G. Cheng, X. Han, Q.R. Jin, D.D. Kim, S.J. Chung, and C.K. Shim. 2009. Enhanced electrostatic interaction between chitosan-modified PLGA nanoparticle and tumor. *Int. J. Pharm.* 371:142–147.

Ye, S.Q., C.Y. Wang, X.X. Liu, Z. Tong, B. Ren, and F. Zeng. 2006. New loading process and release properties of insulin from polysaccharide microcapsules fabricated through layer-by-layer assembly. *J. Control. Rel.* 112:79–87.

Yoo, H.S. 2007. Photo-cross-linkable and thermo-responsive hydrogels containing chitosan and pluronic for sustained release of human growth hormone (hGH). *J. Biomater. Sci. Polym. Ed.* 18:1429–1441.

Yoon, H., M. Moon, H. Park, S. Im, and Y. Kim. 2007. Chitosan oligosaccharide (COS) inhibits LPS-induced inflammatory effects in RAW 264.7 macrophage cells. *Biochem. Biophys. Res. Commun.* 358:954–959.

You, J., F.Q. Hu, Y.Z. Du, and H. Yuan. 2007. Polymeric micelles with glycolipid-like structure and multiple hydrophobic domains for mediating molecular target delivery of paclitaxel. *Biomacromolecules* 8:2450–2456.

Zaharoff, D.A., C.J. Rogers, K.W. Hance, J. Schlom, and J.W. Greiner. 2007. Chitosan solution enhances the immune adjuvant properties of GM-CSF. *Vaccine* 25:8673–8686.

Zhang, C., Y. Cheng, G. Qu, X. Wu, Y. Ding, Z. Cheng, L. Yu, and Q. Ping. 2008a. Preparation and characterization of galactosylated chitosan coated BSA microspheres containing 5-fluorouracil. *Carbohyd. Polym.* 72:390–397.

Zhang, D.Y., X.Z. Shen, J.Y. Wang, L. Dong, Y.L. Zheng, and L.L. Wu. 2008b. Preparation of chitosan–polyaspartic acid-5-fluorouracil nanoparticles and its anti-carcinoma effect on tumor growth in nudemice. *World J. Gastroenterol.* 14:3554–3562.

Zhang, H., S. Mardyani, W.C. Chan, and E. Kumacheva. 2006. Design of biocompatible chitosan microgels for targeted pH-mediated intracellular release of cancer therapeutics. *Biomacromolecules* 7:1568–1572.

Zhang, X.G., H.J. Zhang, Z.M. Wu, Z. Wang, H.M. Niu, and C.X. Li. 2008c. Nasal absorption enhancement of insulin using PEG-grafted chitosan nanoparticles. *Eur.J. Pharm. Biopharm.* 68:526–534.

Zhang, Y., J. Chen, and Y. Pan. 2007. A novel PEGylation of chitosan nanoparticles for gene delivery. *Biotechnol. Appl. Biochem.* 46:197–204.

Zhao, H.P., B. Wu, H. Wu, L. Su, J. Pang, T. Yang, and Y. Liu. 2006. Protective immunity in rats by intranasal immunization with Streptococcus mutans glucan-binding protein D encapsulated into chitosan-coated poly(lactic-co-glycolic acid) microspheres. *Biotechnol. Lett.* 28:1299–1304.

Zhu, B.D., Y.Q. Qie, and J.L. Wang 2007. Chitosan microspheres enhance the immunogenicity of an Ag85B-based fusion protein containing multiple T-cell epitopes of *Mycobacterium tuberculosis. Eur. J. Pharm. Biopharm.* 66:318–326.

Zhu, L., J. Ma, N. Jia, Y. Zhao, and H. Shen. 2009. Chitosan-coated magnetic nanoparticles as carriers of 5-fluorouracil: Preparation, characterization and cytotoxicity studies. *Coll. Surf. B. Biointerfaces* 68:1–6.

Zhu, X.L., Y.Z. Du, R.S. Yu, P. Liu, D. Shi, Y. Chen, Y. Wang, and F.F. Huang. 2013. Galactosylated chitosan oligosaccharide nanoparticles for hepatocellular carcinoma cell-targeted delivery of adenosine triphosphate. *Int. J. Mol. Sci.* 14:15755–15766.

13 Chitosan-Based Delivery of Gene Therapeutics for Cancer

Anish Babu and Rajagopal Ramesh

CONTENTS

13.1 INTRODUCTION

The use of genetic materials, including RNA, oligonucleotides, or DNA, to control cellular processes is the basic treatment strategy employed in cancer gene therapy (Cross and Burmester 2006). Gene therapy tools, such as small interfering RNA (siRNA), short hairpin RNA, or DNA, offer a significant potential in cancer treatment (Devi 2006; Ibraheem et al. 2014). However, nucleic acid therapeutics administered *in vivo* suffer from poor cellular uptake due to their net negative charges and vulnerability to nuclease digestion. They also have limited stability in the bloodstream and are required to cross cellular barriers to reach targets within the cells (Phillips 2001; Wang et al. 2010). Therefore, gene delivery vehicles are required for nucleic acid therapeutics to overcome the hurdles in

351

blood circulation and for cellular internalization (Zhang et al. 2012). A successful gene therapy strategy requires the right choice of gene delivery vehicle. Viral vectors are known to give high transfection efficiencies; however, potential mutagenesis and oncogenic effects limit the use of viral vectors as gene delivery agents (Thomas et al. 2003).

The advent of nanotechnology has put forward a number of nonviral gene delivery vehicles (Li and Huang 2006). Cationic liposomes are routinely used as gene delivery systems for *in vitro* and *in vivo* applications (Simoes et al. 2005). Despite the great success in gene transfection efficiency achieved by cationic liposomes, the use of these liposomes in the clinic setting is limited by their nonspecific toxicity (Audouy et al. 2002; Knudsen et al. 2015). Recently, researchers have shown enormous interest in using natural, biocompatible materials for the safe delivery of therapeutic nucleic acids. Chitosan, a polysaccharide obtained from crustaceans and some fungal sources, is a natural polymer that has been highly investigated as an alternative material for gene delivery (Saranya et al. 2011). Chitosan has numerous attractive qualities, including low toxicity, negligible immunogenicity, biocompatibility, and biodegradability, which suggest that it might provide a safe material for gene delivery (Lee 2007). In this chapter, we highlight the applications of chitosan in gene delivery. Emphasis is given to the properties of chitosan and chitosan-based formulations that facilitate the process of successful gene transfection in mammalian cells. Challenges and future prospects for chitosan formulations for gene therapy are also discussed.

13.2 CHITOSAN CHARACTERISTICS THAT FACILITATE GENE DELIVERY

13.2.1 PHYSICOCHEMICAL PROPERTIES

13.2.1.1 N/P Ratio

The abundance of positively charged free amine groups is the striking feature of chitosan that allows its strong interaction with nucleic acids. These free amine groups electrostatically interact with the negatively charged phosphate groups of nucleic acids to form self-assembled complexes. The amino nitrogen-to-phosphate (N/P) ratio is an important parameter that facilitates the interaction between the chitosan polymer and nucleic acid to form complex. The interaction between free amines and phosphate groups is stonger at acidic pH because the protonation of amines and the solubility of chitosan are more at low pH, which allows the complex formation in nano-sized particles. Disruption of the N/P ratio by a change in pH or lack of proper incubation may result in loosening of siRNA–chitosan complex leading to premature release of siRNA. Therefore it is important to maintain a proper charge-to-charge ratio (N/P ratio) for efficient protection and delivery of siRNA or DNA to mammalian cells.

In addition, the particle size and stability of the complex have been shown to be dependent on the N/P ratio (Alameh et al. 2012). A proper N/P ratio ensures strong binding of the nucleic acids to the chitosan polymer, and averts premature release

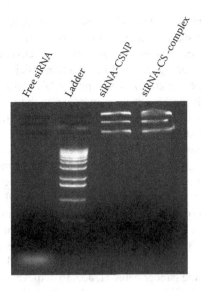

FIGURE 13.1 Electrophoretic gel retardation assay of chitosan–siRNA complex and siRNA-loaded chitosan–TPP nanoparticles. Note the migration of free siRNA compared to chitosan nanoparticle-protected siRNAs, which were retained in the wells of 1.2% agarose gel.

and possible digestion of the nucleic acids by the ubiquitously present nucleases. Figure 13.1 shows the nucleic acid protection efficiency of chitosan in complex and ionotropic gelation formulations, as revealed by gel retardation assay.

13.2.1.2 Molecular Weight and Degree of Deacetylation

The molecular weight (MW) of the chitosan polymer is also important in determining the nucleic acid–chitosan complex formation. Chitosan is categorized into three groups, according to the MW: low (LMW; Average MW 120 KDa), medium (MMW; Average MW 250 KDa), and high (HMW; Average MW 340 KDa; Ribeiro et al. 2014). Studies have shown that gene-carrying ability and transfection efficiency are influenced by the MW (Sato et al. 2001; Moran et al. 2009). Moreover, the MW of chitosan also influences the particle size and cellular uptake. HMW chitosan offers numerous free cationic amines to strongly bind with siRNA or plasmid DNA. This type of strong binding is advantageous for nucleic acids, because strong binding provides stability and protection against degradation in the presence of nucleases. However, strong complexation with HMW chitosan may affect the timely release of the bound nucleic acids within the cell, leading to poor transfection efficiency. This is especially true when the chitosan polymer is cross-linked with anionic polymers or chemical cross-linkers. Hence, MMW or LMW chitosans have gained much attention in research into the development of gene delivery systems.

Recently, Alameh et al. (2012) have highlighted the suitability of LMW chitosan for siRNA delivery. They demonstrated that, at low N/P ratios, LMW chitosan complexed with siRNA could efficiently transfect a range of cell lines under optimal conditions. The influence of the MW on particle size was also clearly demonstrated (Huang et al. 2005). When the MW changed from 213 to 48 kDa, the particle size of chitosan nanocarriers decreased from 181 to 155 nm.

Along with the MW, the degree of deacetylation (DDA) also plays an important role in the stability, cellular uptake, and transfection efficiency of chitosan–nucleic acid complexes (Huang et al. 2005). Knowing the DDA of the chitosan polymer is necessary to calculate the appropriate combination of chitosan and oligonucleotides to achieve proper N/P ratios. It has been shown that similar transfection efficiencies with DNA would be achieved by lowering the DDA and increasing the MW, or lowering the MW and increasing the DDA, of chitosan (Lavertu et al. 2006).

We have synthesized chitosan–tripolyphosphate (TPP) nanoparticles loaded with siRNA targeting human antigen R (*HuR*) gene in lung cancer cells. We formulated nanoparticles with LMW chitosan (~58 KDa) and 85% DDA. The nanoparticles were spherical and homogeneous, with an average 100-nm diameter, as shown in the transmission electron microscopic (TEM) image in Figure 13.2. Our laboratory is conducting an ongoing evaluation of this LMW chitosan as chitosan–siRNA complexes and/or as chitosan-coated polylactic-*co*-glycolic acid (PLGA) nanoparticles for siRNA delivery to lung cancer cells. Hence, to achieve a desirable particle size, stability, and transfection efficiency, one should consider using an appropriate combination of MW and DDA in formulating chitosan-based gene delivery vehicles.

13.2.1.3   siRNA or Plasmid DNA Concentrations

Another key factor that determines successful transfection is the concentration of siRNA or plasmid DNA used in the formulation. In general, nanoparticles that deliver siRNA or microRNA to the cell cytoplasm are inefficient in delivering plasmid DNA to the nucleus, due to the differences in the sizes and charges of siRNA/miRNA and plasmid DNA. Chitosan also presents variability in transfection efficiency between plasmid DNA and siRNA. The ability of chitosan to condense DNA has been reported in several studies (Strand et al. 2005; Amaduzzi et al.

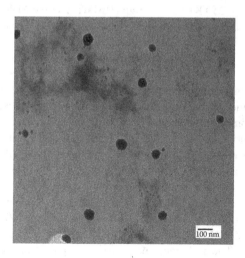

FIGURE 13.2   TEM image of chitosan–TPP nanoparticles loaded with HuR siRNA.

2014). Researchers have also shown that the charge and charge density of chitosan, the size of plasmid DNA, and the pH at which complexation occurs influence the condensation process (Lavertu et al. 2006; Maurstad et al. 2007). Although the ability of chitosan to condense siRNA is known to be variable and depends on the MW, pH, charge density of chitosan, and siRNA concentration, chitosan can potentially integrate siRNA into small discrete particles, leading to enhanced stability (Dehousse et al. 2010). Katas and Alpar (2006) reported that, by optimizing the type, concentration, MW, and preparation method, chitosan can be formulated as a viable vector for siRNA delivery.

13.2.1.4 Formulation Methods and pH Values

The methods selected to formulate chitosan nanocarriers have critically influenced siRNA and DNA transfection efficiency. Simple complexation and coacervation/ ionic gelation are commonly used to achieve gene delivery with chitosan. As mentioned earlier, simple complexation relies on the charge-based interaction between a chitosan polymer and nucleic acids. The complexes are less rigid at physiological pH, causing premature release of the nucleic acids before the complexes enter the cells. Hence, the pH of the transfection medium plays an important role in successful gene delivery using chitosan complexes.

Sato et al. (2001) reported that the transfection using a chitosan–DNA complex at pH 6.9 (acidic; nonphysiological) was more efficient than the transfection at pH 7.4 (physiological). At low pH, the zeta potential of the chitosan polyplexes remains more positive, which ultimately influences the interaction with negatively charged membranes to allow successful transfection (Agirre et al. 2014). Acidic pHs are also known to prevent chitosan aggregation and influence the particle size in the transfection medium (Agirre et al. 2014). Katas and Alpar (2006) suggest that ionic gelation of chitosan in the presence of sodium TPP gives enhanced stability to entrapped siRNA. The enhanced binding capacity and high loading efficiency of siRNA allowed chitosan–TPP nanoparticles to achieve better transfection efficiency than did simple complexation. Coacervation of chitosan with polyguluronate has also been shown to have excellent properties for a suitable siRNA nanocarrier (Lee et al. 2009). The basic principle of coacervation is the same as ionic gelation, because polyguluronate, a sodium alginate derivative, is strongly anionic in nature and binds with chitosan to form nanostructured particles. The particle size and siRNA loading can be easily manipulated by choosing the appropriate weight ratios of chitosan and polyguluronate. Hence, all three methods have yielded successful gene delivery to cancer cells, allowing researchers to choose between formulations for the desired transfection outcome.

13.2.1.5 Chitosan Cross-Linking

Cross-linking of chitosan polymer increases the rigidness of the nanocarrier so that the incorporated nucleic acids are well protected within the entanglement of the chitosan polymer. Csaba et al. (2009) studied ionically cross-linked chitosan for gene delivery in both *in vitro* and *in vivo* models. Their results showed that cross-linked chitosan enhanced the association efficiency of DNA with chitosan, resulting in high and long-lasting gene expression levels *in vitro*. Further, intranasal administration of DNA-loaded chitosan–TPP nanoparticles showed enhanced expression in *in vivo* animal models (Csaba et al. 2009). Raja et al. (2015) reported that the stability and efficiency of siRNA-loaded chitosan nanoparticles depended on the type of cross-linker used in the formulation. Moreover, the particle size, morphology, zeta potential, and entrapment efficiency of chitosan nanoparticles have been reported to vary according to the type of cross-linkers.

Hence, the optimization of physicochemical properties and the assessment of transfection parameters are key to successful gene delivery and efficient transfection with chitosan-based gene delivery carriers. Table 13.1 summarizes several important optimization studies of chitosan nanoparticle synthesis for gene delivery applications published over the past two decades.

13.2.2 FORMULATION METHODS FOR siRNA-/pDNA-LOADED CHITOSAN NANOPARTICLES

Although numerous methods, including emulsification and cross-linking, emulsion droplet coalescence, emulsion solvent diffusion, and reverse micellization, are employed for chitosan nanoparticle formulation (Grenha 2012; Sailaja et al. 2011), self-assembly and ionotropic gelation are most commonly used for gene delivery applications (Calvo et al. 1997; He et al. 2015). These procedures are frequently employed due to their efficiency, mildness, and reproducibility.

13.2.2.1 Self-Assembly

Self-assembled complexation is an easy and mild method to complex siRNA/pDNA with a chitosan polymer. Chitosan forms self-assembled complexes with negatively charged nucleic acid molecules. These complexes are, however, reversible upon changes in the pH of the medium, as mentioned elsewhere. The addition of siRNA or DNA into a chitosan solution in acidic pH, usually between 4.5 and 5.5, results in spontaneous self-assembly and nanoparticle formation at room temperature. Mechanical stirring of chitosan solution during the preparation procedure ensures the formation of small and stable nanoparticles.

13.2.2.2 Ionotropic Gelation/Coacervation

Ionotropic gelation (Calvo et al. 1997) or coacervation of chitosan in the presence of counter ions results in the formation of defined nanostructures in solution. The strong association between chitosan and cross-linker molecules allows the entrapment of siRNA/pDNA with high encapsulation efficiency. For this purpose, an anionic cross-linker is often mixed with nucleic acids and added dropwise to chitosan solution under mild stirring at room temperature, to allow spontaneous gelation of the chitosan polymer in the nanoparticle size range. Ionic cross-linkers, such as thiamine pyrophosphate (Rojanarata et al. 2008), TPP, dextran sulfate (Chen et al. 2007), and poly-D-glutamic acid, are commonly used for chitosan nanoparticle formulation in gene delivery applications (Raja et al. 2015). Figure 13.3 shows a schematic representation of self-assembly complexation and ionotropic gelation techniques employed for siRNA/pDNA-loaded chitosan nanoparticles.

TABLE 13.1
Optimization Studies for Chitosan-Based Gene Delivery Systems

Payload	Formulation/ Techniques	Purpose	Conclusion/Outcome	Reference
pDNA	Polyplex/ complexation	Structure–property relationship of chitosan–pDNA polyplexes	Chitosan is an alternative to other polymers for nontoxic gene delivery.	Koping-Hoggard et al. 2001
pDNA	Chitosan nanoparticles/ complex coacervation and solvent evaporation	Evaluation of physicochemical characteristics	Chitosan–pDNA nanoparticles prepared by complex coacervation could be used as DNA transfection vectors.	Bozkir and Saka 2004
siRNA	Chitosan–TPP nanoparticle/Ionic cross-linking (coacervation)	Optimization study for siRNA delivery *in vitro*	siRNA transfection efficiency was demonstrated in CHO K1 and HEK 293 cells. Ionic gelation showed better stability and transfection efficiency than simple complexation.	Katas and Alpar 2006
siRNA	Folate-conjugated chitosan nanoparticles/ complexation	Optimize the use of LMW chitosan conjugated with folate for targeted gene delivery	The MW of chitosan has a major influence on its biological and physicochemical properties. Folate–chitosan promoted targeting and enhanced gene transfection efficiency.	Fernandes et al. 2012
siRNA	Polyethyleneglycol (PEG)-modified chitosan–PEI–TPP nanoparticles/ionic cross-linking	Improve siRNA transfection efficiency by adding endosomal disrupting agent PEI to chitosan	Addition of PEG improved nanoparticle stability under physiological conditions; PEI enhanced siRNA transfection efficiency *in vitro* and *in vivo*. Use of hyaluronic acid instead of TPP gives more biocompatibility.	Ragelle et al. 2014
siRNA	Polyplex/ complexation (by ultrasonication)	Optimize the process parameters for chitosan–siRNA polyplex formulation	Optimized N/P ratio and sonication parameters for achieving small particle size, optimum polydispersity index, and high siRNA loading efficiency.	Gharehdaghi et al. 2014

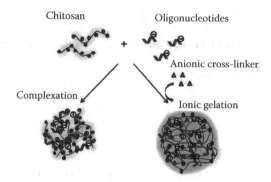

FIGURE 13.3 Commonly used methods for chitosan–oligonucleotide (siRNA or DNA) nanoparticle formulation. Complexation: Cationic chitosan polymer and anionic oligonucleotides are self-assembled when mixed and incubated at acidic pH at room temperature. Ionic (Ionotropic) gelation: Ionic gelation of chitosan is induced by an anionic cross-linker, such as TPP or thiamine pyrophosphate, which is added with negatively charged oligonucleotides under mild stirring.

13.3   CHITOSAN MODIFICATIONS FOR GENE DELIVERY APPLICATIONS

To enhance the solubility of chitosan at physiological pH and to improve its transfection efficiency, derivatives of chitosan have been synthesized and used in many gene delivery applications. The presence of functional groups in chitosan can be exploited for chemical modification to facilitate enhanced gene delivery efficiency. Tong et al. (2009) published an exhaustive review on chitosan and its derivatives in gene therapy applications. Chemical groups with hydrophilic, hydrophobic, and thermo- and pH-sensitive functions, and targeting ligands have been introduced into chitosan polymers to improve transfection efficiency. The addition of glycol and thiol groups to chitosan has improved the nanoparticles' stability and siRNA transfection efficiency in drug-resistant cancer cells. In a typical study, thiolated glycol chitosan, which formed stable nanoparticles via self-cross-linking, was successfully used to deliver poly-siRNA (Yhee et al. 2015). The interaction between siRNA and chitosan was facilitated through disulfide bond formation. Following cellular entry, these functionalized chitosan–siRNA nanoparticles were able to deliver siRNA into the cytoplasm, resulting in knockdown of the targeted gene, P-glycoprotein (*Pgp*). In a different study, Lee et al. (2012) fabricated a self-cross-linking poly-siRNA-glycol chitosan nanoparticle in a similar fashion to knock down target genes in *in vitro* and *in vivo* tumor models.

Increasing the hydrophobicity of chitosan may enhance the cell surface attachment of chitosan via hydrophobic–hydrophobic interaction and subsequent cell uptake (Shi et al. 2011). Moreover, the presence of hydrophobic moieties in chitosan may assist the cytoplasmic release of bound DNA from the chitosan–DNA complex (Kurisawa et al. 2000). Alkylation methods generally followed by quarternization reactions generated many derivatives of chitosan, such as trimethylated chitosan,

N-dodecylated chitosan *N,N*-diethyl *N*-methyl chitosan, and alkyl bromide-modified chitosan. Such chemical modifications contribute to chitosan nanocarriers' improved hydrophobicity, making chitosan carriers more suitable for gene delivery applications (Safari et al. 2012). Thanou et al. (2002) used a quaternized chitosan oligomer for DNA transfection of COS-1 and Caco-2 cell lines. Compared with regular (*N*-[1-(2,3-dioleoyloxy)propyl]-*N,N,N*-trimethylammonium sulfate (DOTAP) lipoplexes, quarternized chitosan oligomer complexes had less transfection efficiency. However, quaternized chitosan showed no toxicity and stability in the presence of fetal calf serum in the transfection medium, compared with toxic and less stable DOTAP lipoplexes (Thanou et al. 2002).

Apart from chemical modification, conjugation of lipophilic molecules to chitosan has improved chitosan's physicochemical properties for the purposes of gene delivery. For example, modification of glycol chitosan using 5β-cholanic acid, a hydrophobic moiety, improved stability and promoted strong hydrophobic interaction with a supportive polymer polyethylene imine to form self-assembled nanoparticles for siRNA delivery (Huh et al. 2010). Further, successful siRNA gene silencing efficiency was achieved in animal models using this 5β-cholanic acid-modified chitosan/polyethelyneamine (PEI)–siRNA complex. In a similar study, 5β-cholanic acid-modified glycol chitosan was used as a platform to co-deliver BCl2 siRNA and doxorubicin to tumors in mice (Yoon et al. 2014).

Chitosan nanoparticles can be tuned to release their nucleic acid payload in response to pH variations in biological systems (Singh et al. 2014). The presence of a pH-sensitive component (negatively charged in physiological pH) in the chitosan nanoparticles' surface could shift the charge of the nanoparticles from negative to positive upon entry into a tumor microenvironment with a weak acidic pH. The negatively charged pH-sensitive component on the surface of the chitosan–nucleic acid complex helps to prevent serum protein interaction and early clearance of chitosan nanoparticles from the circulation. Moreover, this strategy facilitates tumor-targeted delivery of nucleic acid therapeutics. The use of agmatine–chitosan conjugate for the pH-sensitive delivery of siRNA *in vitro* and *in vivo* is a recent example (Li et al. 2015). Agmatine modification allows chitosan–siRNA complexes to minimize serum adsorption and facilitates target cell internalization of siRNA, resulting in remarkable gene silencing efficiency.

To enhance the successful cytoplasmic delivery of nucleic acid payload via endosomal/lysosomal destruction, chitosan nanoparticles are often modified or combined with strongly cationic molecules that exert powerful proton sponge effects. Histidine or imidazole group modification of chitosan is a commonly employed procedure by which the proton sponge property can be enhanced to allow endosomal disruption and efficient release of chitosan–DNA polyplexes into the cytoplasm (Chang et al. 2010). Studies showed that endosomal disruption is made possible by urocanic acid bearing an imidazole group-modified chitosan, resulting in enhanced gene transfection efficiency in *in vitro* (Kim et al. 2003) and *in vivo* cancer models (Jin et al. 2008). Ghosn et al. (2010) reported the use of an imidazole-modified chitosan nanocarrier for siRNA delivery targeting lung and liver tissues. Intranasal delivery of imidazole-chitosan-siRNA resulted in enhanced gene silencing of model gene *GAPDH* (glyceraldehyde phosphate dehydrogenase) in lung tissues, whereas intravenous delivery demonstrated strong GAPDH gene silencing effects in both lung and liver tissues, possibly via enhanced endosomal escape properties conferred by the imidazole moiety in chitosan after the complex entered the cells.

13.4   CHITOSAN-BASED HYBRID NANOPARTICLES IN GENE DELIVERY

The transfection efficiency of chitosan can also be improved by grafting or combining other positively charged polymers or lipids. In a recent study, Poly-L-arginine-grafted chitosan (PLR-CS) was prepared for siRNA transfection *in vivo* (Noh et al. 2010). The PLR-CS–DNA nanoparticles demonstrated higher cellular delivery efficiency of siRNA than did CS or poly-L-arginine alone. Delivery of red fluorescent protein siRNA resulted in efficient target gene knockdown for PLR-CS in mice tumor models, compared with CS or PLR alone. Another study demonstrated that chitosan and poly-L-arginine polymers, when combined together with siRNA in a specific ratio, form stable nanoparticles that are less sensitive to serum binding and efficiently protect siRNA from degradation (Plianwong et al. 2013). Delivery of green fluorescent protein (GFP) siRNA was successful with CS-PLA (poly-L-arginine) in HeLa cells. However, the safety level of CS-PLA-siGFP is questionable, as ~25% cell inhibition was observed.

PEI is another well-known, synthetic, cationic polymer. Grafting linear PEI (LPEI) with chitosan enhances the transfection efficiency of chitosan severalfold in comparison with CS, LPEI, or even the commercial reagent lipofectamine in various cancer cells (Tripathi et al. 2012). Such systems are generally called hybrid polymer nanosystems. CS–PEI hybrid systems benefit from chitosan's biocompatibility and PEI's proton sponge-inducing capability (Jiang et al. 2008). Grafting beta-cyclodextrin-modified PEI with chitosan resulted in enhanced condensation and protection of plasmid DNA and siRNA, which formed compact and spherical nanoparticles upon complexation (Ping et al. 2011). The gene transfection efficiency of native chitosan was increased by beta-cyclodextrin-modified PEI, as evident from siRNA transfection studies in HEK293 and L929 cell lines. The cyclodextrin moieties in these nanoparticles also allowed supramolecular pegylation, resulting in enhanced nanoparticle stability under physiological conditions (Ping et al. 2011).

Chitosan is also a major component in hybrid nanoparticles for delivery of siRNA/pDNA. It forms ternary complexes with lipids and DNA; these complexes have different shapes and structures (Wang et al. 2012). These lipopolyplexes, formed by noncovalent interactions, showed enhanced delivery and transfection efficiency of plasmid DNA, compared with lipid–DNA or chitosan–DNA complexes. Moreover, chitosan enhanced the rapid delivery of pDNA by lipids in the nucleus (Wang et al. 2012). Salva et al. (2014) have recently reported the efficiency of chitosan-coated liposomes in siRNA delivery. They codelivered two siRNAs, siHIF1-α and siVEGF, using chitosan-coated liposomes against breast cancer cell lines. Chitosan coating enhanced the stability, cellular interaction, and transfection efficiency, and reduced the toxicity of the liposomal carrier. Moreover, the codelivery of siRNAs was successful and an efficient gene silencing was observed, suggesting the applicability of chitosan-coated liposomes in siRNA-based gene therapies for cancer (Salva et al. 2014).

In addition, chitosan is used to improve the transfection efficiency and/or drug/gene delivery in combination with other nanoparticles. For instance, chitosan coating is reported to enhance the siRNA delivery efficiency of PLGA nanoparticles (Jagani et al. 2013). Chitosan coating imparts a positive charge to the PLGA nanoparticle, so that the cellular interaction will be enhanced to facilitate sufficient internalization of siRNA-loaded nanoparticles, resulting in enhanced gene silencing efficiency. Chen et al. (2012) used electrospinning to prepare PLGA nanofibers encapsulated with chitosan–siRNA polyplex, in order to achieve slow and controlled siRNA release and efficient gene silencing. In H1299 lung cancer cells, the resulting chitosan–siRNA complex produced an efficient gene transfection and silenced 50% of the target gene, highlighting this complex's potential as a vector for siRNA delivery and sustained release.

Recently, we have showed that successful delivery of a siRNA–pDNA combination is possible with chitosan-coated polylactic acid nanoparticles, resulting in target gene knockdown by siRNA and overexpression of the target protein induced by pDNA expression (Babu et al. 2014). The MMW chitosan served as an adsorption and condensation layer for siRNA/pDNA onto the nanoparticle surface through electrostatic interaction. Concurrent delivery of cisplatin encapsulated in the nanoparticles' core and siRNA/pDNA adsorbed onto its surface resulted in cisplatin sensitivity in a drug-resistant ovarian cancer cell line. Thus, the chitosan coating imparted biocompatibility, enhanced cellular interaction through its positive charge, and allowed complexation with nucleic acid therapeutics for intracellular delivery.

13.5 LIGAND-TARGETED DELIVERY OF CHITOSAN–siRNA/pDNA NANOPARTICLES

Conjugation of cell-specific ligands or antibodies to chitosan nanoparticles is an effective way of targeting nucleic acid therapeutics to the desired tumor sites. The mechanism of targeting molecule/ligand uptake to promote targeting and internalization could improve chitosan nanoparticles' transfection rates. Chitosan offers numerous functional groups that can be exploited to conjugate targeting molecules. Several ligands, such as folic acid (Chan et al. 2007), transferrin (Mao et al. 2001), galactose, and mannose (Kim et al. 2006), have been used to endow chitosan gene delivery vehicles with targeting capability. Among these vehicles, folate-conjugated chitosan appears in a large portion of literature describing targeted gene delivery toward cancer cells that overexpress the folate receptor (Zheng et al. 2009; Zheng et al. 2011).

In a typical study, folate–chitosan–siRNA showed improved transfection efficiency and gene silencing in various cancer cells over chitosan–siRNA (Fernandes et al. 2012). Yang et al. (2014) developed folate–chitosan–TPP nanoparticles for the targeted delivery of siRNA to activated microphages in mouse models. They observed that folic acid conjugation enhanced the cellular uptake and siRNA delivery in activated macrophages *in vivo*. Another study demonstrated the use of folate-conjugated stearic acid-modified chitosan (FA-CS-SA) nanoparticles for the delivery of plasmid DNA to cancer cells (Du et al. 2011). Folate conjugation was achieved via a 1-ethyl-3-(3-dimethylaminopropyl) carbodiimide-coupling reaction. The FA-CS-SA–pDNA complex formed a micellar structure and was efficient in pDNA condensation and targeted delivery of pDNA to folate receptor-overexpressing cancer cells.

Transferrin-modified chitosan gene delivery systems have also been evaluated in transferrin-overexpressing cancer cells. Mao et al. (2001) developed, optimized, and tested transferrin-conjugated chitosan nanoparticles for DNA delivery to cancer cells. In HEK293 and HeLa cells, they observed nearly fourfold enhancement in transfection efficiency by transferrin-conjugated chitosan nanoparticles compared with nontargeted chitosan nanoparticles. A recent study described the efficacy of iron-saturated transferrin-conjugated chitosan in delivering doxorubicin to glio-sarcoma cells (Dufes et al. 2004), suggesting the utility of transferrin–chitosan nanoparticles for targeted gene delivery.

The conjugation of oligonucleotide aptamers with chitosan is an important developing strategy for targeted delivery of gene therapeutics against cancer. Aptamers are single-stranded DNA or RNA oligos that can specifically bind to target molecules and are expressed by cells with high affinity. The interaction between chitosan and oligonucleotide aptamers is charge based, like the interaction between DNA/siRNA and chitosan. A recent study demonstrated the use of DNA aptamer for Mucin 1-conjugated chitosan in targeting the anticancer molecule SN38 in colon cancer cells (Sayari et al. 2014). The efficacy of SN38 was increased in colon cancer cells via MUC 1 aptamer conjugation to a chitosan nanocarrier. Another study reported that chitosan–aptamer nanoparticles target transforming growth factor β (TGFβ) II in glaucoma therapy (Chen et al. 2013). The aptamer S58 was efficiently protected by the chitosan nanocarrier, enabling its prolonged activity and allowing it to efficiently inhibit TGFβ II-induced cell proliferation. Thus, aptamer–chitosan conjugate-based gene delivery strategies show promise in cancer therapy.

13.6   CONCLUSION AND FUTURE PROSPECTS

DNA or RNA interference (RNAi) molecules have recently emerged as potential therapeutic agents for the treatment of cancer and other diseases. Safe and efficient delivery tools are required to translate these experimental gene therapeutic processes to clinical settings. Chitosan has been subjected to intense investigations as a potential nanocarrier for siRNA/pDNA, due to its biocompatibility, low immunogenicity, easy formulation, facile modification, and ability to protect nucleic acids from degradation. Studies revealed that the MW of chitosan used, DDA, pH, N/P ratios, formulation methods, type of cross-linking agents, nucleic acid-releasing properties, and derivation strategies influence the gene transfection efficiency of chitosan-based nanocarriers. The literature has provided significant information regarding the safety and gene transfection efficiency of chitosan and its derivatives.

However, the full potential of chitosan-based gene delivery formulations in animal models is yet to be realized, as many studies are in the developmental stage. Advances in chitosan research, such as the generation of new derivatives, novel chitosan-based hybrid nanoparticle systems, and efficient targeting techniques represent valuable strategies for the future application of chitosan-based gene delivery systems. Such systems must be tested thoroughly in laboratory and preclinical settings before they can be explored in clinical trials. Novel high-throughput technologies, such as microfluidics, would allow the production of consistent batch-to-batch uniform nanoparticle formulations and provide opportunities for large-scale screening (Valencia et al. 2012; Majedi et al. 2013). These approaches offer a way to accelerate the clinical translation of chitosan-based gene delivery systems.

ACKNOWLEDGMENTS

The study was supported in part by a grant received from the National Institutes of Health R01 CA167516 and by funds received from the Jim and Christy Everest Endowed Chair in Cancer Developmental Therapeutics, the University of Oklahoma Health Sciences Center (OUHSC), OK, USA. The authors thank Ms. Kathy Kyler at the Office of the Vice President for Research, the OUHSC, for editorial assistance. Rajagopal Ramesh is an Oklahoma Tobacco Settlement Endowment Trust (TSET) Research Scholar and holds the Jim and Christy Everest Endowed Chair in Cancer Developmental Therapeutics.

REFERENCES

Agirre, M., Zarate, J., Ojeda, E., Puras, G., Desbrieres, J., Pedraz, J. L. 2014. Low molecular weight chitosan (LMWC)-based polyplexes for pDNA delivery: From bench to bedside. *Polymers* 6:1727–55.
Alameh, M., DeJesus, D., Jean, M., et al. 2012. Low molecular weight chitosan nanoparticulate system at low N:P ratio for nontoxic polynucleotide delivery. *Int J Nanomedicine* 7:1399–414.
Amaduzzi, F., Bomboi, F., Bonincontro, A., et al. 2014. Chitosan DNA complexes: Charge inversion and DNA condensation. *Colloids Surf B Biointerfaces* 114:1–10.
Audouy, S. A. L., de Leij, L. F. M. H., Hoekstra, D., Molema, G. 2002. *In vivo* characteristics of cationic liposomes as delivery vectors for gene therapy. *Pharm Res* 19:1599–605.
Babu, A., Wang, Q., Muralidharan, R., Shanker, M., Munshi, A., Ramesh, R. 2014. Chitosan coated polylactic acid nanoparticle-mediated combinatorial delivery of cisplatin and siRNA/Plasmid DNA chemosensitizes cisplatin-resistant human ovarian cancer cells. *Mol Pharm* 11:2720–33.
Bozkir, A. and Saka, O. M. 2004. Chitosan nanoparticles for plasmid DNA delivery: Effect of chitosan molecular structure on formulation and release characteristics. *Drug Deliv* 11:107–12.
Calvo, P., Remunan-Lopez, C., Vila-Jato, J. L., Alonso, M. J. 1997. Chitosan and chitosan/ ethylene oxide-propylene oxide block copolymer nanoparticles as novel carriers for proteins and vaccines. *Pharm Res* 14:1431–6.
Chan, P., Kurisawa, M., Chung, J. E., Yang, Y. Y. 2007. Synthesis and characterization of chitosan-g-poly(ethylene glycol)-folate as a non-viral carrier for tumor-targeted gene delivery. *Biomaterials* 28:540–9.
Chang, K. L., Higuchi, Y., Kawakami, S., Yamashita, F., Hashida, M. 2010. Efficient gene transfection by histidine-modified chitosan through enhancement of endosomal escape. *Bioconjug Chem* 21:1087–95.
Chen, M., Gao, S., Dong, M., et al. 2012. Chitosan/siRNA nanoparticles encapsulated in PLGA nanofibers for siRNA delivery. *ACS Nano* 6:4835–44.
Chen, X., Zhu, X., Li, L., et al. 2013. Investigation on novel chitosan nanoparticle-aptamer complexes targeting TGF-β receptor II. *Int J Pharm* 456:499–507.
Chen, Y., Mohanraj, V. J., Wang, F., Benson, H. A. E. 2007. Designing chitosan-dextran sulfate nanoparticles using charge ratios. *AAPS PharmSciTech* 8:131–9.

Cross, D. and Burmester, J. K. 2006. Gene therapy for cancer treatment: Past, present and future. *Clin Med Res* 4:218–27.

Csaba, N., Kopping-Hoggard, M., Fernandez-Megia, E., Novoa-Carballal, R., Riguera, R., Alonso, M. J. 2009. Ionically crosslinked chitosan nanoparticles as gene delivery systems: Effect of PEGylation degree on in vitro and in vivo gene transfer. *J Biomed Nanotechnol* 5:162–71.

Dehousse, V., Garbacki, N., Jaspart, S., et al. 2010. Comparison of chitosan/siRNA and trimethylchitosan/siRNA complexes behaviour in vitro *J B. Int i ol Macromol* 46:342–9.

Devi, G. R. 2006. siRNA-based approaches in cancer therapy. *Cancer Gene Ther* 13:819–29.

Du, Y.-Z., Cai, L.-L., Li, J., Zhao, M.-D., Chen, F.-Y., Yuan, H., et al. 2011. Receptor-mediated gene delivery by folic acid-modified stearic acid-grafted chitosan micelles. *Int J Nanomedicine* 6: 1559–68.

Dufes, C., Muller, J. M., Couet, W., Olivier, J. C., Uchegbu, I. F., Schatzlein, A. G. 2004. Anticancer drug delivery with transferrin targeted polymeric chitosan vesicles. *Pharm Res* 21:101–7.

Fernandes, J. C., Qiu, X., Winnik, F. M., et al. 2012. Low molecular weight chitosan conjugated with folate for siRNA delivery in vitro: Optimization studies. *Int J Nanomedicine* 2012:5833–45.

Gharehdaghi, E. E., Amani, A., Khoshayand, M. R., et al. 2014. Chitosan nanoparticles for siRNA delivery: Optimization of processing/formulation parameters. *Nucleic Acid Ther* 24:420–7.

Ghosn, B., Singh, A., Li, M., et al. 2010. Efficient gene silencing in lungs and liver using imidazole-modified chitosan as a nanocarrier for small interfering RNA. *Oligonucleotides* 20:163–72.

Grenha, A. 2012. Chitosan nanoparticles: A survey of preparation methods. *J Drug Target* 20:291–300.

He, C., Yin, L., Song, Y., Tang, C., Yin, C. 2015. Glycol chitosan nanoparticles as specialized cancer therapeutic vehicles: Sequential delivery of doxorubicin and Bcl-2 siRNA. *Acta Biomater* 17:98–106.

Huang, M., Fong, C. W., Khorc, E., Lim, L. Y. 2005. Transfection efficiency of chitosan vectors: Effect of polymer molecular weight and degree of deacetylation. *J Control Release* 106:391–406.

Huh, M. S., Lee, S. Y., Park, S. 2010. Tumor-homing glycol chitosan/polyethylenimine nanoparticles for the systemic delivery of siRNA in tumor-bearing mice. *J Control Release* 144:134–43.

Ibraheem, D., Elaissari, A., Fessi, H. 2014. Gene therapy and DNA delivery systems. *Int J Pharm* 459:70–83.

Jagani, H. V., Josyula, V. R., Palanimuthu, V. R., Hariharapura, R. C., Gang, S. S. 2013. Improvement of therapeutic efficacy of PLGA nanoformulation of siRNA targeting anti-apoptotic Bcl-2 through chitosan coating. *Eur J Pharm Sci* 48:611–8.

Jiang, H. L., Kim, T. H., Kim, Y. K., Park, I. Y., Cho, M. H., Cho, C. S. 2008. Efficient gene delivery using chitosan-polyethylenimine hybrid systems. *Biomed Mater* 3: 025013. doi: 10.1088/1748-6041/3/2/025013.

Jin, H., Kim, H. W., Chung, Y. S., et al. 2008. Urocanic acid-modified chitosan-mediated PTEN delivery via aerosol suppressed lung tumorigenesis in K-ras(LA1) mice. *Cancer Gene Ther* 15:275–83.

Katas, H. and Alpar, H. O. 2006. Development and characterisation of chitosan nanoparticles for siRNA delivery. *J Control Release* 115:216–25.

Kim, T. H., Ihm, J. E., Choi, Y. J., Nah, J. W., Cho, C. S. 2003. Efficient gene delivery by urocanic acid-modified chitosan. *J Control Release* 93:389–402.

Kim, T. H., Nah, J. W., Cho, M. H., Park, T. G., Cho, C. S. 2006. Receptor-mediated gene delivery into antigen presenting cells using mannosylated chitosan/DNA nanoparticles. *J Nanosci Nanotechnol* 6:2796–803.

Knudsen, K.B., Northeved, H., Kumar, P.E., et al. 2015. In vivo toxicity of cationic micelles and liposomes. *Nanomedicine* (Lond) 11:467–77.

Koping-Hoggard, M., Tubulekas, I., Guan, H., et al. 2001. Chitosan as a nonviral gene delivery system. Structure-property relationships and characteristics compared with polyethylenimine in vitro and after lung administration in vivo. *Gene Ther* 8:1108–21.

Kurisawa, M., Yokoyama, M., Okano, T. 2000. Transfection efficiency increases by incorporating hydrophobic monomer units into polymeric gene carriers. *J Control Release* 68:1–8.

Lavertu, M., Methot, S., Tran-Khanh, N., Buschmann, M. D. 2006. High efficiency gene transfer using chitosan/DNA nanoparticles with specific combinations of molecular weight and degree of deacetylation. *Biomaterials* 27:4815–24.

Lee, D. W., Yun, K. S., Ban, H. S., Choe, W., Lee, S. K., Lee, K. Y. 2009. Preparation and characterization of chitosan/polyguluronate nanoparticles for siRNA delivery. *J Control Release* 139:146–52.

Lee, K. Y. 2007. Chitosan and its derivatives for gene delivery. *Macromol Res* 15:195–201.

Lee, S. J., Huh, M. S., Lee, S. Y., et al. 2012. Tumor-homing poly-siRNA/glycol chitosan self-cross-linked nanoparticles for systemic siRNA delivery in cancer treatment. *Angew Chem Int Ed* 51:7203–7.

Li, S. D. and Huang, L. 2006. Gene therapy progress and prospects: Non-viral gene therapy by systemic delivery. *Gene Ther* 13: 1313–9.

Li, Y., Yang, J., Xu, B., Gao, F., Wang, W., Liu, W. 2015. Enhanced therapeutic siRNA to tumor cells by a pH-sensitive agmatine-chitosan bioconjugate. *ACS Appl Mater Interfaces* 7:8114–24.

Majedi, F. S., Hasani-Sadrabadi, M. M., Emami, S. H., et al. 2013. Microfluidic assisted self-assembly of chitosan based nanoparticles as drug delivery agents. *Lab Chip* 13:204–7.

Mao, H. Q., Roy, K., Troung-Le, V. L., et al. 2001. Chitosan-DNA nanoparticles as gene carriers: Synthesis, characterization and transfection efficiency. *J Control Release* 70:399–421.

Maurstad, G., Danielsen, S., Stokke, B. T. 2007. The influence of charge density of chitosan in the compaction of the polyanions DNA and xanthan. *Biomacromolecules* 8:1124–30.

Moran, M. C., Laranjeira, T., Ribeiro, A., Miguel, M. G., Lindman, B. 2009. Chitosan-DNA particles for DNA delivery: Effect of chitosan molecular weight on formation and release characteristics. *J Dispersion Sci Technol* 30:1494–9.

Noh, S. M., Park, M. O., Shim, G., et al. 2010. Pegylated poly-l-arginine derivatives of chitosan for effective delivery of siRNA. *J Control Release* 145:159–64.

Phillips, A. J. 2001. The challenge of gene therapy and DNA delivery. *J Pharm Pharmacol* 53:1169–74.

Ping, Y., Liu, C., Zhang, Z., Liu, K. L., Chen, J., Li, J. 2011. Chitosan-graft-(PEI-β-cyclodextrin) copolymers and their supramolecular PEGylation for DNA and siRNA delivery. *Biomaterials* 32:8328–41.

Plianwong, S., Opanasopit, P., Ngawhirunpat, T., Rojanarata, T. 2013. Chitosan combined with Poly-L-arginine as efficient, safe, and serum-insensitive vehicle with RNase protection ability for siRNA Delivery. *BioMed Res Int* 2013: 574136. http://dx.doi.org/10.1155/2013/574136.

Ragelle, H., Riva, R., Vandermeulen, G. 2014. Chitosan nanoparticles for siRNA delivery: Optimizing formulation to increase stability and efficiency. *J Control Release* 176:54–63.

Raja, M. A. G., Katas, H., Wen, T. J. 2015. Stability, intracellular delivery, and release of sirna from chitosan nanoparticles using different cross-linkers. *PLoS One* 10: e0128963. doi:10.1371/journal.pone.0128963.

Ribeiro, L. N., Alcantara, A. C., Darder, M., Aranda, P., Araujo-Moreira, F. M., Ruiz-Hitzky, E. 2014. Pectin-coated chitosan-LDH bionanocomposite beads as potential systems for colon-targeted drug delivery. *Int J Pharm* 463:1–9.

Rojanarata, T., Opanasopit, P., Techaarpornkul, S., Ngawhirunpat, T., Ruktanonchai, U. 2008. Chitosan-thiamine pyrophosphate as a novel carrier for siRNA delivery. *Pharm Res* 25:2807–14.

Safari, S., Zarrintan, M. H., Soleimani, M., et al. 2012. Evaluation and optimization of chitosan derivatives-based gene delivery system via kidney epithelial cells. *Adv Pharm Bull* 2:7–16.

Sailaja, A. K., Amareshwar, P., Chakarvarthy, P. 2011. Different techniques used for the preparation of nanoparticles using natural polymers and their application. *Int J Pharm Pharm Sci* 3:45–50.

Salva, E., Turan, S. O., Eren, F., Akbuga, J. 2014. The enhancement of gene silencing efficiency with chitosan-coated liposome formulations of siRNAs targeting HIF-1α and VEGF. *Int J Pharm* 478:147–54.

Saranya, N., Moorthi, A., Saravanan, S., Devi, M.P., Selvamurugan, N. 2011. Chitosan and its derivatives for gene delivery. *Int J Biol Macromol* 48:234–8.

Sato, T., Ishii, T., Okahata, Y. 2001. In vitro gene delivery mediated by chitosan. Effect of pH, serum, and molecular mass of chitosan on the transfection efficiency. *Biomaterials* 22:2075–80.

Sayari, E., Dinarvand, M., Amini, M., et al. 2014. MUC1 aptamer conjugated to chitosan nanoparticles, an efficient targeted carrier designed for anticancer SN38 delivery. *Int J Pharm* 473:304–15.

Shi, Q., Tiera, M. J., Zhang, X., Dai, K., Benderdour, M., Fernandes, J. C. 2011. Chitosan-dna/sirna nanoparticles for gene therapy, in *Non-viral Gene Therapy*, X. Yuan (Ed.), InTech. Available from: http://www.intechopen.com/books/non-viral-gene-therapy/chitosan-dna-sirna-nanoparticles-for-gene-therapy.

Simoes, S., Filipe, A., Faneca, H., et al. 2005. Cationic liposomes for gene delivery. *Expert Opin Drug Deliv* 2:237–54.

Singh, B., Choi, Y. J., Park, I. K., Akaike, T., Cho, C. S. 2014. Chemical modification of chitosan with pH-sensitive molecules and specific ligands for efficient DNA transfection and siRNA silencing. *J Nanosci Nanotechnol* 14:564–76.

Strand, S. P., Danielsen, S., Christensen, B. E., Vårum, K. M. 2005. Influence of chitosan structure on the formation and stability of DNA-chitosan polyelectrolyte complexes. *Biomacromolecules* 6:3357–66.

Thanou, M., Florea, B. I., Geldof, M., Junginger, H. E., Borchard, G. 2002. Quaternized chitosan oligomers as novel gene delivery vectors in epithelial cell lines. *Biomaterials* 23:153–9.

Thomas, C. E., Ehrhardt, A., Kay, M. A. 2003. Progress and problems with the use of viral vectors for gene therapy. *Nat Rev Genet* 4:346–58.

Tong, H., Qin, S., Fernandes, J. C., Li, L., Dai, K., Zhang, X. 2009. Progress and prospects of chitosan and its derivatives as non-viral gene vectors in gene therapy. *Curr Gene Ther* 9:495–502.

Tripathi, S. K., Goyal, R., Kumar, P., Gupta, K. C. 2012. Linear polyethylenimine-graft-chitosan copolymers as efficient DNA/siRNA delivery vectors in vitro and in vivo. *Nanomedicine* (Lond) 8:337–45.

Valencia, P. M., Farokhzad, O. C., Karnik, R., Langer, R. 2012. Microfluidic technologies for accelerating the clinical translation of nanoparticles. *Nat Nanotechnol* 7:623–9.

Wang, B., Zhang, S., Cui. S., et al. 2012. Chitosan enhanced gene delivery of cationic liposome via non-covalent conjugation. *Biotechnol Lett* 34:19–28.

Wang, J., Lu, Z., Wientjes, G., Au, J. L. S. 2010. Delivery of siRNA therapeutics: Barriers and carriers. *AAPS J* 12:492–503.

Yang, C., Gao, S., Kjems, J. 2014. Folic acid conjugated chitosan for targeted delivery of siRNA to activated macrophages *in vitro* and *in vivo*. *J Mater Chem B* 2: 8608–15.

Yhee, J. Y., Song, S., Lee, S. J., et al. 2015. Cancer-targeted MDR-1 siRNA delivery using self-cross-linked glycol chitosan nanoparticles to overcome drug resistance. *J Control Release* 198:1–9.

Yoon, H. Y., Son, S., Lee, S-J., et al. 2014. Glycol chitosan nanoparticles as specialized cancer therapeutic vehicles: Sequential delivery of doxorubicin and Bcl-2 siRNA. *Sci Rep* 4:6878.

Zhang, Y., Satterlee, A., Huang, L. 2012. In vivo gene delivery by nonviral vectors: Overcoming hurdles? *Mol Ther* 20:1298–304.

Zheng, Y., Cai, Z., Song, X., et al. 2009. Receptor mediated gene delivery by folate conjugated N-trimethyl chitosan in vitro. *Int J Pharm* 382:262–9.

Zheng, Y., Song, X., He, G., et al. 2011. Receptor-mediated gene delivery by folate-poly(ethylene glycol)-grafted-trimethyl chitosan in vitro. *J Drug Target* 19:647–56.

14 Role of Alginate in Drug Delivery Applications

Sougata Jana, Kalyan Kumar Sen, Arijit Gandhi,
Subrata Jana, and Chandrani Roy

CONTENTS

14.1   INTRODUCTION

The release of drugs from an appropriate dosage form at definite time intervals and at predetermined rates is considered as a major challenge among formulation scientists, and, although significant advances have been made in recent years in the area of controlled/modified drug release, many objectives still need to be achieved for successful drug delivery. An ideal drug delivery system should be prepared in such a manner that it reduces dosing frequency to an extent that once daily dose is sufficient for therapeutic management through uniform plasma concentration providing maximum utility of drug with reduction in local and systemic side effects and cure or control condition in the shortest possible time by using the smallest quantity of drug to assure greater patient compliance. In recent years, natural polysaccharides have been extensively used in biomedical and pharmaceutical applications to optimize drug targeting and/or release rate. This is because they are usually abundant, in most cases available from renewable sources, and have a large variety of composition and properties that may allow appropriately tailored chemical modifications, and also due to their sustainability, biodegradability, and biosafety (Coviello et al. 2007, Jana et al. 2011, Liu et al. 2013).

Among the natural polysaccharides, alginate, a naturally occurring anionic polymer typically obtained from brown seaweed, is one of particular interest for a broad range of applications as a biomaterial and especially as the supporting matrix or delivery system and tissue repair and regeneration. Due to its outstanding properties in terms of biocompatibility, biodegradability, non-antigenicity, and chelating ability, alginate has been widely used in a variety of biomedical applications and tissue engineering. As a result of the naturally occurring polysaccharide, alginate exhibits a pH-dependent anionic nature and has the ability to interact with cationic polyelectrolytes and proteoglycans. Therefore, delivery systems for cationic drugs and molecules can be obtained through simple electrostatic interactions. Alginate can be easily modified via chemical and physical reactions to obtain derivatives having various structures, properties, functions, and applications. Tuning the structure and properties such as biodegradability, mechanical strength, gelation property, and cell affinity can be achieved through combination with other biomaterials, immobilization of specific ligands such as peptide and sugar molecules, and physical or chemical cross-linking (Williams 2009, Stevens et al. 2004, Kuo and Ma 2001, Lee and Mooney 2012).

For these reasons, researchers are exploring possible applications of alginates as coating materials for preparation of drug delivery systems such as micro- and nanoparticles, beads, pellets, gels, fibers, and membranes, and also in wound healing, cartilage repair, and bone regeneration.

14.2 STRUCTURE OF ALGINATE

Alginate, a naturally occurring anionic and hydrophilic polysaccharide, contains blocks of (1–4)-linked β-D-mannuronic acid (M) and α-L-guluronic acid (G) monomers (Figure 14.1).

Typically, the blocks are composed of three different forms of polymer segments: consecutive G residues, consecutive M residues, and alternating MG residues. It was seen that alginate could be regarded as a true block composed of homopolymeric regions of M and G, termed M and G blocks, respectively, interspersed with regions of alternating structure (Narayanan et al. 2012, Skjak-Braerk et al. 1989).

Different seaweeds give rise to varying ratios of M, G, and MG groups within the alginic acid, with seasonal changes in the ratio of M and G groups also seen within species. Alginate solutions will react with many divalent or trivalent cations to form gels, with the nature of the gel strongly dependent upon the mix of M, G, and MG groups in the alginate. Alginates that are high in M groups have

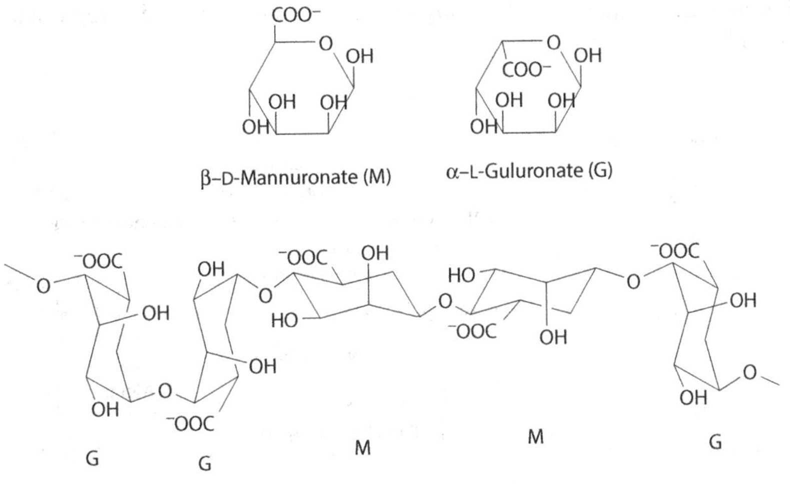

FIGURE 14.1 Chemical structure of G, M, and alternating blocks in alginate.

a flat ribbon-like molecular appearance, whereas areas high in G groups have a much more buckled chain shape. These differences in the molecular appearance affect gel formation: high M alginates form gels quicker, which are softer and more elastic than those produced by G-rich alginates that hold calcium and form gels slowly. G-rich alginates form gels slowly as the buckled shape acts as an *egg box* in which the calcium ions are packed and held strongly (chelated) by the structure of the tetrahydropyran ring of the α-L-guluronic acid monomer and the presence of hydroxyl oxygen atoms (Lee and Mooney 2012, Pawar and Edgar 2012, Lee and Yuk 2007).

14.3 BIOSYNTHESIS OF ALGINATES AND METHOD OF MANUFACTURE

Alginate biosynthesis (Figure 14.2) involves the oxidation of a carbon source to acetyl coenzyme A, which enters the tricarboxylic acid (TCA) cycle to be converted into fructose-6-phosphate via gluconeogenesis. Fructose-6-phosphate then undergoes a series of biosynthetic transformations to be eventually converted into GDP-mannuronic acid, which acts as a precursor to alginate synthesis. GDP-mannuronic acid is polymerized to polymannuronic acid followed by periplasmic transfer. Polymannuronic acid is acetylated at the O-2 and/or O-3 positions by several transacetylases. Epimerization is then performed by a family of epimerase enzymes to convert some nonacetylated M residues into G residues. Finally, alginate is released from the cell through transmembrane porins (Hay et al. 2010, Remminghorst and Rehm 2006).

Alginate is extracted for commercial purposes from various species of kelp, or brown algae, including *Laminaria hyperborean, Ascophyllum nodosum*, and *Macrocystis pyrifera*. Alginates occur in brown algae in the intracellular matrix as gels containing sodium, calcium, magnesium, strontium, and barium ions, such that the counterion composition is determined by the ion-exchange equilibrium with seawater. A schematic of the alginate extraction procedure is represented in Figure 14.3.

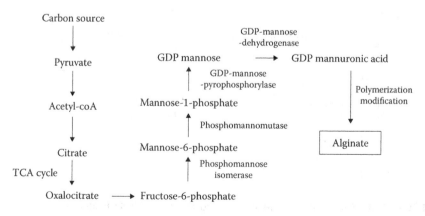

FIGURE 14.2 Biosynthetic pathway of alginate.

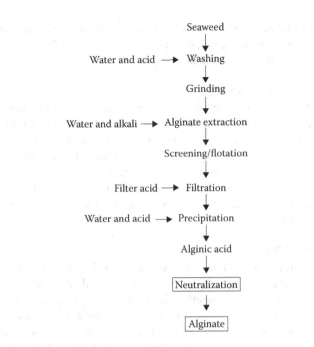

FIGURE 14.3 Extraction process of alginate.

The first step in the extraction process is removal of the counterions by proton exchange using mineral acid. Then insoluble alginic acid is solubilized by neutralization with alkali such as sodium carbonate or sodium hydroxide to form sodium alginate. Rigorous separation processes such as sifting, flotation, centrifugation, and filtration follow in order to remove particulate matter. Sodium alginate is then precipitated directly by alcohol, calcium chloride, or a mineral acid. The product is dried and milled. Alginates obtained using the described procedure contain several mitogens and cytotoxic impurities making them unsuitable for biomedical applications. Ultrapure and amitogenic alginates that are suitable for biomedical purposes have therefore been prepared using more rigorous extraction processes. Free flow electrophoresis was applied as one technique to remove mitogenic impurities from commercial alginates (Zimmermann et al. 1992).

14.4 PROPERTIES OF ALGINATE

14.4.1 PHYSICAL PROPERTIES

14.4.1.1 Solubility
The solubility of alginates in water is governed by three parameters: (1) pH of the solvent, (2) ionic strength of the medium, and (3) presence of gelling ions in the solvent. To make alginates soluble, it is essential that the pH be above a certain critical value and the carboxylic acid groups be deprotonated. The solubility of alginates depends strongly on the state of the backbone carboxylic acid groups. Alginic acid

with its carboxylic acid groups in their protonated form is not fully soluble in any solvent system examined, including water. Na-alginate dissolves in water, but it is not entirely soluble in any organic medium examined.

14.4.1.2 Ionic Cross-Linking

Alginate chelates with divalent cations to form hydrogels. Gel formation is driven by the interactions between G blocks that associate to form tightly held junctions in the presence of divalent cations (Sikorski et al. 2007). In addition to G blocks, MG blocks also participate, forming weak junctions (Donati et al. 2005). Thus, alginates with high G contents yield stronger gels. The affinity of alginates toward divalent ions decreases in the following order: Pb > Cu > Cd > Ba > Sr > Ca > Co, Ni, Zn > Mn (Morch et al. 2006). Ca^{2+} however, is the most commonly used cation to induce alginate gel formation.

14.4.1.3 Gel Formation

A controlled introduction of cross-linking ions is made possible by two fundamental methods for preparing alginate gel: (1) *diffusion* method, in which cross-linking ions diffuse into the alginate solution from an outside reservoir; and (2) *internal setting* method, in which the ion source is located within the alginate solution and a controlled trigger (typically pH or solubility of the ion source) sets off the release of cross-linking ions into solution. The diffusion method yields gels having an ion concentration gradient across the thickness, whereas the internal setting gives gels with uniform ion concentrations throughout (Skjåk-Bræk et al. 1989).

14.4.1.4 Molecular Weight

The molecular weights of commercially available sodium alginates range between 32,000 and 400,000 g/mol. Increasing the molecular weight of alginate can improve the physical properties of resultant gels. However, an alginate solution formed from high-molecular-weight polymer becomes greatly viscous, which is often undesirable in processing. For example, proteins or cells mixed with an alginate solution of high-viscosity risk damage from the high shear forces generated during mixing and injection into the body (LeRoux et al. 1999, Kong et al. 2003).

14.4.2 CHEMICAL PROPERTIES

Alginate undergoes hydrolytic cleavage under acidic conditions, which involves protonation of the glycosidic oxygen. Sodium alginate in the form of dry powder can be stored without degradation in a cool, dry place and away from sunlight for several months. Its shelf life can be extended to several years by storing it in the freezer. Alginic acid degrades more rapidly than the sodium salt form. The enzymatic degradation of alginates by lyase occurs by a β-elimination mechanism resulting in unsaturated compounds. A similar degradation route is followed when they are subjected to strongly alkaline environments. The rate of degradation increases rapidly above pH 10.0 and below pH 5.0. Above a pH of 10.0, the degradation arises mostly from the β-elimination mechanism, whereas below a pH of 5.0, the degradation is mostly due to acid-catalyzed hydrolysis. Alginates are susceptible to chain degradation not only in the presence of acids or bases, but also at neutral pH values in the presence of reducing compounds. Alginates derived from brown algae contain varying amounts of phenolic compounds, depending on the algal species. The rate of degradation in species containing a higher quantity of phenolics was shown to be much greater (Pawar and Edgar 2012).

14.4.3 BIOLOGICAL PROPERTIES

14.4.3.1 Immunogenicity

Research into the immunogenicity of alginate polymer has brought together a consensus that the chemical composition and the mitogenic contaminants found in alginate are the two main reasons for reported immunogenicity. Alginate polymer comes in many different grades commercially, including food or research grade and ultrapure medicinal grade. It has been shown that the impurities found in commercial alginate are responsible for the side effects observed, including cytokine release and inflammatory reactions. However, it is also proven that pure alginate does not contain these impurities and therefore does not induce any side effects. In addition, researchers have proven that there is a correlation between the level of mannuronic acid blocks and cytokine production (Otterlei et al. 1991); therefore, it is recommended that pure alginate rich in α-L-gluronic acid is used for *in vivo* research to avoid inflammatory reactions (Spargo et al. 1994).

14.4.3.2 Bioadhesion

Alginate polymer has a very strong bioadhesive property, which again makes it a viable candidate for mucosal delivery. With carboxyl end groups, alginate is classified as an anionic mucoadhesive polymer. Research has shown that polymers with charge density are strong mucoadhesive agents (Chickering and Mathiowitz et al. 1995). It is believed that penetration of the polymer chain across a polymer–mucosa interface is responsible for the great adhesion (Jabari et al. 1993). Alginate has proven to have the greatest mucoadhesive strength compared with other polymers, including polystyrene, chitosan, carboxy-methylcellulose, and poly (lactic acid). Alginate's strong bioadhesive properties will serve to localize the drug upon release, and therefore would potentially improve the overall drug effectiveness with mucosal delivery.

14.4.3.3 Biocompatibility

Biocompatibility of alginate has been extensively evaluated *in vitro* as well as *in vivo*. However, this property is affected by varying levels of purity in the alginate For example, it has been reported that high M content alginates were immunogenic and approximately 10 times more potent in inducing cytokine production compared with high G alginates (Otterlei et al. 1991). Alginate purified by a multistep extraction procedure to a very high purity did not induce any significant foreign body reaction when implanted into animals (Orive et al. 2002). Similarly, no significant inflammatory response was observed when gels formed from commercially available, highly purified alginates have been subcutaneously injected into mice (Lee and Lee 2009).

14.5 CHEMICAL MODIFICATION OF ALGINATE FOR SUCCESSFUL DRUG DELIVERY

14.5.1 COVALENT CHEMICAL MODIFICATIONS

1-Ethyl-(dimethylaminopropyl) carbodiimide (EDC) as a water-soluble carbodiimide, is widely used to couple carboxylic groups on alginates with molecules containing primary or secondary amines as well as dihydrazides (Gomez et al. 2006) (Figure 14.4).

N-Hydroxysulfosuccinimide (sulfo-NHS) is used as a stabilizer. Hybrid of sodium alginate with other biopolymers would widen the field of applications; such type of products that have shown improved swelling and barrier properties. Alginate beads with ionic properties were synthesized through the conjugation reaction of alginate and tyramine (a monoamine compound derived from the amino acid tyrosine) (Sakai and Kawakami 2007). The mucoadhesive properties of alginate can be improved by the covalent attachment of cysteine (Schnürch et al. 2001). In addition to the improvement in adhesive properties, the swelling behavior and cohesive properties are also improved, making alginate a useful excipient for various dosage forms such as matrix tablets and microparticles, providing an improved stability of the drug delivery system and a prolonged residence time on mucosal tissues (Schnürch et al. 2001).

14.5.2 HYDROPHOBICALLY MODIFIED ALGINATE

Amphiphilic derivatives of sodium alginate, prepared by chemical covalent binding of long alkyl chains onto the polysaccharide backbone via ester functions, form strong hydrogels in aqueous solutions (Leonard et al. 2004). Microparticles were prepared from this hydrophobic alginate by dispersion in sodium chloride solutions. Model proteins, such as bovine serum albumin (BSA), human hemoglobin, and a vaccine protein (*Helicobacter pylori*) urease, were incorporated in this matrix and the release was studied. Encapsulation yields were found to be very high (70%–100%)

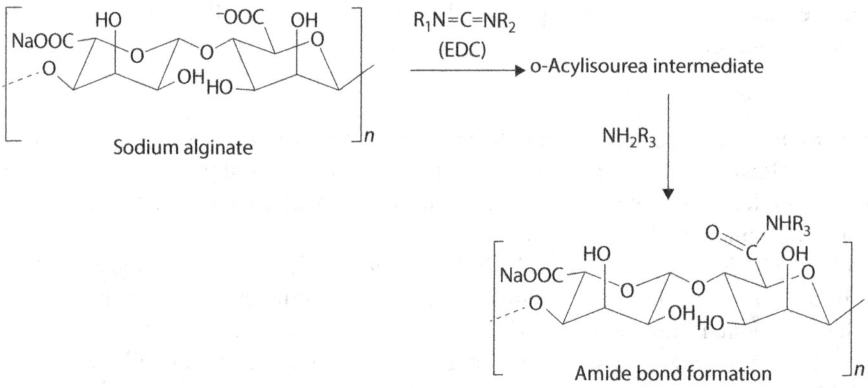

FIGURE 14.4   Mechanism of amide bond formation in the presence of EDC.

in all cases and a highly controlled release protein was obtained. Another study reported the synthesis of hydrophobically modified alginate (Alg-CONH-C8) by coupling n-octylamine to the backbone carboxylic acid groups using 1-ethyl-3-(3-dimethylaminopropyl) carbodiimide hydrochloride (Galant et al. 2006).

14.5.3 PHOSPHORYLATION OF ALGINATES

Recently, the synthesis of phosphorylated alginate derivatives has gained attention. Phosphorylation was performed using urea/phosphoric acid reagent by creating a suspension of alginate in dimethylformamide (Figure 14.5).

Phosphoric acid as a strong acid causes alginate molecular weight degradation. Accordingly, a two- to fourfold reduction in the value of molecular weight was reported for phosphorylated alginates compared to unreacted alginates. It was found that these phosphorylated alginates were found to be incapable of forming Ca-cross-linked ionic gels. The reduction of molecular weight during reaction and conformational changes resulting from phosphorylation were responsible for the inability of these alginate derivatives to form gels. However, Ca-cross-linked gels could be formed by blending unreacted alginate with phosphorylated alginate. Such gels formed using alginate blends showed higher resistance to calcium extraction compared to gels formed using only unreacted alginates (Coleman et al. 2011).

14.5.4 SULFATION OF ALGINATES

Sulfation of polysaccharides can provide blood compatibility and anticoagulant activity. Ronghua et al. first reported the sulfation of sodium alginate using chlorosulfonic acid in formamide. Sulfates with degree of substitution up to 1.41 were obtained. The anticoagulant activity of alginate sulfates was measured using activated partial thrombosis time (APTT), thrombin time (TT) and prothrombin time (PT). Using APTT, the anticoagulant activity of alginate sulfate was found to be comparable to heparin. However, using PT, the activity was very low. Alginate sulfates were found to have a greater influence on the intrinsic coagulation pathway. It is seen that oversulfation is undesirable because it can cause side effects. Therefore, to decrease the anticoagulant activity, alginate sulfates were reacted with 2,3-epoxypropyl trimethylammonium chloride to attach pendent quaternary amine groups. The number of quaternary ammonium groups attached was controlled by the moles of the epoxy reagent added. The reduction of activity was proportional to the number of quaternary ammonium groups attached (Ronghua et al. 2003). Common

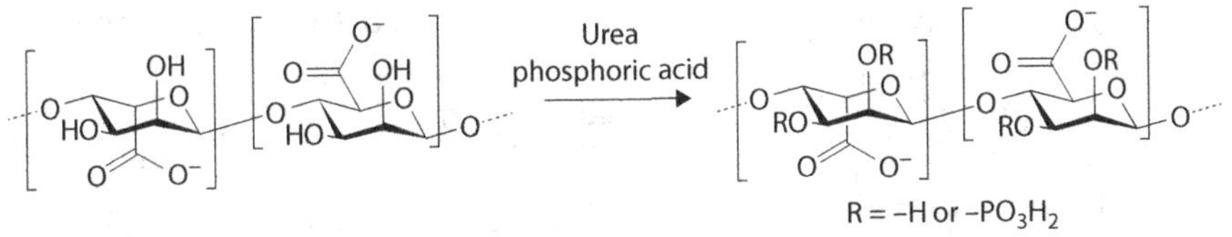

FIGURE 14.5 Phosphorylation of alginate.

sulfation reagents such as sulfuric acid, chlorosulfonic acid, sulfuryl chloride, sulfur trioxide, and sulfamic acid cause hydrolytic degradation of alginates. To overcome this limitation Fan et al. reported the sulfation of alginates by an uncommon reagent prepared using sodium bisulfite and sodium nitrite in an aqueous medium. The reaction was performed in water, wherein the sulfation reagent was first adjusted to the desired pH followed by addition of sodium alginates. An optimum DS value of 1.87 was achieved at pH 9.0, 40°C and 2:1 mole ratio of reagent:uronic acid residue. Anticoagulant activities for the sulfated alginate derivatives were measured. DS, molecular weight, and concentration were found to be the influential factors for anticoagulant activity (Fan et al. 2011).

14.5.5 OXIDATION OF ALGINATE

The introduction of aldehydic groups, more reactive than hydroxyl or carboxylic ones, into sodium alginate via periodate oxidation represents a selected approach to activate the polysaccharide for the successive chemical modifications (Balakrishnan et al. 2005). Periodate oxidation selectively cleaves the vicinal glycols in polysaccharides to form their dialdehyde derivatives (Figure 14.6).

The reaction proceeds with a significant depolymerization of alginate. Depolymerization mainly depends on the primary structure; as a matter of fact, the oxidation is still more degradative when the content of mannuronic and guluronic alternating blocks (MG blocks) is high, as chain scission preferentially takes place at atypical sugar units.

14.5.6 GRAFTING OF ALGINATE

Grafting provides a method of adding certain desirable properties to a polysaccharide without greatly disturbing the strength and other mechanical properties of the polysaccharide. Graft copolymerization usually is accomplished by generating radical sites on the first polymer backbone onto which the monomer of the second polymer is copolymerized. An important advantage of graft polymerization is that the grafted polymer chains are held together by chemical bonding, allowing the two polymers to be intimately associated. The polymer that is grafted is expected to be distributed on the backbone of the substrate polymer and also to impart the beneficial effects on its properties. The grafting of poly(acrylic acid) onto an alginate gives a superabsorbent hydrogel. Poly(N-vinyl-2-pyrrolidone)-grafted sodium alginate hydrogel was used for oral controlled delivery of indomethacin drugs (Isıklan et al. 2008). Partially hydrolyzed

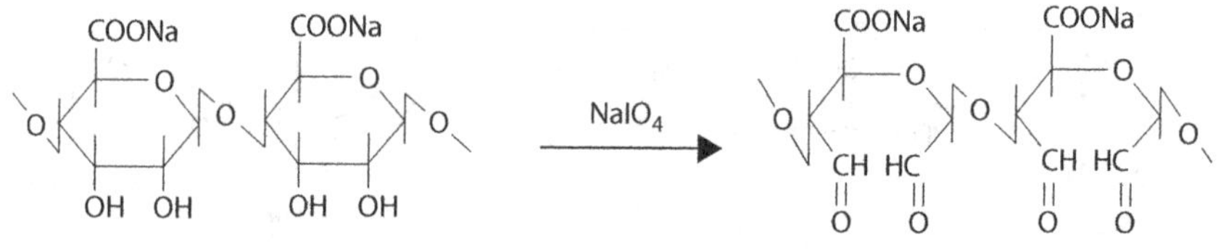

FIGURE 14.6 Periodate oxidation of alginate.

cross-linked alginate-*graft*-polymethacrylamide as a novel biopolymer-based super-absorbent hydrogel having pH-responsive properties (Pourjavadi et al. 2005).

14.5.7   CROSS-LINKING OF ALGINATE

Cross-linked alginate has more capacity to retain the entrapped drugs, and also it shows a more controlled release profile of entrapped drugs. Polymeric blend beads of poly(vinyl alcohol) with sodium alginate were prepared by cross-linking with glutaraldehyde and were used to deliver diclofenac sodium (Sanli et al. 2007), and the authors observed a decrease in the rate of drug release with increasing poly(vinyl alcohol)-to-sodium alginate ratio, drug-to-polymer ratio, and the extent of cross-linking. Poly(ion complex) membrane made by blending chitosan and sodium alginate biopolymers followed by cross-linking with glutaraldehyde was tested for the separation of ethanol–water mixtures (Kanti et al. 2004). Cellulose/alginate blend membranes were successfully cross-linked by Ca^{2+} bridge in 5% $CaCl_2$ (Yang et al. 2000).

14.5.8   PHYSICAL MODIFICATION

This is basically done by mixing or blending the parent polysaccharides with suitable substrates which may be a monomer or an oligomer or even a polysaccharide/polymer. In these cases, the change in the characteristics is brought about not by breaking and/or forming chemical bonds but by virtue of association of compounds facilitated by weak forces (van der Waals forces) and hydrogen bonds as well as charge transfer complexes imparting supramolecular structural orientations. Carbohydrate polymeric blend microspheres of sodium alginate and methylcellulose were prepared for controlled release of nifedipine (Ramesh Babu et al. 2007). In 2008, Rinaudo described some important biomedical applications of alginate blends. One of the applications described in the review involved the thermosensitive gel of calcium alginate and poly(*N*-isopropylacrylamide) (PNIPAAm). The characteristic lower critical solution temperature (LCST) of this blend was tailored to be close to human body temperature by controlling the amount of *N*-isopropylacrylamide and calcium alginate during the synthesis (Rinaudo 2008). Donati et al. (2007) reported the preparation of alginate and a lactose-modified chitosan mixture under physiological conditions and at a semidilute concentration avoiding associative phase separation (Donati et al. 2007).

14.6   METHOD OF PREPARATION OF ALGINATE PARTICLES

14.6.1   ALGINATE HYDROGELS

Hydrogels are three-dimensionally cross-linked networks composed of hydrophilic polymers with high water content. Alginate hydrogels can be formed using chemical or physical cross-linking strategies, ionic methods being the most widely used. Alginate is typically used in the form of a hydrogel in biomedicine, including wound healing, drug delivery, and tissue engineering applications. An overview of some of the cross-linking strategies is provided in Sections 14.6.1.1 through 14.6.1.4.

14.6.1.1 Ionic Cross-Linking

The most commonly used method to prepare hydrogels from an aqueous alginate solution is to combine the solution with ionic cross-linking agents. Cross-linking is achieved through the exchange of sodium ions from guluronic acid units with divalent cations such as calcium (Ca^{2+}), strontium (Sr^{2+}), and barium (Ba^{2+}) (Morch et al. 2006). The guluronate blocks of one polymer then form junctions with the guluronate blocks of adjacent polymer chains in what is termed the egg-box model of cross-linking, resulting in a gel structure (Figure 14.7).

Calcium chloride ($CaCl_2$) is one of the most frequently used agents to ionically cross-link alginate. Ionic cross-linking of alginate can be further obtained by external or internal gelation. External gelation of alginate hydrogels uses soluble salts of divalent cations, such as calcium chloride ($CaCl_2$), as an ionic cross-linker. It is a very simple process that provides an immediate and nontoxic cell entrapment. This method is commonly used to obtain gel beads by dripping a sodium alginate solution into an aqueous solution of calcium ions. However, it typically leads to rapid and poorly controlled gelation due to its high solubility in aqueous solutions (Lee and Mooney 2012).

Internal gelation strategies are being widely investigated with a view to promoting *in situ* hydrogel formation. The most common strategy for promoting the internal gelation of alginate hydrogels consists in using divalent cation salts of low solubility, which enable the gelation rate to be slowed down and hence afford better control over the gelation time. Calcium carbonate ($CaCO_3$) and calcium sulfate ($CaSO_4$) have been widely used for this purpose. They have low solubility in pure water at neutral pH, but are soluble under acidic conditions, allowing their uniform distribution in the alginate solution before gelation occurs. For example, an alginate solution can be mixed with $CaCO_3$, which is not soluble in water at neutral pH. Glucono-δ-lactone is then added to the alginate/$CaCO_3$ mixture in order to dissociate Ca^{2+} from the $CaCO_3$ by lowering the pH. The released Ca^{2+} subsequently initiates the gelation of the alginate solution in a more gradual manner (Crow and Nelson 2006, Oliveira et al. 2008).

The gelation rate is a critical factor in controlling gel uniformity and strength when using divalent cations, and slower gelation produces more uniform structures and greater mechanical integrity (Kuo and Ma 2001). The gelation temperature also influences the gelation rate and the resultant mechanical properties of the gels. At lower temperatures, the reactivity of ionic cross-linkers (e.g., Ca^{2+}) is reduced, and cross-linking becomes slower.

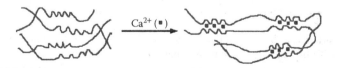

FIGURE 14.7   Alginate hydrogels prepared by ionic cross-linking (egg-box model).

14.6.1.2 Covalent Cross-Linking

Covalent cross-linking of alginate hydrogels can be achieved by a variety of different methods and usually provides more stable and mechanically stronger gels than ionic cross-linking (Zhao et al. 2010). Covalent cross-linking of alginate with poly(ethylene glycol)-diamines of various molecular weights was first investigated in order to prepare gels with a wide range of the mechanical properties (Eiselt et al. 1999). The use of multifunctional cross-linking molecules to form hydrogels provides a wider range and tighter control over degradation rates and mechanical stiffness than bifunctional cross-linking molecules. For example, the physical properties and degradation behavior of poly(aldehyde guluronate) gels prepared with either poly(acrylamide-*co*-hydrazide) as a multifunctional cross-linker or adipic acid dihydrazide as a bifunctional cross-linker were monitored *in vitro* (Lee et al. 2004).

14.6.1.3 Thermal Gelation

Thermo-sensitive hydrogels have been widely investigated to date in many drug delivery applications, due to their adjustable swelling properties in response to temperature changes, leading to on-demand modulation of drug release from the gels. PNIPAAm hydrogels are the most extensively exploited thermo-sensitive gels, and these undergo a reversible phase transition near body temperature in aqueous media (lower critical solution temperature near 32°C). Graft copolymerization of NIPAAm onto the alginate backbone after reaction with ceric ions also provides a useful means to prepare temperature-responsive alginate gels, with sensitivity near body temperature (Roy et al. 2010, Rzaev et al. 2007).

14.6.1.4 Cell Cross-Linking

Specific receptor–ligand interactions have been employed to cross-link alginate hydrogels. They exhibit good biocompatibility. The strategy of cell cross-linking is to introduce ligands, for example, arginine–glycine–aspartic acid (Arg–Gly–Asp, RGD) sequence, onto alginate for cell adhesion by chemical coupling utilizing water-soluble carbodiimide chemistry. Once mammalian cells have been added to this RGD-modified alginate to form a uniform dispersion within the solution, the receptors on the cell surface can bind to ligands of the modified alginate. The RGD-modified alginate solution has been subsequently cross-linked to form network structures via specific receptor–ligand interactions between cell surface and RGD sequences. Although the cell-cross-linked hydrogel shows excellent bioactivities, the network exhibits low strength and toughness, which may limit its practical applications (Lee et al. 2003, Koo et al. 2002).

14.6.2 ALGINATE-BASED INTERPENETRATING POLYMER NETWORKS AND SEMI-INTERPENETRATING POLYMER NETWORKS

An interpenetrating polymer network (IPN) is a composition of at least two polymers, exhibiting varied characteristics, which is obtained when at least one polymer network is synthesized or cross-linked independently in the immediate presence of the other (Myung et al. 2008). On account of high versatility and tailorable mechanical properties of alginate, alginate has been used as one of the most studied building blocks of interpenetrating polymer networks.

14.6.2.1 Temperature-Responsive Alginate IPNs

Thermosensitive polymers have been frequently combined with alginate to yield (semi)-IPNs. These *smart* materials, which are characterized by rapid responses to thermal stimuli, undergo a transition from a hydrophilic to a more hydrophobic material triggered by small changes in environmental temperature. The hydrophilic/hydrophobic (sol/gel) transition is usually reversible, meaning that the material returns to its original initial state by a temperature variation in the opposite direction. For example, IPNs composed of pNIPAAm and alginate have been most frequently used for this purpose (Figure 14.8).

In a study, Muniz et al. studied the effect of temperature on the mechanical properties and permeability of semi-IPNs and IPNs membranes composed of chemically cross-linked pNIPAAm and physically calcium-cross-linked alginate. The authors evaluated the IPN hydrogel strength and observed a synergism of the mechanical performances of the alginate and pNIPAAm networks, both below and above the LCST. The effect was more pronounced above the LCST where the hydrogel uniaxial compressive modulus was much higher than that of plain alginate and pNIMAAm hydrogels (De Moura et al. 2005). Semi-IPNs based on alginate and cellulose derivatives, that is, hydrophobically modified ethyl hydroxyethyl cellulose or hydroxypropyl methyl cellulose, prepared using an emulsification method, were also used for the controlled release of BSA as a model protein and the polysaccharide drug heparin (Nochos et al. 2008, Karewicz et al. 2010). In another study, IPNs were formed by dropping an aqueous solution of alginate, NIPAAm, and the chemical cross-linker N,N'-bis(acryloyl)cystamine into an aqueous $CaCl_2$ and radical polymerization initiator solution, thus immediately and simultaneously the physical gelation of alginate and the polymerization and chemical cross-linking of NIPAAm occurred. The formed beads had a higher concentration of alginate hydrogel on the outer part compared to the core, because the diffusion of Ca^{2+} ions into the droplets is slowed down as the gelation occurs, whereas pNIPAAm was more abundant in the inner core of the beads where reactants were confined during the formation of the beads. Consequently, the resulting IPN was inhomogeneous and could be microscopically visualized by raising the temperature above the LCST of pNIPAAm. Actually, when the temperature was raised up to 37°C, the pNIPAAm network collapsed evidencing the formation of beads with a core–shell structure (Park and Choi 1998).

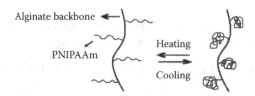

FIGURE 14.8   The temperature-dependent behavior of PNIPAAm-*g*-alginate hydrogels.

14.6.2.2   pH-Responsive Alginate IPNs

Electrolyte and ampholyte polymers can exhibit a sol/gel transition in response to environmental pH changes. A pH sensitive semi-IPN hydrogel was developed by Chen et al., which involved the development of a chemical network that was obtained by cross-linking *N,O*-carboxymethyl chitosan with genipin in the presence of alginate. The obtained semi-IPNs were stable and their swelling was dependent on both pH and polymer concentration. As a result, also the release of an entrapped model protein (BSA) was affected by environmental pH (Chen et al. 2004). Shi et al. studied the effect of pH and temperature on the release of indomethacin, a nonsteroidal anti-inflammatory drug, from semi-IPN beads based on Ca-alginate and pNIPAAm. At pH 2.1 and 37°C, the drug was mainly retained in the beads and less than 10% of the drug was released in 7°hour (burst release), whereas it was fully released within 3 hour at pH 7.4. Also the temperature influenced the drug delivery profiles of the same gel, leading to a faster release at 37°C than at 25°C (Shi et al. 2006). Methoxy poly(ethylene glycol)-grafted carboxymethyl chitosan (mPEG-*g*-CMC) and alginate were chosen as the constituents of hydrogel beads for the construction of a pH-responsive interpenetrating polymer network matrix. A contrast study between the mPEG-*g*-CMC hydrogel and mPEG physically mixed with CMC hydrogel was carried out. BSA as a model for a protein drug was encapsulated in the hydrogel network, and the drug release properties were studied. The hydrogels prepared by these two methods maintained good pH sensitivity; the loading capacity of the mPEG-*g*-CMC/alginate hydrogel was enhanced in comparison with that of the hydrogel prepared by physically mixing mPEG. The burst release of the protein was slightly decreased at pH 1.2, whereas the release at pH 7.4 was improved, suggesting that the mPEG-*g*-CMC/alginate pH-sensitive hydrogel will be promising for a site-specific protein drug delivery in the intestine (Yang et al. 2013).

14.6.3   ALGINATE MICROPARTICLES

Alginate is one of the most commonly used polymers for the formation of (micro) particles. Several methods have been developed to form alginate microparticles of various size ranges. The majority of these methods are based on an external gelation method, where an alginate solution is added dropwise to a bath containing cation, such as in a $CaCl_2$ solution. The material to be encapsulated is often mixed with the alginate solution prior to particle formation and gelation. Alginate can also interact with cationic polymers, such as chitosan, and form a polyelectrolyte complex. Hence, alginate capsules can also be obtained by dripping an alginate solution in a bath containing a cationic polymer (Kailasapathy 2002, Sugiura et al. 2005).

Alginates can readily form gel and solid microspheres methods to be made as delivery systems. Basically, alginate gel spheres are prepared under aqueous conditions via ionic cross-linking, and they are suitable for encapsulation of cells, growth factors, and bioactive proteins. Compared to the gel spheres, alginate solid spheres can be fabricated by emulsion solvent evaporation techniques, which are mainly used to load drugs. Both alginate-based gel and solid microspheres show good biocompatibilities when they are used for regenerative medicine. Drugs can be mixed with the alginate solution evenly, and the mixture should then be emulsified under sonication.

Drug-loaded alginate microspheres can be fabricated by adding the mixture drop-wise to an organic emulsion with constant stirring. The alginate-based carriers can protect drugs from degradation and may improve plasma half-time to ensure transport and release of drugs. In addition to carrying drugs, the alginate-based solid microspheres can also be used as cell microcarriers, another kind of injectable cell scaffold for tissue engineering (Basmanav et al. 2008, Man et al. 2012).

In a study, Ching et al. carried out the pH-dependent adsorption of sodium caseinate onto the surface of micron-sized calcium alginate microgel particles (20–80 µm). z-Potential measurements and protein assay results suggested that protein adsorption occurred due to electrostatic complexation between sodium caseinate and calcium alginate and was pH dependent. Confocal laser scanning and fluorescence microscopy confirmed the presence of protein layer on the surface of alginate microgel particles at pH 3 and 4. Micrographs from transmission electron microscopy revealed a protein coating with a thickness of ~206–240 nm on the gel particle surfaces (Ching et al. 2015). In another study, galactosylated alginate (GA)–chitosan oligomer microcapsule was prepared to provide a sufficient mechanical stability, a selective permeability, and an appropriate three-dimensional (3D) microenvironment for hepatocyte microencapsulation. The stable microcapsule was obtained when GA was lower than 50%, whereas the permeability was increased with an increase of GA. A balance between mechanical stability and permeability was achieved through modulating membrane porosity and thickness. The optimal microcapsule displays a selective permeability allowing an efficient transport of human serum albumin while effectively blocking immunoglobulin G (Tian et al. 2014).

Soni et al. prepared spherical microspheres of theophylline (TP) using sodium alginate to prolong the release. It was observed that the mean particle size of the microspheres increased with an increase in the concentration of polymer. The entrapment efficiency was found to be in the range of 70%–93%. Optimized alginate microspheres were found to possess good sphericity, size, and adequate entrapment efficiency. The *in vitro* release studies were carried out in pH progression media (pH 1.2, 2.5, 4.5, 7, and 7.4 solutions). Results indicated that the percentage of drug release decreased with an increased alginate concentration. TP-loaded alginate microspheres showed extended *in vitro* drug release; thus, the use of microspheres potentially offers a sustained release profile along with improved delivery of TP (Soni et al. 2010). Recently, a novel method called melt coaxial electrospray has been used to produce phase change material (PCM) microcapsules with sodium alginate as the shell and *n*-nonadecane as the core. The effect of production parameters on microcapsule size and structure was studied. The results of Fourier transform infrared spectroscopy and differential scanning calorimetry confirmed the successful melt coaxial electrospraying of PCMs. Careful control of production parameters yielded spherical PCM microcapsules with a diameter lower than 100 µm and a 56% ± 5% encapsulation ratio (Moghaddam et al. 2015). Microparticles containing sunflower oil were produced by ionic gelation using a 1:1 alginate:pectin mixture and were electrostatically coated with whey and egg white proteins. Emulsions of the polysaccharide mixture and the protein solutions were evaluated in terms of their zeta potentials. High encapsulation efficiency (87.6% at pH 3.5 and 90.8% at pH 3.75) was obtained for the microparticles. For the microparticles, an increase in the protein content in solution yielded an increase in the protein content adsorbed, independent of the type of protein used. When 4% protein in solution was used, protein adsorption onto the microparticles (59.2% for whey protein and 45.5% for egg white protein) was significantly higher likely due to the smaller amount of calcium present on the microparticles and the larger surface area of the particles (Aguilar et al. 2015). Bera et al. developed floating–mucoadhesive oil-entrapped alginate beads coated with crosss-linked alginate–sterculiagum gel membrane for gastroretentive risperidone delivery. Oil-entrapped alginate beads containing risperidone as the core were prepared by the ionotropic gelation technique. The biopolymeric-coated optimized beads exhibited an excellent buoyancy, better *ex vivo* mucoadhesion, and slower drug release rate (Bera et al. 2015).

14.6.4 ALGINATE NANOPARTICLES

Nanoaggregates, nanocapsules, and nanospheres are nanosized systems with diameters generally ranging from 10 to 1000 nm in size. These systems can hold enzymes, drugs, and other compounds by dissolving or entrapping them in, or attaching them to the particle's matrix. The method used to obtain the nanoparticles determines whether nanoaggregates, nanocapsules, nanospheres, or nanocapsules with a structured interior are obtained. Nanoaggregates can be described as nanosized colloidal systems in which the drug is physically dispersed and can have different morphologies. Nanocapsules are vesicular systems in which the drug is confined to an oily or aqueous liquid core, surrounded by a polymeric membrane. Nanospheres are spherical particles with a gelled interior in which the entrapped component is physically dispersed (Mora-Huertas et al. 2010, Soppimath et al. 2001).

Alginate is now largely used to prepare nanoparticles. Generally, following intravenous injection, nanoparticles can be rapidly cleared from the blood by the mononuclear phagocyte system. Moreover, it is well known that the cells predominantly involved in this uptake are the macrophages of the liver, the spleen, and circulating monocytes. The more hydrophobic the nanoparticle surface is, the more rapid is their uptake from circulation. This can be modulated by the particle size and surface properties of the nanoparticles. Primarily, alginate nanoparticle formation is based on two methods: complexation and water in oil (w/o) emulsification coupled with the gelation of the alginate emulsion droplet.

For example, gelled nanospheres of alginate were prepared through a single-step technique involving emulsification and gelation. $CaCO_3$ nanoparticles, together with glucono delta-lactone, are dispersed in an alginate solution, which is subsequently dispersed in an oil phase and followed by gelation of the alginate spheres. It was found that nanoparticles of $CaCO_3$ result in smaller alginate spheres and reduce the gelation time significantly, compared to microparticles of $CaCO_3$ (Paques et al. 2014). Core–shell biopolymer nanoparticles were prepared using antisolvent precipitation to form surfactant-stabilized zein core nanoparticles and then electrostatic deposition to form an alginate shell. The particle yield was relatively high (95%). The nanoparticle suspensions had relatively good stability to pH: the particles were stable to aggregation from pH 3 to 8, but aggregated at pH 2 due to loss of charge. They also possess good thermal stability at pH 7. The coreshell biopolymer nanoparticles fabricated in this study have potential to be used as nano-delivery systems for bioactive molecules in food and pharmaceutical formulations (Hu and McClements 2015).

It is seen that using mild conditions and no organic solvents in the preparation of alginate nanoparticles makes them applicable for the entrapment of sensitive materials and for use in pharmaceuticals and foods. The formation of shell layers and the functionalization of the particle surface with certain groups or ligands are useful to obtain specific stability and functionality.

Sarmento et al. prepared insulin-loaded nanoparticles by ionotropic pre-gelation of alginate with calcium chloride followed by complexation between alginate and chitosan. The influence of the pH and stoichiometry relationship between polyelectrolytes providing individual particles with a nanoscale size was assessed by photon correlation spectroscopy. Individual and smaller size nanoparticles, around 800 nm, were obtained at pH 4.7 with an alginate:chitosan mass ratio of 6:1 (Sarmento et al. 2006). Alginate is also used to prepare electrospun nanofibers. An alginate-based nanofiber matrix is similar, with its nanoscaled fibrous extracellular matrix (ECM) proteins, and thus is a candidate ECM-mimetic material. Electrospinning is a facile method to fabricate alginate nanofibrous mats, which have a range of applications extending far beyond regenerative medicine. The feature sizes of electrospun mats, such as fiber diameters, can be tailored by the solution properties (e.g., viscosity, concentration) and process conditions (e.g., flow rate, electric field). The mat thickness is also affected by the total mass of deposited fibers and size of the collector plate. Although alginate-based electrospun mats have shown promise as tissue scaffolds, their feature sizes and topography also have drawbacks. Specifically, electrospun nanofiber mats have a relatively flat topography, limited thickness, and dense fiber packing; as such, when used as tissue scaffolds, cell infiltration is restricted to the top layers of the electrospun mat. Hence, a traditional electrospun nanofiber mat without modification may have limited use in regenerative medicine. For tissue engineering applications, electrospun alginate mat formations have been tailored by a variety of approaches in order to expand their capabilities (Kang et al. 2012, Bonino et al. 2012).

14.7   APPLICATIONS OF ALGINATE

Alginate-based carriers have attracted a lot of interest during the past few decades, because they can deliver low-molecular-weight drugs, as well as large biomacromolecules such as proteins and genes, either in a localized or in a targeted manner (Table 14.1). Alginate has been widely adopted as a carrier to immobilize or encapsulate drugs, bioactive molecules, proteins, and cells.

14.7.1   Delivery of Drugs

14.7.1.1   Oral Drug Delivery

The use of alginate for the systemic and localized delivery by the oral route has increased over the years. Urbanska et al. encapsulated oxaliplatin, a slightly soluble antitumoral drug, within chitosan-coated alginate microparticles for oral

TABLE 14.1

Application Summary of Alginate-Based Drug Delivery

Polymer(s)	Drug or Active Agent	Formulation	Reference
Sodium alginate	TP	Microspheres	Soni et al. (2010)
Alginate + chitosan	Oxaliplatin	Microspheres	Urbanska et al. (2012)
Alginate + locust bean gum	Aceclofenac	IPN microparticles	Jana et al. (2015)
Alginate + gelatin + egg albumin	Cefadroxil	IPN beads	Kulkarni et al. (2001)
Alginate + chitosan	5-Aminosalicylic acid	Microspheres	Mladenovska et al. (2007)
Sodium alginate + PNIPAAm-g-guar gum	Isoniazid	Hydrogel microspheres	Kajjari et al. (2012)
Alginate + poly (lactic-co-glycolic acid)	Silymarin	Nano hydrogel matrices	El-Sherbiny et al. (2011)
Sodium alginate	Gliclazide	Microcapsules	Prajapati et al. (2008)
Alginate + chitosan	Amoxicillin	Nanoparticles	Arora et al. (2011)
sodium alginate	α-Interferon	Microspheres	Saez et al. (2012)
Alginate + poly (lactic-co-glycolic acid)	Insulin	Microparticles	Schoubben et al. (2009)
Alginate + chitosan	Albendazole	Microparticles	Wang et al. (2010)
Sodium alginate + Eudragit S100	Valdecoxib	Microparticles	Thakral et al. (2011)
Alginate + aminopropyl silicate	Bioartificial pancreas	Membranes	Sakai et al. (2002)
Alginate	Plasmid DNA	Microparticles	Nograles et al. (2012)
Alginate	Polymyxin B	Microparticles	Coppi et al. (2004)
Alginate + chitosan	Triamcinolone	Microparticles	Lucinda-Silva et al. (2010)
Alginate	Testosterone	Nanocapsules	Bhowmik et al. (2006)
Alginate + chitosan	Prednisolone	Microparticles	Wittaya-Areekul et al. (2006)

administration in colorectal cancer (Urbanska et al. 2012). The study was complemented with histopathology, where the different gastrointestinal compartments were stained with hematoxylin and eosin. Control groups showed tubular adenomas that protruded into the colon lumen and polypoid adenomas in the small intestine, whereas oxaliplatin groups showed microadenomas.

A strategy to improve the mechanical stability of alginate matrices in aqueous media is to blend it with polycationic polymers (e.g., chitosan, pectin, gelatin) to form polyelectrolyte complexes. Jaya et al. (2009) encapsulated aspirin within alginate/pectin microspheres (90 µm) by means of a homogenization/atomization and calcium cross-linking method and assessed the effect of the composition on the release kinetics (Jaya et al. 2009). The release was slow and controlled in the pH range between 1.2 and 8.2, which covers the conditions of the gastrointestinal tract. In addition, an increase of the pectin content increased the release rate.

The fast release of the encapsulated drugs is a relevant drawback of alginate. To stabilize the matrix and sustain the release, microparticles could be also obtained by forming interpenetrated polymer networks of alginate with other polysaccharides and natural polymers that are cross-linked ionotropically and/or covalently with different coupling agents (Kulkarni et al. 2012). It enables a better control of the matrix porosity and swelling and mechanical properties and consequently of the release rate. In this framework, Kulkarni et al. (2001) developed interpenetrating network beads made of alginate, gelatin, and egg albumin that were cross-linked with glutaraldehyde to increase the half-life of the antibiotic cefadroxil. The encapsulation efficiency was as high as 88% and the burst release was relatively low. Moreover, the release was sustained for at least 7 hour.

The controlled and localized delivery of antineoplastic agents has also been achieved using partially oxidized alginate gels. Multiple drugs can be loaded into alginate-based gels for simultaneous or sequential delivery, as the chemical structure of the drug and mode of incorporation will dramatically alter the release kinetics. For example, methotrexate (noninteractive with alginate) was rapidly released by diffusion, whereas doxorubicin, covalently attached to the alginate, was released via chemical hydrolysis of the cross-linker. Mitoxantrone, ionically complexed to alginate, was only released after the dissociation of the gel (Bouhadir et al. 2001).

Ahmad et al. (2006, 2007) encapsulated the antifungal drugs clotrimazole and econazole and the antituberculosis drugs rifampicin, ethambutol, isoniazid, and pyrazinamide within alginate nanoparticles (Pandey et al. 2005) by means of a modified cation-induced controlled gelification. After oral administration, free drugs were detectable for only 6–24 hour, whereas the encapsulated ones were detectable between 8 and 15 days. The beneficial effect of aginate was also investigated to develop mucopenetrating alginate/chitosan nanoparticles for the release of amoxicillin in the treatment of the infection by *H. pylori*, a pathogen that colonizes the deep gastric mucosa lining (Arora et al. 2011).

Hydrophobic drugs can be incorporated in the form of small crystals homogeneously dispersed in the alginate matrix, as reported for the hypoglycemic drug gliclazide (Prajapati et al. 2008) and the anti-inflammatory prednisolone (Wittaya-Areekul et al. 2006), or encapsulated within nanoparticles of a hydrophobic polymer (e.g., poly[lactide]) and then reencapsulated within alginate, as shown for silymarin (El-Sherbiny et al. 2011).

14.7.1.2 Colon Targeted Drug Delivery

Alginate has also been widely exploited for colon targeted drug delivery. The colon-specific drug delivery system should be capable of protecting the drug *en route* to the colon, that is, drug release and absorption should not occur in the stomach as well as the small intestine, but only released and absorbed once the system reaches the colon. For example, the inhibitor of the cyclooxygenase-2 enzyme, valdecoxib, was encapsulated within Eudragit S100 and sodium alginate microparticles for colonic release (Thakral et al. 2011). More recently, pH- and thermoresponsive microspheres of alginate and poly(*N*-isopropylacrylamide)-*g*-guar gum were obtained by emulsion coupled to chemical cross-linking with glutaraldehyde to encapsulate the antituberculosis drug isoniazid (Kajjari et al. 2012). The release was sustained for at least

12 h with a strong dependence on the pH of the medium; the release increased at pH 7.4 with respect to 1.2. Furthermore, the incorporation of graft copolymer enabled a much better control of the release kinetics with a substantial decrease of the burst effect. The modulation of the release using external stimuli (e.g., electrical current) has also been explored, though not in the case of particles but of macroscopic hydrogels. Coppi et al. produced ALG microparticles of a diameter smaller than 3 μm by spray-drying for the uptake of M cells of the Peyer's patches and the targeting of polymixin B to the gut-associated lymphoid tissue (Coppi et al. 2004). Particles were cross-linked with chitosan and calcium, and they were gastroresistant. The sustained release of TP was achieved from carbon nanotube (CNT)-incorporated alginate microspheres. The addition of CNT enhanced the mechanical stability of gels, without affecting the structure and morphology of the microspheres, and no significant cytotoxicity was observed, indicating potential application as a delivery carrier to the intestine and colon (Zhang et al. 2010).

Multiparticulate systems of alginate and chitosan containing triamcinolone were prepared by a complex coacervation/ionotropic gelation method for colonic drug delivery. A higher swelling degree and faster drug release were observed from the particulate systems in a simulated enteric environment (pH 7.5), compared to a simulated gastric environment (pH 1.2) (Lucinda-Silva et al. 2010). Magnetic alginate-chitosan beads loaded with albendazole (ABZ) were also prepared for passive targeting to the gastrointestinal tract using physical capture mechanisms (e.g., magnetic field, pH). The beads showed unique pH-dependent swelling behaviors and a continuous release of ABZ (Wang et al. 2010). Mladenovska et al. (2007) have developed alginate microparticles loaded with 5-aminosalicylic acid that were cross-linked and coated with calcium and chitosan using a spray-drying technique for application in inflammatory bowel disease. Singh et al. developed a multiparticulate system combining pH-sensitive property and specific biodegradability, which has been investigated to prepare and evaluate ES-100-coated sodium alginate microspheres for colon targeting of Tinidazole. Sodium alginate microspheres were prepared by inotropic gelation method using different ratios of Tinidazole and sodium alginate. Eudragit coating of Tinidazole sodium alginate microspheres was performed by coacervation phase separation technique with different core:coat ratios. The core microspheres sustained the release for 8 h in a pH progression medium mimicking the condition of gastro intestinal tract (GIT). The release studies of coated microspheres were performed in a similar dissolution medium as mentioned previously. In the acidic medium, the release rate was much slower; however, the drug was released quickly at pH 7.4 and their release was sustained up to 24 h (Singh et al. 2012).

14.7.2 DELIVERY OF PROTEINS AND PEPTIDES

One of the major challenges in protein and peptide delivery via the oral route is fast release and degradation in the aggressive gastrointestinal fluids. Alginate is an excellent candidate for delivery of protein drugs, because proteins can be incorporated into alginate-based formulations under relatively mild conditions that minimize their denaturation, and the gels can protect them from degradation until their release. A variety of strategies have been investigated to control the rate of protein release from alginate gels.

Yu et al. (2009) reported on composite pH-sensitive microparticles of alginate, chitosan, and pectin for the encapsulation of BSA as a model protein. The method was shredding and combined tripolyphosphate cross-linking of chitosan, electrostatic complexation by alginate and/or pectin with chitosan, and ionotropic gelation of alginate with calcium ions. The release at pH values of 1.2 and 5.0 was substantially slower than at 7.4, supporting the potential of this system for specific oral delivery. To improve the delivery of α-interferon by the oral route without degradation, Saez et al. (2012) microencapsulated it within alginate microspheres. Interferons are usually injected, and this approach would represent a breakthrough in the immunotherapy with this immunomodulatory, antiproliferative, and antiviral agent. Heparin-binding growth factors such as vascular endothelial growth factor (VEGF) or basic fibroblast growth factor exhibit reversible binding to alginate hydrogels, enabling a sustained and localized release (Silva and Mooney 2010).

Insulin appears as one of the most appealing proteins to investigate the novel drug delivery systems of administration by nonparenteral routes. One approach was the re-encapsulation of bovine insulin-loaded alginate particles within poly(lactic-co-glycolic) acid microparticles. Composite microparticles showed a diameter of ~22 μm and a porous surface, and they sustained the release over 130 days. Thus, these systems are more promising for parenteral than for oral administration (Schoubben et al. 2009).

Other proteins that have been encapsulated within alginate microparticles include the proteases papain (Sankalia et al. 2005) and subtilisin (Simi and Abraham 2007). More recent works have also explored the encapsulation of other sensitive biologicals such as adenoviruses (Park et al. 2012) and plasmid DNA (Nograles et al. 2012).

The low encapsulation efficiency and fast release from alginate gels exhibited by many proteins can also be addressed with various cross-linking or encapsulation techniques, and/or by enhancing proteinhydrogel interactions. For example, insulin-loaded alginate microspheres were prepared by blending alginate with anionic polymers (e.g., cellulose acetate phthalate, polyphosphate, dextran sulfate), followed by chitosan coating in order to protect insulin at gastric pH and obtain its sustained release at intestinal pH (Silva et al. 2006). In order to develop an oral vaccine against schistosomiasis, a parasitic disease, the Smrho protein was encapsulated within chitosan nanoparticles coated with alginate (Oliveira et al. 2012).

Some works also related to the chemical modification of alginate to confer gene transfection capacity or active targeting properties. In this context, alginate nanoparticles loaded with the fluorescent probe protoporphyrin IX were modified with 5-aminolevulinic acid, a ligand that is selectively recognized by cancerous cells that overexpress the folic acid receptor, to confer diagnostic capability by endoscopy. Nanoparticles were endocytosed by colorectal cancer cells, and the probe was released to the intracellular space and accumulated for sensitive photodynamic detection (Yang et al. 2011).

14.7.3 TISSUE REGENERATION WITH PROTEIN AND CELL DELIVERY

Alginate gels have been widely used as a vehicle to deliver proteins or cell populations for regeneration of various tissues and organs in the body. The applications of alginate gels in this area are due to their wide range of gelling approaches, physical properties, cell adhesion, and degradation behavior.

14.7.3.1   Bone Regeneration

In the fields of orthopedics and oral and maxillofacial surgery, bone regeneration remains a clinical challenge. Alginate gels have found potential in bone regeneration by delivery of osteoinductive factors, bone-forming cells, or combination of both. The first studies to report the culture of bone cells in a 3D alginate-based micro-environment were carried out using unmodified hydrogels and cell types, such as the mouse calvarial-3T3 osteoblastic cell line (MC3T3) or primary chick embryo osteoblasts. Majmudar et al. (1991) observed that osteoblasts were kept viable for as long as 8 months within alginate beads

Using an *in situ* gelling strategy, Kuo and Ma (2001) were able to control the gelation rate of alginate hydrogels and successfully entrapped MC3T3 pre-osteoblastic cells (Kuo and Ma 2001). The combination of stem cells with growth factors within a matrix may lead to increased bone formation. To examine this possibility, Simmons et al. investigated whether bone marrow stromal cells (BMSCs) entrapped within 2 wt.% irradiated alginate with RGD could enhance bone regeneration, in the absence or presence of bone morphogenetic protein-2 and/or transforming growth factor (TGF)-β3. The authors observed that only BMSCs transplanted in the presence of both factors produced significant bone tissue. Therefore, the entrapment of cells and growth factors in a single matrix may provide a strategy for bone tissue formation (Simmons et al. 2004). The transplantation of stem cells using alginate hydrogels has been widely explored in bone tissue engineering. The thickness of calcium cross-linked alginate gels was demonstrated to alter the behavior of rat bone marrow cells; however, different geometries did not influence cell differentiation (Barralet et al. 2005). Alginate has also been combined with inorganic materials to enhance bone tissue forma-tion. Alginate/hydroxyapatite composite scaffolds with interconnected porous structures were prepared by a phase separation method, which enhanced the adhe-sion of osteosarcoma cells (Lin and Yeh 2004).

14.7.3.2   Cartilage Regeneration

Repair of damaged or degraded cartilage is still one of the major challenges in the orthopedics field, but tissue engineering approaches have recently shown poten-tial in cartilage regeneration. Alginate gels have proved to be useful for trans-planting chondrogenic cells to restore damaged cartilage in animal models. Human mesenchymal stem cells encapsulated in alginate gel beads have been cultured in serum-free medium with the addition of TGF-β1, dexamethasone, and ascorbate 2-phosphate for more than 1 week, and demonstrated to form cartilage in large osteochondral defects (Igarashi et al. 2010). Dobratz et al. (2009) prepared an injectable *in situ* cross-linking system to produce an engineered cartilage by injecting a CaCl$_2$ solution immediately after mixing a 2% alginate solution with primary perichondrium-derived human chondrocytes. This minimally invasive sys-tem allowed for an *in vivo* molding that maintained its shape for at least 38 weeks after injection (Dobratz et al. 2009).

14.7.3.3 Muscle, Nerve, Pancreas, and Liver Tissue Regeneration

Alginate gels are also being actively investigated for their ability to mediate the regeneration and engineering of a variety of other tissues and organs, including the skeletal muscle, nerve, pancreas, and liver. A combined delivery of VEGF and insulin-like growth factor-1 from alginate gels was used to modulate both angiogenesis and myogenesis. The localized and sustained delivery of both growth factors led to significant muscle regeneration and functional muscle formation (Borselli et al. 2010). Alginate-based highly anisotropic capillary gels, introduced into acute cervical spinal cord lesions in adult rats, were integrated into the spinal cord parenchyma without major inflammatory responses and directed axonal regrowth (Prang et al. 2006). Alginate gels, covalently cross-linked with ethylenediamine, are useful to restore a 50-mm gap in cat sciatic nerves (Hashimoto et al. 2005). Alginate encapsulated pancreatic islet allografts and xenografts were developed to cure type I diabetes. These alginate beads are generally coated with poly(amino acids), such as poly-L-lysine, to decrease the outer pore size, while keeping a liquid core structure (Sakai et al. 2002). Tissue engineering is a potential approach to provide hepatic tissues for replacement of a failing liver. Hepatocytes were transplanted into the liver lobe of Lewis rats using VEGF-releasing porous alginate gels (Kedem et al. 2005).

14.7.3.4 Intervertebral Disk Regeneration

Nucleus pulposus (NP) of the intervertebral disk (IVD) with injectable biomaterials represents a potential treatment strategy for IVD degeneration. For example, when bovine NP cells within alginate beads were cultured in the presence of bovine lactoferricin, there was a decrease in inflammatory mediators involved in degenerative disk disease (cytokine interleukin-1 and endotoxin lipolysaccharide) that mediate the suppression of prostaglandin accumulation (Kim et al. 2013).

14.8 CONCLUSIONS AND FUTURE PERSPECTIVES

In summary, alginate has been extensively utilized as a biomaterial for many biomedical applications, particularly in the areas of wound healing, drug delivery, *in vitro* cell culture, and tissue engineering. The most attractive features of alginate for these applications include biocompatibility, mild gelation conditions, and simple modifications to prepare alginate derivatives with new properties. Alginic acid and sodium and potassium alginates have emerged as one of the most extensively explored mucoadhesive biomaterials owing to very good cytocompatibility and biocompatibility, biodegradation, sol/gel transition properties, and chemical versatility that make possible further modifications to tailor their properties. In future, effort should be made on chemical derivatization of alginate to create next generation alginate biomaterials having enhanced or altogether new properties. A thorough understanding of the chemistry of alginates is vital to this goal. An important challenge that remains is the development of alginate particles, with a narrow size distribution, high mechanical and chemical stability, and feasibility to scale up to industrial scale production volumes.

REFERENCES

Aguilar, K.C., F. Tello, A.C.K. Bierhalz, M.G.G. Romo, H.E.M. Flores, and C.R.F. Grosso. 2015. Protein adsorption onto alginate-pectin microparticles and films produced by ionic gelation. *Journal of Food Engineering* 154: 17–24.

Ahmad, Z., R. Pandey, S. Sharma, and G. K. Khuller. 2006. Pharmacokinetic and pharmaco-dynamic behaviour of antitubercular drugs encapsulated in alginate nanoparticles at two doses. *International Journal of Antimicrobial Agents* 27: 420–427.

Ahmad, Z., S. Sharma, and G.K. Khuller. 2007. Chemotherapeutic evaluation of alginate nanoparticle-encapsulated azole antifungal and antitubercular drugs against murine tuberculosis. *Nanomedicine Nanotechnology, Biology, and Medicine* 3: 239–243.

Arora, S., S. Gupta, R.K. Narang, and R.D. Budhiraja. 2011. Amoxicillin loaded chitosan-alginate polyelectrolyte complex nanoparticles as mucopenetrating delivery system for *H. pylori*. *Scientia Pharmaceutica* 79: 673–694.

Balakrishnan, B., S. Lesieur, D. Labarre, and A. Jayakrishnan. 2005. Periodate oxida-tion of sodium alginate in water and in ethanol–water mixture: A comparative study. *Carbohydrate Research* 340: 1425–1429.

Barralet, J.E., L. Wang, J.T. Lriffitt, P.R. Cooper, and R.M. Shelton. 2005. Comparison of bone marrow cell growth on 2D and 3D alginate hydrogels. *Journal of Materials Science Materials in Medicine* 16: 515–519.

Basmanav, B.F., G.T. Kose, and V. Hasirci. 2008. Sequential growth factor delivery from com-plexed microspheres for bone tissue engineering. *Biomaterials* 29: 4195–4204.

Bera, H., S.G. Kandukuri, A.K. Nayak, and S. Boddupalli. 2015. Alginate–sterculia gum gel-coated oil-entrapped alginate beads forgastroretentive risperidone delivery. *Carbohydrate Polymers* 120: 74–84.

Bhowmik, B.B., B. Sa, and A. Mukherjee. 2006. Preparation and in vitro characterization of slow release testosterone nanocapsules in alginates. *Acta Pharmaceutica* 56: 417–429.

Bonino, C.A., K. Efimenko, S.I. Jeong, M.D. Krebs, E. Alsberg, and S.A. Khan. 2012. Three-dimensional electrospun alginate nanofiber mats via tailored charge repulsions. *Small* 8:1928–1936.

Borselli, C., H. Storrie, F. Benesch-Lee et al. 2010. Functional muscle regeneration with combined delivery of angiogenesis and myogenesis factors. *Proceedings of the National Academy of Sciences of the United States of America-Physical Sciences* 107:3287–3292.

Bouhadir, K.H., E. Alsberg, and D.J. Mooney. 2001. Hydrogels for combination delivery of antineoplastic agents. *Biomaterials* 22: 2625–2633.

Chen, S.C., Y.C. Wu, F.L. Mi, Y.H. Lin, L.C. Yu, and H.W. Sung. 2004. A novel pH-sensitive hydrogel composed of N,O-carboxymethyl chitosan and alginate cross-linked by genipin for protein drug delivery. *Journal of Controlled Release* 96: 285–300.

Chickering, D.E. and E. Mathiowitz. 1995. Bioadhesive microspheres: A novel electro-based method to study adhesive interactions between individual microspheres and intestinal mucosa. *Journal of Controlled Release* 34: 251–261.

Ching, S.H., B. Bhandari, R. Webb, and N. Bansal. 2015. Visualizing the interaction between sodium caseinate and calcium alginate microgel particles. *Food Hydrocolloids* 43: 165–171.

Coleman, R.J., G. Lawrie, L.K. Lambert, M. Whittaker, K.S. Jack, and L. Grøndahl. 2011. Phosphorylation of alginate: Synthesis, characterization, and evaluation of in vitro min-eralization capacity. *Biomacromolecules* 12: 889–897.

Coppi, G., V. Iannuccelli, N. Sala, and M. Bondi. 2004. Alginate microparticles for Polymyxin B Peyer's patches uptake: Microparticles for antibiotic oral administration. *Journal of Microencapsulation* 21: 829–839.

Coviello, T., P. Matricardi, C. Marianecci, and F. Alhaique. 2007. Polysaccharide hydrogels for modified release formulations. *Journal of Controlled Release* 119: 5–24.

Crow, B.B. and K.D. Nelson. 2006. Release of bovine serum albumin from a hydrogel-cored biodegradable polymer fiber. *Biopolymers* 81: 419–427.

De Moura, M.R., M.R. Guilherme, G.M. Campese, E. Radovanovic, A.F. Rubira, and E.C. Muniz 2005. Porous alginate-Ca2+ hydrogels interpenetrated with PNIPAAm networks: Interrelationship between compressive stress and pore morphology. *European Polymer Journal* 41: 2845–2852.

Dobratz, E., S. Kim, A. Voglewede, S.S. Park. 2009. Injectable cartilage: Using alginate and human chondrocytes. *Archives of Facial Plastic Surgery* 11: 40–47.

Donati, I., I.J. Haug, T. Scarpa et al. 2007. Synergistic effects in semidilute mixed solution of alginate and lactose-modified chitosan(chitlac). *Biomacromolecules* 8: 957–962.

Donati, I., S. Holtan, Y.A. Mørch, M. Borgogna, M. Dentini, and G. Skjåk-Bræk. 2005. New hypothesis on the role of alternating sequences in calcium-alginate gels. *Biomacromolecules* 6: 1031–1040.

Eiselt, P., K.Y. Lee, and D.J. Mooney. 1999. Rigidity of two-component hydrogels prepared from alginate and poly(ethylene glycol)-diamines. *Macromolecules* 32: 5561–5566.

El-Sherbiny, I.M., M. Abdel-Mogib, A.A.M. Dawidar, A. Elsayed, and H.D.C. Smyth. 2011. Biodegradable pH-responsive alginate-poly (lactic-co-glycolic acid) nano/micro hydrogel matrices for oral delivery of silymarin. *Carbohydrate Polymers* 83: 1345–1354.

Fan, L., L. Jiang, and Y. Xu. 2011. Synthesis and anticoagulant activity of sodium alginate sulfates. *Carbohydrate Polymers* 83: 1797–1803.

Galant, C., A.L. Kjoniksen, G.T.M. Nguyen, K.D. Knudsen, and B. Nystrom. 2006. Altering associations in aqueous solutions of a hydrophobically modified alginate in the presence of beta-cyclodextrin monomers. *Journal of Physical Chemistry B* 110: 190–195.

Gomez, C.G., G. Chambat, H. Heyraud, M. Villar, and R. Auzély-Velty. 2006. Synthesis and characterization of a β-CD-alginate conjugate. *Polymer* 47: 8509–8516.

Hashimoto, T., Y. Suzuki, K. Suzuki, T. Nakashima, M. Tanihara, and C. Ide. 2005. Peripheral nerve regeneration using non-tubular alginate gel crosslinked with covalent bonds. *Journal of Materials Sciencematerials in Medicine* 16: 503–509.

Hay, I.D., Z.U. Rehman, A. Ghafoor, and B.H.A. Rehm. 2010. Bacterial biosynthesis of alginates. *Journal of Chemical Technology and Biotechnology* 85: 752–759.

Hu, K. and D.J. McClements. 2015. Fabrication of biopolymer nanoparticles by antisolvent precipitation and electrostatic deposition: Zein-alginate core/shell nanoparticles. *Food Hydrocolloids* 44: 101–108.

Igarashi, T., N. Iwasaki, Y. Kasahara, and A. Minami. 2010. A cellular implantation system using an injectable ultra-purified alginate gel for repair of osteochondral defects in a rabbit model. *Journal of Biomedical Materials Research Part A* 94: 844–855.

Isiklan, N., M. Inal, and M. Yiğitoğlu. 2008. Synthesis and characterization of poly(N-Vinyl-2-pyrrolidone) grafted sodium alginate hydrogel beads for the controlled release of indomethacin. *Journal of Applied Polymer Science* 110: 481–493.

Jabari, E., N. Wisniewski, and A. Peppas. 1993. Evidence of mucoadhesion by chain interpretation at a Poly(acrylic acid)/mucin interface using ATR-FTIR spectroscopy. *Journal of Controlled Release* 26: 99–108.

Jana, S., A. Gandhi, K.K. Sen, and S.K. Basu. 2011. Natural polymers and their application in drug delivery and biomedical field. *Journal of Pharmaceutical Science and Technology* 1: 16–27.

Jana S., A. Gandhi, S. Sheet, and K.K. Sen. 2015. Metal ion-induced alginate–locust bean gum IPN microspheres for sustained oral delivery of aceclofenac. *International Journal of Biological Macromolecules* 72: 47–53.

Jaya, S., T.D. Durance, and R. Wang. 2009. Effect of alginate-pectin composition on drug release characteristics of microcapsules. *Journal of Microencapsulation* 26: 143–153.

Kailasapathy, K. 2002. Microencapsulation of probiotic bacteria: Technology and potential applications. *Current Issues in Intestinal Microbiology* 3: 39–48.

Kajjari, P.B., L.S. Manjeshwar, and T.M. Aminabhavi. 2012. Novel pH- and temperature-responsive blend hydrogel microspheres of sodium alginate and PNIPAAm-g-GG for controlled release of isoniazid. *AAPS Pharmaceutical Science and Technology* 13: 1147–1157.

Kang, E., Y.Y. Choi, S.K. Chae, J.H. Moon, J.Y. Chang, and S.H. Lee. 2012. Microfluidic spinning of flat alginate fibers with grooves for cell-aligning scaffolds. *Advanced Materials* 24: 4271–4277.

Kanti, P., K. Srigowri, J. Madhuri, B. Smitha, and S. Sridhar. 2004. Dehydration of ethanol through blend membranes of chitosan and sodium alginate by pervaporation. Separation and Purification Technology. *Separation and Purification Technology* 40: 259–266.

Karewicz, A., K. Zasada, K. Szczubialka, S. Zapotoczny, R. Lach, and M. Nowakowska. 2010. "Smart" alginate–hydroxypropylcellulose microbeads for controlled release of heparin. *International Journal of Pharmaceutics* 385: 163–169.

Kedem, A., A. Perets, I. Gamlieli-Bonshtein, M. Dvir-Ginzberg, S. Mizrahi, and S. Cohen. 2005. Vascular endothelial growth factor-releasing scaffolds enhance vascularization and engraftment of hepatocytes transplanted on liver lobes. *Tissue Engineering* 11: 715–722.

Kim, J.S., M.B. Ellman, D. Yan et al. 2013. Lactoferricin mediates anti-inflammatory and anti-catabolic effects via inhibition of IL-1 and LPS activity in the intervertebral disc. *Journal of Cellular Physiology* 228: 1884–1896.

Kong, H.J., M.K. Smith, and D.J. Mooney. 2003. Designing alginate hydrogels to maintain viability of immobilized cells. *Biomaterials* 24: 4023–4029.

Koo, L.Y., D.J. Irvine, A.M. Mayes, D.A. Lauffenburger, and L.G. Griffith. 2002. Coregulation of cell adhesion by nanoscale RGD organization and mechanical stimulus. *Journal of Cell Science* 115: 1423–1433.

Kulkarni, A.R., K.S. Soppimath, T.M. Aminabhavi, and W.E. Rudzinski. 2001. In-vitro release kinetics of cefadroxil-loaded sodium alginate interpenetrating network beads. *Eur. J. Pharm. Biopharm.* 51: 127–133.

Kulkarni, R.V., S. Mutalik, B.S. Mangond, and U.Y. Nayak. 2012. Novel interpenetrated polymer network microbeads of natural polysaccharides for modified release of water soluble drug: In-vitro and in-vivo evaluation. *Journal of Pharmacy and Pharmacology* 64: 530–540.

Kuo, C.K. and P.X. Ma. 2001. Ionically crosslinked alginate hydrogels as scaffolds for tissue engineering: Part 1. Structure, gelation rate and mechanical properties. *Biomaterials* 22: 511–521.

Lee, J. and K.Y. Lee. 2009. Local and sustained vascular endothelial growth factor delivery for angiogenesis using an injectable system. *Pharmaceutical Research* 26: 1739–1744.

Lee, K.Y., K.H. Bouhadir, and D.J. Mooney. 2004. Controlled degradation of hydrogels using multi-functional cross-linking molecules. *Biomaterials* 25: 2461–2466.

Lee, K.Y., H.J. Kong, R.G. Larson, and D.J. Mooney. 2003. Hydrogel formation via cell cross-linking. *Advanced Materials* 15: 1828–1832.

Lee, K.Y. and D.J. Mooney. 2012. Alginate: Properties and biomedical applications. *Progress in Polymer Science* 37: 106–126.

Lee, K.Y. and S.H. Yuk. 2007. Polymeric protein delivery systems. *Progress in Polymer Science* 32: 669–697.

Leonard, M., M.R. Boisseson De, P. Hubert, F. Dalencon, and E. Dellacherie. 2004. Hydrophobically modified alginate hydrogels as protein carriers with specific controlled release properties. *Journal of Control Release* 98: 395–405.

LeRoux, M.A., F. Guilak, and L.A. Setton. 1999. Compressive and shear properties of alginate gel: Effects of sodium ions and alginate concentration. *Journal of Biomedical Materials Research* 47: 46–53.

Lin, H.R. and Y.J. Yeh. 2004. Porous alginate/hydroxyapatite composite scaffolds for bone tissue engineering: Preparation, characterization, and in vitro studies. *Journal of Biomedical Materials Research PartB* 71: 52–65.

Liu, W., W.D. Wu, C. Selomulya, and X.D. Chena. 2013. On designing particulate carriers for encapsulation and controlled release applications. *Powder Technology* 236: 188–196.

Lucinda-Silva, R.M., H.R.N. Salgado, and R.C. Evangelista. 2010. Alginate-chitosan systems: In vitro controlled release of triamcinolone and in vivo gastrointestinal transit. *Carbohydrate polymers* 81: 260–268.

Majmudar, G., D. Bole, S.A. Goldstein, and J. Bonadio. 1991. Bone cell culture in a threedimensional polymer bead stabilizes the differentiated phenotype and provides evidence that osteoblastic cells synthesize type III collagen and fibronectin. *Journal of Bone and Mineral Research* 6: 869–881.

Man, Y., P. Wang, Y. Guo. 2012. Angiogenic and osteogenic potential of platelet-rich plasma and adipose-derived stem cell laden alginate microspheres. *Biomaterials* 33: 8802–8811.

Mladenovska, K., O. Cruaud, P. Richomme et al. 2007. 5-ASA loaded chitosan-Ca-alginate microparticles: Preparation and physicochemical characterization. *International Journal of Pharmaceutics* 345: 59–69.

Moghaddam, M.K., S.M. Mortazavi, and T. Khayamian. 2015. Preparation of calcium alginate microcapsules containing n-nonadecane by a melt coaxial electrospray method. *Journal of Electrostatics* 73: 56–64.

Mora-Huertas, C.E., H. Fessi, and A. Elaissari. 2010. Polymer-based nanocapsules for drug delivery. *International Journal of Pharmaceutics* 385: 113–142.

Morch, Y.A., I. Donati, and B.L. Strand. 2006. Effect of Ca^2+, Ba^2+, and Sr^2+ on alginate microbeads. *Biomacromolecules* 7: 1471–1480.

Myung, D., D. Waters, M. Wiseman et al. 2008. Progress in the development of interpenetrating polymer network hydrogels. *Polymers for Advanced Technologies* 19: 647–653.

Narayanan, R.P., G. Melman, N.J. Letourneau, N.L. Mendelson, and A. Melman. 2012. Photodegradable iron(III) cross-linked alginate gels. *Biomacromolecules* 13: 2465–2471.

Nochos, A., D. Douroumis, and N. Bouropoulos. 2008. In vitro release of bovine serum albumin from alginate/HPMC hydrogel beads. *Carbohydrate Polymers* 74: 451–457.

Nograles, N., S. Abdullah, M.N. Shamsudin, N. Billa, and R. Rosli. 2012. Formation and characterization of pDNA-loaded alginate microspheres for oral administration in mice. *Journal of Bioscience and Bioengineering* 113: 133–140.

Oliveira, S.M., C.C. Barrias, I.F. Almeida et al. 2008. Injectability of a bone filler system based on hydroxyapatite microspheres and a vehicle with in situ gel-forming ability. *Journal of Biomedical Materials Research B* 87B: 49–58.

Oliveira, C.R., C.M.F. Rezende, M.R. Silva, A.P. Pego, O. Borges, and A.M. Goes. 2012. A new strategy based on Smrho protein loaded chitosan nanoparticles as a candidate oral vaccine against schistosomiasis. *PLOS Neglected Tropical Diseases* 6: e1894.

Orive, G., S. Ponce, R.M. Hernandez, A.R. Gascon, M. Igartua, and J.L. Pedraz. 2002. Biocompatibility of microcapsules for cell immobilization elaborated with different type of alginates. *Biomaterials* 23: 3825–3831.

Otterlei, M., K. Ostgaard, G. Skjak-Brack, O. Smidsrod, P. Soon-Shiong, and T. Espevik. 1991. Induction of cytokine production from human monocytes stimulated with alginate. *Journal of Immunotherapy* 10: 286–291.

Pandey, R., Z. Ahmad, S. Sharma, and G.K. Khuller. 2005. Nanoencapsulation of azole antifungals: Potential applications to improve oral drug delivery. *International Journal of Pharmaceutics* 301: 268–276.

Park, H., P.H. Kim, T. Hwang et al. 2012. Fabrication of cross-linked alginate beads using electrospraying for adenovirus delivery. *International Journal of Pharmaceutics* 427: 417–425.

Park, T.G. and H.K. Choi. 1998. Thermally induced core–shell type hydrogel beads having interpenetrating polymer network (IPN) structure. *Macromolecular Rapid Communications* 19: 167–172.

Paques, J.P., L.M.C. Sagis, C.J.M. van Rijn, and E. van der Linden. 2014. Nanospheres of alginate prepared through w/o emulsification and internal gelation with nanoparticles of CaCO$_3$. *Food Hydrocolloids* 40: 182–188.

Pawar, S.N. and K.J. Edgar. 2012. Alginate derivatization: A review of chemistry, properties and applications. *Biomaterials* 33: 3279–3305.

Pourjavadi, A., M.S. Amini-Fazl, and H. Hosseinzadeh. 2005. Partially hydrolyzed crosslinked alginate-graft-polymethacrylamide as a novel biopolymer-based superabsorbent hydrogel having pH-responsive Properties. *Macromolecular Research* 13: 45–53.

Prajapati, S.K., P. Tripathi, U. Ubaidulla, and V. Anand. 2008. Design and development of gliclazide mucoadhesive microcapsules: In vitro and in vivo evaluation. *AAPS Pharmaceutical Science and Technology* 9: 224–230.

Prang, P., R. Muller, A. Eljaouhari et al. 2006. The promotion of oriented axonal regrowth in the injured spinal cord by alginate-based anisotropic capillary hydrogels. *Biomaterials* 27: 3560–3569.

Ramesh Babu, V., M. Sairam, K.M. Hosamani, and T.M. Aminabhavi. 2007. Preparation of sodium alginate-methylcellulose blend microspheres for controlled release of nifedipine. *Carbohydrate Polymers* 69: 241–250.

Remminghorst, U. and B.H. Rehm. 2006. Bacterial alginates: From biosynthesis to applications. *Biotechnology Letters* 28: 1701–1712.

Rinaudo, M. 2008. Main properties and current applications of some polysaccharides as biomaterials. *Polymer International* 57: 397–430.

Ronghua, H., D. Yumin, and Y. Jianhong. 2003. Preparation and in vitro anticoagulant activities of alginate sulfate and its quaterized derivatives. *Carbohydrate Polymers* 52: 19–24.

Roy, D., J.N. Cambre, and B.S. Sumerlin. 2010. Future perspectives and recent advances in stimuliresponsive materials. *Progress in Polymer Science* 35: 278–301.

Rzaev, Z.M.O., S. Dincer, and E. Piskin. 2007. Functional copolymers of Nisopropylacrylamide for bioengineering applications. *Progress in Polymer Science* 32:534–595.

Saez, V., J. Ramón, C. Peniche, and E. Hardy. 2012. Microencapsulation of alpha interferons in biodegradable microspheres. *Journal of Interferon & Cytokine Research* 32: 299–311.

Sankalia, M.G., R.C. Mashru, J.M. Sankalia, and V.B. Sutariya. 2005. Papain entrapment in alginate beads for stability improvement and site-specific delivery: Physicochemical characterization and factorial optimization using neural network modelling. *AAPS Pharmaceutical Science and Technology* 6: E209–E222.

Sanli, O., N. Ay, and N. Isiklan. 2007. Release characteristics of diclofenac sodium from poly(vinyl alcohol)/sodium alginate and poly(vinyl alcohol)-grafted-poly(acrylamide)/ sodium alginate blend beads. European *Journal of Pharmaceutics and Biopharmaceutics* 65: 204–214.

Sakai, S. and K. Kawakami. 2007. Synthesis and characterization of both ionically and enzymatically crosslinkable alginate. *Acta Biomaterials* 3: 495–501.

Sakai, S., T. Ono, H. Ijima, and K. Kawakami. 2002. In vitro and in vivo evaluation of alginate/ sol-gel synthesized aminopropyl silicate/alginate membrane for bioartificial pancreas. *Biomaterials* 23: 4177–83.

Sarmento, B., D. Ferreira, F. Veiga, and A. Ribeiro. 2006. Characterization of insulin-loaded alginate nanoparticles produced by ionotropic pre-gelation through DSC and FTIR studies. *Carbohydrate Polymers* 66: 1–7.

Schnürch, A.B., C.E. Kast, and M.F. Richter. 2001. Improvement in the Mucoadhesive properties of alginate by the covalent attachment of cysteine. *Journal of Control Release* 71: 277–285.

Schoubben, A., P. Blasi, S. Giovagnoli, L. Perioli, C. Rossi, and M. Ricci. 2009. Novel composite microparticles for protein stabilization and delivery. *European Journal of Pharmaceutical Sciences* 36: 226–234.

Shi, J., N.M. Alves, and J.F. Mano. 2006. Drug release of pH/temperature-responsive calcium alginate/poly(N-isopropylacrylamide) semi-IPN beads. *Macromolecular Bioscience* 6: 358–363.

Sikorski, P., F. Mo, G. Skjåk-Bræk, and B.T. Stokke. 2007. Evidence for egg-box-compatible interactions in calcium-alginate gels from fiber X-ray diffraction. *Biomacromolecules* 8: 2098–2103.

Silva, C.M., A.J. Ribeiro, D. Ferreira, and F. Veiga. 2006. Insulin encapsulation in reinforced alginate microspheres prepared by internal gelation. *European Journal of Pharmaceutical Sciences* 29: 148–159.

Silva, E.A. and D.J. Mooney. 2010. Effects of VEGF temporal and spatial presentation on angiogenesis. *Biomaterials* 31: 1235–1241.

Simi, C.K. and T.E. Abraham. 2007. Encapsulation of crosslinked subtilisin microcrystals in hydrogel beads for controlled release applications. *European Journal of Pharmaceutical Sciences* 3: 217–223.

Simmons, C., E. Alsberg, S. Hsiong, W. Kim, and D. Mooney. 2004. Dual growth factor delivery and controlled scaffold degradation enhance in vivo bone formation by transplanted bone marrow stromal cells. *Bone* 35: 562–569.

Singh, S.K., A.K. Singh, A.A. Mahajan et al. 2012. Formulation and evaluation of colon targeted drug delivery of an anti-amoebic drug. *International Journal of Pharmaceutical Innovations.* 2: 138–152.

Skjåk-Bræk, G., H. Grasdalen, and O. Smidsrød. 1989. Inhomogeneous polysaccharide ionic gels. *Carbohydrate Polymers* 10: 31–54.

Spargo, B.J., A.S. Rudolph, and F.M. Rollwagen. 1994. Recruitment of tissue resident cells to hydrogel composites: In vivo response to implant materials. *Biomaterials* 15: 853–858.

Soni, M.L., M. Kumar, and K.P. Namdeo. 2010. Sodium alginate microspheres for extending drug release: Formulation and in vitro evaluation. *International Journal of Drug Delivery* 2: 64–68.

Soppimath, K.S., T.M. Aminabhavi, A.R. Kulkarni, and W.E. Rudzinski. 2001. Biodegradable polymeric nanoparticles as drug delivery devices. *Journal of Controlled Release* 70: 1–20.

Stevens, M.M., H.F. Qanadilo, R. Langer, and V.P. Shastri. 2004. A rapid-curing alginate gel system: Utility in periosteum-derived cartilage tissue engineering. *Biomaterials* 25: 887–894.

Sugiura, S., T. Oda, Y. Izumida et al. 2005. Size control of calcium alginate beads containing living cells using micro-nozzle array. *Biomaterials* 26: 3327–3331.

Thakral, N.K., A.R. Ray, D. Bar-Shalom, A.H. Eriksson, and D.K. Majumdar. 2011. The quest for targeted delivery in colon cancer: Mucoadhesive valdecoxib microspheres. *International Journal of Nanomedicine* 6: 1057–1068.

Tian, M., B. Han, H. Tan, and C. You. 2014. Preparation and characterization of galactosylated alginate–chitosanoligomer microcapsule for hepatocytes microencapsulation. *Carbohydrate Polymers* 112: 502–511.

Urbanska, A.M., E.D. Karagiannis, G. Guajardo, R.S. Langer and D.G. Anderson. 2012. Therapeutic effect of orally administered microencapsulated oxaliplatin for colorectal cancer. *Biomaterials* 33: 4752–4761.

Wang, F.Q., P. Li, J.P. Zhang, A.Q. Wang, and Q. Wei. 2010. A novel pH-sensitive magnetic alginate—Chitosan beads for albendazole delivery. *Drug Development and Industrial Pharmacy* 36: 867–877.

Williams, D.F. 2009. On the nature of biomaterials. *Biomaterials* 30: 5897–5909.

Wittaya-Areekul, S., J. Kruenate, and C. Prahsarn. 2006. Preparation and in vitro evaluation of mucoadhesive properties of alginate/chitosan microparticles containing prednisolone. *International Journal of Pharmaceutics* 312: 113–118.

Yang, G., L. Zhanga, T. Penga, and W. Zhongb. 2000. Effects of Ca^{2+} bridge cross-linking on structure and pervaporation of cellulose/alginate blend membranes. *Journal of Membrane Science* 175: 53–60.

Yang, J., J. Chen, D. Pan, Y. Wan, and Z. Wang. 2013. pH-sensitive interpenetrating network hydrogels based on chitosan derivatives and alginate for oral drug delivery. *Carbohydrate Polymers* 92: 719–725.

Yang, S.J., F.H. Lin, H.M. Tsai et al. 2011. Alginate-folic acidmodified chitosan nanoparticles for photodynamic detection of intestinal neoplasms. *Biomaterials* 32: 2174–2182.

Yu, C.Y., B.C. Yin, W. Zhang, S.X. Cheng, X.Z. Zhang, and R.X. Zhuo. 2009. Composite microparticle drug delivery systems based on chitosan, alginate and pectin with improved pH-sensitive drug release property. *Colloids and Surfaces B: Biointerfaces* 68: 245–249.

Zhang, X.L., Z.Y. Hui, D.X. Wan et al. 2010. Alginate microsphere filled with carbon nanotube as drug carrier. *International Journal of Biological Macromolecules* 47: 389–395.

Zhao, X.H., N. Huebsch, D.J. Mooney, and Z.G. Suo. 2010. Stress-relaxation behaviour in gels with ionic and covalent crosslinks. *Journal of Applied Physics* 107: 1–5.

Zimmermann, U., G. Klöck, K. Federlin et al.1992. Production of mitogen-contamination free alginates with variable ratios of mannuronic acid to guluronic acid by free flow electrophoresis. *Electrophoresis* 13: 269–274.

15 Marine Biopolymers in Bone Tissue Repair and Regeneration

Jayachandran Venkatesan, Baboucarr Lowe,
Sukumaran Anil, Kranti Kiran Reddy Ealla,
and Se-Kwon Kim

CONTENTS

15.1 INTRODUCTION

The limited number of organ donors have surpass demand resulting to a global shortage to meet existing transplantation demands; this is due to the increasing number of organ failure cases. For example, in the United States, 1 patient is added to the waiting list every 10 minutes, whereas an average of 18 deaths per day is the result of organ donor shortage (Liu et al. 2013). Hence, the development of new therapeutic technologies to replace, restore, and or repair defect tissues, and improve the quality of lives of patients became eminent. Tissue engineering strategies serve as reliable options to overcome the dire shortage and long waiting time for organ transplantation. Approximately 15 million global fracture cases have been reported (O'Keefe and Mao 2011). Thus, bone is one of the most transplanted tissues in the world (Salgado et al. 2004).

15.2   BONE AND PROPERTIES

By nature, bone is a highly organized composite material existing at various hierarchical levels. Structurally, bone is made of two main parts: a compact (cortical) bone and a spongiosa or trabecular bone—a porous core. The amalgamation is such that the dense shear stress-resisting shell and the inner cellular structure provide a typical relative mass-to-volume ratio (0.05 and 0.3) that averts buckling and results in a thin core analogous to a sandwich structure with excellent bending resistance (Pschyrembel and Dornblüth 2004; Gibson 2005; Meng et al. 2013). Bone disorders are an increasing health concern due to the increase in our population. Bone grafting is one of the therapeutic options used to restore damage bone tissues. Biomaterials have been an alternative source of therapeutics largely defined by the fabrication of biomimetic hydrogels or scaffold, which are bioactive and bioresorbale to enhance tissue formation and growth (Bose et al. 2012; Pereira et al. 2012; Venkatesan et al. 2015). For a scaffold to be applicable in bone tissue engineering, one of the primary requirements is *biocompatibility*, a term that has been described in many ways. For a scaffold to be degraded and biocompatible, its ability to support normal cellular activity without systemic toxic effect needs to be satisfied (Khan et al. 2008). Hence, as simply put by Williams (1987), biocompatibility refers to the ability of a material to perform with an appropriate host response in a specific situation. Further, the scaffold should also have a minimal strength capable of hosting bone tissues especially in load-bearing ones. For reference, this should be in close proximity to Young's modulus of 15–20 GPa for cortical bone and 0.1–2 GPa for cancellous bone. However, the compressive strength is between 100 and 200 MPa and 2 and 20 GPa for cortical and cancellous bones, respectively. (Olszta et al. 2007). Detailed discussions about the mechanical properties of the bone have been reported in the works of Currey (1990, 2003), Currey et al. (1995), Nalla et al. (2005), Thompson et al. (2001), and Vashishth (2004). An interconnected porous scaffold allows successful diffusion of essential nutrients and oxygen for cell survival. A pore size of at least 100 μm proves to be essential for the supply of oxygen and nutrients. Otherwise, it is often limited by diffusion processes that can only supply cells in close proximity to 100–200 μm to the next capillary (Rouwkema et al. 2008). Meanwhile, a mean pore size of 325 μm is reportedly found to be optimal for bone tissue ingrowth (Murphy et al. 2010). The degradability of the scaffold with time *in vivo* is an essential requirement in bone tissue engineering. This, via the controlled resorption rate, allows the growing new tissue to colonize the template provided by the scaffold. Therefore, the degradation rate should also correspond to the site of application, for example, 9 months or more in spinal fusion or 3–6 months in crano-maxillofacial applications (Olszta et al. 2007). Meanwhile, the successful integration of these important properties is still a great challenge in research for application purposes in bone defects (Lichte et al. 2011; Bose et al. 2012).

15.3   NATURAL BIOPOLYMERS

Marine-derived biopolymers used in tissue engineering form a part of the growing number of materials being studied and applied as suitable regenerative therapeutic options for the treatment of bone defects and/or restoration of the damaged bone function. They are readily available in nature and can be isolated using specific methods. They have different properties ideal for use in the development of bioengineering-based technologies for clinical applications.

15.3.1 Chitosan

Chitosan can be isolated from chitin through N-deacetylation process. It is a linear polysaccharide composed of β(1→4)-linked D-glucosamine and N-acetyl-D-glucosamine units (Yin et al. 2003), stemming the crustacean shells and insects' exoskeleton. Depending on the degree of deacetylation, source, and preparation method employed, chitosan may have molecular weights ranging from 300 to >1000 kDa. It is readily soluble in dilute acid (pH < 6.0), and the protonated free amino acids of the glucosamine enhance the solubility of the molecule (Domish et al. 2001; Madihally et al. 1999; Di Martino et al. 2005). Further, the presence of N-acetyl-D-glucosamine and β(1→4)-linked D-glucosamine subunits in its structure is linked to biological activities such as being a biocompatible polymer with low toxicity, biodegradability, antimicrobial and hemostatic maintenance (wound healing) through the modulation of inflammatory cell (neutrophils, macrophages, fibroblasts, and endothelial cells) function, and promotion of the formation and organization of granulation tissue (Levengood and Zhang 2014; Figure 15.1).

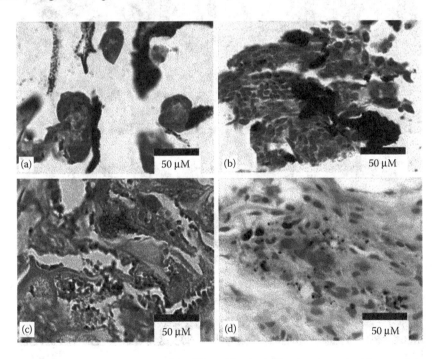

FIGURE 15.1 Optical images of Von Kossa histological stain assay on chitosan–alginate scaffolds after (a) 10 days and (b) 28 days of culture *in vitro*, and (c) 4 weeks and (d) 8 weeks after implantation *in vivo*. (Reproduced with permission from Li, Z. et al., *Biomaterials*, 26, 3919–3928, 2005.)

These primary properties are exploited for other biomedical application purposes; thus, chitosan can be chemically modified through its amino and hydroxyl groups to form complexes for introducing the functionalities for targeted purposes (Sashiwa and Aiba 2004; Ho et al. 2005; Jiang et al. 2006). It is an important material used in tissue engineering. Chitosan is not the most ideal material for bone tissue engineering. As a result, it is usually combined with other bioactive materials to improve its application capabilities for bone tissue repair and/or regeneration (Kong et al. 2006); this suitability pack has yielded promising results for further considerations in reconstruction of large bone defects (Figure 15.2).

The developed composites materials can mimic the natural function of bone and also allow the cell adhesion, proliferation and differentiation (Frohbergh et al. 2012). Considering this, biomimetic chitosan–nano-hydroxyapatite scaffold is used to mimic the natural bone fabricated via *in situ* hybridization by ionic diffusion process (Hu et al. 2004), freeze drying and lyophilization (Kong et al. 2006), and coprecipitation and mineralization via double diffusion (Rusu et al. 2005).

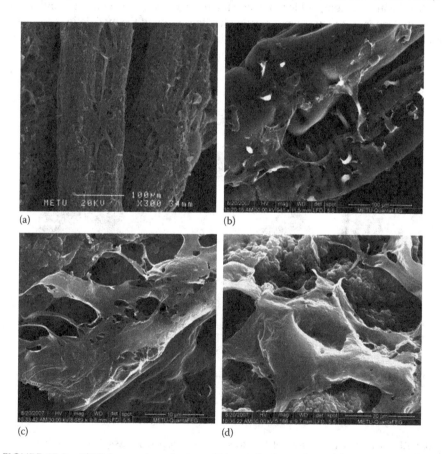

FIGURE 15.2 MSC (mesenchymal stem cells) attachment and spreading on (a, b) CHI4–HAc2 and (c, d) CHI4–PEO2–HAc5 scaffolds after 21 days of incubation. (Reproduced with permission from Yilgor, P. et al., *Biomaterials*, 30, 3551–3559, 2009.)

Macroporous calcium phosphate–chitosan composite scaffold shows increased bioactivities of alkaline phosphatase (ALP) and osteocalcin (OC) in 11 days using MG63 cells; enhancing the mechanical strength of the composite and degradation rate (Zhang et al. 2003). Chitosan/hydroxyapatite/alginate provides a bio-inspired microenvironment defined by an interconnected pore size and mechanical stability triggering osteoblastic differentiation confirmed via ALP activity and mineralization (Kim et al. 2015). Chitosan–gelatin scaffold engrafted with simvastatin-loaded poly(lactic-co-glycolic acid) (PLGA) microparticles for localized controlled release of simvastatin has been studied for bone tissue engineering applications. The scaffold that loads simvastatin enhance cell proliferation and mineralization (Gentile et al. 2016). Chitosan sponges can be used as a suitable scaffold for tissue engineering showing bone formation *in vitro* and *in vivo* for transplantation of bone tissue regeneration (Seol et al. 2004).

15.3.2 Fucoidan

During the past few decades, many carbohydrate polymers have been shown to have biological effects either by themselves or inducing a specific effect through complex reaction cascades (Paulsen 2002). The use of fucoidan in bone tissue regeneration is increasing due to exceptional biological properties. The seaweed-derived polysaccharide is reported to have an inducing role in osteoblast formation in mesenchymal stem cells. This Functional property is largely associated with its anionic nature and presence of fucose and sulfate ester groups (Li et al. 2008; Jin and Kim 2011; Bilan et al. 2002; Chizhov et al. 1999) and position of the sulfated group (Wijesinghe and Jeon 2012). Fucoidan can be isolated from marine invertebrates such as sea urchins and sea cucumber. Fucoidan has extensively been studied for many biological activities (Jin and Kim 2011) as in anticoagulatory, antithrombotic, antiviral, antitumor and immunomodulatory, anti-inflammatory, blood lipids reducing, antioxidant and anticomplementary properties against hepatopathy, uropathy and renalpathy, gastric protective effects and therapeutic potential in surgery (Jin and Kim 2011). Algal polysaccharides are heterogeneously branched with sometimes additional monosaccharide constituents of acetyl groups. The orders of the Chordariales and Laminariales (Phaeosporophyceae) contain polysaccharides with linear backbones made up of $(1\rightarrow3)$-linked α-L-fucopyranose residues (Chizhov et al. 1999; Nagaoka et al. 1999) with Fucales (Cyclosporophyceae, e.g., *Fucus evanescens*, *Ascophyllum nodosum*, and *F. vesiculosus*) having alternating $(1\rightarrow3)$- and $(1\rightarrow4)$-linked α-L-fucopyranose residues. This structural difference has been elucidated in the work of Bilan et al. (2004). Fucoidan is also composed of uronic acids, galactose, xylose, and sulfated fucose (Rioux et al. 2007). Murakami et al. (2010) reported a hydrogel blend of chitin/chitosan and fucoidan; fucoidan has the functional property to stabilize and activate other heparin-binding cytokines in exudates that induce angiogenesis and wound repair, and thus, it is useful for healing-impaired wounds bearing a nontoxic behavior on tissues (Murakami et al. 2010). Poly(ε-caprolactone) (PCL)/fucoidan composite showed higher mineralization than PCL scaffold via a control release mechanism in to the composite with majority of the fucoidan release in 24 h (Jin and Kim 2011). Chitosan–alginate–fucoidan composite reported by Venkatesan et al. (2014) showed

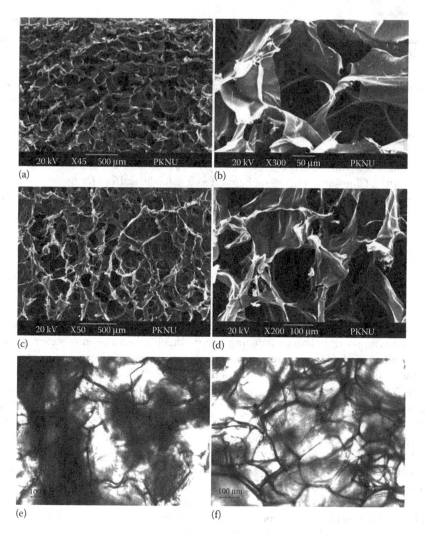

FIGURE 15.3 High- and low-magnification scanning electron microscopy (SEM) images of (a, b) chitosan-alginate, (c, d) chitosan-alginate-fucoidan, and optical microscopic images of (e) chitosan-alginate and (f) chitosan-alginate-fucoidan. (Reproduced with permission from Venkatesan, J. et al., *Mar. drugs*, 12, 300–316, 2014.)

better bioactivity for use in bone tissue regeneration to enhance protein adsorption and increase mineralization in MG63 cell lines (Figure 15.3).

15.3.3 ALGINATE

Alginate has been reported extensively in tissue engineering, cell transplantation, and cell encapsulation due to its biocompatibility, biodegradability, mass transports, and ability to be injected into defect areas (Hwang et al. 2009). The structural framework of alginate is made of (1–4)-linked β-D-mannuronic acid (M units) and α-L-guluronic acid (G units) monomers, which vary in amount and sequential distribution along the polymer chain depending on the source (Martinsen et al. 1989). Several authors have reported the use of alginate in bone tissue engineering applications. Zhao et al. (2010) reported injectable calcium phosphate–alginate hydrogel–umbilical cord mesenchymal stem cell paste for bone tissue engineering in which alginate was used to encapsulate and protect the cells. The encapsulated human umbilical cord mesenchymal stem cells (hUCMSCs) differentiated into osteogenic lineage showing elevated ALP, OC, collagen I and Osterix expression, ALP protein synthesis, and mineralization (Zhao et al. 2010; Figure 15.4).

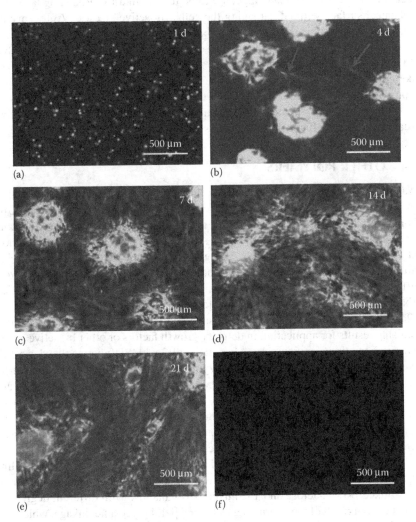

FIGURE 15.4 Typical fluorescent live/dead staining images for the oxidized alginate-fibrin microbeads (type 3). Live cells (a) 1, (b) 4, (c) 7, (d) 14, and (e) 21 days. (f) Dead cells at 21 days. (Reproduced with permission from Zhou, H., Xu, H.H.K., *Biomaterials*, 32, 7503–7513, 2011.)

Porous alginate/hydroxyapatite fabricated by phase separation showed excellent cell attachments (rat osteosarcoma UMR 106 cells) providing interconnected porous structures of >82% with an average size of 150 μm (Lin and Yeh 2004). Stem cell-guided differentiation is promising for use in bone tissue engineering through sinister-specific biochemical cascades to producing osteoblast lineages (Jansen et al. 2005; Benoit et al. 2006; Reilly et al. 2007; Sarugaser et al. 2005; Varghese et al. 2010). Similarly, Zhou and Xu (2011) reported that stem cell-encapsulating alginate-fibrin microbeats encapsulated hUCMSCs and showed excellent proliferation and osteogenic differentiation, and synthesized bone minerals, of which a fibrin concentration of 0.1% alginate appeared to be the optimal for producing a suitable mechanical surface without damaging the cells. Bioactive glasses (Vrouwenvelder et al. 1994) and ceramic surface enhance bone formation with capacities of bonding the surrounding bone tissue *in vivo* (Hupa et al. 2010; Yao et al. 2005) showing bioactivities essential for use in bone tissue engineering applications. Erol et al. (2012) reported alginate cross-linked copper ions in coated bioactive glass consisting of boron with nominal composition (wt.%) 65 SiO_2, 15 CaO, 18.4 Na_2O, 0.1 MgO, and 1.5 B_2O_3 prepared via the foam replica method. Results of scanning microscopy revealed profound cell attachment on the scaffold surface.

15.4 OTHER POLYMERS

Ulvan an anionic sulfated polysaccharide that is water soluble and semicrystalline in nature (Alves et al. 2012a, b) extractable from the cell walls of green algae (*Ulva lactuca*) in pure form (Alves et al. 2010) is a biodegradable polymer used in bone tissue engineering. Ulvan is composed of sugar subunits such as sulfated rhamnose and idurionic acid in its backbone. Using poly-D,L-lactic acid (PDLLA) enriched with Ulvan particles, Alves et al. (2012a) prepared a novel three-dimensional porous scaffold loaded with dexamethasone within the PDLLA matrix using a subcritical carbon dioxide sintering process (Figure 15.5).

The successful loading of dexamethasone within the PDLLA matrix produced promising results for application in delivery growth factors or other bioactive agents for use in bone tissue engineering (Alves et al. 2012a, b). Biofunctionalized crossed-linked Ulvan hydrogel using natural enzyme ALP inducers was investigated for osteogenic cellular activities. The homogenized hydrogel showed mineralization and ALP mineral formation, which are important parameters for application purposes in bone tissue engineering (Dash et al. 2014). Carboxymethylation of ulvan and chitosan as bone cement showed a noncytotoxic behavior and a strong compressive strength for bone tissue engineering applications (Barros et al. 2013).

Carrageenan is also a marine-derived polymer that has an expressive gelling property. It has a linear primary structure made up of alternating copolymers of 1,3-linked β-D-galactose and 1,4-linked α-D-galactose with different degrees of sulfatation as a result of the alternating α-1,3 and β-1,4 glycosidic linkage, which fills the backbone of carrageenan making anionic polymer (Francis et al. 2004; Abad et al. 2003; Chronakis et al. 1996). There are three common types of carrageenan: traditionally labeled kappa (κ), iota (γ), and lambda (λ) (Maolin et al. 2000). Carrageenans have an extraordinary biocompatibility because they do not induce a toxic reaction

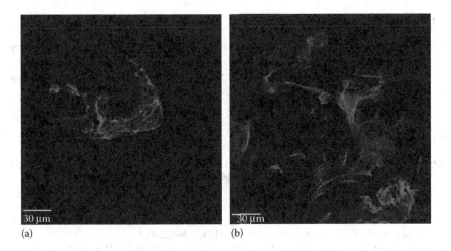

FIGURE 15.5 Confocal laser scanning microscopy (CLSM) micrographs of MC3T3 × 10⁻¹ cells cultured on (a) Ulvan-methacrylate (UMA) blank scaffolds and (b) Ulvan-methacrylate (UMA) 5 scaffolds at 20× magnification. (Reproduced with permission from Dash, M. et al., *ACS Appl. Mater. Interfaces*, 6, 3211–3218, 2014.)

(Cohen and Ito 2002). Carrageen-based hydrogel was studied for the control delivery of platelet derived growth factor (PDGF-BB) in bone tissue engineering by Santo et al. (2009); results of the investigation showed that κ-carrageenan is a suitable carrier system delivery of encapsulated growth factors for tissue engineering showing a release kinetics and thermogelling properties suitable for delivering cells (Santo et al. 2009). Carrageenan has a strong resemblance with glycosaminoglycan, which is one of the main component of the extracellular matrix. In a study reported by Mihaila et al. (2014), chitosan-reinforced κ-carrageenan produced a stable fiber owing to the presence of chitosan by controlling the swelling rate. This fiber network supported encapsulated cells during longer culture periods and cell delivery system was also suitable for the independently heterotypic cell-containing hydrogels (Mihaila et al. 2014).

15.5 CONCLUSION

Extractable marine polymers have huge contribution in tissue engineering by virtue of their functional properties, nontoxic nature, biodegradability, and gelling properties. Hence, they become desirable for use in tissue engineering applications and development of bone grafts. Marine biopolymers with bioceramics-based biocomposite materials have the capacity to induce several important bone-related markers such as alkaline phosphatase (ALP), Osteocalcin (OC), and Osteopontin (OP). They continue to be studies along with other polymers to increase their efficacies and meet the mechanical stability of bone-substituted materials. The utilization of marine biomaterials will continue to model in the future of regenerative medicine especially in bone tissue engineering.

ACKNOWLEDGMENTS

This chapter was supported by research funds from Pukyong National University in 2015 and a grant from the Marine Bioprocess Research Center of the Marine Biotechnology Program, funded by the Ministry of Oceans and Fisheries, The Republic of Korea.

REFERENCES

Abad, L.V., L.S. Relleve, C.T. Aranilla, and A.M. Dela Rosa. 2003. Properties of radiation synthesized PVP-kappa carrageenan hydrogel blends. *Radiation Physics and Chemistry* 68 (5):901–908.

Alves, A., S.G. Caridade, J.F. Mano, R.A. Sousa, and R.L. Reis. 2010. Extraction and physico-chemical characterization of a versatile biodegradable polysaccharide obtained from green algae. *Carbohydrate Research* 345 (15):2194–2200.

Alves, A., A.R.C. Duarte, J.F. Mano, R.A. Sousa, and R.L. Reis. 2012a. PDLLA enriched with ulvan particles as a novel 3D porous scaffold targeted for bone engineering. *The Journal of Supercritical Fluids* 65:32–38.

Alves, A., E.D. Pinho, N.M. Neves, R.A. Sousa, and R.L. Reis. 2012b. Processing ulvan into 2D structures: Cross-linked ulvan membranes as new biomaterials for drug delivery applications. *International Journal of Pharmaceutics* 426 (1):76–81.

Barros, A.A.A., A. Alves, C. Nunes, M.A. Coimbra, R.A. Pires, and R.L. Reis. 2013. Carboxymethylation of ulvan and chitosan and their use as polymeric components of bone cements. *Acta Biomaterialia* 9 (11):9086–9097.

Benoit, D.S.W., C.R. Nuttelman, S.D. Collins, and K.S. Anseth. 2006. Synthesis and characterization of a fluvastatin-releasing hydrogel delivery system to modulate hMSC differentiation and function for bone regeneration. *Biomaterials* 27 (36):6102–6110.

Bilan, M.I, A.A. Grachev, N.E. Ustuzhanina, A.S. Shashkov, N.E. Nifantiev, and A.I. Usov. 2002. Structure of a fucoidan from the brown seaweed Fucus evanescens C. Ag. *Carbohydrate Research* 337 (8):719–730.

Bilan, M.I., A.A. Grachev, N.E. Ustuzhanina, A.S. Shashkov, N.E. Nifantiev, and A.I. Usov. 2004. A highly regular fraction of a fucoidan from the brown seaweed Fucus distichus L. *Carbohydrate Research* 339 (3):511–517.

Bose, S., M. Roy, and A. Bandyopadhyay. 2012. Recent advances in bone tissue engineering scaffolds. *Trends in biotechnology* 30 (10):546–554.

Chizhov, A.O., A. Dell, H.R. Morris, S.M. Haslam, R.A. McDowell, A.S. Shashkov, N.E. Nifant'ev, E.A. Khatuntseva, and A.I. Usov. 1999. A study of fucoidan from the brown seaweed Chorda filum. *Carbohydrate Research* 320 (1):108–119.

Chronakis, I.S., L. Piculell, and J. Borgström. 1996. Rheology of kappa-carrageenan in mixtures of sodium and cesium iodide: Two types of gels. *Carbohydrate Polymers* 31 (4):215–225.

Cohen, S.M., and N. Ito. 2002. A critical review of the toxicological effects of carrageenan and processed eucheuma seaweed on the gastrointestinal tract. *CRC Critical Reviews in Toxicology* 32 (5):413–444.

Currey, J.D. 1990. Biomechanics of mineralized skeletons. *Skeletal Biomineralization: Patterns, Processes and Evolutionary Trends*:11–25. 10.1029/SC005p0011.

Currey, J.D. 2003. Role of collagen and other organics in the mechanical properties of bone. *Osteoporosis International* 14 (5):29–36.

Currey, J.D., P. Zioupos, and A. Sedman. 1995. Microstructure–property relations in vertebrate bony hard tissues: Microdamage and toughness. *Biomimetics Design and Processing of Materials*. AIP Press, Woodbury, New York.

Dash, M., S.K. Samal, C. Bartoli, A. Morelli, P.F. Smet, P. Dubruel, and F. Chiellini. 2014. Biofunctionalization of ulvan scaffolds for bone tissue engineering. *ACS Applied Materials and Interfaces* 6 (5):3211–3218.

Di Martino, A., M. Sittinger, and M.V. Risbud. 2005. Chitosan: A versatile biopolymer for orthopaedic tissue-engineering. *Biomaterials* 26 (30):5983–5990.

Domish, M., D. Kaplan, and Ø. Skaugrud. 2001. Standards and guidelines for biopolymers in tissue-engineered medical products. *Annals of the New York Academy of Sciences* 944 (1):388–397.

Erol, M.M., V. Mouriño, P. Newby, X. Chatzistavrou, J.A. Roether, L. Hupa, and A.R. Boccaccini. 2012. Copper-releasing, boron-containing bioactive glass-based scaffolds coated with alginate for bone tissue engineering. *Acta Biomaterialia* 8 (2):792–801.

Francis, S., Manmohan Kumar, and Lalit Varshney. 2004. Radiation synthesis of superabsorbent poly (acrylic acid)–carrageenan hydrogels. *Radiation Physics and Chemistry* 69 (6):481–486.

Frohbergh, M.E., A. Katsman, G.P. Botta, P. Lazarovici, C.L. Schauer, U.G. Wegst, and P.I. Lelkes. 2012. Electrospun hydroxyapatite-containing chitosan nanofibers crosslinked with genipin for bone tissue engineering. *Biomaterials* 33 (36):9167–9178.

Gentile, P., V.K. Nandagiri, J. Daly, V. Chiono, C. Mattu, C. Tonda-Turo, G. Ciardelli, and Z. Ramtoola. 2016. Localised controlled release of simvastatin from porous chitosan–gelatin scaffolds engrafted with simvastatin loaded PLGA-microparticles for bone tissue engineering application. *Materials Science and Engineering: C* 59:249–257.

Gibson, L.J. 2005. Biomechanics of cellular solids. *Journal of biomechanics* 38 (3):377–399.

Ho, M.H., D.M. Wang, H.J. Hsieh, H.C. Liu, T.Y. Hsien, J.Y. Lai, and L.T. Hou. 2005. Preparation and characterization of RGD-immobilized chitosan scaffolds. *Biomaterials* 26 (16):3197–3206.

Hu, Q., B. Li, M. Wang, and J. Shen. 2004. Preparation and characterization of biodegradable chitosan/hydroxyapatite nanocomposite rods via in situ hybridization: A potential material as internal fixation of bone fracture. *Biomaterials* 25 (5):779–785.

Hupa, L., K.H. Karlsson, M. Hupa, and H.T. Aro. 2010. Comparison of bioactive glasses in vitro and in vivo. *Glass Technology-European Journal of Glass Science and Technology Part A* 51 (2):89–92.

Hwang, Y.S., J. Cho, F. Tay, J.Y. Heng, R. Ho, S.G. Kazarian, D.R. Williams, A.R. Boccaccini, J.M. Polak, and A. Mantalaris. 2009. The use of murine embryonic stem cells, alginate encapsulation, and rotary microgravity bioreactor in bone tissue engineering. *Biomaterials* 30 (4):499–507.

Jansen, J.A., J.W.M. Vehof, P.Q. Ruhe, H. Kroeze-Deutman, Y. Kuboki, H. Takita, E.L. Hedberg, and A.G. Mikos. 2005. Growth factor-loaded scaffolds for bone engineering. *Journal of Controlled Release* 101 (1):127–136.

Jiang, T., W.I. Abdel-Fattah, and C.T. Laurencin. 2006. In vitro evaluation of chitosan/poly (lactic acid-glycolic acid) sintered microsphere scaffolds for bone tissue engineering. *Biomaterials* 27 (28):4894–4903.

Jin, G., and G.H. Kim. 2011. Rapid-prototyped PCL/fucoidan composite scaffolds for bone tissue regeneration: design, fabrication, and physical/biological properties. *Journal of Materials Chemistry* 21 (44):17710–17718.

Khan, Y., M.J. Yaszemski, A.G. Mikos, and C.T. Laurencin. 2008. Tissue engineering of bone: Material and matrix considerations. *The Journal of Bone & Joint Surgery* 90 (1):36–42.

Kim, H.L., G.Y. Jung, J.H. Yoon, J.S. Han, Y.J. Park, D.G. Kim, M. Zhang, and D.J Kim. 2015. Preparation and characterization of nano-sized hydroxyapatite/alginate/chitosan composite scaffolds for bone tissue engineering. *Materials Science and Engineering: C* 54:20–25.

Kong, L., Y. Gao, G. Lu, Y. Gong, N. Zhao, and X. Zhang. 2006. A study on the bioactivity of chitosan/nano-hydroxyapatite composite scaffolds for bone tissue engineering. *European Polymer Journal* 42 (12):3171–3179.

Levengood, S.K.L., and M. Zhang. 2014. Chitosan-based scaffolds for bone tissue engineering. *Journal of Materials Chemistry B* 2 (21):3161–3184.

Li, B., F. Lu, X. Wei, and R. Zhao. 2008. Fucoidan: Structure and bioactivity. *Molecules* 13 (8):1671–1695.

Li, Z., H.R. Ramay, K.D. Hauch, D. Xiao, and M. Zhang. 2005. Chitosan–alginate hybrid scaffolds for bone tissue engineering. *Biomaterials* 26 (18):3919–3928.

Lichte, P., H.C. Pape, T. Pufe, P. Kobbe, and H. Fischer. 2011. Scaffolds for bone healing: Concepts, materials and evidence. *Injury* 42 (6):569–573.

Lin, H.-R., and Y.-J. Yeh. 2004. Porous alginate/hydroxy apatite composites scaffolds for bone tissue engineering: Preparation, characterization, and in vitro studies. *Journal of Biomedical Materials Research Part B: Applied Biomaterials* 71 (1):52–65.

Liu, Y., J. Lim, and S.-H. Teoh. 2013. Review: Development of clinically relevant scaffolds for vascularised bone tissue engineering. *Biotechnology Advances* 31 (5):688–705.

Madihally, S.V., and H.W.T. Matthew. 1999. Porous chitosan scaffolds for tissue engineering. *Biomaterials* 20 (12):1133–1142.

Maolin, Z., H. Hongfei, F. Yoshii, and K. Makuuchi. 2000. Effect of kappa-carrageenan on the properties of poly (N-vinyl pyrrolidone)/kappa-carrageenan blend hydrogel synthesized by γ-radiation technology. *Radiation Physics and Chemistry* 57 (3):459–464.

Martinsen, A., G. Skjak-Braek, and O. Smidsred. 1989. Alginate as immobilization material: I. Correlation between chemical and physical properties of alginate gel beads. *Biotechnology and Bioengineering* 33 (1):79–89.

Meng, J., B. Xiao, Y. Zhang, J. Lei, H. Kong, Y. Huang, Z. Jin, N. Gu, and H. Zu. 2013. Superparamagnetic responsive nanofibrous scaffolds under static magnetic field enhance osteogenesis for bone repair in vivo. *Scientific Reports* 3:2655.

Mihaila, S.M., E.G. Popa, R.L. Reis, A.P. Marques, and M.E. Gomes. 2014. Fabrication of endothelial cell-laden carrageenan microfibers for microvascularized bone tissue engineering applications. *Biomacromolecules* 15 (8):2849–2860.

Murakami, K., H. Aoki, S. Nakamura, M. Takikawa, M. Hanzawa, S. Kishimoto, H. Hattori, Y. Tanaka, T. Kiyosawa, Y. Sato, and M. Ishihara. 2010. Hydrogel blends of chitin/chitosan, fucoidan and alginate as healing-impaired wound dressings. *Biomaterials* 31 (1):83–90.

Murphy, C.M., M.G. Haugh, and F.J. O'Brien. 2010. The effect of mean pore size on cell attachment, proliferation and migration in collagen–glycosaminoglycan scaffolds for bone tissue engineering. *Biomaterials* 31 (3):461–466.

Nagaoka, M., H. Shibata, I. Kimura-Takagi, S. Hashimoto, T. Kimura, R. Aiyama, S. Ueyama, and T. Yokokura. 1999. Structural study of fucoidan from Cladosiphon okamuranus TOKIDA. *Glycoconjugate journal* 16 (1):19–26.

Nalla, R.K., J.J. Kruzic, J.H. Kinney, and R.O. Ritchie. 2005. Mechanistic aspects of fracture and R-curve behavior in human cortical bone. *Biomaterials* 26 (2):217–231.

O'Keefe, R.J., and J. Mao. 2011. Bone tissue engineering and regeneration: From discovery to the clinic—An overview. *Tissue Engineering Part B: Reviews* 17 (6):389–392.

Olszta, M.J., X. Cheng, S.S. Jee, R. Kumar, Y.Y. Kim, M.J. Kaufman, E.P. Douglas, L.B. Gower. 2007. Bone structure and formation: A new perspective. *Materials Science and Engineering: R: Reports* 58 (3):77–116.

Paulsen, B.S. 2002. Biologically active polysaccharides as possible lead compounds. *Phytochemistry Reviews* 1 (3):379–387.

Pereira, T.F., M.A.C. Da Silva, M.F. Oliveira, I.A. Maiab, J.V.L. Silvab, M.F. da Costa, and R.M.S.M. Thireal. 2012. Effect of process parameters on the properties of selective laser sintered Poly (3-hydroxybutyrate) scaffolds for bone tissue engineering: This paper analyzes how laser scan spacing and powder layer thickness affect the morphology and mechanical properties of SLS-made scaffolds by using a volume energy density function. *Virtual and Physical Prototyping* 7 (4):275–285.

Pschyrembel, W., and O. Dornblüth. 2004. Pschyrembel Klinisches Wörterbuch:(... enthält... 330 Tabellen). Berlin (ua). de Gruyter.

Reilly, G.C., S. Radin, A.T. Chen, and P. Ducheyne. 2007. Differential alkaline phosphatase responses of rat and human bone marrow derived mesenchymal stem cells to 45S5 bioactive glass. *Biomaterials* 28 (28):4091–4097.

Rioux, L.-E., S.L. Turgeon, and M. Beaulieu. 2007. Characterization of polysaccharides extracted from brown seaweeds. *Carbohydrate Polymers* 69 (3):530–537.

Rouwkema, J., N.C. Rivron, and C.A. van Blitterswijk. 2008. Vascularization in tissue engineering. *Trends in biotechnology* 26 (8):434–441.

Rusu, V.M., C.-H. Ng, M. Wilke, B. Tiersch, P. Fratzl, and M.G. Peter. 2005. Size-controlled hydroxyapatite nanoparticles as self-organized organic–inorganic composite materials. *Biomaterials* 26 (26):5414–5426.

Salgado, A.J., O.P. Coutinho, and R.L. Reis. 2004. Bone tissue engineering: State of the art and future trends. *Macromolecular Bioscience* 4 (8):743–765.

Santo, V.E., A.M. Frias, M. Carida et al. 2009. Carrageenan-based hydrogels for the controlled delivery of PDGF-BB in bone tissue engineering applications. *Biomacromolecules* 10 (6):1392–1401.

Sarugaser, R., D. Lickorish, D. Baksh, M.M. Hosseini, and J.E. Davies. 2005. Human umbilical cord perivascular (HUCPV) cells: A source of mesenchymal progenitors. *Stem cells* 23 (2):220–229.

Sashiwa, H., and S.-I. Aiba. 2004. Chemically modified chitin and chitosan as biomaterials. *Progress in Polymer Science* 29 (9):887–908.

Seol Y.J., J.Y. Lee, Y.J. Park, Y.M. Lee, Y.K., I.C. Rhyu, S.J. Lee, S.B. Han, and C.P. Chung. 2004. Chitosan sponges as tissue engineering scaffolds for bone formation. *Biotechnology Letters* 26 (13):1037–1041.

Thompson, J.B., J.H. Kindt, B. Drake, H.G. Hansma, D.E., Morse, and P.K. Hansma. 2001. Bone indentation recovery time correlates with bond reforming time. *Nature* 414 (6865):773–776.

Varghese, S., N.S. Hwang, A. Ferran, A. Hillel, P. Theprungsirikul, A.C. Canve, Z. Zhang, J. Geahart, J. Elisseeff. 2010. Engineering musculoskeletal tissues with human embryonic germ cell derivatives. *Stem Cells* 28 (4):765–774.

Vashishth, D. 2004. Rising crack-growth-resistance behavior in cortical bone: Implications for toughness measurements. *Journal of Biomechanics* 37 (6):943–946.

Venkatesan, J., I. Bhatnagar, and S.K. Kim. 2014. Chitosan-alginate biocomposite containing fucoidan for bone tissue engineering. *Marine drugs* 12 (1):300–316.

Venkatesan. J., B. Lowe, P. Manivasagan, K.H. Kang, E.P. Chalisserry, S. Anil, D.G. Kim, and S.K. Kim. 2015. Isolation and characterization of nano-hydroxyapatite from salmon fish bone. *Materials* 8 (8):5426–5439.

Vrouwenvelder, W.C.A., C.G. Groot, and K. De Groot. 1994. Better histology and biochemistry for osteoblasts cultured on titanium-doped bioactive glass: Bioglass 45S5 compared with iron-, titanium-, fluorine-and boron-containing bioactive glasses. *Biomaterials* 15 (2):97–106.

Wijesinghe, W.A.J.P., and Y.-J. Jeon. 2012. Biological activities and potential industrial applications of fucose rich sulfated polysaccharides and fucoidans isolated from brown seaweeds: A review. *Carbohydrate Polymers* 88 (1):13–20.

Williams, D.F. 1987. *Definitions in Biomaterials: Proceedings of a Consensus Conference of the European Society for Biomaterials, Chester, England, March 3–5, 1986.* Vol. 4, Elsevier Science Limited, New York.

Yao, J., S. Radin, P.S. Leboy, and P. Ducheyne. 2005. The effect of bioactive glass content on synthesis and bioactivity of composite poly (lactic-co-glycolic acid)/bioactive glass substrate for tissue engineering. *Biomaterials* 26 (14):1935–1943.

Yilgor, P., K. Tuzlakoglu, R.L. Reis, N. Hasirci, and V. Hasirci. 2009. Incorporation of a sequential BMP-2/BMP-7 delivery system into chitosan-based scaffolds for bone tissue engineering. *Biomaterials* 30 (21):3551–3559.

Yin, Y., F. Ye, J. Cui, F. Zhang, X. Li, and K. Yao. 2003. Preparation and characterization of macroporous chitosan-gelatin/-β tricalcium phosphate composite scaffolds for bone tissue engineering. *Journal of Biomedical Materials Research Part A* 67 (3):844–855.

Zhang, Y., M. Ni, M. Zhang, and B. Ratner. 2003. Calcium phosphate-chitosan composite scaffolds for bone tissue engineering. *Tissue engineering* 9 (2):337–345.

Zhao, L., M.D. Weir, and H.H.K. Xu. 2010. An injectable calcium phosphate-alginate hydrogel-umbilical cord mesenchymal stem cell paste for bone tissue engineering. *Biomaterials* 31 (25):6502–6510.

Zhou, H., and H.H.K. Xu. 2011. The fast release of stem cells from alginate-fibrin microbeads in injectable scaffolds for bone tissue engineering. *Biomaterials* 32 (30):7503–7513.

16 Marine Microbial Biopolymers and Biomedical Applications

Busi Siddhardha and Sairengpuii Hnamte

CONTENTS

16.1 INTRODUCTION

There is an increase demand for the use of biopolymers as a biomaterial. Biopolymers are a brick of monomeric units produced by microorganisms intracellularly or extracellularly. They differ based on the nature of their monomeric composition and are of high molecular weight. They are produced by a variety of microorganisms, plants, and animals. Biopolymers can be grouped into four classes depending on the origin of biopolymers: (1) natural and (2) synthetic (conventionally and chemically synthesized) biopolymers from biomass, (3) synthetic biopolymers from microbes, and (4) synthetic (conventionally and chemically synthesized) bioplymers from petroleum products. Synthetic biopolymers such as polylactic acid, polycaprolactone, polyhydroxyalkano-ates (PHAs), polyglycolic acid, and polyvinyl alcohol possess unique properties such as biocompatibility and biodegradability. Microbial biopolymers can be further distributed into biodegradable and nonbiodegradable depending on their degradation properties (Tian et al. 2012). Polysaccharides such as chitosan, cellulose, dextran, pullulan, hyaluronan, chondroitin sulfate (CS), and alginate are naturally occurring biopolymers (Payne and Raghavan 2007, Stern and Jedrzejas 2008). These natural polysaccharides have a wide range of applications in food, pharmaceutical, and other industries. Alginates, hyaluronan, and chitosan are widely used in biomedical field.

16.2 MARINE MICROBIAL BIOPOLYMERS

Biopolymers from marine microorganisms are embellished with a rich diversity of unexploited resources. A vast array of biopolymers is being isolated from aquatic organisms, which can be classified into three classes: polysaccharides, proteins, and nucleic acids (McNaught et al. 1997). Polysaccharides and proteins are derived biologically, whereas nucleic acids are synthetic biopolymers (Nair and Laurencin 2007). Due to their biodegradability, biocompatibility, and bioresorbability, they are extensively used in biomedical fields (Tian et al. 2012). Some of the important microbial biopolymers are discussed in Sections 16.2.1 through 16.2.7.

16.2.1 SODIUM ALGINATE

Sodium alginate was first reported from a seaweed in 1940. It is the sodium salt of alginic acid, composed of guluronic acid (G) and mannuronic acid, generally recognized as safe (GRAS) by the FDA (Goh et al. 2012, Nayak and Pal 2011). Alginate as a biomaterial has found its tremendous applications in engineering and medical fields Otari et al.(2013) due to its unique properties such as biocompatibility, low toxicity, low cost, and ability to mild gently; its biomedical uses include pharmaceutical applications such as delivery of small chemical drugs, wound dressings in cell culture, and protein delivery. They are used in tissue regeneration with protein and cell delivery in blood vessels, cartilage, muscles, nerve, pancreas, liver, and bone (Lee and Mooney 2012). They are widely used for the treatment of acute or chronic wounds as a wound dressing material (Zimmermann et al. 2007)

The source of alginate is given in Table 16.1.

TABLE 16.1
Alginate and Its Marine Microbial Source

Biopolymer	Source	Reference
Alginate	Extracted from brown algae (Phaeophyceae), *Laminaria hyperborea*, *Laminaria digitata*, *Laminaria japonica*, *Ascophyllum nodosum*, and *Macrocystis pyrifera*	Smidsrod and Skjak-Braek (1990)

16.2.2 FUCOIDAN

In 1913, Kylin first isolated "fucoidin" from marine brown algae and which was later named as "fucoidan". It is a sulfated polysaccharide mainly composed of fucose and sulfate (Li et al. 2008a). It is found mostly in brown algae such as wakame, hijiki, derwrack, komby, mozuku, and sea cucumber. Depending on different algal sources, the structure and chemical composition of fucoidan varies significantly. Structural properties play an important role as the biological activity and biomedicine strongly depend on it (Mourao 2004). Due to their unique property and interesting characteristics, fucoidans have been widely used in biomedical applications due to their antithrombic, anticoagulant, antioxidant, and antiviral properties (Silva et al. 2005). Sinurat and dan Rosmawaty (2015) extracted fucoidan from brown seaweed *Sargassum crassifolium* and evaluated its bioactivity as antigastric ulcers in mice. Due to its complexity in structure and deficiency of suitable functional groups, there has been a difficulty in incorporating fucidon into biomaterials. Keeping this in mind, however, Mattias et al. (2014) developed an assay for synthesis of fucoidan-mimetic glycopolymers by cyanoxyl-mediated free-radical polymerization, a technique that is appropriate for subsequent linkage to biomaterials (Tengdelius et al. 2014).

16.2.3 CARRAGEENAN

Carrageenans are a family of water-soluble, sulfated, linear polymers consisting of a backbone derived from galactose. They are extracted from *Chondrus*, *Gigartina*, *Eucheuma*, and *Iridaea*, which belong to the phylum Rhodophyta (Silva et al. 2012). Distantina et al. (2013) extracted hydrogel-based carrageenans from *Kappaphycus alvarezii*. They have successfully prepared Kappa carrageenan hydrogel membranes by cross-linking with gluteraldehyde solution (Distantina et al. 2013). Carrageenan has been widely used in food industry due to its interesting characteristics such as thickening, emulsifying, stabilizing, and jelling abilities, and it has been used for improving cottage cheese texture, binders, and stabilizers in the industry of processing meat (Campo et al. 2009). In recent years, researchers have showed much interest in pharmaceutical field. Carrageenans have potent pharmaceutical properties, including antioxidant, antihyperlipidimic, anticoagulant, antitumor, immunomodulatory, and antiviral activities (Wijesekara et al. 2011). They have also reported that carrageenans possess the antiviral activities *in vitro* by inhibiting the replication of hepatitis A viruses (Girond et al. 1991).

16.2.4 AGAR

Agar is a complex polysaccharide present in the cell wall of red algae, agarophytes, including species belonging to the genera *Gelidium* and *Gracilaria* (Li et al. 2008). *Gelidium* and *Gracilaria* agars are the two types of agar that have a remarkable difference in their gelling temperature—*Gracilaria* at 40°C and *Gelidium* at 30°C—and their methoxyl content (Guiseley 1989). One unique feature of this polysaccharide is that even at low concentration, it has the capacity to produce strong gels (Duckworth and Yaphe 1971) and is reversible thermally and independent of cation

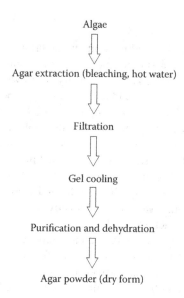

Algae

Agar extraction (bleaching, hot water)

Filtration

Gel cooling

Purification and dehydration

Agar powder (dry form)

FIGURE 16.1   Schematic representation of agar production.

gels (Rochas and Lahaye 1989, Guiseley 1989). Different factors such as sulfate content, molecular weight and distribution of molecular weight, chemical substituents, alga species, and methods of extraction greatly influenced agar viscosity and properties of forming gels (Murano et al. 1992, El-Sayed 1983). Applications of agar and agarose are reported by various researchers. Agarose is used as a medium for the growth of microorganisms, and in gel electrophoresis, it is used to support macroporous gels (Stellwagen and Stellwagen 1994).

A schematic diagram of agar production is shown in Figure 16.1.

16.2.5   CHONDROITIN SULFATE

CS is an important component in the connective tissue of extracellular matrix, and it plays an important role in different biological processes such as hemostasis and inflammation, regulation of cell development, cell adhesion, proliferation, and differentiation. It consists of hexosamine and hexuronic acid units that are arranged in alternating unbranched sequence in a disaccharide basic unit(Vazquez et al. 2013, Schiraldi et al. 2010a). Classification of CS depends on molecular weight, chain length, and sulphate substitution position. CS has been isolated from different sources such as terrestrial and marine species (Cassaro and Dietrich 1977, Lamari et al. 2006, Luo et al. 2002). Marine sources include whale (Michelacci and Dietrich 1986), king crab (Kitagawa et al. 1997), skate (Lignot et al. 2003), salmon (Majima et al. 2001), sea cucumber (Vieira and Mourao 1988), and so on. It has been extracted from microbial sources such as *Escherichia coli* K4, *Bacillus subtilis* natto, *E. coli* 05:K4:H4, and *Pasteurella multocida* (Schiraldi et al. 2010b).

Due to its unique features such as high biocompatibility and its use in engineering of biological tissues associated with the process of bone repair, cutaneous wood, and cartilage, CS demand in the number of commercial applications is increased. Acceleration to regenerate damaged structures is being studied in combination with other biopolymers such as hyaluronic acid (HA), proteoglycans, and collagen (Pipitone 2003, Chang et al. 2003). From various studies, CS is known to be a potent antiviral (Cai et al. 2005).

Fucosylated CS (CS-F) isolated from sea cucumber inhibits adenocarcinoma growth in lungs using mouse as a model system (Borsig et al. 2007). In terms of food preservatives, purified CS is also widely used as a food preservative with emulsifying properties (Hamano et al. 1989). However, the most profitable commercial products of CS are those associated with cartilage regeneration, osteoarthritis, and anti-inflammatory activities (Conte et al. 1995, Volpi 2009).

16.2.6 HYALURONIC ACID

HA is a high-molecular-weight unbranched and non-sulfated glucosaminoglycan, distributed in connective tissues such as cartilage, vitreous of the human eye, umbilical cord, and synovial fluid. It is a major macromolecular component of the intercellular matrix (Hardingham 2004, Liao et al. 2005). HAs are found in the marine environment in vitreous humour and cartilaginous of different fish species. They are produced in large scales through microbial production by *Streptococcus* bacteria (Kim et al. 2006b, Rangaswamy and Jain 2008, Liao et al. 2005). They have been extracted from microbial sources such as group A and C *Streptococci* (*Streptococcus equi* subsp. *equi*, *S. equi* subsp. *zooepidemicus*), *S. pyogenes*, and *S.* uberis (Chong et al. 2005, Schiraldi et al. 2010b). The main source of HA in marine organism is the vitreous humor present in the eyeball of fish and in the cartilage of chondrichthyes (Murado et al. 2012). Due to their uniform and simple primary structure, HA polymers have a wide range of interesting biological functions based on the size of their molecules (Tammi et al. 2002). Their biotechnological applications include antiaging cosmetics, arthritis treatment, major burns, intraocular surgery, and joint injection (Schiraldi et al. 2010a).

16.2.7 MARINE EXOPOLYSACCHARIDE

Exopolysaccharides (EPSs) with their potential applications have been extracted from different sources, of which marine source is of great concern and attractive to researchers due to their unique properties. Different EPSs have enormous applications in different fields. They have been used in several applications such as in pharmaceutical and food industry because of their interesting biological activity (Laurienzo 2010). Recently, polysaccharide-based biomaterials are of great interest and have been used in different biomedical applications such as drug delivery device, tissue engineering, and gel entrapment methods. There are several reports on EPS-producing strains and have been extensively studied. Nichols et al. (2005) isolated a marine bacterium *Pseudoalteromona* CAM025 from ice sea sample and studied the effects of incubation on growth and their production. Mehta et al. (2014) isolated an extracellular polysaccharide from the marine strain of *Alteromonas macleodii*. They reported that the purified polysaccharide has the ability to produce spherical shaped silver nanoparticles, which have been characterized by ultraviolet–visual spectroscopy, dynamic light scattering, and transmission electron microscopy.

16.3   CHEMISTRY OF MICROBIAL BIOPOLYMERS

Bacteria, fungi, and algae are the bioactive polymers produced naturally by microorganisms that are nontoxic, biocompatible, and biodegradable. These bioactive polymers that have been extracted from marine organisms are being extensively used in the field of dentistry, pharmacology, medicine, and so on. Recently, various modification methods have been employed to modify their structure stability on account of their momentous contributions in pharmaceutical and biomedical fields. Microbial polymers are usually chemically modified for the improvement in their biological activity and physical property. Commercially available poly(propylene imine) dendrimers have been modified with 32 surface primary amine groups by Chen et al. (2000), thereby introducing the quaternary ammonium function on the dendrimer. The antimicrobial properties of the modified dendrimers were evaluated using a bioluminescence method. The results clearly show that higher dendrimers possess higher antibacterial activities. The modern advances in polar chemistry bestow an ideal system for microbial biopolymer. Biopolymers exhibit tremendously diverse characteristics in favor of their shape and mechanical properties such as elasticity, toughness, robustness, and strength. They repeatedly require transformative solutions for the concept of new materials (Gronau et al. 2012).

Chemically novel biomaterials are obtained by hydroxylation, esterification, sulfation, and halogenation. The most commonly chemicals that are produced naturally by microorganisms are fumaric, malic, itaconic, and succinic acids. These acids can be used as monomers for synthesizing different polymers such as poly(propylene fumarate), poly(butylenes succinate), and poly(acrylate-co-itaconate). Commercialization by microbial fermentation has been a keen interest particularly for succinic, lactic, and itaconic acids as they have a wide range of applications in polymer industry (Lee et al. 2011). Chemical properties of various biopolymers have been reported by several researchers. Thanh et al. (2013) studied chemical and conformational structures of fucoidan extracted from brown seaweed *Turbinaria ornata*. Electrospray ionization mass spectroscopy revealed that fucoidans have a sulfate content of 25.6% and are mainly composed of fucose and galactose residues (Thanh et al. 2013). Praiboon et al. (2006) have studied agar polysaccharides extracted from Thai and Japanese species of *Gracilaria*. They have been analyzed by the physical and chemical properties of agar polysaccharides. They reported that alkali treated with agar had a lower content of sulfate than the native one. The native agar *Gymnopilus edulis* had a sulfate content of 7.54% w/w, and the 3,6-anhydrogalactose content of *Gracilaria* sp. was the highest after treatment of alkali. CS is a type of glycosaminoglycan. According to its sulfation pattern, CS can be grouped as CS-O, CS-A, CS-B, CS-C, CS-D, CS-E, CS-F, and CS-K (CS-A [GlcAβ1-3GalNAc(4S)], CSC [GlcAβ1-3GalNAc(6S)], CS-D [GlcA(2S)β1-3GalNAc(6S)], CS-E [GlcAβ1-3GalNAc(4S,6S)], CS-F [GlcA(α1-3Fuc)β1-3GalNAc(4S)], CS-O [GlcAβ1-3GalNAc]) (Schiraldi et al. 2010b).

16.4 ISOLATION AND CHARACTERIZATION OF MICROBIAL BIOPOLYMER

Several techniques have been used by researchers for isolation of microbial biopolymer. Selection of a substrate from different sources is of crucial factor in biopolymer production as the type of polymer produced highly depends on the nature of microbes and the type of nutrient supplied (Sivakumara et al. 2013). The methods used for isolation of CS from marine cartilage include chemical hydrolysis, proteoglycan core breakdown, protein elimination, recovery, and purification (Roden et al. 1972, Chascall et al. 1994, Sumi et al. 2002). Guiyan et al. (2014) isolated fucoidans from five brown algae, characterized, and evaluated their antioxidant activities. Fucoidan extraction was performed by solvent extraction and centrifugation. For characterization, they used various methods such as chemical composition analysis, determination of molecular weight by high-performance gel permeation chromatography, and monosachharide composition analysis by high-performance liquid chromatography. Viswanathan and Nallamuthu (2014) extracted sodium alginate from selected seaweeds. They used 2% $CaCl_2$ for extraction, and, based on their physical properties such as their ash and water content, and gelling and melting temperature, performed biochemical analysis such as estimation of proteins, carbohydrates, and lipids. HAs have been isolated from liver marine stingray *Aetobatus narinari* by Sadhasivam et al. (2013). The types of biopolymers and their sources are given in Table 16.2.

The characterization of biopolymers comprises the evaluation of their biological, chemical, and physical properties, which are a key factor to perceive their nature and behavior in different environments, enabling to prognosticate their potential applications (Poli et al. 2011). Physical properties concern the appearance and solubility; chemical properties include the identification of their repeating units,

TABLE 16.2
Marine Microbial Biopolymers and Their Sources

Name of Microorganism	Type of Biopolymer	Source	Reference
Saccharococcus thermophilus	polyhydroxybutyrate (PHB)	Marine soil	Kalaivani and Sukumaran (2013)
Bacillus sonorensis and *Halomonas hydrothermalis*	PHA	Soil and marine environment	Shrivastav et al. (2010)
Bacillus and *Pseudomonas*	PHB	Rhizosphere soil	Sathianachiyar and Devaraj (2013)
Pseudomonas aeruginosa CMG607w and CMG1421	PHA	Sediments of Lyari outfall to Arabian Sea-marine source	Jamil and Ahmed (2008)
Vibrio spp. (strains M11, M14, M20, and M31)	PHB	Marine environment	Chien et al. (2007)
Alcaligenes eutrophus, *A. latus*, and *Hydrogenophaga* sp.	PHA	Soil	Tanamool et al. (2013)

sugar residues, and chain group constituents; and biological activity is linked with their applications. Numerous techniques have been used for characterizing microbial biopolymers: determination of molecular weight, molecular structure, fourier transform infrared spectroscopy (FTIR) and nuclear magnetic resonance (NMR) characterization, characterization of thermal and mechanical properties, gas chromatography-mass spectrometry (GC-MS), and elemental sulfur analysis (Reddy et al. 2015, Lustke-Eversloh et al. 2001).

16.5 BIOMEDICAL APPLICATION OF MICROBIAL BIOPOLYMER

16.5.1 ANTIMICROBIAL ACTIVITY

Microbial infection hindrance is a conspicuous topic in modern society. In 1965, Cornell and Dundra prepared 2-methacryloxytroponones that eradicate bacteria; since then, antimicrobial polymers have been acknowledged (Cornell and Donaruma 1965). The emergence of multidrug-resistant bacterial strains that reduced the susceptibility to antibiotics is increased. Therefore, there is a need to search for a new biomaterial to terminate microbial infection. Antimicrobial biopolymer, a class of biocides, can be used as a substitute for antibiotics. There are some characteristics that an ideal antimicrobial polymer should acquire: (1) nontoxic, (2) capable of regeneration after loss of activity, (3) nonvolatile, (4) chemically stable, and (5) not soluble in water in case of water-disinfectant application (Kenawy et al. 2007). An application of antimicrobial polymers is in a flourishing field. They can help in diminishing the problems of using conventional antimicrobial agents. Polymers with active functional groups act as a carrier system for antimicrobial agents (Alamri et al. 2012). Alamri prepared amine-terminated polyacrylonitrile that can be used as a novel polymeric carrier for benzaldehyde derivatives and inhibits the growth of microorganisms that enhance applications for biomedical and water treatment. Screening of the antimicrobial potential of chitosan and its derivatives has currently gained momentum due to its wide applications in dentistry (Ikinci et al. 2002), ophthalmology (Felt et al. 2000), food preservation (Rhoades and Roller 2000), and the manufacture of wound dressings (Ueno et al. 2001). A quaternized amino-rich biopolymer has been isolated from *Klebsiella terrigena* by Khaira et al. (2014) in 2014. The purpose of their study is to evaluate the antibacterial activity. The biopolymer isolated from bacteria is capable of inhibiting against all the selected bacterial pathogens such as *Listeria monocytogenes* ATCC 19111, *Aeromonas hydrophila* ATCC 35654 and *Escherichia coli* 0157: H7 ATCC 32150 suggesting the application as an effective disinfectant in water (Khaira et al. 2014). A glycogen biopolymer encapsulated with silver nanoparticles and its antimicrobial properties have been reported by Bozanic et al. (2011).

Glycogen from bovine liver has been used as a stabilizing agent for the growth of silver nanoparticles. Two different methods have used in the preparation of samples: fast (using microwave radiation) and slow (conventional) heating of the reaction mixtures, of which the former showed more peaks than the latter. *Staphylococcus aureus*, *Escherichia coli* and *Candida albicans* were used for the antimicrobial activity; the results showed that with an increase in silver content, the microbial growth gradually increased. The number of cells also significantly reduced after a 2-hour exposure to the nanocomposites.

16.5.2 ANTIOXIDANT ACTIVITY

Antioxidants can be natural or man-made substances that prevent or delay the types of cell damage. These molecules are capable of suppressing or protecting the cells from the damage caused by free radicals. Seaweeds and sponges have abundant sources of natural antioxidants and antimicrobials (Ngo et al. 2012), which have potential applications and contain significant quantities of proteins, lipids, vitamins, and minerals that are beneficial to human health (Newman and Cragg 2004). Polyphenolic compounds such as flavonoids, cinnamic acid, quercetin, gallic acid, benzoic acid, and phlorotannins are the antioxidants produced by marine organisms (Al-Saif et al. 2014). Algal sulfate polysaccharides are of great concern as they have the ability to scavenge free radicals and antioxidants in preventing oxidative damage in living organisms (Bultel-Ponce et al. 1998). The antioxidant activities of different derivatives of levan, that is, acetylated levan, phosphorylated levan, and benzylated levan, from *Paenibacillus polymyxa* EJS-3 have been determined by Liu et al. (2012). Derivatized levan exhibits higher reducing power and scavenging activity against superoxide radical and hydroxyl radical than the natural polysaccharide EPS-1. They suggested that the derivatives could be explored as a promising antioxidant agent (Liu et al. 2012). Abdel-Fattah et al. (2012) also studied the antioxidant activities of levan and its derivatives from *B. subtilis* NRC1aza, the uniqueness being able to produce the two types of levan with different molecular weights. From their findings, levan and its derivatives (SL1 and SL2) exhibit a strong free radical scavenging activity with 2,2-diphenyl-1-1-picrylhydrazyl (DPPH), which is recommended as a stronger antioxidant. An EPS (EPS-3) isolated from *Lactobacillus plantarum* LP6, purified by ion exchange and gel chromatography, is shown to be an effective antioxidant. The study reveals that EPS-3 could enhance the activities of the antioxidant enzyme system, which inhibits the lipid peroxidation maintaining the integrity of cell that prevents from external reactive oxygen species (ROS). This study could lay the foundation for utilization of lactic acid bacteria source resulting in its application of food systems (Li et al. 2013). Raza et al. (2012) also found a new natural antioxidant, extracellular polysaccharide extracted from *Pseudomonas fluorescens* WR-1, optimized, and reported for its antioxidant activity. The EPS exhibited a good hydrogen scavenging activity in a concentration dependent manner which was 11% higher than the ascorbic acid, the assay of reducing capacity increased with 45% higher than the EPS and the free radical scavenging activity also increased with 27% lower than the ascorbic acid of the radical scavenging activity. Sun et al. (2014) have reported a novel marine EPS from deep-sea bacterium *Zunongwangia profunda* SM-A87. They have purified and evaluated their rheological properties and antioxidant activity. They reported a novel microbial synthesis of catalytically active Ag-alginate (Ag-Alg) by using immobilized organism in alginate beads. Aqueous silver nitrate reduced to silver nanoparticles by the microorganisms present in the polymer, which get trapped in the polymer to form Ag-Alg biohydrogel. This biohydrogel exhibits the antimicrobial activity against fungi and pathogenic bacteria.

16.5.3 Anticancer/Cytotoxic Activity

Cancer is one of the most dreadful diseases that threaten human lives. There is an increasingly attempt to explore the anticancer activity from microbial biopolymers as due to their nontoxic, non-mutagenic, non-carcinogenic nature; therefore, they have been extensively used in medical applications such as wound healing, targeted drug/gene delivery, and tissue engineering, and also in diagnostic applications such as receptor, perfusion, and vascular compartment imaging using as quantum dots. A biopolymer, pullulan, that is purified from the fermentation medium of *Aureobasidium pullulans* is a highly water-soluble linear polysaccharide that can be used as a drug delivery carrier. Pullulans have various types of inert bioconjugates possibly acting as anticancer and anti-inflammatory, which are synthesized by pullulan derivatization with either doxorubicin or folic acid (Mishra et al. 2011, Mishra and Vuppu 2012). Oda et al. (1983) have reported an antitumor EPS produced by *Lactobacillus helveticus* ssp. *jugurti*. They used ascites Sarcoma -180 as a model and injected it in the EPS preparation. They concluded that host-mediated actions might be responsible for the antitumor activity of EPS. There is a need to search for an antitumor agent because cancer therapy drugs are toxic and affect normal cells. It has been reported that fucoidans extracted from brown algae *Eclonia cava*, *Sargassum hornery*, and *Costaria costata* are known to be effective tumor agents as they play an inhibitory role in human in colony formation of human melanoma SK-MEL-28 and colon cancer DLD-1 cells (Ermakova et al. 2011). The molecular weight of fucoidans highly depends on their anticancer activity. Yang et al. (2008) studied the effects of molecular weight and hydrolysis conditions on the anticancer activity of fucoidans from sporophyll of *Undaria pinnatifida*. There is a drastic change in the anticancer activity of 37.6% to 75.9% when hydrolyzed in boiling water with HCl for 5 minutes. This clearly shows that lowering their molecular weight greatly enhanced the anticancer activity of fucoidans. Salah et al. (2013) have reported high antitumor effect of low-molecular-weight (LMW) chitin. In this study, the anticancer activities of chitin, chitosan, and LMW chitin were evaluated using a human monocyte leukemia cell line THP-1, which concluded that LMW chitin has an important role in anticancer drug development.

16.5.4 Antidiabetic Activity

A chronic metabolic disorder that continues to be a global leading problem is diabetes mellitus, which influences ~4% of the population globally and presumes to increase by 5.4% in 2025 (Kim et al. 2006). A number of studies show that in the antioxidant defense system, oxidative stress leads to an increased production of ROS including superoxide radical, hydroxyl radical, and hydrogen peroxide, which are often associated with diabetes (Rahimi et al. 2005, Rudge et al. 2007). Dahecha et al. (2011) studied microbial levan and evaluated hypoglycemic and antioxidant activities in the alloxan-induced diabetic rats, which revealed that polysaccharide levan helps in reducing the oxidative stress in rats with diabetes mellitus. Yeo et al. (2007) have reported the antidiabetic effects of a novel biopolymer (PGB) 1 extracted from a new *Enterobacter* sp. BL-2. They used db/db mice as a model system being divided into normal control, rosiglitazone, low PGB1, and high PGB1 groups. Their results showed that the onset and progression of type 2 diabetes are prevented by high PGB1 and stimulate insulin secretion, thereby enhancing the hepatic glucose-metabolizing enzyme activities. Hayashi and Ito (2002) have studied the LMW chitosan and its antidiabetic activity in genetically obese diabetic mice. The main purpose of their study is to clear up the effects of LMW chitosan on hypoglycemia, hyperinsulinemia, and hypertriglyceridemia in genetically obese diabetic male KK-Ay mice. The serum glucose levels are lowered by LMW chitosan in a dose-dependent manner. They concluded that LMW chitosan may be beneficial for the treatment of obesity type 2 diabetes. Yang et al. (2002) investigated the hypoglycemic effects of exo- and endo-biopolymers produced from the submerged mycelial culture of *Ganoderma lucidum* in streptozotocin-induced diabetic rats. The hypoglycemic effects are seen in both exo- and endo-biopolymers, with the exo-biopolymer being more potent. The results suggest that exo-biopolymer may alleviate the blood glucose level by increased insulin secretion.

16.5.5 Cholesterol-Lowering Activity

Cholesterol can be claimed as excellent or poor based on its concentration, accumulation, abnormal deposition, and circulation within the body; however, a complex mechanism of sterol absorption, anabolism, excretion, and catabolism maintains cholesterol homeostasis (Yu Chen et al. 2011). Arteriosclerosis may occur due to an increase of plasma cholesterol (Wald and Law 1995). Soh et al. (2003) studied the total cholesterol adsorbed by polysaccharide by a new *in vitro* assay, that is, by enzymatic reaction and polysaccharide precipitation procedure. They compared the total adsorption cholesterol capacities, in a mixture of polysaccharides and total cholesterol, for apple pectin, xanthan gum, gelrite gellan gum, citrus pectin, high-viscous pectin, low-viscous pectin, zooglan, and dextran. Cholesterol-lowering and antioxidant activities of microbial gum have been studied by Rico et al. (2011) using C57BL/6N mice fed with a high-fat diet as a model system. For a period of 7 weeks, the mice were fed with a normal control, a high-fat diet, or a high-fat diet supplement with microbial gum. The results illustrated that microbial gum may be useful for preventing and treating high-fat diet-induced obesity and reducing the risk of obesity-related disease; hence, it possesses the cholesterol-lowering and antioxidant activities. Cholesterol-lowering effect on human trial has been reported by various researchers. Maezakia et al. (1993) investigated the hypocholesterolemic effect of chitosan in adult males. Total serum cholesterol significantly decreased when 3–6 g/day of chitosan was given in the diet to eight healthy males. Moreover, the ingestion of chitosan significantly increased serum HDL cholesterol. It has been observed that ingestion of as little as 3 g/day of chitosan controls serum cholesterol level, which makes it a great interest. Application of diets can be expected from the aspect of preventive medicine. Ylitalo et al. (2002) reviewed the cholesterol-lowering properties and the safety of chitosan. From their study, chitosan is claimed to control obesity and to lower serum cholesterol as a dietary supplement.

16.5.6 DRUG DELIVERY

Nowadays, microbial biopolymers are of great concern and receiving more attention in drug delivery field. Biopolymers from marine sources, particularly polysaccharides, are being used in the advancement of biomaterials technology (Baldwin et al. 2010). Chitosan and alginate have been extensively studied by various researchers due to their unique properties, which build them to be promising biomaterials for drug delivery system. Chitosan has the ability to form colloidal particles and enables to entrap bioactive molecules through various mechanisms such as ionic cross-linking and chemical cross-linking. Chemical modification of chitosan enables to associate with bioactive molecules to polymer, thereby enhancing to control the profile of drug release (Prabaharan and Mano 2005). Among the most versatile biopolymers, alginates have interesting characteristics such as thickening, stabilizing, and gelling properties, which play an important role in drug delivery system as these properties depend on the drug products as an excipient (Tonnesen and Karlsen 2002). Chitosan and alginate can be used in various forms such as beads, capsules, and films. Chitosan-alginate beads can be used for drug delivery together or separately to modify the release beads of the drug-loaded form (Bhattarai et al. 2011). For more effective beads, alginate and chitosan may be used together in drug delivery; their polyelectrolyte complex is of highly useful and has been extensively used for obtaining devices for controlled release of drug (Xu et al. 2007). Shi et al. (2008) prepared chitosan coated with alginate beads, which contain poly(N-isopropylacrylamide) to be used as a drug delivery system. They have investigated that the efficiency of drug loading of the beads coated with the polyelectrolyte complex is higher than the one uncoated. These findings proved the application as an effective temperature/pH delivery system.

16.5.7 TISSUE ENGINEERING AND NANOBIOTECHNOLOGY

Tissue engineering has also been a compelling area in developing artificial organs. To develop artificial organs, various materials such as natural and synthetic materials have been used. Natural biopolymers are of great interest in tissue engineering, which are being supportive in cell adhesion and function of their biological activity; however, due to their poor mechanical properties, improvement in their mechanical strength and biological is still required for the betterment in bone tissue engineering (Sahoo et al. 2013). Synthesized polymers are also extensively used and studied in bone tissue engineering for the preparation of nanocomposite (Zhang et al. 2009). Chitosans have been widely used in tissue engineering and play a crucial role because of their appealing properties such as nontoxicity, biodegradability, biocompatibility, intrinsic antibacterial nature, and minimal reactions of foreign body (Venkatesan and Kim 2010). Duan et al. (2006) used an electrospinning method for investigating a nanofibrous membrane of PLGA-chitosan, which has shown a good candidate for skin substitutes in tissue engineering. Pereira et al. (2009) established an injectable gel system for cartilage tissue regeneration. They have used a combined polysaccharide carrageenan with fibrin/HA-based hydrogel and have investigated that the vehicle used for human articular chondrocytes has the ability to fix and regenerate bovine articular cartilage of lesion experimentally made; hence, they are proved as a promising delivery system of cells in tissue engineering applications of cartilage. Nowadays, biopolymer-based materials are gaining a rapid interest. In 2013, Muller et al. (2013) have investigated an appealing and interesting biopolymer bacterial nanocellulose as a drug delivery system) using protein albumin as a model. Their findings concluded that bacterial nanocellulose has the capability of controlling and releasing products.

16.5.8 Other Techniques

Antimicrobial, antioxidant, anticancer, antidiabetic, and cholesterol properties and their activities have been described briefly. In addition, microbial biopolymers have a wide range of applications in different fields due to their unique and interesting characteristics. Other techniques include anti-inflammatory and immunomodulatory activities, tissue engineering, wound healing, drug delivery applications, bioseparation, diagnostic applications, hydrogels, membranes, food packaging, and water treatment. A new approach arises in the advancement of biomaterials regarding bioseparation and diagnostic applications. For this, a biomaterial should have ideal properties such as compatibility with denaturation and reduction of nonspecific absorption, ability to amplify and transmit signals, and favorable in high-throughput screening (Goddard and Hotchkiss 2007). Polymer surface modification or surface-coated functional polymers are useful for the preparation of biochips, which find their applications in diagnostics, food industry, and environmental monitoring. To improve biocompatibility and immobilization of the targeted analyte, surface modifications of polymers such as wet chemical, organosilanization, ionized gas treatments, and ultraviolet irradiation are highly useful (Gautam et al. 2014). There are several reports on microbial EPS and its immunomodulatory activity. Xu et al. (2009) have studied an EPS enriched with selenium with immunomodulatory activity extracted from *Enterobacter cloacae* Z0206. From their findings, selenium-enriched EPS could be used as a useful immunomodulatory agent. As already mentioned, the marine environment is well endowed with rich sources of diversified organisms. Recently, marine organism-derived biomaterials for wound healing and tissue engineering are of great concern. Thus, there are numerous ongoing studies to identify and isolate an ideal material for healing wound and substitute for tissue-engineered as a remedial agent (Gautam et al. 2014, Nwe et al. 2010).

16.6 FUTURE PERSPECTIVE

Biopolymers and their applications within the medical fields had greatly reduced and minimized the diseases of human beings offering a healthy life. A large number of novel compounds/biopolymers are being extracted from marine sources with a wide range of applications including textile industry, waste treatment, health care products, artificial organs, and bone replacement and implants. It has been proved that marine environment is well embellished with a diversity of unexploited resources, but there is a need to develop biomaterials and explore more of them. Modification of biopolymer is an extensively and widely used approach that allows marine-derived polymers to enhance their biological activity and improve their physical and chemical property, and used in terms of applications especially in tissue engineering, biomass production, and tissue delivery. The development of marine microbial biopolymers may open up a comprehensive utilization as biomaterials in different fields. Further studies and exploration are important to investigate the maximum potential of marine microbial biopolymers.

REFERENCES

Abdel-Fattah, A. M., Gamal-Eldeenb, A. M., Helmya, W. A., and M. A. Esawy. 2012. Antitumor and antioxidant activities of levan and its derivative from the isolate *Bacillus subtilis* NRC1aza. *Carbohyd Polym* 89:314–322.

Alamri, A., El-Newehy, M. H., and I. S. S. Al-Deyab. 2012. Biocidal polymers: Synthesis and antimicrobial properties of benzaldehyde derivatives immobilized onto amine-terminated polyacrylonitrile. *Chem Cent J* 6:111.

Al-Saif, S. S., Abdel-Raouf, N., El-Wazanani, H. A., and I. A. Aref. 2014. Antibacterial substances from marine algae isolated from Jeddah coast of Red sea, Saudi Arabia, Saudi. *J Biol Sci* 21:57–64.

Baldwin, A. D., and K. L. Kiick. 2010. Polysaccharide-modified synthetic polymeric biomaterials. *Biopolymers* 94(1):128–40.

Bhattarai, R. S., Dhandapani, N. V., and A. Shrestha. 2011. Drug delivery using alginate and chitosan beads: An Overview. *Chron Young Sci* 2(4):192–196.

Borsig, L., Wang, L., Cavalcante, M. C., Cardilo-Reis, L., Ferreira, P. L., Mourao, P. A., Esko, J. D., and M. S. Pvao. 2007. Selectin blocking activity of a fucosylated chondroitin sulphate glycosaminoglycan from sea cucumber. Effect on tumor metastasis and neutrophil recruitment. *J Biol Chem* 282:14984–14991.

Bozanic, D. K., Dimitrijevic-Brankovic, S., Bibic, N., Luyt, A. S., and V. Djokovic. 2011. Silver nanoparticles encapsulated in glycogen biopolymer: Morphology, optical and antimicrobial properties. *Carbohydr Polymer* 83 (2):883–890.

Bultel-Ponce, V. V., Debitus, C., Berge, J. P., Cerceau, C., and M. Guyot. 1998. Metabolites from the sponge associated bacterium Micrococcus luteus. *J Mar Biotechnol* 6:233–236.

Cai, S., Liu, Y., Shu, X. Z., and G. D. Prestwich. 2005. Injectable glycosaminoglycan hydrogels for controlled release of human basic fibroblast growth factor. *Biomaterials* 26: 6054–6067.

Campo, V. L., Kawano, D. F., Silva, D. B. Jr., and D. I. Carvalho. 2009. Carrageenans: Biological properties, chemical modifications and structural analysis—A review. *Carbohydr Polymer* 77:167–180.

Cassaro, C. M., and C. P. Dietrich. 1977. Distribution of sulfated mucopolysaccharides in invertebrates. *J Biol Chem* 252(7):2254–2261.

Chang, C. H., Liu, H. C., Lin, C. C., Chou, C. H., and F. H. Lin. 2003. Gelatin–chondroitin–hyaluronan tri-copolymer scaffold for cartilage tissue engineering. *Biomaterials* 24:4853–4858.

Chascall, V., Calabro, A., Midura, R. J., and M. Yanagishita. 1994. Isolation and characterization of proteoglycans. In *Methods in Enzymology*. Lennarz, W. J., Hart, G. W., Eds., Academic Press: San Diego, CA, Volume 230, pp. 390–417.

Chen, C. Z., Beck-Tan, N. C., Dhurjati, P., Van Dyk, T. K., LaRossa, R. A., and S. L. Cooper. 2000. Quaternary ammonium functionalized poly (propylene imine) dendrimers as effective anti-microbials: Structure-activity studies. *Biomacromolecules* 1(3):473–480.

Chien, C. C., Chen, C. C., Choi, M. H., Kung, S. S., and Y. H. Wei. 2007. Production of poly-β-hydroxybutyrate (PHB) by *Vibrio* spp. Isolated from marine environment. *J Biotechnol* 132(3):259–63.

Chong, B. F., Blank, L. M., Mclaughlin, R., and L. K. Nielsen. 2005. Microbial hyaluronic acid production. *Appl Microbiol Biotechnol* 66:341–351.

Conte, A., Volpi, N., Palmieri, L., Bahous, I., and G. Ronca. 1995. Biochemical and pharmaco-kinetic aspects of oral treatment with chondroitin sulphate. *Arzneim Forsch* 45:918–925.

Cornell, R. J., and L. G. Donaruma. 1965. 2-Methacryloxytroponones. Intermediates for synthesis of biologically active polymers. *J Med Chem* 8:388–390.

Dahecha, I., Belghitha, K. S., Hamdenb, K., Feki, A., Belghithc H., and H. Mejdouba. 2011. Antidiabetic activity of levan polysaccharide in alloxan-induced diabetic rats. *Int J Biol Macromo* 49:742–746.

Distantina, S., Rochmadi, M. Fahrurrozi, and Wiratni. 2013. Hydrogels Based on Carrageenan Extracted from Kappaphycus alvarezii. *Proc World Acad Sci Eng Tech* 7:06–22.

Duan, B., Yuan, X., Zhu, Y., Zhang, Y., Li, X., Zhang, Y. and K. Yeo. 2006. A nanofibrous composite membrane of PLGA-Chitosan/PVA prepared by electrospinning. *Eur Polym J* 42:2013–2022.

Duckworth, M., and W. Yaphe. 1971. The structure of agar: Part I. Fractionation of a complex mixture of polysaccharides. *Carbohydr Res* 16 (1):189–197.

El-Sayed, M. M. 1983. Purification and characterization of agar from digenea simplex. *Carbohydr Res* 118:119–126.

Ermakova, S., Sokolova, R., Kim, S. M., Um, B. H., Isakov, V., and T. Zvyagintseva. 2011. Fucoidans from brown seaweeds *Sargassum hornery, Eclonia cava, Costaria costata*: Structural characteristics and anticancer activity. *Appl Biochem Biotechnol* 164:841–850.

Felt, O., Carrel, A., Baehni, P., Buri, P., and R. Gurny. 2000. Chitosan as tear substitute. A wetting agent endowed with antimicrobial efficacy. *J Ocul Pharmacol Ther* 16:261–270.

Gautam, M. K., Purohit, V., Agarwal, M., Singh, A., and R. K. Goel. 2014. In vivo healing potential of aegle marmelos in excision, incision, and dead space wound models. *Sci World J* 2014: 9.

Girond, S., Crance, J. M., Van Cuyck-Gandre, H., Renaudet, J., and R. Deloince. 1991. Antiviral activity of carrageenan on hepatitis A virus replication in cell culture. *Res Virol* 142:261–270.

Goddard, J. M., and J. H. Hotchkiss. 2007. Polymer surface modification for the attachment of bioactive compounds. *Prog Polym Sci* 32:698–725.

Goh, C. H., Heng, P. W. S., and L. W. Chan. 2012. Alginates as a useful natural polymer for microencapsulation and therapeutic applications *Carbohydr Polym* 88:1–12.

Gronau, G., Sreevidhya, T., Krishnaji, S. T., Kinahan, M. E., Giesa, T., Wong, J. Y., Kaplan, D. L., and M. J. Buehler. 2012. A review of combined experimental and computational procedures for assessing biopolymer structure–process–property relationships. *Biomaterials* 33(33):8240–8255.

Guiseley, K. B. 1989. Chemical and physical properties of algal polysaccharides used for cell immobilization. *Enzyme Microb Technol* 11 (11):706–716.

Guiyan, Q. U., Xu, L. U., Dongfeng, W., Yi, Y., and H. Lijun. 2014. Isolation and characterization of fucoidans from five brown algae and evaluation of their antioxidant activity. *J Ocean Univ China* 5:851–856.

Hamano, T., Mitsuhashi, Y., Acki, N., Yamamoto, S., Tsuji, S., Ito, Y., and Y. Oji. 1989. High-performance liquid chromatography assay of chondroitin sulfate in food products. *Analyst* 114:891–893.

Hardingham, T. 2004. Solution Properties of Hyaluronan. In *Chemistry and Biology of Hyaluronan*. Garg, H. G., Hales, C. A., Eds., Elsevier: Oxford, UK, pp. 1–16.

Hayashi, K., and M. Ito. 2002. Antidiabetic action of low molecular weight chitosan in genetically obese diabetic KK-AY mice. *Biol Pharmaceut Bull* 25:188:192.

Ikinci, G., Senel, S., Akincibay, H., Kas, S., Ercis, S., Wilson C. G., and A. A Hincal. 2002. Effect of chitosan on a periodontal pathogen Porphyromonas gingivalis. *Int J Pharm* 235:121–127.

Jamil, N., and N. Ahmed. 2008. Production of biopolymers by *Pseudomonas aeruginosa* isolated from marine source. *Braz Arch Biol Tech* 51(3):457–464.

Kalaivani, R., and V. Sukumaran. 2013. Isolation and identification of new strains to enhance the production of biopolymers from marine sample in Karankura, Tamil Nadu. *Eur J Exp Biol* 3(3):56–64.

Kenawy, E. R., Worley, S. D., and R. Broughton. 2007. The chemistry and applications of antimicrobial polymers: A state-of-the-art review. *Biomacromolecules* 8(5): 1359–1384.

Khaira, G. K., Ganguli, A., and M. Ghosh. 2014. Synthesis and evaluation of antibacterial activity of quaternized biopolymer from Klebsiella terrigena. *J Appl Microbiol* 116(3):511.

Kim, S. H., Hyun, S. H., and S. Y., Choung. 2006. Anti-diabetic effect of cinnamon extract on blood glucose in db/db mice. *J Ethnol* 104:119–123.

Kim, S. J., Park, S. Y., and C. W. Kin. 2006. A novel approach to the production of hyaluronic acid by Streptococcus zooepidemicus. *J Microbiol Biotechnol* 16:1849–1855.

Kitagawa, H., Tanaka, Y., Yamada, S., Seno, N., Haslam, S. M., Morris, H. R., Dell, A., and K. Sugahara. 1997. A novel pentasaccharide sequenceGlcA(3-sulfate)(b1–3)GalNAc(4-sulfate)(b1–4)(Fuca1-3)GlcA(b1-3)GalNAc(4-sulfate) in the oligosaccharides isolated from king crab cartilage chondroitin sulfate K and its differential susceptibility to chondroitinases and hyaluronidase. *Biochemistry* 36(13):3998–4008.

Lamari, F. N., Theocharis, A. D., Asimakopoulou, A. P., Malavaki, C. J., and N. K. Karamanos. 2006. Metabolism and biochemical/physiological roles of chondroitin sulfates: Analysis of endogenous and supplemental chondroitin sulfates in blood circulation. *Biomed Chromatogr* 20 (6–7):539–550.

Laurienzo, P. 2010. Marine polysaccharides in pharmaceutical applications: An overview. *Mar Drugs* 8(9):2435–2465.

Lee, J. W., Kim, H. U., Choi, S., Yi, J., and S. Y. Lee. 2011. Microbial production of building block chemicals and polymers. *Curr Opin Biotechnol* 22(6):758–67.

Lee, K. Y., and J. D. Mooney. 2012. Alginate: Properties and biomedical applications. *Progr Polymer Sci* 37:106–126.

Li, B., Lu, F., Wei, X., and R. Zhao. 2008a. Fucoidan: Structure and bioactivity. *Molecules* 13:1671–169.

Li, H. Y., Yu, X. J., Jin, Y., Zhang, W., and Y. L. Liu. 2008b. Development of an eco-friendly agar extraction technique from the red. Seaweed gracilaria lemaneiformis. *Bioresour Technol* 99(8):3301–3305.

Li, J. Y., Jin, M. M., Meng, J., Gao, S. M., and R. R. Lu. 2013. Exopolysaccharide from *Lactobacillus planterum* LP6: Antioxidation and the effect on oxidative stress. *Carbohydr Polym* 98(1):1147–1152.

Liao, Y. H., Jones, S. A., Forbes, B., Martin, G. P., and M. B. Brown. 2005. Hyaluronan: Pharmaceutical characterization and drug delivery. *Drug Deliv* 12(6):327–342.

Lignot, B., Lahogue, V., and P. Bourseau. 2003. Enzymatic extraction of chondroitin sulfate from skate cartilage and concentrationdesalting by ultrafiltration. *J Biotechnol* 103 (3): 281–284.

Liu, J., Luo, J., Ye, H., and X. Zeng. 2012. Preparation, antioxidant and antitumor activities in vitro of different derivatives of levan from endophytic bacterium Paenibacillus polymyxa EJS-3. *Food Chem Toxicol* 50(3–4):767–772.

Luo, X. M., Fosmire, G. H., and R. M. Leach Jr. 2002. Chicken keel cartilage as a source of chondroitin sulphate. *Poult Sci* 81(7):1086–1089.

Lustke-Eversloh, T., Bergander, K., Luftmann, H., and A. Steinbuchel. 2001. Identification of a new class of biopolymer: Bacterial synthesis of a sulfur-containing polymer with thioester linkages. *Microbiology* 147:11–19.

Maezakia, Y., Tsujib, K., Nakagawac, Y., Kawaid, Y., Akimotod, M., Tsugitae, T., Takekawaf, W., Teradag, A., Harag, H., and T. Mitsuokag. 1993. Hypocholesterolemic Effect of Chitosan in Adult Males. *Biosci Biotech Biochem* 57(9):1439–144.

Majima, M., Takagaki, K., Sudo, S. I., Yoshihara, S., Kudo, Y., and S. Yamagishi. 2001. Effect of proteoglycan on experimental colitis. *Int Cong Ser* 1223:221–224.

Mattias, T., Chyan-Jang, L., Magnus, G., May, G., Peter, P., and K. Peter. 2014. Synthesis and Biological Evaluation of Fucoidan-Mimetic Glycopolymers through Cyanoxyl-Mediated Free-Radical Polymerization. Biomacromolecules 15 (7): 2359–2368.

McNaught, A. D., Wilkinson, A., and A. Jenkins. 1997. *Compendium of Chemical Terminology (The Gold Book)*. Blackwell Scientific Publications: Oxford 2nd edn. p. B0066.

Mehta, A., Sidhu, C., Pinnaka, A. K., Roy and A. Choudhury A. 2014. Extracellular polysaccharide production by a novel osmotolerant marine strain of *Alteromonas macleodii* and its application towards biomineralization of silver. *PLoS One* 9(6):e98798. doi:10.1371/journal.pone.0098798.

Michelacci, Y. M., and C. P. Dietrich. 1986. Structure of chondroitin sulphate from whale cartilage: Distribution of 6- and 4-sulphated oligosaccharides in the polymer chains. *Int J Biol Macromol* 8(2):108–113.

Mishra, B., and S. Vuppu. 2012. The microbial pullulan as therapeutic tool in Medicine. *IJAHM* 2(1):180–186.

Mishra, B., Vuppu, S., and K. Rath. 2011. The role of microbial pullulan, a biopolymer in pharmaceutical approaches: A review. *Int Res J Pharmaceut Appl Sci* 1(6):45–50.

Mourao, P. A. S. 2004. Use of sulfated fucans as anticoagulant and antithrombotic agents: Future perspectives. *Curr Pharmaceut* 10:967–981.

Muller, A., Ni, Z., Hessler, N., Wesarg, F., Muller, F. A., Kralisch, D., and D. Fischer. 2013. The biopolymer bacterial nanocellulose as drug delivery system: Investigation of drug loading and release using the model protein albumin. *J Pharm Sci* 102(2):579–92.

Murado, M. A., Montemayor, M. I., Cabo, M. L., Vazque, J. A., and M. P. Gonzalez. 2012. Optimization of extraction and purification process of hyaluronic acid from fish eyeball. *Food Bioprod Proc* 90:491–498.

Murano, E., Toffanin, R., Zanetti, F., Knutsen, S. H., Paoletti, S., and R. Rizzo. 1992. Chemical and macromolecular characterisation of agar polymers from *Gracilaria dura* (C. Agardh) J. Agardh (Gracilariaceae, Rhodophyta). *Carbohydr Polym* 8(3):171–178.

Nair, L. S., and C. T. Laurencin. 2007. Biodegradable polymers as biomaterials. *Prog Polym Sci* 32:762–98.

Nayak, A. K., and D. Pal. 2011. Development of pH-sensitive tamarind seed polysaccharide-alginate composite beads for controlled diclofenac sodium delivery using response surface methodology. *Int J Biol Macromol* 49:784–793.

Newman, D. J., and G. M. Cragg. 2004. Marine natural products and related compounds in clinical and advanced preclinical trials. *J Nat Prod* 67:1216–1238.

Ngo, D. H., Vo, T. S., Ngo, D. N., Wijesekara, I., and S. K. Kim. 2012. Biological activities and potential health benefits of bioactive peptides derived from marine organisms. *Int J Biol Macromol* 51:378–383.

Nichols, C. M., Bowman, J. P., and J. Guezennec 2005. Effects of incubation temperature on growth and production of exopolysaccharides by an Antarctic Sea ice bacterium grown in batch culture. *Appl Environ Microbiol* 71:3519–3523.

Nwe, N., Furuike, T., and H. Tamura. 2010. Selection of a biopolymer based on attachment, morphology and proliferation of fibroblast NIH/3T3 cells for the development of a biodegradable tissue regeneration template: Alginate, bacterial cellulose and gelatin. *Process Biochem* 45(4):457–466.

Oda, M., Hasegawa, H., Komatsu, S., Kambe, M., and F. Tsuchiya 1983. Anti-tumor polysaccharide from LactoBacillus spp. *Agric Biol Chem* 47:1623–1625.

Otari, S. V., Patil, R. M., Waghmare, S. R., Ghosh, S. J., and S. H. Pawar. 2013. A novel microbial synthesis of catalytically active Ag-alginate biohydrogel and its antimicrobial activity. *Dalton Trans* 42(27):9966–9975.

Payne, G. F., and S. R. Raghavan. 2007. Chitosan: A soft interconnect for hierarchical assembly of nano-scale components. *Soft Matter* 3:521–7.

Pereira, R. C., Scaranari, M., Castagnola, P., Grandizio, M., Azevedo, H. S., Reis, R. L., Cancedda, R., and C. Gentili. 2009. Novel injectable gel (system) as a vehicle for human articular chondrocytes in cartilage tissue regeneration. *J Tissue Eng Regen Med* 3(2):97–106.

Pipitone, V. R. 2003. Chondroprotection with chondroitin sulphate. *Drugs Exp Clin* 17:3–7.

Poli, A., Donato, P. D., Abbamondi, G. R., and B. Nicolaus. 2011. Synthesis, production, and biotechnological applications of exopolysaccharides and polyhydroxyalkanoates by archaea. *Archaea* 2011:1–13.

Prabaharan, M., and J. F. Mano. 2005. Chitosan-based particles as controlled drug delivery systems. *Drug Deliv* 12(1):41–57.

Praiboon, J., Chirapart, A., Akakabe, Y., Bhumibhamond, O., and T. Kajiwarac. 2006. Physical and chemical characterization of agar polysaccharides extracted from the Thai and Japanese species of gracilaria. *ScienceAsia* 32(1):11–17.

Rahimi, R., Nikfar, S., Larijani, B., and M. Abdollahi. 2005. A review on the role of anti-oxidants in the management of diabetes and its complications. *Biomed Pharmacother* 59(7):365–373.

Rangaswamy, V., and D. Jain. 2008. An efficient process for production and purification of hyaluronic acid from *Streptococcus equi* subsp. Zooepidemicus. *Biotechnol Lett* 30:493–496.

Raza, W., Yang, W., Jun, Y., Shakoor, F., Huang, Q., and Q. Shen. 2012. Optimization and characterization of a polysaccharide produced by Pseudomonas fluorescens WR-1 and its antioxidant activity. *Carbohydr Polym* 90(2):921–9.

Reddy, C. H., Siddartha, G., Ramaiah, M. J., and K. B. Uppuluri. 2015. Review on production, characterization and applications of microbial levan. *Carbohydr Polym* 120(20):102 –114.

Rhoades, J., and S. Roller. 2000. Antimicrobial actions of degraded and native chitosan against spoilage organisms in laboratory media and foods. *Appl Environ Microbiol* 66:80–86.

Rico, C. W., Shin, J. H., Um, I. C., and M. Y. Kang. 2011. Cholesterol-lowering action and antioxidative effects of microbial gum in C57BL/6N mice fed a high fat diet. *Biotechnol Bioproc Eng* 16:167–172.

Rochas, C., and Lahaye, M. 1989. Average molecular weight and molecular weight distribution of agarose and agarose-type polysaccharides. *Carbohydr Polym* 10(4):289–298.

Rudge, M. V., Damasceno, D. C., Volpato, G. T., Almeida, F. C., Calderon, I. M., and I. P. Lemonica. 2007. Effect of Ginkgo biloba on the reproductive outcome and oxidative stress biomarkers of streptozotocin-induced diabetic rats. *Braz J Med Biol Res* 40:1095–1099.

Sadhasivam, G., Muthuvel, A., Pachaiyappan, A., and B. Thangavel. 2013. Isolation and characterization of hyaluronic acid from the liver of marine stingray *Aetobatus narinari*. *Int J Biol Macromo* 54:84–89.

Sahoo, N. G., Pan, Y. Z., Li, L., and C. B. He. 2013. Nanocomposites for bone tissue regeneration. *Nanomedicine* 8(4):639–653.

Salah, R., Michaud, P., Mati, F., Harrat, Z., Lounici, H., Abdi, N., Drouiche, N., and N. Mameri. 2013. Anticancer activity of chemically prepared shrimp low molecular weight chitin evaluation with the human monocyte leukaemia cell line, THP. *Int J Biol Macromo* 52:333–339.

Sathianachiyar, S., and A. Devaraj. 2013. Biopolymer production by bacterial species using Glycerol, a byproduct of biodiesel. *IJSRP* 3(8):2250–3153.

Schiraldi, C., Cimini, D., and M. de Rosa. 2010a. Production of chondroitin sulphate and chondroitin. *Appl Microbiol Biotechnol* 87:1209–1220.

Schiraldi, C., La Gatta, A., and M. De Rosa. 2010b. Biotechnological production and application of hyaluronan. In *Biopolym.* Elnashar, M, ed., InTech, Rijeka: Croatia, pp. 387–412.

Shi, J., Alves., N. M., and J. F. Mano. 2008. Chitosan coated alginate beads containing poly (N-isopropylacrylamide) for dual-stimuli-responsive drug release. *J Biomed Mater Res B Appl Biomater* 84(2):595–603.

Shrivastav, A., Mishra, S. K., Shethia, B., Pancha, I., Jain, D., and S. Mishra. 2010. Isolation of promising bacterial strains from soil and marine environment for polyhydroxyalkanoates (PHAs) production utilizing Jatropha biodiesel byproduct. *Int J Biol Macromol* 47(2010):283–287.

Silva, T. H., Alves, A., Ferreira, B. M., Oliveira, J. M., Reys, L. L., Ferreira, R. J. F., Sousa, R. A., Silva, S. S., Mano, J. F., and R. L. Reis. 2012. Materials of marine origin: A review on polymers and ceramics of biomedical interest. *Int Mater Rev* 57(5):276–306.

Silva, T. M. A., Alves, L. G., Queiroz, K. C. S., Santos, M. G. L., Marques, C. T., Chavante, S. F., Rocha, H. A. O., and E. L. Leite. 2005. Partial characterization and anticoagulant activity of a heterofucan from the brown seaweed Padina gymnospora. *Braz J Med Biol* 38:523–533.

Sinurat, E., and P. dan Rosmawaty. 2015. Evaluation of fucoidan bioactivity as anti gastric ulcers in mice. *Procedia Environ Sci* 23:407–411.

Sivakumara, N., Bahryb, S. A., and H. S. Al-Battashic. 2013. Screening of biopolymer producing bacteria isolated from some brassica plants. *APCBEE Procedia* 5:333–338.

Roden, L., Baker, J. R., Cifonelli, J. A., and M. B. Mathews. 1972. Isolation and characterization of connective tissue polysaccharides. *Methods Enzymol* 28:73–140.

Smidsrod, O., and G. Skjak-Braek. 1990. Alginate as immobilization matrix for cells. *Trend Biotechnol* 8:71–8.

Soh, H. S., Kim, C. S., and S. P. Lee. 2003. A new in vitro assay of cholesterol adsorption by food and microbial polysaccharides. *J Med Food* 6(3):225–30.

Stellwagen, J., and N. C. Stellwagen. 1994. Transient electric birefringence of agarose gels. II. Reversing electric fields and comparison with other polymer gels. *Biopolymers* 34:1259.

Stern, R., and M. J. Jedrzejas. 2008. Carbohydrate polymers at the center of life's origins: The importance of molecular processivity. *Chem Rev* 108:5061–85.

Sumi, T., Ohba, H., Ikegami, T., Shibata, M., Sakaki, T., Salay, I., Park, S. S. Method for the preparation of chondroitin sulfate compounds. U.S. Patent 6,342,367, January 29, 2002.

Sun, M. L., Liu, S. B., Qiao, L. P., Chen, X. L., Pang, X., Shi, M., Zhang, X. Y., Qin, Q. L., Zhou, B. C., Zhang, Y. Z., and B. B. Xie. 2014. A novel exopolysaccharide from deep-sea bacterium Zunongwangia profunda SM-A87: Low-cost fermentation, moisture retention, and antioxidant activities. *Appl Microbiol Biotechnol* 98(17):7437–45.

Tammi, M. I., Day, A. J., and E. A. Turley. 2002. Hyaluronan and homeostasis: A balancing act. *J Biol Chem* 277(7):4581–4584.

Tanamool, V., Imai, T., Danvirutai, P., and P. Kaewkannetra. 2013. Biopolymer generation from sweet sorghum juice: Screening, isolation, identification, and fermentative polyhydroxyalkanoate production by Bacillus aryabhattai. *Turk J Biol* 37:259–264.

Tengdelius, M., Lee, C. J., Grenegard, M., Griffith, M., Pahlsson, P., and P. Konradsson. 2014. Synthesis and biological evaluation of fucoidan-mimetic glycopolymers through cyanoxyl-mediated free-radical polymerization. *Biomacromolecules* 15:2359–2368.

Thanh, T. T. T., Tran, V. T. T., Yuguchi, Y., Bui, L. M., and T. T. Nguyen. 2013. Structure of fucoidan from brown seaweed *Turbinaria ornata* as studied by electrospray ionization mass spectrometry (ESIMS) and small angle X-ray scattering (SAXS) techniques. *Mar Drugs* 11(7):2431–2443.

Tian, H., Tang, Z., Zhuang, X., Chen, X., and X. Jing. 2012. Biodegradable synthetic polymers: Preparation, functionalization and biomedical application. *Progr Polymer Sci* 37(2):237–280.

Tonnesen, H. H., and J. Karlsen. 2002. Alginate in drug delivery systems. *Drug Dev Ind Pharm* 28(6):621–30.

Ueno, H., Mori, T., and T. Fujinaga. 2001. Topical formulations and wound healing applicaions of chitosan. *Adv Drug Deliv Rev* 52:105–115.

Vazquez, J. A., Amado, I. R., Montemayor, M. I., Fraguas, J., Gonzalez, M. P., and M. A. Murado. 2013. Chondroitin sulfate, hyaluronic acid and chitin/chitosan production using marine waste sources: Characteristics, applications and eco-friendly processes: A review. *Mar Drugs* 11:747–774.

Venkatesan, J., and S. K. Kim. 2010. Chitosan composites for bone tissue engineering–an overview. *Mar Drugs* 8(8):2252–66.

Vieira, R. P., and P. A. Mourao. 1988. Occurrence of a unique fucosebranched chondroitin sulfate in the body wall of a sea cucumber. *J Biol Chem* 263(34):18176–18183.

Viswanathan, S., and T. Nallamuthu. 2014. Extraction of sodium alginate from selected seaweeds and their physiochemical and biochemical properties. *IJIRSET* 3(4):10998–1003.

Volpi, N. 2009. Quality of different chondroitin sulphate preparations in relation to their therapeutic activity. *J Pharm Pharmacol* 61:1271–1277.

Wald, N. J., and M. R. Law. 1995. Serum cholesterol and ischemic heart disease. *Atherosclerosis* 118:1–5.

Wijesekara, I., Pangestuti, R., and S. K. Kim. 2011. Biological activities and potential health benefits of sulfated polysaccharides derived from marine algae. *Carbohydr Polym* 84:14–21.

Xu, C. L., Wang, Y. Z., Jin, M. L., and X. Q. Yang. 2009. Preparation, characterization and immunomodulatory activity of selenium-enriched exopolysaccharide produced by bacterium Enterobacter cloacae Z0206. *Bioresource Technol* 100:2095–2097.

Xu, Y., Zhan, C., Fan, F., Wang, L., and H. Zheng. 2007. Preparation of dual crosslinked alginate-chitosan blend gel beads and in vitro controlled release in oral site-specific drug delivery system. *Int J Pharm* 336:329–37.

Yang, C., Chung, D., Shin, I. S., Lee, H., Kim, J., Lee, Y., and S. You. 2008. Effects of molecular weight and hydrolysis conditions on anticancer activity of fucoidans from sporophyll of Undaria pinnatifida. *Int J Biol Macromo* 43(5):433–7.

Yang, Keuni, B., Jeong, S. C., and C. H. Song. 2002. Hypolipidemic effect of exo- and endo-biopolymers produced from submerged mycelial culture of ganoderma lucidum in rats. *J Microbiol Biotechnol* 12(6):872–877.

Yeo, J., Lee, Y. H., Jeon, S. M., Jung, U. J., Lee, M. K., Jung, Y. M., and M. S. Choi. 2007. Supplementation of a novel microbial biopolymer, PGB1, from new Enterobacter sp. BL-2 delays the deterioration of type 2 diabetic mice. *J Microbiol Biotechnol* 17(12):1983–90.

Ylitalo, R., Lehtinen, S., Wuolijoki, E., Ylitalo, P., and T. Lehtimaki. 2002. Cholesterol-lowering properties and safety of chitosan. *Arzneimittelforschung* 52(1):1–7.

Yu Chen, Z., Ma, K. Y., Liang, Y., Peng, C., and Y. Zuo. 2011. Role and classification of cholesterol-lowering functional foods. *J Funct Foods* 3(2):61–69.

Zhang, P. B., Hong, Z. K., Yu, T., Chen, X. S., and X. B. Jing. 2009. In vivo mineralization and osteogenesis of nanocomposite scaffold of poly (lactide-coglycolide) and hydroxyapatite surface-grafted with poly(l-lactide). *Biomaterials* 30:58–70.

Zimmermann, H., Shirley, S., and U. Zimmermann. 2007. Alginate-based encapsulation of cells: Past, present, and future. *Curr Diab Rep* 7:314–20.

17 Electrospinning of Marine-Origin Biopolymers toward Tissue Regeneration

Ana L.P. Marques, Tiago H. Silva, and Rui L. Reis

CONTENTS

17.1 INTRODUCTION

The aquatic environment, such as oceans, rivers, or lakes, is rich in biodiversity: fishes, marine sponges, jellyfishes, molluscs, crustaceans, or algae, among many others (including a huge and mostly unknown multiplicity of microorganisms). This variety turns out to be a gold mine in terms of natural biopolymers diversity. The exploitation of marine compounds for biological and biomedical applications is an area being explored more intensely in the latest years, in order to take advantage of all these abundant and underexplored marine resources. The idea is the valorization of underexplored marine organisms, such as seaweeds, or of by-products as consequence of the activity of fish processing industries. This involves, for instance, marine organisms that are caught by mistake on sea net fishes (by-catches) and are not used for food purpose, or fish processing by-products from industries. Indeed, ~75% of fish weight is discarded as processing leftovers such as skins, bones, fins, heads, guts, and scales, from which arises a huge potential for conversion into valuable products. Those natural polymers can be classified into proteins (collagen, gelatin, keratin, etc.), polysaccharides (agar, alginate, carrageenan, chitin, fucoidan, chondroitin sulfate, hyaluronic acid, etc.), and nucleic acids. Also bioceramics (hydroxyapatite, biosilica, calcium carbonates, etc.) take part in the constitution of some marine organisms (Ratner et al. 2004). Recent researches have arisen with the successful development of methods for isolation, purification, and characterization of these compounds from several marine sources, envisaging their application in many different industrial fields (Percival 1979; Nagai et al. 1999; Nagai and Suzuki 2000; Kinoshita-Toyoda et al. 2004; Abdou et al. 2008; Li et al. 2008).

A significant issue that has been under discussion lately when considering the use of natural polymers in health is the risk of posing diseases from animals to humans. In particular, bovine and porcine origins are common sources used to isolate natural polymers, and these have that inherent risk of transmitting diseases, such as bovine spongiform encephalopathy, to humans, a disease that attacked a huge area worldwide. Moreover, there are the constraints regarding some consumers due to their religious beliefs (halal and kosher markets). In this way, marine biopolymers can overcome such issues, because there is, until now, no evidence of disease risk from marine organisms to humans; therefore, they can be consumed by everyone, despite religious beliefs.

In this context, biopolymers from marine origin have gained an increased interest in the market of different fields. Paul Scheuer (University of Hawaii) was the first chemist to study marine natural products in 1950s until his death in 2003. With this starting research on marine toxin structures, other works in this area led to the discovery of biologically active molecules, which had potential to be used in human pharmaceutical agents. A high importance has been given to pharmaceutical science for drug delivery purposes, because there are several compounds with different bioactivities, including antitumor. For instance, extracted marine bioactive peptides have shown several biological functions such as anticancer, antihypertensive, antioxidative, antimicrobial, antithrombotic, antihypercholesterol, immunomodulatory, prebiotic, opioid agonistic, and mineral-binding activities, without the potential side effects of the developed synthetic drugs (Kim et al. 2013). Other potential applications have arisen in others fields, with the evolution of extraction, purification, and processing techniques. For example, improvement in solubility of marine food proteins is explored so they can be used as food supplements, along with chemical and enzymatic modifications. Natural bioactive compounds are mostly required for beauty purposes, which are used to maintain a young appearance with the use of new cosmetics. So, there is an increasing need of using natural products, which are safe and inexpensive ingredients, so far. With this growing interest, it is very likely that the use of by-products to extract marine compounds is instilling a new commercial value to them. Regarding this, the valorization of by-products can be exploited for this purpose, giving them a new meaning with great economic and environmental advantages (Dutta et al. 2004; Silva et al. 2012).

17.2 MARINE BIOPOLYMERS IN HEALTH AND WELL-BEING SECTORS

Several marine-origin compounds are already well established and commercialized in pharmaceutical, cosmetic, and food industries. There are two main classes—proteins and polysaccharides—with biopolymers well known for their good features in different science fields being currently the components in numerous products.

17.2.1 PROTEINS

Collagen, a general term that defines a group of proteins composed of a triple helix of polypeptide chains (α-chains), exists in several tissues in the body, such as the bone, skin, and tendon (mainly type I), cartilage (type II), and blood vessel wall (type III), among others, constituting approximately 30% of total protein of human body. There are, until now, 28 known collagen types existing in nature, type I (Figure 17.1) being the most abundant, and playing a structural and mechanical function.

Commercial sources of this type I collagen are commonly rat tail, pig skin, cow bones, and other bovine and porcine sources. Marine type I collagen is a promising alternative to these ones, with several methods already established to isolate collagen type I from marine sources, especially from fish skins, scales, or fish bones, representing an abundant discard from fisheries and fish processing industries (Silva et al. 2014). Just like mammal collagen, marine collagen can be used to apply in food, cosmetics, or pharmaceutics industry, and also, in tissue engineering (Simpson et al. 2012; Silva et al. 2014). As this protein is the principal component of the skin, it is incorporated in lotions and creams, aiming at maintaining a youth and healthy skin, being present in the life of millions of people. Several nutraceutical products include it as well, promoting the properties of collagen for the well-being. In several of those products, fish collagen is used first, instead of bovine and porcine ones, particularly in Asia where the market seems to be more developed for this kind of products. Illustrative examples of nutraceutical and cosmetic products can be found in Neocell (http://neocell.com/splash/index.php) and Natural Collagen Inventia (https://collagenshop.net/products/inventia-pure-gold-mask-with-native-fish-collagen), respectively.

It is also used in the medical field to promote regeneration of damaged skin by burns and other trauma. In fact, it has a lot of possibilities that it can be used in the medical area, due to its ubiquitous presence in the human body, and due to its very good properties of biocompatibility, biodegradability, and low antigenicity, collagen is a big candidate for tissue engineering and regenerative medicine applications.

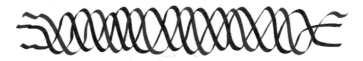

FIGURE 17.1   Type I collagen molecule. Results obtained from the association of two α1(I) and one α2(I) chains. (Adapted from Marques, C.G. et al., Colagénio marinho: Valorização de subprodutos marinhos com vista à regeneração de tecidos, in C.G. Sotelo et al. (eds.), *Valorización de Recursos Marinos: Biomateriales en Regeneración de Tejidos y Liberación de fármacos*, IIM-CSIC, Vigo, Spain, pp. 49–77, 2015.)

Kim et al. (2013) addressed that gelatin is a biopolymer derived from collagen, corresponding to the denaturated form of the protein, sometimes also hydrolyzed into smaller peptides. Denaturation causes separation of the collagen chains due to the destruction of hydrogen bonds, thus leading to the loss of triple helix conformation. Just like its precursor, gelatin is extracted from bovine and porcine sources, having the very same concerns about its consumption. Fish and poultry sources of gelatin, such as skins and bones, have been increasing, but its commercial production still generates low yields. The use of such raw materials is increasing, but currently it is still limited to 1% of the annual world gelatin production, even if research on the subject have started back in the 1950s (Songchotikunpan et al. 2008; Karim and Bhat 2009). Nevertheless, several fish sources—such as cold-water species, including, cod, hake, Alaska Pollock, or salmon, and warm-water species, including, tuna, catfish, tilapia, Nile perch, or shark—have been researched for this purpose (Karim and Bhat 2009).

Gelatin is well known by the final consumer, being commonly used in food, pharmaceutical, and cosmetic industries, but also in the photographic industry, where it is used in the production of films. In food-related products, it is widely used as a gelling agent, giving texture, foam stabilization, and creaminess, forming complexes with other proteins. It is used in desserts, yogurts, ham coatings, and fruit toppings for pastry, among others. In pharmaceutical and cosmetic fields, it is used in the production of capsules for oral administration. It can also be used in medicine, along with collagen, for the production of matrix and coatings of implants; in the formulation of microspheres for the controlled drug delivery of a drug; or in wound care devices (Karim and Bhat 2008).

17.2.2 POLYSACCHARIDES

Polysaccharides are another kind of biopolymers found abundantly in marine organisms also exhibiting a wide field of application possibilities. Besides the widespread chitin and chitosan, sulfated polysaccharides found in seaweeds are receiving growing attention due to the several bioactivities being described in the scientific literature (Zubia et al. 2009; Raposo et al. 2015; Springer Handbook of Marine Biotechnology 2015).

Chitin (Figure 17.2) is a natural polysaccharide—the second most abundant polymer in nature—extracted from the organic matrix of exoskeletons of arthropods such as crustaceans (shells of shrimps, crabs, and lobsters) and from the endoskeleton of

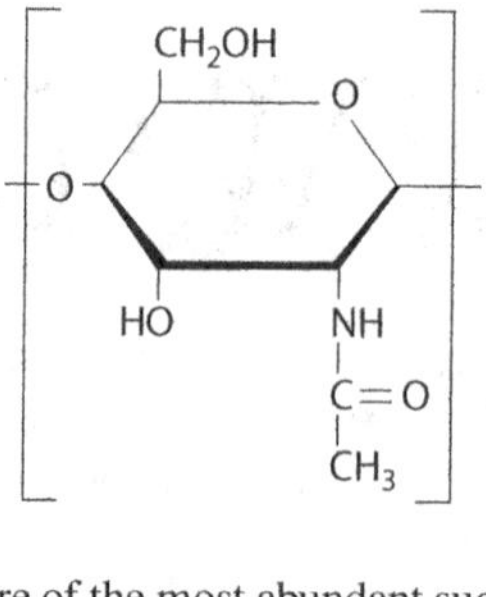

FIGURE 17.2 Molecular structure of the most abundant sugar in chitin: *N*-acetylglucosamine.

molluscs, structures where reinforcement and strength are necessary, and where they occur as ordered crystalline micro fibrils (Rinaudo 2006; Silva et al. 2014).

Chitin has strong inter- and intramolecular hydrogen bonds, which lead to a specific chain arrangement, with two allomorphs α- and β-chitins, the α-chitin being the most abundant (present in crustaceans).

Although chitin is widely available, its very low solubility in common organic solvents is a limitative step for further use. A derivative of chitin, named chitosan, is one of the most used polysaccharides used in biomedical applications. Chitosan is obtained by partial deacetylation of chitin in the solid state under alkaline conditions, or by enzymatic hydrolysis, to reach a degree of deacetylation (number of non-acetylated sugars in respect to the total number of sugars) higher than 50%. The removal of the acetyl group leaves free amino groups, which turn chitosan into a positively charged polyelectrolyte in acidic pH, allowing its solubility. Despite its use in cosmetic and pharmaceutical industries, among other industrial fields, chitosan has been extensively studied for tissue engineering. It has very good biocompatibility, biodegradability, and the ability for cell binding; fosters wound healing; and has hemostatic, antibacterial, and antifungal properties, being proposed as a component of several matrices for cell culture (Lee et al. 2009; Reys et al. 2013).

Carrageenan corresponds to a family of linear sulfated polymers and is extracted from red algae, being up to 60%–80% of its dry weight. Commercially, three main types of carrageenans are identified, classified according to the number of sulfated groups in each disaccharide basic unit after alkaline modification: κ (kappa), ι (iota), and λ (lambda), having one, two, and three sulfate groups, respectively (Silva et al. 2012).

Alginate is a polysaccharide present in the cell wall of brown algae, being up to 45% of its dry weight. Its jellifying properties make it a useful compound for textile, food, and cosmetic industries. For tissue engineering purposes, alginate can be combined with other polymers to produce suitable scaffolds, with acceptable mechanical properties and changing hydrophilic behavior, important for absorption of body fluids and transportion of nutrients. Brown algae are also rich in sulfated polysaccharides, in which fucoidan is the most common and representative sulfate polysaccharide. Fucoidan is used as an ingredient in nutraceutical products being known to have anticoagulant, antithrombotic, anti-inflammatory, antitumor, contraceptive, and antiviral activities (Ponce et al. 2003, with illustrative examples being found in Swanson Health Products [https://www.swansonvitamins.com/swanson-greenfoods-formulas-fucoidan-brown-seaweed-extract-500-mg-60-veg-caps] and Immukare [http://www.immukare.com/product_fucoidan-pro]).

17.3 ELECTROSPINNING OF MARINE BIOPOLYMERS FOR TISSUE ENGINEERING

17.3.1 TISSUE ENGINEERING AND MARINE BIOPOLYMERS

Tissue engineering is regarded as a new resolution of medicine. A new path is being drawn with the development of bioengineering methods to trigger and support the regeneration of human tissues. By joining engineering, materials science, and biology approaches, natural and synthetic materials are being combined with cells towards "living constructs" aiming the recovery of a damaged tissue, changing to a new paradigm of tissue regeneration. With this, the recovery of a damaged tissue is possible, by inducing the creation of a new tissue. At this point, it is necessary to work at macro and also at nano level, to control the bioactivity between material and cells. Natural and synthetic polymers are used in tissue engineering, single or in combination, according to biological and mechanical properties, aiming at replacing partially or completely a damaged tissue. Natural materials offer the advantages of biocompatibility and biodegradability. Looking in particular into the marine environment, some of its natural proteins and polysaccharides are already being used in this field, including the ones abovementioned, chitosan and fucoidan.

Research has been conducted to test the adaptability of marine proteins in the production of scaffolds, membranes, or drug delivery systems. For instance, collagen from the scales of freshwater fish has been tested in the development of scaffolds to be used in tissue engineering, demonstrating very good results due to its nonimmunogenic properties (Pati et al. 2012). Collagen from salmon skin has been tested to be used in bone tissue regeneration, showing promising results due to its cytocompatibility exhibited during *in vitro* assays and its capacity to produce porous scaffolds (Hoyer et al. 2012).

A well-known technique to process polymers in tissue-engineered membranes is electrospinning, a technique that mimics the tissue structures such as the extracellular matrix (ECM). In fact, this technique allows the production of two-dimensional (2D) nanofiber membranes from polymer solutions or blends. With a relatively simple apparatus, it uses an electrical field that will elongate fibers and create a fibrous matrix, whose fiber diameter is in the range of nano- to micrometers. Fibers are accommodated in the collector, and the membranes are very porous, mimicking the structure of the ECM. Biologically, they are suitable for a variety of tissues such as the skin, bone, blood vessels, nerve, and cartilage, among others, because these tissues are, in their basic constitution, organized from the nano to the macro scale in a hierarchical fashion. Thus, electrospun membranes provide a particular environment where cells can attach, develop, and proliferate, creating a new tissue over time, where the expression of new ECM polymers is followed by the biodegradation of the electrospun fibers (corresponding to the general strategy of tissue engineering based on biodegradable polymers).

17.3.2 Electrospinning Process

Electrospinning relies essentially on three factors: polymer solution properties (concentration, molecular weight, viscosity, and surface tension), process parameters (applied potential/voltage, flow rate, distance needle collector and collector geometry), and ambient conditions (humidity and temperature). All these factors affect the properties of the electrospun fibers. Exemplifying on how these parameters can affect the processing, polymer concentration is related to the capacity of producing regular fibers (suitable concentration) or fibers with beads or particles (low concentration). Viscosity also plays a key role, because a low-viscosity solution will form electrospun polymer spheres. Furthermore, the molecular weight of the polymer plays an important role in the morphology of the fibers: for the same concentration, using a polymer with low molecular weight leads to the formation of beads within the fibers; on the contrary, using a high-molecular-weight polymer will lead to the production of zigzag ribbon-like fibers (Zhenyu Li and Ce Wang 2010).

Ambient parameters also affect the fiber morphology. Several studies done on this issue show that at higher ambient temperatures, electrospun fibers are thinner. Temperature and humidity influence the evaporation of the solvent: a lower level of humidity induces a faster solvent evaporation, obtaining dry fibers, and thus avoiding fiber joint formation due to the presence of solvent.

Regarding the processing itself, electrospinning is highly dependent on four parameters, which need to be adjusted for the collection of suitable fibers: (1) flow rate, (2) applied potential/voltage, (3) distance between the needle and the collector, and (4) collector geometry. Each one of these is addressed in further detail in sections

1. *Flow rate*: It is the rate at which the polymer is ejected from the syringe. The higher the flow rate, the higher the diameter of the fiber. However, it is related to the applied voltage: if the flow rate is increased and the applied voltage is too low, a drop will appear at the edge of the needle, because the electrical field is not enough for stretching the drop and creating a fiber.

2. *Applied voltage*: A high-voltage supply is used to produce an electrical field between the needle and the collector (which is connected to the ground). With the applied voltage, the polymer is positively charged, resulting in an increase in charge repulsion within polymer, balanced by the electrical field established between the needle and the collector. A drop is formed at the edge of the needle, with a meta-equilibrium between charge repulsion and surface tension. To overcoming the superficial tension, the drop starts to stretch, obtaining the conformation of a cone, called Taylor cone, and a nanofiber is created from that small droplet. The higher the applied voltage, the higher will be the electrical field. It also influences the diameter of the fiber.

3. *Distance between the needle and the collector*: With a certain applied voltage, the electrical field is dependent on the distance between the needle and the collector (Ohm's law):

$$V_n - V_g = \int_g^n E.dl \qquad (17.1)$$

where:
   n is the needle
   g is the ground
   V is the voltage or potential
   E is the electrical field
   l is the distance between the needle and the ground

4. *Collector geometry*: According to the final application in the biological tissue, fiber orientation may play an important role. To acquire fibers with

random orientation, a simple plane collector can be used, as shown in Figure 17.3. However, if the goal is to obtain fibers with some kind of orientation (parallels, crossed, etc.), a different collector is needed. A rotatory cylinder or parallel stripes can be used to align fibers. When there is a rotatory movement, the cylinder pulls the fibers that will suffer some stretch, becoming thinner and aligned around the cylinder (Figure 17.4). When there are two parallel electrodes, fibers will align between electrodes, providing an aligned fiber mesh.

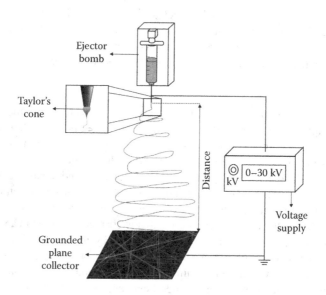

FIGURE 17.3 Electrospinning apparatus to acquire random fiber orientation.

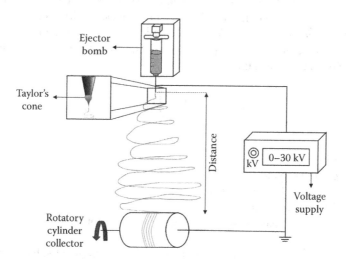

FIGURE 17.4 Electrospinning apparatus to acquire aligned fiber orientation.

Thus, conjugating all these factors, smooth and regular fibers are produced giving origin to 2D membranes. Fiber morphology can be adjusted, regarding the application, from several micrometers to tens of nanometers.

This technique has been growing, being used to process not only polymers, but also ceramics and composite materials, into thin fibers with adjustable characteristics. Its evolution leads to set up an assembly in specific ways to create hollow or core–shell fibers, random and aligned fibers, or even layer-by-layer films. Thus, all this development leads to a wide range of applications, with different materials (Li and Xia 2004). Researchers have studied their application not only applied in tissue engineering, but also in textile industry for protective clothing, or as barriers to liquid penetration in protective clothing systems for agricultural workers, for example (Gorji et al. 2012; Lee and Obendorf 2007).

17.3.3 ELECTROSPINNING OF MARINE POLYMERS

Natural polymers are, generally, polyelectrolytes in nature, increasing their ability to carry charge under the influence of an electric field. Due to this characteristic, it is very difficult to do electrospinning of natural polymers. Nevertheless, there are some procedures that can be used to overcome such bottleneck. For instance, the addition of salts, such as KH_2PO_4 or NaCl, or the combination with another polymer have been already explored for the electrospinning of natural polymers. (Li and Ce Wang 2013; Angammana and Jayaram 2008).

Scaffolds and membranes from natural polymers tend to have weak mechanical properties in aqueous environments (when prepared by electrospinning, with natural polymers being polyelectrolytes, high conductivity leads to very thin fibers). However, synthetic polymers such as polycaprolactone (PCL) demonstrate very good results regarding the mechanical properties of electropsun membranes. Thus, the addition of other polymer(s) is a way to facilitate the electrospinning process (e.g., by reducing the overall conductivity), to improve the mechanical properties of the membranes, and to possess additional properties that are desired according to the final goal (Chakrapani et al. 2012).

The processing of the main marine biopolymers by electrospinning to render structures for tissue engineering will be addressed in more detail, giving particular attention to the ones highlighted previously.

Due to its ubiquitous presence in the human body, collagen is a key choice as a building block for tissue engineering approaches. Nevertheless, when considering electrospinning, collagen is quite difficult to process. Its lower denaturation temperature and low-melting point are the main obstacles to electrospun this protein. Most of the research that has been done on electrospinning of collagen is related to type I acid-soluble collagen. The two solvents mostly used are hexafluro-2-propanol (HFP) and acetic acid solution (Chakrapani et al. 2012; Yang et al. 2008). The fluoroalcohol HFP is a strong H-bonding solvent, widely used as a solvent for collagen and its blends, for example, with chondroitin-6-sulfate, elastin, or silk fibroin (Hofman et al. 2012). Given its high toxicity, other solvents are being pursued, or alternatively, at least assure the complete removal of toxic solvent from the produced membranes. In addition, it has been also reported that this solvent may induce denaturation of the collagen molecule, even before the electrospinning process. Thus, some properties that make collagen an unique biopolymer in tissue engineering might be lost during electrospinning, also due to high tension applied during processing (Zeugolis et al. 2008). A careful characterization of the solubilized collagen, as well as the produced systems, should hence be performed to assess the preservation of collagen biochemical features. Aiming at circumventing the drawbacks associated with the use of HFP, a mixture of phosphate-buffered saline and ethanol was tested as a solvent for collagen, demonstrating a noteworthy efficacy (Dong et al. 2009). This water/alcohol/salt system enables the production of a collagen solution and its further electrospinning, apparently, without denaturation of collagen. Another alternative to HFP is the use of acetic acid, widely used by the research community for the solubilization of collagen, because it is less harmful and has a less influence on the protein denaturation (Liu et al. 2010; Chakrapani et al. 2012). It is rather beneficial than HFP, taking also into account that collagen extraction from marine by-products is carried out mostly by using this acid.

Type I collagen can be used for electrospinning to create nanofiber membranes, whereas structural collagens such as types III and IV that were already studied can be used as blends, adding functionalities to the membranes regarding the final application (Sell et al. 2009).

Promising results have been particularly achieved when collagen is conjugated with other polymers, especially synthetic polymers. It has been commonly reported that the addition of synthetic polymers forms a blend in order to facilitate the electrospinning of a collagen solution and to improve properties of the final membranes, whether in HFP or acetic acid solution (Sell et al. 2009; Powell and Boyce 2009). Poly(ethylene oxide) (PEO) and PCL are the polymers widely used to tailor the morphology and mechanical properties of collagen-based membranes. The higher the PEO concentration, the higher the viscosity of the solution, which, at a certain point, improves the process, reducing the presence of beads in the fibers (Huang et al. 2001). In its turn, PCL/collagen blend is a good option, if the mechanical properties of membranes need to be improved. The diameter of the fibers increases and the tensile strength and elasticity are more adequate, when the final goal is the development of vascular grafts, showing also a good environment for vascular cell growth (Lee et al. 2008).

Although both mammal and fish collagens face the same challenges in electrospinning, the marine counterpart seems to exhibit some properties that may be of benefit, particularly the denaturation temperature. Marine organisms in general live at a lower environmental temperature than humans, and the denaturation temperature of their constituting collagens is typically lower, related to the inferior content of hydroxyproline. In fact, this special amino acid plays an important role in the stabilization of the triple helix. The characteristics of the fish individuals selected for collagen extraction are also quite relevant, being easier to solubilize collagen from younger animals, resulting in structures with lower tensile strength, due to lower cross-linking compared with collagen in older individuals. The cross-linking levels are, nevertheless, increased significantly if the animals suffer from starvation (Benjakul et al. 2012).

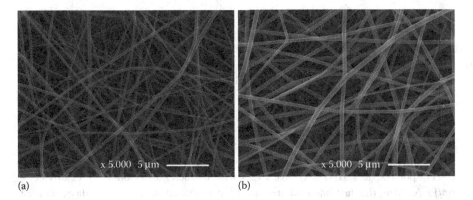

(a)   (b)

FIGURE 17.5   Membranes of collagen-based nanofibers, produced with (a) pure collagen or with (b) a 50:50 (w/w) blend of collagen and PCL. Collagen has been extracted from the skin of squid *Illex argentinus*.

To illustrate the possibility of producing fibrillar membranes using marine-origin collagen, skins of squid *Illex argentinus* have been selected as raw material and collagen has been extracted using a mixture of acetic acid and pepsin. From the results illustrated in Figure 17.5, one can observe an increment and harmonization of the fiber diameter when collagen was blended with PCL (50:50 w/w), compared with collagen only. Moreover, the use of pure collagen solution renders quite irregular membranes, often characterized by the presence of aggregates and other types of defects.

This type of collagen membranes can find their application in diverse sites and structures of human body, such as on the development of blood vessels, in cornea regeneration, in the treatment of skin wounds—because the nanofiber structure mimics the morphological features of ECM—or even in combination with other scaffolds, providing a hierarchical structure (Tuzlakoglu et al. 2011). Membranes can also be conjugated with a bioactive compound, aiming at achieving a sustained drug delivery in the specific site of action.

Gelatin has been also widely studied for tissue engineering, due to its similar composition to collagen, biodegradability, and biocompatibility. Similar to collagen, the attempts to produce nanofibers of gelatin by electrospinning involve the use of organic solvents, such as 2,2,2-trifluoroethanol, HFP, *N,N*-dimethylformamide, or the acetic or formic acid (Correia et al. 2013). However, this polymer has a hydrophilic behavior, in which the fiber structure is affected by moisture, resulting in membranes with poor mechanical properties. To overcome this, cross-linking strategies have been explored, such as the use of glutaraldehyde vapor, 1-Ethyl-3-(3-dimethylaminopropyl) carbodiimide (EDC), or genipin, as well as dehydrothermal treatment, resulting in a reduced loss of mass according to the cross-linking time reaction (Gomes et al. 2013; Rose et al. 2014). The combination of gelatin with other polymers has been explored as well to enhance the mechanical properties of the final membrane, with the resulting structures being proposed for wound dressings or drug release (An et al. 2010).

Synthetic polymers such as PCL or poly(vinyl alcohol) (PVA) are usually tested to create copolymers, with very good results toward tissue engineering, by mimicking the ECM, where gelatin seems to have a bioactive behavior, promoting the increase of cell growth (Chiou et al. 2013). According to the origin of gelatin, the processing by electrospinning may be facilitated, with gelatin obtained from cold-water fish exhibiting lower gelation temperature compared with collagen obtained from warm-water fish or mammalian collagen (Chiou et al. 2013). Despite, not even with the use of another polymer to produce a blend, aiming at improvinge the physicochemical properties of produced membranes, the success of the electrospinning process cannot be assured (An et al. 2010). As an example, electrospun fibers of copolymer solution of gelatin/PVA or poly(lactic acid) (PLA) have a very wide diameter distribution, especially gelatin/PLA. Also, this last one remains intact when soaked in water for 3 days, without any cross-linking, whereas gelatin/PVA completely dissolved after 1 day, thus requiring a cross-linking treatment to be more stable, which clearly exhibits the complexity and peculiarities of this processing technique when using proteins (Chiou et al. 2013).

Besides collagen and derivatives, marine-origin polysaccharides have gained a substantial attention among tissue engineering professionals, due to their characteristics similar to those of glycosaminoglycans of human ECM. The mostly studied one is probably chitosan, which exhibits attractive biocompatibility and biodegradability, while supporting cell binding (Lee et al. 2009). However, electrospinning chitosan is not an easy task. Its polycationic nature, revealed in acidic conditions due to the protonation of the free amino groups, increases solution surface tension that affects the morphology of the produced fibers, with a high voltage being required for a successful fiber formation. Just like collagen and gelatin, chitosan alone renders structures with poor mechanical properties. To improve the performance of the produced membranes to tensile stimuli, a cross-linking agent or another polymer to form a blend is used as a valuable alternative. PEO was the first polymer to be used in the electrospinning of a chitosan blend. This polymer helped in the production of nanofibers with a diameter ranging from 40 to 290 nm (Spasova et al. 2004). At low concentration, a regular fiber cannot be formed, whereas at high concentration, a too viscous solution is obtained, also hindering the electrospinning of chitosan. To better control it, blending with PVA, PLA, silk, or collagen is being explored. Another option is the use of specific solvents that can reduce interactions between chitosan chains. However, some of those solvents are environmentally harmful, as is the case of trifluoroacetic acid, with the associated toxicity hampering their use for the development of biomedical applications (Koosha and Mirzadeh 2015).

Other marine polysaccharides were also processed by electrospinning to produce fibers and featuring membranes. Iota-carrageenan was used in a blend with PCL to produce electrospun membranes, with carrageenan showing the influence on the morphology of the produced fibers. These membranes have been tested *in vivo*, and no evidence of adverse inflammation on mice has been observed (Basilia et al. 2008). Although quite common in biomedical and microbiology laboratories, agar could not be successfully processed with electrospinning. Neither using low or high concentration nor the combination with PVA (50/50 w/w) was a valid option to produce regular fibers (Sousa et al. 2015). The incorporation of agar in polyacrylonitrile, aiming at inducing attachment of silver nanoparticles to the surface of polyacrylonitrile nanofibers due to the abundance of hydroxyl groups, has however shown similar result (Yang et al. 2015). Alginate has been also explored for tissue engineering purposes, being combined with other polymers to produce suitable scaffolds, with acceptable mechanical properties and changing hydrophilic behavior, important for absorption of body fluids and transportion of nutrients. Although PCL alone possesses good mechanical properties but a totally hydrophobic behavior, the incorporation of alginate improves radically this property, even in small quantities, which is quite beneficial regarding the biological performance of the developed scaffolds, in which viability of pre-osteoblasts (MC3T3-E1 cells) was higher than the one observed in PCL only (Kim and Kim 2014). More recently, fucoidan has been studied as structural polymer in matrices for application in biomedical purposes, in addition to its well established use in nutraceutics and pharmaceutics based in the numerous bioactivities reported for this biopolymer. It has been added in small quantities to a pullulan/dextran solution, improving the interactions between vascular endothelial growth factor and the fibers, promising an enhanced biological behavior of the derived biomedical product regarding its vascularization (Rujitanaroj et al. 2014).

17.4   FINAL REMARKS

Marine organisms represent a yet unknown fount of bioactive compounds, which are receiving now a growing attention among biomedical scientists and engineers. Although significant progress is clearly observed and a few examples of marine biomaterials are already presented in advanced preclinical studies, besides some bioactive compounds that are already in the market as active pharmaceutical ingredients, there is still a long path to be taken. Particularly, regarding electrospinning, most of the marine biopolymers mentioned throughout this chapter still lack deeper study before being considered as established and validated building blocks for the production of biomaterials using this processing technique, despite the steps already given with marine collagen and chitosan. Even though they are naturally derived compounds, they show some adequate properties for their use in tissue engineering, such as biodegradability and biocompatibility, which are strong features that need to be taken with extreme importance for this field.

Natural polymers in general and marine biopolymers in particular have some characteristics that, on one hand, make them desired materials to be used in tissue engineering, but, on the other hand, raise some obstacles related to their processing, resulting in several challenges for researchers. Suitable efforts to overcome such drawbacks and bottlenecks pass through the combination of these marine biopolymers with other polymers, such as the ones obtained by chemical synthesis, the use of cross-linking strategies to increase the stability of the final structure, and the choice of an adequate solvent. Thus, all these features of solutions need to be taken into consideration, along with process and ambient parameters, for the successful electrospinning of marine biopolymers. All these factors will influence the final characteristics of the nanofibers, whether in terms of fibers morphology or in terms of cellular behavior. It is a tough challenge faced by biomedical scientists, but nothing less is expected from them.

ACKNOWLEDGMENTS

The authors acknowledge the funding from european regional development fund (ERDF) through POCTEP 2007–2013 Project 0687_NOVOMAR_1_P, from the European Union's Seventh Framework Programme (FP7/2007–2013) under grant agreement number REGPOT-CT2012-316331-POLARIS and from the European Research Council under grant agreement number ERC-2012-ADG 20120216-321266 for project ComplexiTE.

REFERENCES

Abdou, E.S., K.S.A. Nagy, and M.Z. Elsabee. 2008. Extraction and characterization of chitin and chitosan from local sources. *Bioresource Technology* 99(5): 1359–1367.

An, K.J., H. Liu, S. Guo, D.N. Kumar, and Q. Wang. 2010. Preparation of fish gelatin and fish gelatin/poly(L-lactide) nanofibers by electrospinning. *International Journal of Biological Macromolecules* 47(3): 380–388.

Angammana, C.J., and S.H. Jayaram. 2008. Analysis of the effects of solution conductivity on electro-spinning process and fiber morphology. *Industry Applications Society Annual Meeting, IAS '08*, 5–9 October, Alberta, Canada. IEEE.

Basilia, B.A., A.P. Robes, K.A. Ledda, and K.B. Dagbay. 2008. In-vitro and In-vivo screenings of electrospun polycaprolactone-carrageenan nanofibrous scaffolds for tissue engineering. *NSTI Nanotechnology Vol 2, Technical Proceedings*, ed. M. Laudon and B. Romanowicz, Austin, Texas pp. 306–309.

Benjakul, S., S. Nalinanon, and F. Shahidi. 2012. *Fish Collagen, in Food Biochemistry and Food Processing*. Wiley-Blackwell Publishing, Hoboken, New Jersey, pp. 365–387.

Chakrapani, V.Y., A. Gnanamani, V.R. Giridev, M. Madhusoothanan, and G. Sekaran. 2012. Electrospinning of type I collagen and PCL nanofibers using acetic acid. *Journal of Applied Polymer Science* 125(4): 3221–3227.

Chiou, B.S., H. Jafri, R. Avena-Bustillos, K.S. Gregorski, P.J. Bechtel, S.H. Imam, G.M. Glen, and W.J. Orts. 2013. Properties of electrospun pollock gelatin/poly(vinyl alcohol) and pollock gelatin/poly(lactic acid) fibers. *International Journal of Biological Macromolecules* 55: 214–220.

Correia, D.M., J. Padrão, L.R. Rodrigues, F. Dourado, S. Lanceros-Méndez, and V. Sencadas. 2013. Thermal and hydrolytic degradation of electrospun fish gelatin membranes. *Polymer Testing* 32(5): 995–1000.

Dong, B., O. Arnoult, M.E. Smith, and G.E. Wnek. 2009. Electrospinning of collagen nanofiber scaffolds from benign solvents. *Macromolecular Rapid Communications* 30(7): 539–542.

Dutta, P.K., J. Dutta, and V.S. Tripathi. 2004. Chitin and chitosan: Chemistry, properties and applications. *Journal of Scientific and Industrial Research* 63(1): 20–31.

Gomes, S.R., G. Rodrigues, G.G. Martins, C.M.R. Henriques, and J.C. Silva. 2013. In vitro evaluation of crosslinked electrospun fish gelatin scaffolds. *Materials Science & Engineering C* 33(3): 1219–1227.

Gorji, M., A.A.A. Jeddi, and A.A. Gharehaghaji. 2012. Fabrication and characterization of polyurethane electrospun nanofiber membranes for protective clothing applications. *Journal of Applied Polymer Science* 125(5): 4135–4141.

Hofman, K., N. Tucker, J.J. Stanger, M. Staiger, S. Marshall, and B. Hall. 2012. Effects of the molecular format of collagen on characteristics of electrospun fibres. *Journal of Materials Science* 47(3): 1148–1155.

Hoyer, B., A. Bernhardt, S. Heinemann, I. Stache, M. Meyer, and M. Gelinsky. 2012. Biomimetically mineralized salmon collagen scaffolds for application in bone tissue engineering. *Biomacromolecules* 13(4): 1059–1066.

Huang, L., K. Nagapudi, R.P. Apkarian, and L. Elliot. 2001. Engineered collagen-PEO nanofibers and fabrics. *Journal of Biomaterials Science, Polymer Edition* 12(9): 979–993.

Karim, A.A., and R. Bhat. 2008. Gelatin alternatives for the food industry: Recent developments, challenges and prospects. *Trends in Food Science & Technology* 19(12): 644–656.

Karim, A.A., and R. Bhat. 2009. Fish gelatin: Properties, challenges, and prospects as an alternative to mammalian gelatins. *Food Hydrocolloids* 23(3): 563–576.

Kim, M.S., and G. Kim. 2014. Three-dimensional electrospun polycaprolactone (PCL)/alginate hybrid composite scaffolds. *Carbohydrate Polymers* 114: 213–221.

Kim, S.-K., D.-H. Ngo, T.-S. Vo, and B. Mi Ryu. 2013. Industry perspectives of marine-derived proteins as biomaterials, in *Marine Biomaterials: Characterization, Isolation and Applications*, S.-K. Kim, Ed., CRC Press: Boca Raton, FL, pp. 737–746.

Kinoshita-Toyoda, A., S. Yamada, S.M. Haslam, K.H. Khoo, M. Suguira, H.R. Morris, A. Dell, and K. Sugahara. 2004. Structural determination of five novel tetrasaccharides containing 3-O-sulfated D-glucuronic acid and two rare oligosaccharides containing a beta-D-glucose branch isolated from squid cartilage chondroitin sulfate E. *Biochemistry* 43(34): 11063–11074.

Koosha, M., and H. Mirzadeh. 2015. Electrospinning, mechanical properties, and cell behavior study of chitosan/PVA nanofibers. *Journal of Biomedical Materials Research Part A* 103(9): 3081–3093.

Lee, K.Y., L. Jeong, Y.O. Kang, S.J. Lee, and W.H. Park. 2009. Electrospinning of polysaccharides for regenerative medicine. *Advanced Drug Delivery Reviews* 61(12): 1020–1032.

Lee, S., and S.K. Obendorf. 2007. Use of electrospun nanofiber web for protective textile materials as barriers to liquid penetration. *Textile Research Journal* 77(9): 696–702.

Lee, S.J., J. Liu, S.H. Oh, S. Soker, A. Atala, and J.J. Yoo. 2008. Development of a composite vascular scaffolding system that withstands physiological vascular conditions. *Biomaterials* 29(19): 2891–2898.

Li, D., and Y.N. Xia. 2004. Electrospinning of nanofibers: Reinventing the wheel. *Advanced Materials* 16(14): 1151–1170.

Li, H.Y., X.J. Yu, Y. Jin, W. Zhang, and Y.L. Liu. 2008. Development of an eco-friendly agar extraction technique from the red seaweed Gracilaria lemaneiformis. *Bioresource Technology* 99(8): 3301–3305.

Liu, T., W.K. Teng, B.P. Chan, and S.Y. Chew. 2010. Photochemical crosslinked electrospun collagen nanofibers: Synthesis, characterization and neural stem cell interactions. *Journal of Biomedical Materials Research Part A* 95(1): 276–282.

Marques, A. L. P., C.G. Sotelo, G.S. Diogo, J. Moreira-Silva, M. Blanco, T.H. Silva, R.I. Pérez- Martín, and R.L. Reis. 2015. Colagénio Marinho: valorizaçao de subprodutos marinhos com vista a regeneraçao de tecidos. In C.G. Sotelo et al.(eds), *Valorización de recursos marinos: biomateriales en regeneración de tejidos y liberación de fármacos*, IIM-CSIC, Vigo, Spain, pp49–77.

Nagai, T., and N. Suzuki. 2000. Isolation of collagen from fish waste material—Skin, bone and fins. *Food Chemistry* 68(3): 277–281.

Nagai, T., O. Tomoe, and N. Nagashi. 1999. Collagen of edible jellyfish exumbrella. *Journal of the Science of Food and Agriculture* 79(6): 855–858.

Pati, F., P. Datta, B. Adhikari, S. Dhara, K. Ghosh, and P.K. Das Mohapatra. 2012. Collagen scaffolds derived from fresh water fish origin and their biocompatibility. *Journal of Biomedical Materials Research Part A* 100(4): 1068–1079.

Percival, E. 1979. Polysaccharides of green, red and brown seaweeds—Their basic structure, biosynthesis and function. *British Phycological Journal* 14(2): 103–117.

Ponce, N.M., C.A. Pujol, E.B. Damonte, M.L. Flores, and C.A. Stortz. 2003. Fucoidans from the brown seaweed Adenocystis utricularis: Extraction methods, antiviral activity and structural studies. *Carbohydrate Research* 338(2): 153–165.

Powell, H.M., and S.T. Boyce. 2009. Engineered human skin fabricated using electrospun Collagen-PCL blends: Morphogenesis and mechanical properties. *Tissue Engineering Part A* 15(8): 2177–2187.

Raposo, M.F.D., A.M.B. de Morais, and R.M.S.C. de Morais. 2015. Marine polysaccharides from algae with potential biomedical applications. *Marine Drugs* 13(5): 2967–3028.

Reys, L.L., S.S. Silva, J.M. Oliveira, S.G. Caridade, J.F. Mano, T.H. Silva, and R.L. Reis. 2013. Revealing the potential of squid chitosan-based structures for biomedical applications. *Biomedical Materials*. 8(4): 045002.

Rinaudo, M. 2006. Chitin and chitosan: Properties and applications. *Progress in Polymer Science* 31(7): 603–632.

Rose, J.B., S. Pacelli, A.J. El Haj, H.S. Dua, A. Hopkinson, L.J. White, and F.R.A.J. Rose. 2014. Gelatin-based materials in ocular tissue engineering. *Materials* 7(4): 3106–3135.

Ratner, B.D., A.S. Hoffman, F.J. Schoen, and J.E. Lemons. 2004. *Biomaterials Science: An Introduction to Materials in Medicine*. Elsevier Science. San Diego, California.

Rujitanaroj, P., A. Rachida, S.C. Yian, and L.V. Catherine. 2014. Polysaccharide electrospun fibers with sulfated poly(fucose) promote endothelial cell migration and VEGF-mediated angiogenesis. *Biomaterials Science* 2(6): 843–852.

Sell, S.A., M.J. McClure, K. Garg, P.S. Wolfe, and G.L. Bowlin. 2009. Electrospinning of collagen/biopolymers for regenerative medicine and cardiovascular tissue engineering. *Advanced Drug Delivery Reviews* 61(12): 1007–1019.

Silva, T.H., J. Moreira-Silva, A.L.P. Marques, A. Domingues, Y. Bayon, and R.L. Reis. 2014. Marine origin collagens and its potential applications. *Marine Drugs* 12(12): 5881–5901.

Silva, T.H., A. Alves, B.M. Ferreira, J.M. Oliveira, L.L. Reys, R.J.F. Ferreira, R.A. Sousa, S.S. Silva, J.F. Mano, and R.L. Reis. 2012. Materials of marine origin: A review on polymers and ceramics of biomedical interest. *International Materials Reviews* 57(5): 276–307.

Simpson, B.K., L.M.L. Nollet, F. Toldra, S. Benjakul, G. Paliyath, and Y.H. Yui. 2012. *Food Biochemistry and Food Processing*. Wiley. Hoboken, New Jersey.

Songchotikunpan, P., J. Tattiyakul, and P. Supaphol. 2008. Extraction and electrospinning of gelatin from fish skin. *International Journal of Biological Macromolecules* 42(3): 247–255.

Sousa, A.M.M., H.K. Silva Souza, J. Uknalis, S.C. Liu, M.P. Goncalves, and L.S. Liu. 2015. Electrospinning of agar/PVA aqueous solutions and its relation with rheological properties. *Carbohydrate Polymers* 115: 348–355.

Spasova, M., N. Manolova, D. Paneva, and I. Rashkov. 2004. Preparation of chitosan-containing nanofibres by electrospinning of chitosan/poly(ethylene oxide) blend solutions. *E-Polymers* 56: 1–12.

Se-Kwon, K. (Ed.) *Springer Handbook of Marine Biotechnology*. 2015. Springer-Verlag: Berlin, Germany.

Tuzlakoglu, K., M.I. Santos, N. Neves, and R.L. Reis. 2011. Design of nano- and microfiber combined scaffolds by electrospinning of collagen onto starch-based fiber meshes: A man-made equivalent of natural extracellular matrix. *Tissue Engineering Part A*. 17(3–4): 463–473.

Yang, L., C.F. Fitie, K.O. van der Werf, M.L. Bennink, P.J. Dijkstra, and J. Feijen. 2008. Mechanical properties of single electrospun collagen type I fibers. *Biomaterials* 29(8): 955–962.

Yang, T., H. Yang, S.J. Zhen, and C.Z. Huang. 2015. Hydrogen-Bond-Mediated in situ fabrication of AgNPs/Agar/PAN electrospun nanofibers as reproducible SERS substrates. *Acs Applied Materials & Interfaces* 7(3): 1586–1594.

Zeugolis, D.I., S.T. Khew, E.S.Y. Yew, A.K. Ekaputra, Y.W. Tong, L.Y.L. Yung, D.W. Hutmacher, C. Sheppard, and M. Raghunath. 2008. Electro-spinning of pure collagen nano-fibres—Just an expensive way to make gelatin. *Biomaterials* 29(15): 2293–2305.

Zhenyu Li., and Ce Wang. 2013. *One-Dimensional Nanostructures: Electrospinning Technique and Unique Nanofibers.* 1 ed. Springer Briefs in Materials. Springer: Heidelberg, Germany.

Zubia, M., M. Sophie Fabre, V. kerjean, K. Le Lann, V. Stiger-Pouvreau, M. Fauchon, and E. Deslandes. 2009. Antioxidant and antitumoural activities of some Phaeophyta from Brittany coasts. *Food Chemistry* 116(3): 693–701.

18 Biomedical Applications of Alginate Biopolymer

J. Annie Kamala Florence, Govindasamy Rajakumar, Ill-Min Chung, and Barur R. Rajeshkumar

CONTENTS

18.1 INTRODUCTION

The marine species have been a valuable resource during the past few decades for the active pharmaceutical ingredients. Large number of compounds are being isolated from aquatic organisms and proposed as novel products for health-related applications ranging from bioactive ingredients to medical devices (Paterson and Anderson 2005). Biopolymers of marine products are involved in terms of drug development, which led to extensive preclinical studies, clinical trials in several therapeutic areas, including cancer, and for several biomedical applications (Dembitsky et al. 2005). Biomaterials are the materials intended to interface with biological systems to evaluate, treat, augment, or replace any tissue, organ, or function of the body (Williams 2009). The design of new biomaterials is now focused on mimicking many functions of the extracellular matrices (ECMs) of body tissues, as these can regulate host responses in a well-defined manner, and with their inherent biocompatibility.

The marine organisms synthesize a variety of biopolymers, which are grouped as three main classes: polysaccharides, proteins, and nucleic acids. Polysaccharides are biopolymers constituted by carbohydrate monomers (hexose) linked by glycosidic bonds. The most representative polysaccharides in marine environment are agar, alginate, carrageenans, and chitin. All the polysaccharides have similar chemical structures, but the apparently small differences are responsible for distinct properties of the polymers. Chitin and its derivative chitosan in the presence of an amine ($-NH_2$) group are protonated and the polymer will bear positive charge, whereas the others are neutral or negatively charged. In other polymers, the nature of the negative charge is also a difference: in carrageenans, it is due to sulfate groups and in alginate, it is due to carboxylate (COO^-), whereas agar is neutral.

18.2   ALGINATE

Alginate is a naturally occurring anionic polymer typically obtained from brown seaweed, and has been extensively investigated and used due to its relatively low cost, biodegradable, mucoadhesive, hemocompatible, nontoxic, nonimmunogenic, and mild gelation properties by addition of divalent cations such as Ca^{2+} (Gombotz and Wee 1998), which make it an interesting polymer for biomedical applications (Motwani 2008; Yao 2010). The British chemist E. C. C. Stanford first described alginate (the preparation of algic acid from brown algae) with a patent dated January 12, 1881 (Standford 1881).

Alginate is present in the cell wall of brown algae, as part of a wide family of glycans that form this group of organisms. These glycans are laminaran, cellulose, sulfated hexouronoxylofucans, fucoidan, and alginate. Among these, alginate is quantitatively the major polysaccharide in brown algae, building up to 45% of the dry weight of these seaweeds. It is responsible for its flexibility, having mechanical and structural functions, and ionic exchange roles (Rinaudo 2008).

18.2.1   PHYSICAL AND CHEMICAL PROPERTIES OF ALGINATE

Commercially, sodium alginate is extracted from giant brown seaweed (*Macrocystis pyrifera*), horsetail kelp (*Laminaria digitata*), and sugar kelp (*Laminaria saccharina*), and recognized as an unbranched anionic copolymer composed of two monomers: (1→4)-linked β-D-mannuronic acid (M) and α-L-guluronic acid (G). Both D-mannuronic (M) and L-guluronic (G) acids are stereoisomers, differing in the configuration of the carboxyl group, linked by β-1,4-glycosidic linkage in such a way that the carboxyl group of each unit is free, whereas the aldehyde group is shielded by the glycosidic linkage. The position of each unit can vary so they can occur in blocks of separate (M or G) or mixed (MG) sequences (Siew et al. 2005; Figure 18.1).

The relative amount of each block type can vary between different alginates. This variability at the molecular level strongly affects the physicochemical and rheological properties of alginate. Brown algae can be used as a source of alginate; high contents of G are generally found in polysaccharide sugar units sequence in alginates prepared from stipes of old blade material from brown algae, whereas alginates from

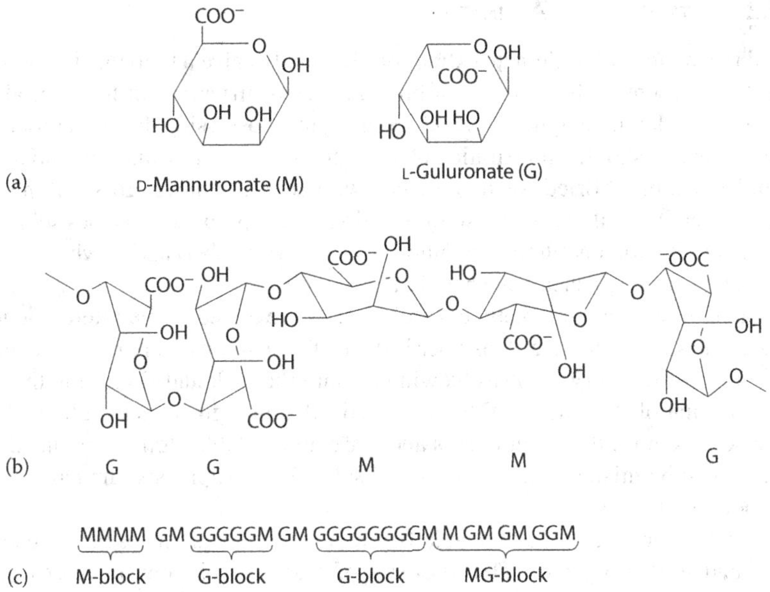

FIGURE 18.1 Structural characteristics of alginates: (a) alginate monomers, (b) chain conformation, and (c) block distribution.

younger blades are characterized by low content of G blocks and low gel strength (McKee et al. 1992). Compositional differences between different types of alginates reflect the relationship between the structure and the function. These differences are correlated with the physicochemical properties of alginate, which depend on the distribution of M and G units along the polysaccharidic chain and overall M/G ratio.

Alginate rich in α-L-guluronic acid will give transparent, stiffer, and more brittle gels in the presence of divalent cations. These types of alginates possess a low M/G ratio. Alginates with higher content of β-D-mannuronic acid or MG blocks will form flexible gels, with low elastic moduli (Drury et al. 2004).

Gelation is an important characteristic of alginates and is determined by various factors, such as solution viscosity, molecular weight and molecular structure of alginates, that is, M/G ratio and molecular sequence, and gelation agent concentration (d'Ayala et al. 2008) through hydrogen bonding at low pH, or by ionic interactions with di- or trivalent ions. G-rich alginate is prone to ionic gelation due to ionic bridge formation between polymer chains and chain association with egg box mechanism.

Although algal alginate is used for commercial purposes, some bacteria are able to produce alginate-like polysaccharides as an extracellular material. Bacterial alginate, produced by *Pseudomonas* and *Azotobacter* is abundant in vegetatively growing cells and is involved in cyst formation (Rehm and Valla 1997). The main difference between algal and bacterial alginates at the molecular level is the acetylation of mannurate units in bacterial alginate.

18.2.2 EXTRACTION OF ALGINATES

A good raw material for alginate extraction should also give a high yield of alginate. Alginate is present in the cell wall of brown algae as different salt forms of alginic acid, such as calcium, magnesium, and sodium salts, possessing different properties. The two processes for the preparation of alginates are extraction and calcium precipitation. Extraction of dried weed is washed with acid to remove cross-linking ions, then dissolved in alkali, typically sodium hydroxide, to produce a viscous solution of alginate. The solution is filtered to remove the cell wall debris and maybe treated to remove color leaving a clear, clean alginate solution.

In calcium precipitation method, calcium salts are added to the filtered liquor to produce a fibrous precipitate. This fiber is then left to harden before being recovered. One method of recovery involves blowing air into the tank and skimming the floating fibrous mat off the surface. The recovered calcium alginate is then treated with more acid to remove the calcium ions and leave an insoluble alginic acid fiber. This fiber can then be mixed with various alkali salts, for example, sodium carbonate to form sodium alginate.

The molecular weight of commercially available sodium alginates ranges between 32,000 and 400,000 g/mol. The viscosity of alginate solutions increases as pH decreases and reaches a maximum around pH = 3–3.5, as carboxylate groups in the alginate backbone become protonated and form hydrogen bonds. Increasing the molecular weight of alginate increases viscosity, which is often undesirable in processing (LeRoux et al. 1999).

18.2.3 MODIFICATION FOR BIOCOMPATIBILITY

Alginate is inherently nondegradable in mammals, as it lacks the enzyme (i.e., alginase), which can cleave the polymer chains, but ionically cross-linked alginate gels can be dissolved by release of the divalent ions cross-linking the gel into the surrounding media due to exchange reactions with monovalent cations such as sodium ions. Even if the gel dissolves, the average molecular weights of many commercially available alginates are higher than the renal clearance threshold of the kidneys, and likely will not be completely removed from the body (Al-Shamkhani and Duncan 1995).

Alginate's properties such as degradability, hydrophobicity, and biological characteristics can be altered by functionalizing available free hydroxyl and carboxyl groups or interfering with carbon–carbon bonds. Alginate is made degradable in physiological conditions by partial oxidation and potential as a delivery vehicle of drugs and cells for various applications. It is typically oxidized with sodium periodate that cleaves the carbon–carbon bond of the *cis*-diol group in the urinate residue and alters the chair conformation to an open-chain adduct, which enables degradation of the alginate backbone that lowers the molecular weight (West et al. 2007). Further partial oxidation of alginate creates acetal groups to hydrolysis, which increases the degree of oxidation and increases degradability of the resulting alginate gel in physiological conditions (Boontheekul et al. 2005).

Alginate is also modified by sulfation; the reaction of alginate with chlorosulfuric acid in formamide gives alginate a structural similarity to heparin and therefore promotes high blood compatibility. Another common modification of alginate, especially for cell encapsulation purposes, is amidation, in which carbodiimide chemistry is used to form amide linkages between amine-containing molecules and the carboxylic acid functional groups of the alginate polymer backbone (Yang et.al. 2011). This is useful for covalently linking specific peptides to the alginate backbone to promote cell–matrix interactions, as cell adhesion is often a strict requirement for cell viability and proliferation.

18.3 BIOMEDICAL APPLICATIONS

Alginates have found great industrial use due to their ability to form a gel with divalent cations such as calcium and strontium. Due to its biocompatibility and low toxicity, alginate is commonly used in food industry as a thickening agent to increase the quality of foods, such as ice cream and wound dressings (Andersen et al. 2012). It has been widely used in the pharmaceutical industry as a drug or protein delivery agent; alginate gels can release macromolecules in a controlled manner and can be orally administered or injected. Recently, alginate research has been extended to tissue engineering applications with relatively low cost and gentle gelation process. Specifically, alginate hydrogels are favorable for cell transplantation or immobilization (Lee and Mooney 2001). Alginate gels have previously been used for the encapsulation and culture of a variety of cell types, including articular chondrocytes (Ab-Rahim et al. 2013), skeletal myoblasts (Hill et al. 2006), and neural stem cells (Purcell et al. 2009); and as a three-dimensional (3D) ECM for the *in vitro* culture of organs and embryos, for the purpose of developmental studies (Elsheikh et al. 1997), disease simulation (Subramanian et al. 2010), and advanced *in vitro* fertilization techniques (Xu et al. 2006).

Calcium alginate is reputed to be a hemostatic agent that stimulates the clotting of blood *in situ*, which is subsequently absorbed in the tissue (Verbitski et al. 2004). Sodium alginate is reported to be a useful adjuvant in immunization against two strains of influenza virus. It is also found effective in diminishing hypercalciuria in urolithiasis and found useful in the treatment of esophagitis. The most significant property of sodium alginate is the ability to remove strontium 85 and strontium 87 from the body without seriously affecting the availability of Ca, Na, or K in the body (Dominguez et al. 1992). The applications of alginates are linked to their ability to retain water, and their gelling, viscosifying, and stabilizing properties. Their unique, gentle, and almost temperature-independent sol/gel transition in the presence of multivalent cations (Ca^{2+}) makes alginates highly suitable as an immobilization matrix for living cells.

18.3.1 ALGINATE WOUND DRESSINGS

Generally gauze wound dressings have provided mainly a barrier function—keeping the wound dry by allowing evaporation of wound exudates and preventing the entry of pathogen into the wound. Modern alginate dressings maintained a physiologically moist environment; they are highly absorbent, which limit wound secretions and minimize bacterial contamination that promotes healing and the formation of granulation tissue. The alginate fibers trapped in a wound are readily biodegraded, and wound healing facilitated (Queen et al. 2004). In addition, they are able to reduce wound pain, lower the bio-burden of the wound, reduce odor, and absorb protein-ases (Opanson et al. 2010; Chrisman 2010; Sweeney et al. 2012). The selection of an alginate dressing is to manage wound exudates as it can absorb 15–20 times its own weight in wound fluid (MA Healthcare Ltd. *Wound Care Handbook 2011–2012*, London). Alginate dressings are produced by ionic cross-linking of calcium ions to form gels, freeze-dried foam porous sheets, and fibrous nonwoven dressings. The mechanism of an alginate dressing is when it comes into contact with wound exudate, there is an ion exchange between the calcium ions in the alginate and the sodium ions in the blood or exudate. When sufficient calcium ions are replaced by sodium ions, the alginate fibers swell, partially dissolve, and form a gel.

Alginate dressings absorb wound fluid to re-gel, and the gels supply water to a dry wound, which promotes granulation tissue formation, rapid epithelialization, and healing. Alginates can be rinsed away with saline irrigation, so removal of the dress-ing is painless and does not interfere with healing granulation tissue. The chemi-cal composition of the alginate impacts on the dressing's ease of removal from the wound. Dressings high in G alginates will only swell slightly during use and can be removed as an intact dressing, whereas dressings high in M alginates will swell to a greater extent and dissolve, allowing them to be removed through irrigation. Alginate dressings can be left in place for 5–7 days, and the dressing should be changed when it has reached its capacity for absorbing wound exudate.

The first commercially available alginate wound dressing was launched in 1983. Alginates also have been useful as hemostatic agents for cavity wounds (Berry et al. 1996). A study confirmed the effects of calcium- and zinc-containing algi-nate dressings had the greatest potentiating effect on prothrombotic coagulation and platelet activation. Various alginate dressings, including Algicell™ (Derma Sciences, NewYork), AlgiSite M™ (Smith & Nephew, London, UK), Kaltostat™ (ConvaTec, Greensboro), and Sorbsan™ (UDL Laboratories, Illinois), are commercially available (Balakrishnan et al. 2006). The addition of silver and zinc ions into alginate dress-ings also enhanced the antioxidant capacity and antimicrobial effects increased the levels of endogenous growth factors (Wiegand et al. 2009). Blends of alginate, chitin/ chitosan, and fucoidan gels have been reported to provide a moist healing environment in rats, with an ease of application and removal (Murakami et al. 2010). Alginates are used in a variety of wound types where exudate is present, including pressure ulcers, venous leg ulcers, diabetic foot ulcers, postoperative wounds, cavity wounds, traumatic wounds, malignant wounds, pilonidal sinus wounds, donor sites, and partial thickness burns (Clark and Bradbury 2010; Harris and Holloway 2012).

Chitin–calcium alginate-covered wound sites underwent normal wound healing with reepithelialization (in rat model) wound healing studies (Shamshina et al. 2014).

18.3.2 Cell Culture

In the cost-efficient development of new drugs, the significance of *in vitro* cell culture studies are of great consideration, in time-efficient treatment of cancer patients, and an understanding of developmental biology and mechanisms of stem cell differentiation. Appropriate cell models would also reduce the need for animal trials, especially for toxicity assays (Prestwich 2008). A wide range of biomaterials have demonstrated the applicability as matrices providing a biologically more relevant environment for cells mimicking several characteristics of the ECM such as physical, mechanical, and biological properties. 3D cell culture can be defined as when cells are embedded in a scaffold or matrix and signals from the scaffold and surrounding cells can be received from all directions. There are several formats and materials available that enable 3D cell culture to better predict the clinical outcome of medical treatments such as chemotherapy and the selection of drugs can be optimized based on the response from isolated cancer cells of the patient. Polymer hydrogels are considered well suited for 3D cell culture as they have similarities to natural ECM. Examples of synthetic materials with the capability of forming hydrogels are polyethylene glycol (PEG), poly(hydroxyethyl methacrylate), polyvinyl alcohol, and polycaprolactone (PCL). Natural polymers (and proteins) able to form hydrogels are alginate, chitosan, hyaluronan, dextran, collagen, and fibrin, where alginate hyaluronan (as a product of bacterial fermentation) and dextran represent non-animal-derived materials. Despite the homogeneous nature of synthetic polymers, their use as cell-entrapping materials has to some extent been avoided due to harsh polymerization conditions (Lee et al. 2008).

Alginate gels are used as a model system for mammalian cell culture in biomedical studies. The gels serve as either two-dimensional (2D) or more physiologically relevant 3D culture systems. The lack of mammalian cell receptors for alginate, combined with the low-protein adsorption to alginate gels, allows these materials to serve in many ways as an ideal blank slate, upon which highly specific and quantitative modes for cell adhesion can be incorporated. Due to the biocompatibility and easy introduction of alginate into the body, the findings of *in vitro* studies can be readily translated *in vivo*. The arginine–glycine–aspartic acid (RGD) peptide sequence is found in ECM proteins. RGD-modified alginate gels have been most frequently used as *in vitro* cell culture substrates to date. The presence of RGD peptides in alginate gels allows one to control the phenotype of interacting myoblasts, chondrocytes (Degala et al. 2011), osteoblasts (Evangelista et al. 2007), ovarian follicle (Kreeger et al. 2006), and bone marrow stromal cells (Bidarra et al. 2010).

The alginate gels have recently been formed in a microfluidic device through light-triggered release of caged calcium using DM-nitrophen™ (Sigma-Aldrich, Canada) compounds and used as a 3D cell culture substrate. Preosteoblasts (MC3T3-E1) and human umbilical vein endothelial cells were co-cultured in the microfluidic device using photo-patterning of alginate hydrogels, and this system may provide a useful means for integrating 3D culture microenvironments into microfluidic systems.

The microscopic images of primary human fibroblasts cultured on alginate gels (2D) modified with either (1) RGDSP or (2) G_{12}RGDSP, and cells encapsulated within the same two types of gels (3D) were shown. Synthesis of alginate derivatives presenting appropriate cyclic RGD peptides capable of promoting stem cell differentiation may enhance tissue regeneration by reducing the need for exogenous soluble factors. Cyclic RGD peptides are more resistant to proteolysis and have higher binding affinity for cellular receptors important to cell response and selectivity than linear RGD peptides (Liu 2006). Study has been conducted using alginate gels presenting cyclic

RGD peptides (glycine$_4$–cystine–arginine–glycine–aspartate–serine–proline–cystine; G$_4$CRGDSPC), which enhanced osteogenic differentiation of stem cells (primary human bone marrow stromal cells and mouse bone marrow stromal D1 cell line) better than gels modified with linear RGD peptides (Hsiong et al. 2009).

Alginate gels as 3D cell culture substrates have revealed key insights regarding stem cell and cancer biology. The cells of nanoscale actively reorganized on the adhesion ligands presented from the gels (Huebsch et al. 2010). Cancer cell signaling and tumor vascularization in the 3D culture microenvironment using alginate gels have also been studied; this finding may lead to the development of new anti-angiogenic cancer therapies (Fischbach et al. 2009).

18.3.3 PROTEIN DELIVERY

The progress in tissue engineering allows the delivery of functional and active proteins to act as chemical cues for desired biological purposes. Regeneration of functional tissues and incorporation of new tissues require adhesion, migration, proliferation, and organization of new and old cells at the injured site. In order to maintain and regulate the complex cellular activities, delivery of signaling proteins and functional peptides is needed.

Alginate gels have been used as a vehicle to deliver proteins or cell populations that can direct the regeneration or engineering of various tissues and organs in the body. Alginate is an excellent candidate for the delivery of protein drugs, because proteins can be incorporated into alginate-based formulations under relatively mild conditions that minimize their denaturation, and the gels can protect them from degradation until their release.

Generally, the release rate of proteins from alginate gels is rapid, due to the inherent porosity and hydrophilic nature of the gels. However, heparin-binding growth factors such as vascular endothelial growth factor (VEGF) exhibit similar, reversible binding to alginate hydrogels, enabling a sustained and localized release (Silva and Mooney 2010).

Ionically cross-linked alginate microspheres efficiently encapsulated high pI proteins such as lysozyme and chymotrypsin; these proteins appear to physically cross-link the sodium alginate, allowing for more sustained release (Wells and Sheardown 2007). Amino group-terminated poly((2-dimethylamino) ethyl methacrylate) has also been reacted with oxidized alginate without using a catalyst, and gel beads have been prepared by dropping the aqueous solution of the alginate derivative into an aqueous CaCl$_2$ solution to form particles for oral delivery of proteins (Gao et al. 2009). Alginate was also used as a building block in the synthesis of a tetrafunctional acetal-linked polymer network for stimuli-responsive gels with adjustable pore sizes. The gels protected acid-labile proteins such as insulin from denaturation in the gastric environment (pH 1.2), while releasing the loaded protein at near zero-order kinetics in neutral pH (Chan and Neufeld 2010).

The insulin-loaded alginate microspheres were prepared by blending alginate with anionic polymers (e.g., polyphosphate, dextran sulfate), followed by chitosan coating in order to protect insulin at gastric pH and obtain its sustained release at intestinal pH. Alginate microspheres have also been coated with *Bombyx mori* silk fibroin using layer-by-layer deposition techniques, which provided mechanically stable shells and a diffusion barrier to the encapsulated proteins (Wang et al. 2007). A combination of microspheres that serve as a depot for proteins and alginate hydrogel also enables sustained protein release. Hydrogel microspheres were prepared by encapsulation of a suspension of poly(D,L-lactide-*co*-glycolide) (PLGA) microspheres in alginate prior to ionic cross-linking. The release of bovine serum albumin (BSA), a model protein, from this combination delivery system was primarily controlled by the mixing ratio of PLGA microspheres and alginate hydrogel, independent of total BSA studied (Lee and Lee 2009).

18.3.4 TISSUE REGENERATION WITH PROTEIN AND CELL DELIVERY

Regeneration of functional tissues and incorporation of new tissues require adhesion, migration, proliferation, and organization of new and old cells at the injured site. Insulin proteins like other hormones and synthetic vaccines have been widely used to manage poorly controlled diseases (Habraken et al. 2007). Growth factors are one type of proteins that have the ability to regulate cell signaling, which can stimulate or inhibit growth of cells. Delivery of growth factors has become a valuable tool for directing cell proliferation, differentiation, migration, and angiogenesis in tissues. The use of synthetic or conjugated peptides has also been proven to effectively guide and facilitate cellular activities owing to their improved penetration abilities into cells (Bickel et al. 2001). Key parameters in designing a protein delivery vehicle include localization of delivered proteins, targeting appropriate cells, optimal time period for protein administration, and appropriate doses of protein needed at different times and incorporating desired proteins into polymeric matrices. Protein release from biodegradable matrices is not only dependent on the diffusion of protein, but also on the degradation rate of the polymers. Biodegradable polymers, such as poly(lactide-*co*-glycolide) (PLG), poly(glycolic poly(lactide-*co*-glycolide) (PLG), poly(glycolic acid) (PGA), poly(lactic acid) (PLA), and poly(lactic-*co*-glycolic acid)), and PCL, have become attractive polymers for protein delivery.

Alginate polymer was shown to have mucoadhesion properties, which makes alginate a good candidate for drugs or proteins needed to be delivered via mucosal tissues. Alginate beads formed by a calcium-induced gelation process have been widely used for tissue engineering applications, such as cell encapsulation, and nucleic acid, drug, and protein delivery. Large alginate beads can be produced by dropping alginate solution into calcium chloride ($CaCl_2$) solution (Rousseau et al. 2004).

Molecules too large to have significant diffusion-based release can still be delivered if the gel degrades. For example, condensed plasmid DNA (Ali and Mooney 2008) can be released from degrading alginate gels, and antibody might be released from alginate gels by the same mechanism.

18.3.5 BONE

Treatment of bone injuries is still limited due to poor healing, but alginate gels have found potential in bone regeneration by delivery of osteoinductive factors and bone-forming cells. Alginate gels have advantages for bone and cartilage regeneration, due to their ability to be introduced into the body in a minimally invasive manner, their ability to fill irregularly shaped defects, and the ease of chemical modification with adhesion ligands (e.g., RGD) and controlled release of tissue induction factors compared with other materials. Alginate gels have proven useful in animal models for the delivery of growth factors that can effectively drive bone regeneration (e.g., bone morphogenetic proteins [BMPs]). DNA-encoding BMPs have also demonstrated that significant bone tissue can be regenerated by alginate gel delivery (Lopiz-Morales et al. 2010). The delivery of multiple factors, either in combination or sequence, is also being explored for BMP-2 and BMP-7 using alginate gels that enhanced osteogenic differentiation of bone marrow-derived stem cells *in vitro* (Basmanav et al. 2008). Alveolar bone defects in dogs repaired with calcium cross-linked alginate gels (Weng et al. 2006). Alginate/chitosan gels entrapping mesenchymal stem cells (MSCs) and BMP-2 showed potential for trabecular bone formation in mice (Park et al. 2005).

Alginate with inorganic materials enhanced bone tissue formation. Alginate/ hydroxyapatite composite scaffolds enhanced the adhesion of osteosarcoma cells (Lin and Yeh 2004). Cell-encapsulating alginate gel beads with calcium phosphate cement showed potential for bone tissue engineering under moderate stress-bearing conditions (Weir et al. 2006). Also alginate gels containing collagen type I and β-tricalcium phosphate enhanced adhesion and proliferation of human bone marrow stromal cells that do not readily attach or proliferate on pure alginate gels.

18.3.6 CARTILAGE

In orthopedics field, repair of damaged or degraded cartilage is still one of the major challenges faced, but alginate gels have proved to be useful for transplanting chondrogenic cells to restore damaged cartilage in animal models. Alginate solution was mixed with calcium sulfate and injected into molds of facial implants in order to produce preshaped cartilage, and the constructs formed cartilage with 3D shape retention after 30 weeks of subcutaneous implantation into mice and sheep (Chang et al. 2001 and 2003). The macroporous alginate gels with predefined geometries were compressed into a significantly smaller form (dry state) and introduced into mice through a small catheter, which allowed cartilage formation in mice with the desired geometry (Thornton et al. 2004).

The cartilage regeneration by the use of stem cells is very attractive. Encapsulation in alginate has been hypothesized that chondrogenesis of stem cells is related to the morphology of the encapsulated round-shaped cells (Dashtdar et al. 2011), and alginate gels promote a rounded morphology that may promote the cellular differentiation process. Cartilage formed in large osteochondral defects by human MSCs encapsulated in alginate gel beads cultured in serum-free medium with the addition of transforming growth factor (TGF)-β1, dexamethasone, and ascorbate 2-phosphate for more than 1 week.

18.3.7 REGENERATION OF ORGANS

Alginate gels have found potential for their ability to mediate the regeneration and engineering of a variety of other tissues and organs, including the skeletal muscle, nerve, pancreas, and liver. A combined delivery of VEGF and insulin-like growth factor-1 from alginate gels was used to modulate both angiogenesis and myogenesis. Due to satellite cell activation and proliferation, and cellular protection from apoptosis by the sustained delivery of growth factors led to significant muscle regeneration and functional muscle formation (Borselli et al. 2010). RGD-alginate gels enhanced the outward migration of primary myoblasts into damaged muscle tissue *in vivo* by the sustained delivery of hepatocyte growth factor and fibroblast growth factor 2 from the gels.

Alginate-based highly anisotropic capillary gels, introduced into acute cervical spinal cord lesions in adult rats, directed axonal regrowth, were studied for the repair of the central and peripheral nerve systems. Alginate gels, covalently cross-linked with ethylenediamine, were used to restore a 50-mm gap in cat sciatic nerves (Hashimoto et al. 2005) and promoted the outgrowth of regenerating axons and astrocyte reactions at the stump of transected spinal cords in young rats (Kataoka et al. 2004). They were used as glue for repair of peripheral nerve gaps that could not be sutured. They may be useful for cell-based neural therapies, as mouse-derived neural stem cells cultured in calcium alginate beads maintained their capacity for multilineage differentiation into neurons (Li et al. 2006).

The alginate gels encapsulating hepatocytes may offer a suitable platform for developing a bio-artificial liver as they are easily manipulated (Koizumi et al. 2007). The hydrophilic nature of alginate gels processed to exhibit an interconnected porous structure allows an efficient seeding of hepatocytes into the gels, while maintaining high hepatocellular functions. Hepatocyte engraftment was improved when hepatocytes were transplanted into the liver lobe of Lewis rats using VEGF-releasing porous alginate gels (Kedem et al. 2005).

In tissue engineering, the first application of alginate gels involved the transplantation of encapsulated pancreatic islet allografts and xenografts in an effort to cure type I diabetes. The gel was used to provide protection from the host immune system. This approach has been successfully used to treat animal models of type I diabetes without the use of immunosuppressive drugs (Calafiore 2003).

18.3.8 DELIVERY OF SMALL CHEMICAL DRUGS

Nanoporous alginate gels have been investigated for the delivery of a variety of low-molecular-weight drugs leading to rapid diffusion of small molecules through the gel. For example, the release of flurbiprofen from ionically cross-linked, partially oxidized alginate gels is almost complete in 1.5 hour; incorporation into beads formed from partially oxidized alginate in the presence of both calcium ions and adipic acid dihydrazide led to a prolonged release due to the increased cross-links and reduced swelling (Maiti et al. 2009). The controlled and localized delivery of antineoplastic agents has also been achieved using partially oxidized alginate gels. For example, methotrexate (noninteractive with alginate) was rapidly released by diffusion, whereas doxorubicin, covalently attached to the alginate, was released via chemical hydrolysis of the cross-linker. Mitoxantrone, ionically complexed to alginate, was only released after the dissociation of the gel (Bouhadir et al. 2001).

The hydrophobic drugs were released with alginate gels. The drug release was complete within 2 hour for alginate-g-PCL/Ca^{2+} beads but in 1 hour for alginate/Ca^{2+} beads (Colinet et al. 2009).The sustained release of theophylline was also achieved from carbon nanotube (CNT)-incorporated alginate microspheres as CNT enhanced the mechanical stability of gels, without affecting the structure and morphology of the microspheres, and no significant cytotoxicity was observed on a delivery carrier to the intestine and colon (Zhang et al. 2010).

The system of alginate and chitosan containing triamcinolone was prepared by a complex ionotropic gelation method for colonic drug delivery. A higher swelling degree and faster drug release were observed from the particulate systems in a simulated enteric environment (pH 7.5). Magnetic alginate-chitosan beads loaded with albendazole (ABZ) were also prepared for passive targeting to the gastrointestinal tract using physical capture mechanisms and showed the release of ABZ (Wang et al. 2010). Chitosan-treated alginate microparticles containing all-*trans* retinoic acid (ATRA) have also been shown to enhance dermal localization and achieved the sustained release of ATRA into the skin.

Amoxicillin-loaded chitosan/poly(γ-glutamic acid) nanoparticles have been incorporated into alginate/Ca^{2+} hydrogels for effective treatment of *Helicobacter pylori* infection. The alginate gel outer layer protected the amoxicillin-loaded nanoparticles in the gastric environment and facilitated amoxicillin interactions specifically with intercellular spaces, which is the infection site of *H. pylori* (Chang et al. 2010).

Pharmaceutical applications include studies on composite alginate/poly(lactic-co-glycolic) microparticles for insulin delivery (Schoubben et al. 2009), coated chitosan-alginate beads for oral delivery of the antibiotic drug cefaclor (Rasool and Fahmy 2013), and tamoxifin-loaded nanoparticles for the treatment of breast cancer (Martinez et al. 2012).

18.3.9 ALGINATE ANTACIDS

Acid reflux occurs when stomach acid leaks back up into your oesophagus and irritates its lining. Antacids containing alginate help to relieve indigestion caused by acid reflux. Chemistry in which the antacid (sodium alginate, sodium hydrogen carbonate, and calcium carbonate) play a role is as follows: soluble sodium alginate reacts with stomach acid to form insoluble alginic acid, which helps to form a barrier that floats on top of the acid in the stomach. This barrier helps prevent stomach acid from moving up into the esophagus, an acid reflux. Calcium carbonate dissolves in the stomach contents releasing calcium ions (Ca^{2+}). The sodium hydrogen carbonate and calcium carbonate react with a little of the stomach acid, forming carbon dioxide gas. The carbon dioxide lifts the raft so that it floats on top of the stomach contents preventing reflux into the oesophagus. The alginate raft will not remain in the stomach permanently, but it is broken down over time by the mechanical action of stomach contractions. Both *in vitro* and *in vivo* studies have demonstrated that alginate-based rafts can entrap carbon dioxide, and antacid components contained in some formulations, thus providing a relatively pH-neutral barrier. Alginate-based raft-forming formulations can additionally provide longer lasting relief than that of traditional antacids. Their unique nonsystemic mechanism of action provides rapid and long-duration relief of heartburn and acid reflux symptoms (Mandel et al. 2000). Gaviscon (Slough, UK) can eliminate or displace the *acid pocket* in gastroesophageal reflux disease (GERD) patients. And suggested that the alginate-antacid formulation to be an appropriately targeted postprandial GERD therapy by neutralizing and/or displacing the acid pocket in GERD patients with low-density gel *raft* that floats on top of gastric contents (Kwiatek et al. 2011).

18.4   CONCLUSION

Alginate has proved to be of great utility and a good biomaterial for many biomedical applications, particularly in the areas of wound healing, drug delivery, *in vitro* cell culture, and tissue engineering. Due to their biocompatibility, mild gelation conditions, and simple modifications to prepare derivatives with new properties, alginates find more applications. Recent studies of alginates in a multidisciplinary approach including islet transplantation for treatment of type 1 diabetes and diabetic foot ulcer treatment. As one looks to the future, the alginate-based materials used in medicine are likely to evolve more considerably. Further understanding of the fundamental properties of alginate and developing new types of cell and tissue-interactive alginate gels may enable future advances in biomedical science, tissue, and genetic engineering applications.

REFERENCES

Ab-Rahim, S., L. Selvaratnam, H.R.B. Raghavendran, and T. Kamarul. 2013. Chondrocyte-alginate constructs with or without TGF-beta 1 produces superior extracellular matrix expression than monolayer cultures. *Mol Cell Biochem* 376: 11–20.

Andersen, T., B. Strand, K. Formo, E. Alsberg and B. Christensen. 2012. Alginates as biomaterials in tissue engineering. *J Carbohyd Chem* 37: 227–258.

Ali, O.A., and D.J. Mooney. 2008. Sustained GM-CSF and PEI condensed pDNA presentation increases the level and duration of gene expression in dendritic cells. *J Control Release* 132: 273–278.

Al-Shamkhani A., and R. Duncan. 1995. Radio iodination of alginate via covalently-bound tyrosin amide allows monitoring of its fate in vivo. *J Bioact Compat Polym* 10: 4–13.

Balakrishnan, B., M. Mohanty, A.C. Fernandez, P.V. Mohanan, and A. Jayakrishnan. 2006. Evaluation of the effect of incorporation of dibutyryl cyclic adenosine mono phosphate in an in situ forming hydrogel wound dressing based on oxidized alginate and gelatin. *Biomaterials* 27: 1355–1361.

Basmanav, F.B., G.T. Kose, and V. Hasirci. 2008. Sequential growth factor delivery for complexed microspheres for bone tissue engineering. *Biomaterials* 29: 4195–420.

Berry, D.P., S. Bale, and K.G. Harding. 1996. Dressings for treating cavity wounds. *J Wound Care* 5: 10–17.

Bickel, U., T. Yoshikawa, and W.M. Pardridge. 2001. Delivery of peptides and proteins through the blood-brain barrier. *Adv Drug Delivery Rev* 46(1–3): 247–279.

Bidarra, S.J., C.C. Barrias, M.A. Barbosa, R. Soares, and P.L. Granja. 2010. Immobilization of human mesenchymal stem cells within RGD-grafted alginate microspheres and assessment of their angiogenic potential. *Biomacromolecules* 11: 1956–1964.

Boontheekul, T., H.J. Kong, and D.J. Mooney. 2005. Controlling alginate gel degradation utilizing partial oxidation and bimodal molecular weight distribution. *Biomaterials* 26(15): 2455–2465.

Borselli, C., H. Storrie, F. Benesch-Lee, D. Shvartsman, C. Cezar, J.W. Lichtman, H.H. Vandenburgh, and D.J. Mooney. 2010. Functional muscle regeneration with combined delivery of angiogenesis and myogenesis factors. *Proc Natl Acad Sci* 107: 3287–3292.

Bouhadir, K.H., E. Alsberg, D.J. Mooney. 2001. Hydrogels for combination delivery of antineoplastic agents. *Biomaterials* 22: 2625–2633.

Calafiore, R. 2003. Alginate microcapsules for pancreatic islet cell graft immune protection: Struggle and progress towards the final cure for type 1 diabetes mellitus. *Exp Opin Biol Ther* 3: 201–205.

Chang, S.C.N., J.A. Rowley, G. Tobias, N.G. Genes, A.K. Roy, D.J. Mooney, C.A. Vacanti, and L.J. Bonassar. 2001. Injection molding of chondrocyte/alginate constructs in the shape of facial implants. *J Biomed Mater Res* 55: 503–511.

Chang, S.C.N., G. Tobias, A.K. Roy, C.A. Vacanti, and L.J. Bonassar. 2003. Tissue engineering of autologous cartilage for craniofacial reconstruction by injection molding. *Plast Reconstr Surg* 112: 793–799.

Chang, C.H., Y.H. Lin, C.L. Yeh, Y.C. Chen, S.F. Chiou, Y.M. Hsu, Y.S. Chen, and C.C. Wang. 2010. Nanoparticles incorporated in pH-sensitive hydrogels as amoxicillin delivery for eradication of *Helicobacter pylori*. *Biomacromolecules* 11: 133–142.

Chan, A.W., and R.J. Neufeld. 2010. Tuneable semi-synthetic network alginate for absorptive encapsulation and controlled release of protein therapeutics. *Biomaterials* 31: 9040–9047.

Chrisman, C.A. 2010. Care of chronic wounds in palliative care and end-of- life patients. *Int Wound J* 7(4): 214–35.

Clark, R., and S. Bradbury. 2010. Silvercel non-adherent made easy. *Wounds Int* 1(5): 1–6.

Colinet, I., V. Dulong, G. Mocanu, L. Picton, and D. Le Cerf. 2009. New amphiphilic and pH-sensitive hydrogel for controlled release of a model poorly water-soluble drug. *Eur J Pharm Biopharm* 73: 345–350.

Dashtdar, H., H.A. Rothan, T. Tay, R.E. Ahmad, R. Ali, L.X. Tay, P.P. Chong, and T. Kamarul. 2011. A preliminary study comparing the use of allogenic chondrogenic pre-differentiated and undifferentiated mesenchymal stem cells for the repair of full thickness articular cartilage defects in rabbits. *J Orthop Res* 29(9): 1336–42.

d'Ayala, G.G., M. Malinconico, and P. Laurienzo. 2008. Marine derived polysaccharides for biomedical applications: Chemical modification approaches. *Molecules* 13(9): 2069–2106.

Degala, S., W.R. Zipfel, and L.J. Bonassar. 2011. Chondrocyte calcium signaling in response to fluid flow is regulated by matrix adhesion in 3-D alginate scaffolds. *Arch Biochem Biophys* 505: 112–117.

Dembitsky, V.M., T.A. Gloriozova, and V.V. Poroikov. 2005. Novel antitumor agents: Marine sponge alkaloids, their synthetic analogs and derivatives. *Mini-Rev Med Chem* 5(3): 319–336.

Dominguez, J. N., A. Taddei, M. Cordero, and I. Blanca. 1992. Synthesis of C(10)-halogenated prostaglandins. I. *J Pharm Sci* 83: 472.

Drury, J.L., R.G. Dennis, and D.J. Mooney. 2004. The tensile properties of alginate hydrogels. *Biomaterials* 25(16): 3187–3199.

Elsheikh, A.S., Y. Takahashi, M. Hishinuma, M.S. Nour, and H. Kanagawa. 1997. Effect of encapsulation on development of mouse pronuclear stage embryos in vitro. *Anim Reprod Sci* 48(2–4): 317–324.

Evangelista, M.B., S.X. Hsiong, R. Fernandes, P. Sampaio, H.J. Kong, C.C. Barrias, R. Salema, M.A. Barbosa, D.J. Mooney, and P.L. Granja. 2007. Upregulation of bone cell differentiation through immobilization with in a synthetic extracellular matrix. *Biomaterials* 28: 3644–3655.

Fischbach, C., H.J. Kong, S.X. Hsiong, M.B. Evangelista, W. Yuen, and D.J. Mooney. 2009. Cancer cell angiogenic capability is regulated by 3D culture and integrin engagement. *Proc Natl Acad Sci* 106: 399–404.

Gao, C.M., M.Z. Liu, S.L. Chen, S.P. Jin, and J. Chen. 2009. Preparation of oxidized sodium alginate-graft poly((2-dimethylamino) ethyl methacrylate) gel beads and in vitro controlled release behavior of BSA. *Int J Pharm* 371: 16–24.

Gombotz, W.R., and S.F. Wee. 1998. Protein release from alginate matrices. *Adv Drug Deliv Rev* 31(3): 267–285.

Habraken, W.J.E.M., J.G.C. Wolke, and J.A Jansen. 2007. Ceramic composites as matrices and scaffolds for drug delivery in tissue engineering. *Adv Drug Deliver Rev* 59(4–5): 234–248.

Harris, C.L., and S. Holloway. 2012. Development of an evidence—Based protocol for care of pilonidal sinus wounds healing by secondary intent using a modified Reactive Delphi procedure. Part 2: Methodology, Analysis and Results. *Int Wound J* 9(2): 173–188.

Hashimoto, T., Y. Suzuki, K. Suzuki, T. Nakashima, M. Tanihara, and C. Ide. 2005. Peripheral nerve regeneration using non-tubular alginate gel crosslinked with covalent bonds. *J Mater SciMater Med* 16: 503–509.

Hill, E., T. Boontheekul, and D.J. Mooney. 2006. Designing scaffolds to enhance transplanted myoblast survival and migration. *Tissue Eng* 12(5): 1295–1304.

Hsiong, S.X., T. Boontheekul, N. Huebsch, and D.J. Mooney. 2009. Cyclic arginine-glycine-aspartate peptides enhance three-dimensional stem cell osteogenic differentiation. *Tissue Eng Part A* 15: 263–272.

Huebsch, N., P.R. Arany, A.S. Mao, D. Shvartsman, O.A. Ali, S.A. Bencherif, J. Rivera-Feliciano, and D.J. Mooney. 2010. Harnessing traction-mediated manipulation of the cell/matrix interface to control stem-cell fate. *Nat Mater* 9: 518–526.

Kataoka, K., Y. Suzuki, M. Kitada, T. Hashimoto, H. Chou, H.L. Bai, M. Ohta, S. Wu, K. Suzuki, and C. Ide. 2004. Alginate enhances elongation of early regenerating axons in spinal cord of young rats. *Tissue Eng* 10: 493–504.

Kedem, A., A. Perets, I. Gamlieli-Bonshtein, M. Dvir-Ginzberg, S. Mizrahi, and S. Cohen. 2005. Vascular endothelial growth factor-releasing scaffolds enhance vascularization and engraftment of hepatocytes transplanted on liver lobes. *Tissue Eng* 11: 715–722.

Koizumi, T., T. Aoki, Y. Kobayashi, D. Yasuda, Y. Izumida, Z.H. Jin, N. Nishino, Y. Shimizu, H. Kato, N. Murai, T. Niiya, Y. Enami, K. Mitamura, T. Yamamoto, and M. Kusano. 2007. Long-term maintenance of the drug transport activity in cryopreservation of micro-encapsulated rat hepatocytes. *Cell Transplantation* 16: 67–73.

Kreeger, P.K., J.W. Deck, T.K. Woodruff, and L.D. Shea. 2006. The invitro regulation of ovarian follicle development using alginate-extracellular matrix gels. *Biomaterials* 27: 714–723.

Kwiatek, M.A., S. Roman, A. Fareeduddin, J.E. Pandolfino, and P.J. Kahrilas. 2011. An alginate-antacid formulation (Gaviscon Double Action Liquid) can eliminate or displace the postprandial "acid pocket" in symptomatic GERD patients. *Aliment Pharmacol Ther* 34(1): 59–66.

Lopiz-Morales, Y., A. Abarrategi, V. Ramos, C. Moreno-Vicente, L. Lopez-Duran, J.L. Lopez-Lacomba, and F. Marco. 2010. In vivo comparison of the effects of rhBMP-2 and rhBMP-4 in osteochondral tissue regeneration. *Eur Cells Mater* 20: 367–378.

Lee, K.Y., and D.J. Mooney. 2001. Hydrogels for tissue engineering. *Chem Rev* 101(7): 1869–1880.

Lee, J., M.J. Cuddihy, and N.A. Kotov. 2008. Three-dimensional cell culture matrices: State of the art. *Tissue Eng Part B-Rev* 14: 61–86.

Lee, J., and K.Y. Lee. 2009. Injectable microsphere/hydrogel combination systems for localized protein delivery. *Macromol Biosci* 9: 671–676.

LeRoux, M.A., F. Guilak, and L.A. Setton 1999. Compressive and shear properties of alginate gel: Effects of sodium ions and alginate concentration. *J Biomed Mater Res* 47: 46–53.

Li, X.Q., T.Q. Liu, K.D. Song, L.S. Yao, D. Ge, C.Y. Bao, X.H. Ma, and Z.F. Cui. 2006. Culture of neural stem cells in calcium alginate beads. *Biotechnol Prog* 22: 1683–1689.

Lin, H.R., and Y.J. Yeh. 2004. Porous alginate/hydroxyapatite composite scaffolds for bone tissue engineering: Preparation, characterization, and in vitro studies. *J Biomed Mater Res Part B* 71: 52–65.

Liu, S. 2006. Radiolabeled multimeric cyclic RGD peptides as integrin $\alpha v \beta 3$ targeted radiotracers for tumor imaging. *Mol Pharm* 3: 472–487.

MA Health Care Ltd. *Wound Care Handbook 2011–2012*. MA Healthcare Ltd, London.

Maiti, S., K. Singha, S. Ray, P. Dey, and B. Sa. 2009. Adipic acid dihydrazide treatedpartially oxidized alginate beads for sustained oral delivery of flurbiprofen. *Pharm Develop Technol* 14: 461–470.

Mandel, K.G., B.P. Daggy, D.A. Brodie, and H.I. Jacoby. 2000. Review article: Alginate-raft formulations in the treatment of heartburn and acid reflux. *Aliment Pharmacol Ther* 14(6): 669–90.

Martinez, A., E. Muniz, I. Iglesias, J.M. Teijón, and M.D. Blanco. 2012. Enhanced preclinical efficacy oftamoxifen developed as alginate–cysteine/disulfide bond reduced albumin nanoparticles. *Int J Pharm* 436: 574–581.

McKee, J.W.A., L. Kavalieris, D.J. Brasch, M.T. Brown, and L.D. Melton. 1992. Alginate content and composition of Macrocystis pyrifera from New Zealand. *J Appl Phycol* 4(4): 357–369.

Motwani, S.K. 2008. Chitosan–sodium alginate nanoparticles as submicroscopic reservoirs for ocular delivery: Formulation, optimisation and in vitro characterisation. *Eur J Pharm Biopharm* 68(3): 513–525.

Murakami, K., H. Aoki, S. Nakamura, S. Nakamura, M. Takikawa, M. Hanzawa, S. Kishimoto, H. Hattori, Y. Tanaka, T. Kiyosawa, Y. Sato, and M. Ishihara. 2010. Hydrogel blends of chitin/chitosan, fucoidan and alginate as healing-impaired wound dressings. *Biomaterials* 31: 83.

Opasanon, S., P. Muangman, and N. Namviriyachote. 2010. Clinical Ectiveness of silver alginate dressing in outpatient management of partial-thickness burns. *Int Wound J* 7(6): 467–71.

Park, D.J., B.H. Choi, S.J. Zhu, J.Y. Huh, B.Y. Kim, and S.H. Lee. 2005. Injectable bone using chitosanalginate gel/mesenchymal stem cells/BMP-2 composites. *J Cranio Maxill Surg* 33: 50–54.

Paterson, I., and E.A. Anderson. 2005. The renaissance of natural products as drug candidates. *Sci* 310(5747): 451–453.

Prestwich, G.D. 2008. Evaluating drug efficacy and toxicology in three dimensions: Using synthetic extracellular matrices in drug discovery. *Acc Chem Res* 41: 139–148.

Purcell, E.K., A. Singh, and D.R. Kipke. 2009. Alginate composition effects on a neural stem cell-seeded scaffold. *Tissue Eng Part C Methods* 15(4): 541–550.

Queen, D., H. Orsted, H. Sanada, and G. Sussman. 2004. A dressing history. *Int Wound J* 1: 59–77.

Rasool, B.K., and S.A. Fahmy. 2013. Development of coated beads for oral controlled delivery of cefaclor: In vitro evaluation. *Acta Pharm* 63(1): 31–44.

Rehm, B.H.A., and S. Valla. 1997. Bacterial alginates: Biosynthesis and applications. *Appl Microbiol Biotechnol* 48 (3): 281–288.

Rinaudo, M. 2008. Main properties and current applications of some polysaccharides as biomaterials. *Polym Int* 57(3): 397–430.

Schoubben, A., P. Blasi, S. Giovagnoli, L. Perioli, C. Rossi, and M. Ricci. 2009. Novel composite microparticles for protein stabilization and delivery. *Eur J Pharm Sci.* 36(2–3): 226–234.

Rousseau, I., D. Le Cerf, L. Picton, J.F. Argillier, and G. Muller. 2004. Entrapment and release of sodium polystyrene sulfonate (SPS) from calcium alginate gel beads. *Eur Polym J* 40(12): 2709–2715.

Shamshina, J.L., G. Guru, L.E. Block, K. Hansen, C. Dingee, A. Walters, and R.D. Rogers. 2014. Chitin–calcium alginate composite fibers for wound care dressings spun from ionic liquid solution. *J Mater ChemB* 2: 3924–3936.

Siew, C.K., P.A. Williams, and N.W.G. Young. 2005. New insights into the mechanism of gelation of alginate and pectin: Charge annihilation and reversal mechanism. *Biomacromolecules* 6(2): 963–969.

Silva, E.A., and D.J. Mooney. 2010. Effects of VEGF temporal and spatial presentation on angiogenesis. *Biomaterials* 31: 1235–1241.

Stanford, E.C.C. 1881. British patent 142.

Subramanian, B., D. Rudym, C. Cannizzaro, R. Perrone, J. Zhou, and D.L. Kaplan. 2010. Tissue-engineered three-dimensional in vitro models for normal and diseased kidney. *Tissue Eng Part A* 16(9): 2821–2831.

Sweeney, I.R., M. Miraftab, and G. Collyer. 2012. A critical review of modern and emerging absorbent dressings used to treat exuding wounds. *Int Wound J* 9: 601–612.

Thornton, A.J., E. Alsberg, M. Albertelli, and D.J. Mooney. 2004. Shape-defining scaffolds for minimally invasive tissue engineering. *Transplant* 77: 1798–1803.

Verbitski, S.M., J.E. Mullally, and F.A. Fitzpatrick. 2004. Punaglandins, chlorinated prostaglandins, function as potent Michael receptors to inhibit ubiquitin isopeptidase activity. *J Med Chem* 47: 2062.

Wang, X., E. Wenk, X. Hu, G.R. Castro, L. Meinel, X. Wang, C. Li, H. Merkle, and D.L. Kaplan. 2007. Silk coatings on PLGA and alginate microspheres for protein delivery. *Biomaterials* 28: 4161–4169.

Wang, F.Q., P. Li, J.P. Zhang, A.Q. Wang, and Q. Wei. 2010. A novel pH-sensitive magnetic alginate74 chitosan beads for albendazole delivery. *Drug Dev Ind Pharm* 36: 867–877.

Weir, M.D., H.H.K. Xu, and C.G. Simon. 2006. Strong calcium phosphate cement-chitosan-mesh construct containing cell-encapsulating hydrogel beads for bone tissue engineering. *J Biomed Mater Res Part A* 77: 487–496.

Wells, L.A., and H. Sheardown. 2007. Extended release of high pI proteins from alginate microspheres via a novel encapsulation technique. *Eur J Pharm Biopharm* 65: 329–335.

Weng, Y.L., M. Wang M, W. Liu, X.J. Hu, G. Chai, Q.M. Yan, L. Zhu, L. Cui, and Y.L. Cao. 2006. Repair of experimental alveolar bone defects by tissue-engineered bone. *Tissue Eng* 12: 1503–1513.

West, E.R., M. Xu, T.K. Woodruff, and L.D. Shea. 2007. Physical properties of alginate hydrogels and their effects on in vitro follicle development. *Biomaterials* 28(30): 4439–4448.

Williams, D.F. 2009. On the nature of biomaterials. *Biomaterials* 30: 5897–5909.

Wiegand, C., T. Heinze, and U.C. Hipler. 2009. Comparative in vitro study on cytotoxicity, antimicrobial activity, and binding capacity for pathophysiological factors in chronic wounds of alginate and silver-containing alginate. *Wound Repair Regen* 17: 511–521.

Xu, M., P.K. Kreeger, L.D. Shea, and T.K. Woodruff. 2006. Tissue-engineered follicles produce live, fertile offspring. *Tissue Eng* 12(10): 2739–2746.

Yang, J.S., Y.J. Xie, and W. He. 2011. Research progress on chemical modification of alginate: A review. *Carbohyd Polym* 84(1): 33–39.

Yao, B. 2010. Hydrophobic modification of sodium alginate and its application in drug controlled release. *Bioprocess Biosyst Eng* 33(4): 457–463.

Zhang, X.L., Z.Y. Hui, D.X. Wan, H.T. Huang, J. Huang, H. Yuan, and J.H. Yu. 2010. Alginate microsphere filled with carbon nanotube as drug carrier. *Int J Biol Macromol* 47: 389–395.

Section IV

Industrial Wastewater Treatment Applications of the Biopolymers

19 Biocomposites and Polymer Blends for Wastewater Treatment

R. Nithya, P. Angelin Vinodhini, P.N. Sudha, and J. Vinoth

CONTENTS

19.1 INTRODUCTION

Water is undoubtedly the most precious natural resources, comprising more than 70% of the earth's surface. Water pollution is a major global problem. It has been documented that pollution of water is one of the leading worldwide causes of deaths and diseases (Pink 2006; West 2006) and that it accounts for the death of more than 14,000 people daily.

Water is typically referred to as polluted when it is unfit for drinking and other uses. Any modifications or change in the chemical, physical, and biological properties of water that can cause any harmful effects on living things and the environment

473

is known as water pollution. The water pollution is caused mainly due to increase in population, growth of industries, urbanization, loss of forest cover, lack of environmental awareness, untreated effluent discharge from industries and municipalities, use of nonbiodegradable pesticides/fungicides/herbicides/insecticides, use of chemical fertilizers instead of organic manures, and so on.

The polluted water may have undesirable color, odor, taste, turbidity, organic matter contents, harmful chemical contents, toxic heavy metals, pesticides, oily matters, industrial waste products, and radioactive materials. Water contains various inorganic, organic, and biological contaminants that are of environmental significance. These contaminants can create health hazards if discharged into streams or oceans without proper care and treatment (Mamta 1999). Contamination of wastewater includes chemical–organic, chemical–inorganic, biological, and physical forms (Table 19.1).

19.1.1 HEAVY METAL POLLUTION

Among the different sources of water pollution, heavy metal contamination has been a critical problem. Toxic heavy metal pollution is of significant environmental and occupational concern because of the tendency of heavy metals to enter the food chain (Sikder et al. 2014). Many industrial processes can generate heavy metal pollution in a large number of ways. The primary sources of these metals are the burning of fossil fuels, the mining and smelting of metalliferous ores, municipal wastes, fertilizers, pesticides, and sewage (Yoon et al. 2006). Examples of heavy metals include mercury (Hg), cadmium (Cd), arsenic (As), chromium (Cr), thallium (Tl), lead (Pb), copper (Cu), zinc (Zn), cobalt (Co), nickel (Ni), and iron (Fe). Heavy metals are classified into the following three categories: toxic metals (Hg, Cr, Pb, Zn, Cu, Ni, Cd, As, Co, and Sn), precious metals (Pd, Pt, Ag, Au, and Ru) and radionuclides [Radium (Ra) and Americium (Am)] (Bishop 2002; Table 19.2).

19.1.2 REMOVAL OF HEAVY METALS FROM WASTEWATER

The present situation of heavy metal pollution in many developing countries is even more serious, largely attributed to their low environmental consciousness and also to their desire of excess economic benefits (Harrison 1990). Hence, the proper management of global environment is increasingly becoming an important issue. Different types of methods have been developed for removing heavy metal ions from

TABLE 19.1
Sources of Different Pollutants

Different Pollutants	Sources
Chemical–organic pollutants	Trace organic, biodegradable, and floating material
Chemical–inorganic pollutants	Nutrients, trace metals, and gaseous inorganic
Biological pollutants	Pathogenic bacteria
Physical pollutants	Suspended solids and dissolved solids

TABLE 19.2

Sources of Metal Pollution from Industries and Their Toxic Effects

Metals	Major Industries	Toxic Effects
Chromium	Leather tanning and finishing, pulp, paper mills, petroleum refining, fertilizers, textile mills, power plant, and metal coatings	Causes allergic reactions, such as skin rash, respiratory problems, weakened immune systems, kidney and liver damage, alteration of genetic material, lung cancer, and death
Copper	Paper mills, electronics, plating, electrical wires, paper, textiles, rubber, printing, plastic, petroleum refining, motor vehicles, and aircraft plating	Causes serious toxicological concerns, such as vomiting, cramps, convulsions, or even death; fibrosis; and epidemiological diseases such as Wilson's disease
Mercury	Paints, pulp and paper, oil refining, rubber processing and fertilizer, batteries, thermometers, fluorescent light tubes and high-intensity street lamps, pesticides, cosmetics, and pharmaceuticals	Causes deformities in the offspring, abnormal distribution of chromosome, impairment of pulmonary function and kidney, chest pain, and dyspnea
Nickel	Electroplating, silver refineries, petroleum refining, zinc-base casting, and storage battery industries	Causes headache, dizziness, nausea and vomiting, chest pain, tightness of the chest, dry cough and shortness of breath, and cancers of lungs, nose and bone
Lead	Pulp, paper mills, paper boards, petrochemicals, basic stall work foundries, fertilizers, aircraft plating and finishing, Fuel additive, batteries, pigments, roofing, and fishing weights	Causes problems in the synthesis of hemoglobin, kidney disease, mental retardation, anemia, and acute or chronic damage to the nervous system
Zinc	Steam generation, power plant, meat processing, fat rendering, fish processing, bakery, miscellaneous foods, brewery, soft drinks and flavorings, and ice creams	Causes eminent health problems, such as stomach cramps, skin irritations, vomiting, nausea, and anemia
Cadmium	Laundrettes, electroplating workshops, plastic manufacturing, pigments, enamels, and paints	Cadmium, for instance, can cause cancer. Also causes a disease "Itai Itai" in Japan, which results in multiple fractures in the body

aqueous solution. Conventional techniques commonly applied for the removal of heavy metals from wastewater are chemical precipitation, coagulation/flocculation and solvent extraction, ion exchange, filtration, adsorption, reverse osmosis, electrochemical treatment, and evaporative recovery (Rengaraj et al. 2001; Yurlova et al. 2002; Benito and Ruiz 2002; Table 19.3).

TABLE 19.3

The Main Advantages and Disadvantages of the Various Physicochemical Methods for Water Treatment

Treatment Methods	Advantages	Disadvantages
Chemical precipitation	Simplicity, inexpensive capital cost, and economical, established method, and most widely used method, particularly at community level	High cost, not applicable for all cases, requires operation and maintenance, requires power, may generate a waste product, and is ineffective when metal ion concentration is low
Coagulation–flocculation	High efficiency and relatively economic, simple, and economically feasible	Involves chemical consumption and has high sludge production, handling, and disposal problems
Electrodialysis	High separation selectivity	High operational cost due to membrane fouling and energy consumption
Lime precipitation	Relatively inexpensive and bulk removal	Nonselective
Ion exchange	Multiple ion-exchange resins High specificity for heavy metal Several sorption and desorption cycles, no sludge production, effective good surface area, and excellent selectivity toward aromatic solutes	High capital and operating costs; economic cost of these processes depends on energy price and the amount of electricity used per treated volume of solution, has economic constraints, and is not effective for disperse dyes
Solvent extraction	High selectivity	Incomplete metal removal, produces large volume of sludge, and is not suitable for dilute metal ion solutions
Membrane filtration	High efficiency, easy, highly effective technique, no chemicals are required, no interference by other ions Works under wide pH range Removes all dye types and produces a high-quality treated effluent	High cost, is a pressure-operated, electrical-assisted technique, and depends on membrane size; relatively higher cost; not suitable for water with high salinity; total dissolved solid (TDS); incapable of treating large volumes; small space requirement; and high separation selectivity

19.1.3 ADSORPTION

In addition to other conventional methods, adsorption is an effective and widely used method used to remove heavy metal ions, especially at medium to low concentrations. Adsorption is a process that occurs when a gas or liquid solute accumulates on the surface of a solid or a liquid (the adsorbent), forming a molecular or atomic film (the adsorbate). Adsorption technology has a good potential to treat water and industrial residues, because it is cost-effective, easy for application, and efficient in various kinds of heavy metal removal. However, traditional adsorbents are activated carbons, clays, polymeric synthetic resins, metal oxides, and some natural materials.

Adsorption effectively removes contaminants in wastewater with high solute loadings and even at dilute concentrations (<100 mg/L). It is an effective technique for purification and separation used in industries, especially in water and wastewater treatments (Al-Asheh et al. 2003). Various low-cost adsorbents, derived from agricultural waste, industrial by-products, natural materials, or modified biopolymers, have been recently developed and applied for the removal of heavy metals from metal-contaminated wastewater.

There are many factors that are affecting the efficiency of adsorption. The factors are initial concentration of metal ion solution, adsorbent dose, pH of the metal solution, temperature, agitation speed, and contact time. In addition, the nature of the adsorbent such as functional groups, porosity, active sites, size, and charges on the surface will participate in the adsorption process.

19.1.4 Biosorption

Biosorption, a sub-branch of adsorption, aims to use cheaper materials of biological origin as adsorbents. Biosorption (adsorption by biomass) can be defined as a nondirected physicochemical interaction that may occur between metal species and microbial cells (Bhuvaneshwari et al. 2011). In other words, biosorption is a passive nonmetabolically mediated process. It removes metals or metalloid species, compounds, and particulates from solution, by materials of living or dead biomass (Gadd 2001). It has several advantages such as low operating cost, minimization of volume of chemicals and biological sludge to be disposed of, and high efficiency in detoxifying very dilute effluents. Many natural materials have been studied as biosorbents because of their capability to adsorb heavy metals and their low cost (Romero-Gonzalez et al. 2001; Klimmek and Stan 2001; Evans et al. 2002; Jodra and Mijangos 2003). Biopolymers can be classified as natural biopolymers such as carbohydrates and protein (e.g., starch, cellulose, chitosan, alginate, soy protein, collagen, and casein), chemically synthesized biodegradable polymers (e.g., polylactic acid [PLA], polygycolic acid [PGA], polyvinyl alcohol [PVA], polybutylene succinate [PBS], and poly [ε-caprolactone] [PCL]), and microbial polyesters (e.g., polyhydroxybutyrate [PHB] and polyhydroxyalkanoates [PHA]) (Bordes et al. 2009).

19.1.4.1 Advantages of Biosorbents
- Cost-effective, and their sources are abundant.
- Minimize volume of chemicals and biological sludge to be disposed of.
- The adsorption capacities can be competitive with commercial-grade absorbents.
- The improvement of their adsorption capacity by diverse treatments is feasible.
- High efficiency in detoxifying very dilute effluents.

19.2 BIOSORBENTS FROM MARINE ORIGIN

19.2.1 CHITIN

Chitin is natural polysaccharide composed of β-(1→4) linked 2-acetamido 2-deoxy β-D-glucose (N-acetylglucosamine) (Dutta et al. 2004). It is the second most abundant natural polymer in nature after cellulose, and it is found in the structure of a wide number of invertebrates such as crustaceans' exoskeleton; insects' cuticles; and the cell walls of fungi, fishes, shrimps, and cockroaches (Aranaz et al. 2009). On account of its availability, biodegradability, and biocompatibility, chitin and its derivatives have been used for a variety of applications such as water treatment, textile and paper, cosmetics, food supplements, drug delivery, agriculture, and biotechnology (Tanodekaew et al. 2004). Chitin can be hydrolyzed into oligomers and monomers by acid hydrolysis, and these oligochitins have been proposed as antimicrobial agents, promoters of plant growth, elicitors of plant resistance, enhancers of the immune response, and agents against malignant growth (Ilankovan et al. 2006).

Chitin exists in different crystalline forms known as α-, β-, and γ-chitins, which have different physicochemical properties (Kramer and Koga 1986). β-Chitin has lesser intramolecular hydrogen bonding than α-chitin, which may result in intracrystalline swelling and solvent absorption (Pillai et al. 2009). However, chitin is soluble in a mixture of N, N-dimethylacetamide (DMAc)/lithium chloride (LiCl) or in a mixture of N-methyl pyrrolidinone (NMP)/lithium chloride (LiCl) (Yilmaz and Bengisu 2003). It is insoluble in common solvents due to the existence of intra- and intermolecular hydrogen bonds and its highly crystalline structure. This strongly restricts many applications of chitin (Liu et al. 2008).

19.2.2 CHITOSAN

Chitosan is a modified carbohydrate polymer derived from chitin. It occurs principally in the organisms of the phylum arthropoda and outer skeleton of insects, crabs, and lobsters, including *Pandalus borealis,* and cell walls of fungi (Nekram and Urmila 2013). Its chemical name is 2-amino-2-deoxy-β-D-glucopyranose and molecular formula is $(C_6H_{11}O_4N)n$. Chitosan is synthesized by the deacetylation of chitin by using sodium hydroxide in excess as a reagent and water as a solvent (Gavhane et al. 2013). It is odorless, biocompatible, nontoxic and biodegradable, and it is a semi-crystalline polymer. It is a heteropolymer with high content of amine ($-NH_2$) functional group. Chitosan has three types of reactive functional groups, an amino group, as well as both primary and secondary hydroxyl groups at the C-2, C-3, and C-6 positions, respectively. Its chemical structure allows specific modifications without too many difficulties, especially at the C-2 position (Rinaudo 2006). The physicochemical properties of chitosan depend on various parameters such as deacetylation, polymer weight, and so on (Guibal 2004). Chitosan has different structural conditions, that is, it is in different forms such as chitosan flakes, powder, membranes, gel beads, fibers and hollow fibers, and inorganic immobilized support.

Owing to these advantages such as biocompatibility, biodegradability, nontoxicity, good film-forming capacity, and excellent chemical-resistant behavior, chitosan has been widely used in membranes for ultrafiltration, reverse osmosis, and evaporation (Chanachai et al. 2000); clinics (Badawy et al. 2000); surfactants (Ngimhuang et al. 2004); drug-delivery systems (Sashiwa et al. 2003); and solid polyelectrolytes formations (Wan et al. 2003). Chitosan is mainly used in water purification plants to remove oil, grease, heavy metals, and the fine particulate matter that cause turbidity in wastewater streams (Varma et al. 2004). The reactive amino group selectively binds to all group III transition metal ions but does not bind to groups I and II (alkali and alkaline earth metal ions) (Muzzarelli 1973).

Chitosan has also been approved as a food additive in Korea and Japan since 1995 and 1983, respectively (Weiner 1992; KFDA 1995; No et al. 2002). Chitosan might bind to some dietary lipids. It may also bind to the fat-soluble vitamins A, D, E, and K, as well as to flavonoids, carotenoids, and some minerals, such as zinc, found in foods (Koide 1998).

19.2.3 ALGINATE

Alginate is a binary, water-soluble, linear heteropolysaccharide containing one-, four-linked α-L-glucuronic acid and β-D-mannuronic acid (Smidsrod and Skjak-Brcek 1990). Alginate is extracted from brown seaweed, and it is also present in the cell wall of brown algae. Alginates are also synthesized by some bacteria (e.g., *Azotobacter* and *Pseudomonas* species). The alginate molecules provide the plant with both flexibility and strength, which are necessary for plant's growth in the sea. Types of alginate include alginic acid, sodium, calcium, ammonium and potassium salts, and propylene glycol alginate, an ester of alginic acid.

Sodium alginate is the main form of alginate used (McHugh 2003). Calcium alginate is insoluble in water and organic solvents but soluble in sodium citrate (Shilpa et al. 2003). Alginates can be formulated into soft elastic gels, fibers, foams, composites, and nanoparticles. This has been widely used in the field of controlled release, ion exchange, adsorption, and the vapor-permeation membrane-separation technique (Kalyani et al. 2008). Alginates were also used in the manufacture of paper and cardboard pharmaceutical, cosmetic creams, and processed foods (Chapman 1987). The graft copolymers are also prepared with alginate, and these copolymers have find applications in diverse fields such as pharmaceutical, biomedical, agriculture, and environmental.

19.2.4 MARINE ALGAE

Algae are one of the biosorbents in which researchers have shown interest nowadays, because of their high sorption capacity and availability in large quantities in seas and oceans (Rincon et al. 2005; Brinza et al. 2007). Algae have low nutrient requirements, and being autotropic, they produce a large biomass. They are nontoxic and biodegradable. Algae are eukaryotic in nature (Prescott et al. 2002), which means that their cells have a membrane-enclosed nucleus and many membranous organelles. Most algae contain chlorophyll and are thus green in color and carry out oxygenic photosynthesis.

The groups of algae are as follows:

- Microalgae or Chlorophyta (green algae or freshwater algae)
- Euglenophyta (euglenoids, also considered with the protozoa)
- Macroalgae or Phaeophyta (brown algae or marine algae)
- Chrysophyta (golden-brown algae, diatoms)
- Pyrrophyta (dinoflagellates)
- Rhodophyta (red algae)

Alginate contributes to the strength and flexibility of the cell wall of brown algae (Wang and Chen 2009). The extracellular polysaccharides (such as alginates and fucoidans) are the main components of cell walls which are responsible for the metal uptake (Davis et al. 2003). Cellulose exists in the cell walls of almost all plants as well as in marine algae. On account of their high content of such polysaccharides, brown algae may have a higher uptake capacity than other algae (Herrero et al. 2006). The principal mechanisms involved in biosorption by algae are (i) ion exchange, wherein ions such as Na, Mg, and Ca become displaced by heavy metal ions, and (ii) adsorption by physical forces, electrostatic interactions (Han et al. 2006), chelation, complexation (Li et al. 2006), and microprecipitation (Gupta et al. 2006).

19.3   COMPOSITES

Composites can be defined as natural or synthesized materials made from two or more materials with significantly different physical and chemical properties, which remain separate and distinct at the microscopic or macroscopic scale within the material (Adeeyo and Bello 2014). Polymer composites in which at least one component is biobased or biodegradable are called biocomposites (Barton et al. 2014). Broadly defined, biocomposites are composite materials made from natural biofiber and/or biodegradable polymers (PLA and PHA). Most composites are made of two materials. One is the matrix or binder and another is reinforcement. Matrix is a binding material that binds the reinforcement together. Reinforcements are fibers or textile structures that give strength to the materials.

Need of biocomposites: Regular polymer composites are nonbiodegradable and pollute the environment. Hence, in order to reduce environmental pollution, biocomposites are used. The uses of biopolymers are as follows:

- They help utilize the agricultural waste.
- They help attain sustainable development.
- They reduce depletion of petroleum reserves.
- They help in the reduction of fossil fuel use and lower greenhouse gas emissions.
- They have functional benefits, with adequate tensile strength, stiffness, as well as competitive costs.

19.3.1 CHITIN/CHITOSAN COMPOSITES FOR WASTEWATER TREATMENT

Recently, chitosan composites have been developed for the adsorption of heavy metals from wastewater. Different kinds of substances have been used to form composites with chitosan. Chitosan–zeolite (CZ) composite was prepared by using zeolite and chitosan for the adsorption of Cu (II) ions from the treated wastewater (Ngah et al. 2012). A novel magnetic cellulose–chitosan composite microsphere was synthesized, and this composite's microspheres exhibited porous structure and large surface area, leading to the efficient uptake capacity of Cu(II) ions (Peng and Meng 2014). A natural biopolymer biocomposite chitin/bentonite has been used as an adsorbent for the sorption process of chromium from aqueous solution. The maximum adsorption occurred at the optimum pH of 4.0 (Saravanan et al. 2013).

Chitosan/polypyrrole composite (CS/PPy) was synthesized and used as an adsorbent for the first time to remove the Cr(VI) ions from aqueous solution. The maximum Cr (VI) removal capacity of CS/PPy composite was 78.61 mg/g at 303 K (Karthik and Meenakshi 2014). Florence et al. (2011) prepared kenaf dust-filled chitosan biocomposite for the adsorption of metal ion Cu^{2+}. The maximum adsorption capacity of the adsorbent for Cu^{2+} was in the range of 232 ± 134 mg/g. A novel biocompatible composite (chitosan–zinc oxide nanoparticle) was used to adsorb the dyes such as AB26 and DB78. It was concluded that the since CS/n-ZnO is a biocompatible, ecofriendly, and low-cost adsorbent, it might be a suitable alternative for elimination of dyes from colored aqueous solutions (Raziyeh et al. 2010). A novel composite foam of poly(vinyl alcohol) (PVA) and chitosan (CS), that is, PVA/CS composite, was prepared as an adsorbent for the removal of malachite green (MG) and Cu^{2+} from aqueous solution. The introduction of CS improved significantly the adsorption capacities of Cu^{2+} and MG (Li et al. 2012).

Chitosan–aluminum oxide composite material was prepared and used as an adsorbent for the removal of Zn^{2+}, and the adsorption of Zn^{2+} onto composite material was found to follow pseudo-second-order kinetic model (Ma et al. 2011). The alumina/chitosan (AlCS) composite was prepared, and it was used to remove chromium by means of electrostatic adsorption-coupled reduction and complexation. The alumina/chitosan (AlCS) composite possesses an enhanced chromium sorption capacity (SC) of 8.62 mg/g, as compared with the original alumina and chitosan flakes, which possess the SCs of 3.7 and 0.67 mg/g, respectively (Gandhi et al. 2010). Chitosan/ceramic alumina composites were used to remove cationic heavy metals such as As(II) and Cu(II) (Boddu et al. 2008a, 2008b). Only few works have been carried out with chitosan/magnetite composite for the removal of heavy metals in wastewater (Huang et al. 2009; Liu et al. 2009; Tran et al. 2010).

Chitosan–clay composites have been developed nowadays to treat wastewater by adsorption method. The organic–inorganic hybrid of chitosan and nanoclay was synthesized by Pandey and Mishra (2011), and this nanobiocomposite was used as an adsorbent for the removal of chromium from aqueous solutions showing an uptake of 357.14 mg/g. Chitosan–clay composite beads were prepared to remove Pb(II) ions from aqueous solution. The maximum adsorption capacity of Pb(II) was observed at pH 4.5 as 7.93 mg/g, according to the Langmuir isotherm model (Tirtom et al. 2012). Chitosan and nanoclay (Cloisite 10A) was chosen to develop chitosan/clay nanocomposite (CCN) by solvent casting method. This was found to be the most efficient in adsorbent behavior of Cr (VI), and the adsorption showed pseudo-second-order kinetics (Pandey and Mishra 2011). Modified ball clay (MBC) and chitosan composite (MBC–CH) was prepared, and its application for the adsorption of methylene blue (MB) from aqueous solution was investigated. The findings of this study revealed that MBC–CH is a potential adsorbent for cationic dye pollution (Auta and Hameed 2014).

Cross-linked chitosan (CCS)/bentonite (BT) composite was prepared by the intercalation of chitosan in bentonite and the crosslinking reaction between chitosan and glutaraldehyde. The adsorption characteristics of CCS/BT were assessed by using an azo dye (Amido Black 10B), and the maximum adsorption capacity was 323.6 mg/g at 293 K and pH 2 (Liu et al. 2015). Chitosan–poly(vinyl alcohol)/bentonite (CTS–PVA/BT) nanocomposites, with high adsorption selectivity for Hg(II) ions, were synthesized by introducing BT into the CTS–PVA polymer matrix. The results revealed that BT content has a great influence on the microstructure of the nanocomposites (Wang et al. 2014). A novel triethylene–tetramine grafted magnetic chitosan composite was synthesized via a combination of chitosan and magnetic nanoparticles and was used for the removal of Pb(II) ions from aqueous solution (Kuang et al. 2013). An uptake of Pb(II) was found to be 370.63 mg/g. The superabsorbent composite of chitosan-g-poly (acrylic acid-co-acrylamide) was prepared by radical polymerization method, and the adsorption of heavy metal cations such as Cu(II), Cd(II), Ni(II), and Pb(II) from aqueous solution was investigated by Khairkar and Raut (2014).

A series of chitosan-g-poly (acrylic acid)/vermiculite hydrogel composites was synthesized, and these composites were used as adsorbents for the removal of methylene blue (MB) from aqueous solution. The adsorption kinetics of MB onto the hydrogel composite followed pseudo-second-order kinetics (Liu et al. 2010). Chitosan–montmorillonite (KSF–CTS) bead composite was prepared by crosslinking with pentasodium tripolyphosphate (TPP). Montmorillonite (KSF–Na), CTS, and KSF–CTS biocomposite were used to remove Cu(II) from aqueous solutions. The maximum adsorption capacity followed the order CTS > KSF–CTS > KSF–Na (Pereira et al. 2013). The magnetic composite microspheres (MCMs), consisting of Fe_3O_4 nanoparticles and poly(acrylic acid) (PAA)-blended chitosan (CS), were prepared successfully by coprecipitation of the compounds in alkaline solution. Then, the MCM materials were employed as absorbents for removal of Cu(II). Experimental results revealed that the CS/PAA–MCM had greater adsorption capacity than CS–MCM (Yan et al. 2012).

A series of chitosan-g-(N-vinyl pyrrolidone)/montmorillonite hydrogel composites was synthesized by *in situ* intercalative polymerization and used for the adsorption of a water-soluble cationic dye rhodamine 6G (Rh6G) (Vanamudan et al. 2014). Polymethacrylic acid-grafted chitosan–bentonite nanocomposite (MACB) was synthesized. The MACB nanocomposite was employed for the adsorption of mercury, cadmium, and lead ions from aqueous solution, and the order of adsorption capacity of MACB nanocomposite for metal ions was Hg^{2+} > Pb^{2+} > Cd^{2+} (Abdel Khalek et al. 2012). Anirudhan and Rijith (2012) prepared a novel adsorbent, poly(methacrylic acid)-grafted chitosan/bentonite composite, through graft copolymerization reaction of methacrylic acid and chitosan in the presence of bentonite and N,N'-methylene bisacrylamide as crosslinking agents. The equilibrium uranium(VI) sorption capacity was estimated to be 117.2 mg/g at 303K. The ammonium ions (NH_4^+) were removed from aqueous solution by using a hydrogel composite chitosan-grafted poly(acrylic acid)/rectorite prepared from *in situ* copolymerization. Rectorite (REC) is a regularly interstratified clay mineral with alternate pairs of dioctahedral mica-like layers (nonexpansible) and dioctahedral montmorillonite-like layers (expansible) in a 1:1 ratio (Zheng and Wang 2009).

Recent researches on chitosan application have focused on imparting magnetic property to chitosan-based adsorbents for facile recovery after treatment. The composite chitosan magnetite microparticles for the removal of Co^{2+} and Ni^{2+} ions in aqueous solution have been evaluated by Hritcu et al. (2012). A magnetic composite was synthesized with chitosan, nanomagnetite, and heulandite to remove Cu(II) and As(V) from aqueous solution (Cho et al. 2012). Novel nanoporous magnetic cellulose–chitosan composite microspheres were prepared by sol–gel transition method by using ionic liquids as solvents for the sorption of Cu(II) (Peng et al. 2014). A new type of composite flocculant, polysilicate aluminum ferric–chitosan, was prepared. The performance was analyzed by testing the removal efficiency of Cu^{2+}, Ni^{2+}, Zn^{2+}, Cd^{2+}, and Cr^{6+} of heavy metals wastewater. For different heavy metal ions, the best removal efficiencies were found to be 100% and 82.2% for Cr^{6+} and Ni^{2+}, respectively (Jun et al. 2010).

Cellulose is immobilized on chitosan to form chitosan–cellulose composite beads; this adsorbent was investigated for the removal of Cu(II), Zn(II), Ni(II), Pb(II), and Cr(VI) (Sun et al. 2009). Hydroxyapatite/chitosan (HApC) composite has been prepared by precipitation method and used for the removal of heavy metals (Cr^{6+}, Zn^{2+}, and Cd^{2+}) from aqueous solution (Kusrini et al. 2013). Aliabadi et al. (2013) reported the performance of chitosan/hydroxyapatite (Cs/HAp) composite nanofiber membrane prepared by electrospinning process for the removal of lead, cobalt, and nickel ions from aqueous solution.

Siraj et al. (2012) reported that a biocomposite of chitosan coated on charcoal was used for the removal of Cr from industrial effluents. Hameed et al. (2008) prepared crosslinked chitosan/oil palm charcoal composite beads to remove reactive blue 19. The silica was immobilized with chitosan on its surface, and the silica–chitosan composite was synthesized by crosslinking adsorbed biopolymer with glutaraldehyde. This composite showed adsorption activity toward microquantities of Zn(II), Cd(II), Pb(II), Cu(II), Fe(III), Mo(VI), and V(V) ions in the aqueous medium. The highest sorption capacity was observed with respect to zinc (0.46 mmol/g) (Budnyak et al. 2014). A generation of layer-by-layer silicate–chitosan composite biosorbent was prepared, and its capability in the removal of Cd(II), Cr(III), and Cr(VI) from an aqueous solution was studied. The results revealed that the silicate–chitosan films with a final layer of silicate demonstrated chitosan retention and had better sorption capacities than those without it (Copello et al. 2008).

19.3.2 ALGINATE COMPOSITES FOR WASTEWATER TREATMENT

Allspice berries are harvested from *Pimenta dioica* L. Merrill, a tree native to central and south America, which belongs to the family Myrtaceae. Allspice–alginate biocomposite beads were prepared and evaluated for the adsorption of Pb(II) in both batch and column operations. According to the Langmuir model, the maximum adsorption capacity of Pb(II) was found to be 6.6 mg/g wet mass, equivalent to 132 mg/g dry mass. The use of allspice residue in combination with alginate in the form of beads lowers the amount of alginate necessary for adsorption beads by 43%, resulting in lower cost (Barrera-Díaz et al. 2015). The removal of Pb(II) ions from aqueous solution by mangrove–alginate composite bead (MACB) was investigated by Abas et al. (2015) by performing batch adsorption studies to evaluate the performances of the bead.

The sorption of Pb(II), Cd(II), and Ni(II) toxic metal ions from aqueous solution by composite alginate–bentonite and alginate was investigated. The adsorption experiment was done for both types of samples. The maximum sorption capacity for each toxic metal ion increased for alginate–bentonite as compared with that for alginate, and also, this composite shortens the duration required for complete sorption (Tzu et al. 2013). Layered clay (pristine clay)–alginate composites with varying amount of sodium alginate (MgAl–Alg) were prepared by Sebastian et al. (2014). Adsorption characteristics of the synthesized composites (MgAl–Alg) were studied for the adsorption of anthraquinone dyes, acid green 25 (AG 25) and acid green 27 (AG 27). The dye adsorption capacity of pristine clay (MgAl) increased considerably on formation of composite with sodium alginate (Alg) and was dependent on the alginate concentration of the composite. The investigation of alginate/polyvinyl alcohol–kaolin composite for the removal of methylene blue from aqueous solutions was carried out. The maximum adsorbed amount of methylene blue was 30.8 mg/g (Abd El-Latif et al. 2010).

The alginate–chitosan hybrid gel beads were prepared, and it is used to adsorb divalent metal ions (Gotoh et al. 2004). Hassan et al. (2014a) used calcium alginate/activated carbon composite beads for the sorption and removal of arsenic(V). The maximum sorption capacity was found to be 66.7 mg/g of the composite at 30°C. Hassan et al. (2014b) also prepared three adsorbents: calcium alginate beads (AB), sodium hydroxide-activated carbon-based coconut shells (C), and calcium alginate/activated carbon composite beads (ACB), and the adsorption experiments were conducted to remove methylene blue.

A novel bead composite was fabricated through a sol–gel reaction by trapping and condensing amorphous silica into the network structures of calcium ion crosslinked alginate (CA)–xanthan gum (XG) gel beads. The reinforced silica/CA–XG composite was found to be a very promising adsorbent for lead removal and recovery from aqueous solutions, with remarkable advantages in terms of biocompatibility, recyclability, ease of operation, and low cost (Zhang et al. 2013)

Alginate–calcium carbonate composite material was prepared in the form of beads. The adsorption of Cd^{2+} ions was studied through batch experiments. The kinetic studies showed that the adsorption of Cd^{2+} ions followed pseudo-first-order kinetics (Mahmood et al. 2015). Alginate–SBA-15 (ALG–SBA-15) was synthesized by encapsulation of the nanoporous SBA-15 in the biopolymeric matrix of calcium alginate. This adsorbent showed the maximum sorption capacity of 222.22 mg/g of lead on ALG–SBA-15 (Cheraghali et al. 2013). A novel environmental friendly material, calcium alginate–immobilized kaolin (kaolin/CA), was prepared by using a sol–gel method and was used as an adsorbent of Cu^{2+} (Li et al. 2011). Algothmi et al. (2013) studied Ca-alginate/graphene oxide (prepared using sol–gel chemistry technique) as a novel composite for the removal of Cu(II) ions from wastewater.

Biopolymer composite beads composed of fly ash and sodium alginate proved to be an effective adsorbent for the removal of Zn(II) ions from aqueous solutions (Nadeem and Datta 2014). A new hydrogel composite, sodium alginate graft poly (acrylic acid-co-2-acrylamido-2-methyl-1-propane sulfonic acid)/attapulgite, was prepared, and the adsorption of heavy metal ions onto the composite was studied (Zhu et al. 2014a). A series of polymer–clay composite beads that consist of Na-alginate and montmorillonite clay were prepared by using $CaCl_2$ as a crosslinker. The prepared composite beads were studied to remove lead from aqueous. Lead adsorption was found to be strongly pH-dependent and displayed a maximum uptake capacity (244.6 mg/g) at pH 6 and minimum uptake capacity (76.6 mg/g) at pH 1 (Shawky 2011).

Kaolin has been widely used as an adsorbent to remove heavy metal ions from aqueous solutions. However, the lower heavy metal adsorption capacity of kaolin limits its practical application. A new composite, kaolin/sodium alginate-grafted poly(acrylic acid-co-2-acrylamido-2-methyl-1-propane sulfonic acid) (KL/SA-g-P(AA-co-AMPS)), was synthesized by intercalation graft polymerization by using ammonium persulfate as an initiator and N,N'-methylene bisacrylamide as a crosslinker. Sorption behavior of heavy metal ions such as lead (Pb^{2+}), cadmium (Cd^{2+}), and zinc (Zn^{2+}) on (KL/SA-g-P(AA-co-AMPS) was investigated (Zhu et al. 2014b). A novel environmental friendly material, calcium alginate-immobilized kaolin (kaolin/CA) composite, was prepared by using a sol–gel method. The Langmuir isotherm was used to describe the experimental adsorption; the maximum Cu^{2+} adsorption capacity of the kaolin/CA composite reached up to 53.63 mg/g (Li et al. 2011).

Cr(III) ionic-imprinted composite membrane adsorbent (Cr(III)-PVA/SA) was prepared by blending sodium alginate (SA) with polyvinyl alcohol (PVA). Cr(III)-PVA/SA exhibited the maximum Cr(III) ions uptake capacity of 59.9 mg/g. Competitive adsorption studies of the binary system of Cr(III)/Cu(II) and Cr(III)/Cd(II) and the ternary system of Cr(III)/Cu(II)/Cd(II) were also investigated by using Cr(III)–PVA/SA, the results of which indicated that selectively adsorbed amount of Cr(III) ion on Cr(III)–PVA/SA is significantly higher than that of Cu(II) and Cd(II) ions (Chen et al. 2010).

19.4 POLYMER BLENDS

Polymer blending is one of the effective ways to obtain materials with specific properties. Polymer blends are a mixture of at least two polymers or copolymers (Utracki 1988). In other words, polymer blending is actually a physical mixing of two polymers in order to produce a new material with desired properties (Allcock et al. 2003). The usual objective for preparing a novel blend of two or more polymers is not to change the properties of the components drastically but to capitalize on the maximum possible performance of the blend.

The advantages of the blending technology are listed below (Utracki 1988):

- Better processability leads to improved product with uniformity and scrap reduction.
- Product may be easily tailorable to specific needs.
- It quick formulation changes, so better flexibility and high productivity.
- Blending reduces capital investment.
- Blends prepared are recyclable, and hence, it is reused many times.

19.4.1 POLYMER BLENDS FOR WASTEWATER TREATMENT

Several methods have been used to modify natural chitosan. Chitosan can be molded in several shapes, such as membranes, microspheres, gel beads (Guibal et al. 1999), fibers (Vincent and Guibal 2000), and films, and is able to provide a surface-area-to-mass ratio that maximizes the adsorption capacity and minimizes hydrodynamic limitation effects. The electrons present in the amino and N-acetylamino groups forms dative bonds with transition metal ions, and some of the hydroxyl groups in these biopolymers may act as donors. Hence, deprotonated hydroxyl groups can be involved in the coordination with metal ions (Lerivrey et al. 1986).

Novel, functional materials based on chitin of marine origin and lignin were prepared and employed for the adsorption of nickel and cadmium. These chitin/lignin biosorbents showed high efficiency of nickel and cadmium adsorption (88.0% and 98.4%, respectively). Mechanism of chitin modification by lignin is based on formation of hydrogen bonds between chitin and lignin (Wysokowski et al. 2014). Alginate/phosphorylated chitin (P-chitin) blend films were prepared by mixing 2% of alginate and P-chitin in water and then crosslinking with 4% $CaCl_2$ solution. The blended films were investigated for the adsorption of Ni^{2+}, Zn^{2+}, and Cu^{2+} onto alginate/P-chitin blend. The maximum adsorption capacity of alginate/P-chitin blend films for Ni^{2+}, Zn^{2+} and Cu^{2+} at pH 5.0 were found to be 5.67 mg/g, 2.85 mg/g, and 11.7 mg/g, respectively (Jayakumar et al. 2009). Polymer blend films of chitin and bentonite were prepared, and this blended polymer was used as an adsorbent for the removal of copper and chromium from the dye effluent (Saravanan et al. 2011). The adsorption of Cu^{2+} on the chitin surface has been studied by Gonzalez-Davila and Millero (1989).

Modified chitosan gel beads with phenol derivatives were found to be effective in the adsorption of cationic dye, such as crystal violet and bismarck brown (Chao et al. 2004). Chitosan beads were crosslinked with epichlorohydrin (ECH) in order to obtain sorbent that is insoluble in aqueous, acidic, and basic mediums, resulting in improvement of swelling behavior. The adsorption of Cr(VI) ions onto chitosan and crosslinked chitosan beads has been investigated at different pH values and at different time intervals. The uptake of Cr(VI) ions on chitosan and chitosan–ECH beads was 52% to 80% and 48% to 78%, respectively, at different time intervals (Jassal et al. 2010). Crosslinking with glutaraldehyde is a typical example of chemical-mediated structural modification. The adsorption capacity of natural and glutaraldehyde-crosslinked chitosan was evaluated by a static method on membranes and spheres. In order to obtain Hg(II) ions in a more concentrated form, adsorption by the dynamic method and desorption by the batch method were performed by Vieira and Beppu (2006). The spherical chitosan–tripolyphosphate chelating resins were used as sorbents for the removal of Cu(II) (Lee 2001).

Chitosan bead is a good adsorbent for the removal of Congo red from its aqueous solution, and 1 g of chitosan in the form of hydrogel beads can remove 93 mg of the dye at pH 6 (Chatterjee et al. 2007). The removal of arsenic (As) species, such as As(III) and As(V), from water by molybdate-impregnated chitosan beads (MICB) in both batch and continuous operations was studied by Chen et al. (2008). The ability of polyvinyl alcohol/chitosan (PVA/CS) binary dry blend as an adsorbent for the removal of Mn(II) ion from aqueous solution was investigated by Abdeen et al. (2015). Polyvinyl alcohol (PVA)-blended chitosan and carboxylated cellulose nanofibrils (CCNFs) were used for the preparation of magnetic hydrogel beads (m-CS/PVA/CCNFs) and also used as adsorbents for the removal of Pb(II) ions (Zhou et al. 2014).

Crown ether-bound chitosan will have a strong complexing capacity and better selectivity for metal ions because of the synergistic effect of high molecular weight. Crown ether-bound chitosan with Schiff's base type was prepared to test its adsorption capacities for metal ions Pb^{2+}, Au^{3+}, Ag^+, and Pd^{2+} in the presence of Cu^{2+} and Hg^{2+} (Tang et al. 2002). The potential suitability of chitosan-coated bentonite (CCB) as an adsorbent in the removal of indium ions from aqueous solution was studied by Calagui et al. (2014). The chitosan film seems to be a good sorbent for Cr(VI) at pH 4, but its physical instability suggests the need for a more resilient support. Owing to this fact, zeolite was added to the chitosan matrix in solutions and a chitosan/zeolite (CS/Zeo) film was thus prepared for the removal of Cr(VI) ions from solutions by Batista et al. (2011).

The adsorption of Cr(VI) ions from aqueous solution by ethylenediamine-modified crosslinked magnetic chitosan resin (EMCMCR) was studied by Hu et al. (2011). A chitosan/cellulose acetate/polyethylene glycol ultrafiltration membrane was prepared, with dimethyl formamide (DMF) as the solvent. It was focused to be efficient in removing chromium from artificial and tannery effluent wastewater. The highest rejection rate was responding (Sudha et al. 2008). A terpolymer of chitosan–melamine–glutaraldehyde was prepared and was quaternized with glycidyltrimethylammonium chloride (GTMAC), and it was found to be effective for the removal of nitrate and phosphate oxyanions. The nitrate and phosphate adsorption capacities of the quaternized chitosan-melamine-glutaraldehyde resin (QCMGR) from 1000 mg/L of respective solutions were 97.5 and 112.5 mg/g, respectively (Sowmya and Meenakshi 2014). Chitosan/carboxymethyl cellulose/silica hybrid membrane (CS/CMC/silica) was prepared by using chitosan and carboxymethyl cellulose in the presence of 3-glycidoxypropyltrimethoxysilane (GPTMS) as the crosslinking agent and was used to remove Cr(VI) ions in the effluent. The pseudo-second-order model fitted the kinetic data well (He et al. 2015).

The use of chitosan beads, chitosan–GLA 1:1 and 2:1 ratio beads, and chitosan–alginate beads for the removal of Cu(II) ions from aqueous solution was investigated. Chitosan beads and chitosan–GLA 1:1 and 2:1 ratio beads agreed well with the nonlinear Freundlich isotherm, with an adsorption capacity of 64.62 mg/g, 31.20 mg/g, and 19.51 mg/g, respectively. Chitosan–alginate beads showed a better fit to the nonlinear Langmuir isotherm, giving an adsorption capacity of 67.66 mg/g (Ngah and

Fatinathan 2008). The combined use of alginic acid and chitosan was expected to form a rigid matrix due to anionic interaction between amino groups of chitosan and carboxyl groups of alginic acid, and the crosslinking between the two successfully takes place through glutaraldehyde. This alginate–chitosan hybrid gel beads were used for the adsorption of Cu(II), Co(II), and Cd(II) ions under acidic conditions (Gotoh et al. 2004). When used in combination, sodium alginate and chitosan were efficient in removing Cu(II) ions from aqueous solutions. Chitosan and sodium alginate can precipitate each other with electrostatic interaction (Qin et al. 2006).

A novel adsorbent chitosan-coated sand (CCS) and calcium alginate (ca–Alg) bead was used as an adsorbent for the removal of heavy metal ions (mostly chromium and iron) and organic acid anions. The maximum uptake capacity for chitosan-coated sand was found to be 59.88 µg/g for iron and 38.022 µg/g for chromium (Priyabrata Pal et al. 2014). Horseradish peroxidase (HRP) encapsulated in calcium alginate for the purpose of phenol removal by one-step encapsulation method for immobilization of HRP in a semi-permeable alginate membrane showed the possibility of continuous phenol removal (Alemzadeh et al. 2009). By combining alginate gel and activated carbon, an activated carbon-containing alginate bead (AC–AB) adsorbent was developed and successfully used to remove heavy metal ions (Pb^{2+}, Mn^{2+}, Cd^{2+}, Cu^{2+}, Zn^{2+}, Fe^{2+}, Al^{3+}, and Hg^{2+}) and toxic organics (p-toluic acid), and it was found that the AC–AB adsorbent has enormous potential for application in drinking water treatment technologies (Park et al. 2007).

A millimeter-sized sorbent was prepared by encapsulating the $BaSO_4$–APRB (weak acidic pink red B) hybrid into calcium alginate gel (Alg–$BaSO_4$–APRB hybrid gels). The selectivity and mechanism of adsorption were studied by investigating the adsorption performance of two anionic (reactive brilliant red K–2BP and weak acid green GS) and three cationic dyes (ethyl violet [EV], methylene blue [MB], and cationic red 3R [CR3R]) (Yu-Lin et al. 2010). A porous membrane adsorbent, 3-aminopropyl-triethoxysilane (APTEOS)-functionalized sodium alginate (SA) (APTEOS/SA) was prepared, and its adsorption performance was tested for the removal of Cr(III) ions (Chen et al. 2013).

The sorption efficiency of elimination of Cu(II) ions by adsorption onto polyvinyl alcohol–alginate-bound nanomagnetite microspheres [PVA–ANM] from water has been investigated for the removal of Cu^{2+} ions from water (Alka and Kathane 2015) Zero-valent iron nanoparticles (nZVI) have been successfully entrapped in biopolymer calcium (Ca)—alginate beads and have demonstrated the potential use in environmental remediation by using nitrate as a model contaminant. Based on scanning electron microscopy images, it can be inferred that the alginate gel cluster acts as a bridge that binds the nZVI particles together. Statistical analysis indicated that there was no significant difference between the reaction rates of bare and entrapped nZVI, and no significant decrease in the reactivity of nZVI toward the nitrate contaminant was observed after the entrapment (Bezbaruah et al. 2009).

A comparison was made for the sorption of manganese and cobalt ions onto alginate beads (ABs) and thermally activated nanocarbon beads encapsulated with alginate (NCBs). Recovery of Mn(II) and Co(II) was greater than 99% with 0.1 N HCl, and NCB could be repeatedly utilized for Mn(II) and Co(II) sorption, with negligible loss in sorption capacity. Elemental analysis confirmed that divalent calcium replacement with heavy metal ions might be a possible sorption mechanism (Khan et al. 2014).

A new biosorbent—*Sargassum* sp. encapsulated with epichlorohydrin (ECH) crosslinked chitosan (CS)—was investigated for the removal of nickel ions. The biosorption kinetics was well fitted by the diffusion-controlled model. The biosorption capacity of nickel on CS was much higher than that of cross-linked chitosan (CLC) bead and lower than that of raw algae due to encapsulation (Yang et al. 2011). Kathiravan et al. (2010) studied the external mass transfer effects on the reduction of hexavalent Cr(VI) by using calcium alginate-immobilized *Bacillus* sp. in a recirculated packed bed batch reactor (RPBR).

The biosorption of Pb(II) by fruiting bodies of *Pleurotus ostreatus* immobilized in calcium alginate was studied by Xiangliang et al. (2005). The maximum adsorption capacity (q_{max}) onto *P. ostreatus* immobilized in calcium alginate was 121.21 mg/g for Pb(II). The fourier transform infrared spectroscopy (FT-IR) analysis showed that the mechanism involved in biosorption of Pb(II) by fruiting bodies of *P. ostreatus* was mainly attributed to Pb(II) binding of amide I group. Alginate extracted from the macroalgae *Sargassum sinicola* was chosen as a raw material for cell immobilization for wastewater treatment and plant growth promotion (Yabur et al. 2007). Hydrogel based on sodium alginate, extracted from the brown marine alga *Turbinaria decurrens*—grafted polymerized with poly(itaconic acid), NaAlg/IA—was employed in studies on the adsorption kinetic of Pb^{+2} in aqueous solution (Mahmoud and Mohamed 2012).

Biopolymer-based membranes present novel systems for the removal of herbicides from contaminated water. The adsorption behavior of the herbicides diquat, difenzoquat, and clomazone on biopolymer membranes prepared with alginate and chitosan (pristine and multilayer model) for contaminated water was studied. Herbicides were adsorbed in either pure alginate, pure chitosan, or a bilayer membrane composed of chitosan/alginate. No adsorption of clomazone was observed on any of the membranes, which was due to a lack of electrostatic interactions between the herbicide and the membranes. Diquat and difenzoquat were adsorbed only on alginate and chitosan/alginate membranes, which indicated that the adsorption takes place in the alginate layer (de Moraes et al. 2013).

Marine algae have been found to be potential suitable sorbents because of their low cost, relatively high surface area, and high binding affinity. The use of marine algae for heavy metal removal has been reported by several authors (Kumar et al. 2007; Deng et al. 2007; Ozer et al. 2009). Marine algae *Gelidium* and algal composite material were investigated for the continuous removal of Cu(II) from aqueous solution in a packed bed column (Vilar et al. 2008). Biosorption of Pb(II) by green algae *Cladophora fascicularis* was investigated, and the biosorption kinetics followed the pseudo-second-order model. The maximum adsorption capacity was 198.5 mg/g at 298 K and pH 5.0. Infrared (IR) spectrum analysis suggested that amido or hydroxyl could combine intensively with Pb(II) (Deng et al. 2007).

Algae–silica hybrid materials for biosorption purposes were prepared by using sol–gel technology. The resulting biological ceramics (biocers) were applied for the biosorption for heavy metals Cr, Ni, Cu, and Pb. Comparative equilibrium sorption experiments were performed batch-wise with 13 different microalgae and macroalgae powders, and the corresponding algae biocers using waters loaded with either concentrations of nickel below 3 mg/L or a mixture of different heavy metals. The silica matrix itself was involved in the sorption of metals. The metal-binding capability of embedded macroalgae biomass was unaffected by immobilization in the silica matrix (Ulrich et al. 2010). Loofa sponge (LS)-immobilized biomass of *Chlorella sorokiniana* (LSIBCS) was investigated as a new biosorbent for the removal of Cr(III) from aqueous solution. A comparison of the biosorption of Cr(III) by LSIBCS and free biomass of *C. sorokiniana* (FBCS) was made, and the results showed an increase in the uptake of 17.79% when the microalgal biomass was immobilized onto loofa sponge. Maximum biosorption capacities for LSIBCS and FBCS were found to be 69.26 and 58.80 mg Cr(III)/g biosorbent, respectively (Akhtar et al. 2008).

Chromium removal efficiency of *Padina tetrastromatica* Hauck (brown algae), *Gracilaria edulis* S. G. Gmelin (red algae), and *Ulva reticulata* Forsskal (green algae) were compared. Maximum of 50.85% of chromium removal was exhibited by *P. tetrastromatica*, which is higher than the powdered biomass of the other two seaweeds. Protonation of powdered biomass of seaweeds enhanced the biosorption rates from 18% to 30% (Abirami et al. 2013).

Five green marine macroalgae, namely, *Cladophora fascicularis, Ulva lactuca, Chaetomorpha* sp., *Caulerpa sertularioides,* and *Valoniopsis pachynema,* were screened for their metal uptake capacities for Cd, Hg, and Pb. Cadmium reduction was found to be the highest at 20 mg/L for all the marine algae, except *C. sertularioides.* The values of cadmium uptake in the different species were in the order *Chaetomorpha* sp. > *C. sertularioides* > *C. fascicularis* > *V. pachynema* > *U. lactuca.* Mercury uptake values followed the sequence *C. sertularioides* > *U. lactuca* > *C. fascicularis* > *V. pachynema* > *Chaetomorpha* sp. The metal uptake values for lead displayed the order *V. pachynema* > *Chaetomorpha* sp. > *C. fascicularis* > *U. lactuca* > *C. sertularioides* (Kumar et al. 2009).

19.5   CONCLUSION

Wastewater with heavy metal ions has been of great concern because of its increased discharge, toxic effects, and some other bad effects on human beings or the environment. In recent years, a wide range of treatment technologies such as chemical precipitation, adsorption, membrane filtration, electrodialysis, and photocatalysis have been developed for heavy metal removal from contaminated wastewater. Although many techniques can be employed for the treatment of wastewater, it is important to select the most suitable treatment for environmental impact and economics parameters such as the capital investment and operational costs. Biosorption is one of the convenient methods for the removal of heavy metals. Biocomposites have become emerging technique for the adsorbtion of heavy metal ions and dyes. In this chapter, the biocomposites and polymer blends of different marine-based biopolymers were discussed. We expect that this chapter will provide insights on the use of these natural polysaccharides for researchers working to discover new materials with new properties for valuable applications.

ACKNOWLEDGMENT

The authors are grateful to authorities of DKM College for Women and Thiruvalluvar University, Vellore, Tamil Nadu, India, for the support. They are also thankful to the editor for the opportunity to review such an innovating field.

REFERENCES

Abas, S. N. A., M. H. S. Ismail, S. I. Siajam, and M. L. Kamal. 2015. Development of novel adsorbent-mangrove-alginate composite bead (MACB) for removal of Pb(II) from aqueous solution. *Journal of the Taiwan Institute of Chemical Engineers* 50:182–189.

Abd El-Latif, M. M., M. F. El-Kady, A. M. Ibrahim, and M. E. Ossman. 2010. Alginate/polyvinyl alcohol—Kaolin composite for removal of methylene blue from aqueous solution in a batch stirred tank reactor. *Journal of American Science* 6(5):280–292.

Abdeen, Z., S. G. Mohammad, and M. S. Mahmoud. 2015. Adsorption of Mn (II) ion on polyvinyl alcohol/chitosan dry blending from aqueous solution. *Environmental Nanotechnology, Monitoring & Management* 3:1–9.

Abdel Khalek, M. A., G. A. Mahmoud, and N. A. El-Kelesh. 2012. Synthesis and characterization of poly-methacrylic acid grafted chitosan-bentonite composite and its application for heavy metals recovery. *Chemistry and Materials Research* 2(7):1–7.

Abirami, S., S. Srisudha, and P. Gunasekaran. 2013. Comparative study of chromium biosorption using brown, red and green macro algae. *International Journal of Biological & Pharmaceutical Research* 4(2):115–129.

Adeeyo, R. O., and O. S. Bello. 2014. Use of composite sorbents for the removal of copper (II) ions from aqueous solution. *Pakistan Journal of Analytical and Environmental Chemistry* 15(2):2.

Akhtar, N., M. Iqbal, S. I. Zafar, and J. Iqbal. 2008. Biosorption characteristics of unicellular green alga Chlorella sorokiniana immobilized in loofa sponge for removal of Cr(III). *Journal of Environmental Sciences* 20:231–239.

Al-Asheh, S., F. A. Banat, and L. Abu-Aitah. 2003. Adsorption of phenol using different types of activated bentonites. *Separation and Purification Technology* 33:1–10.

Alemzadeh, I., S. Nejatib, and M. Vossoughi. 2009. Removal of phenols from wastewater with encapsulated horseradish peroxidase in calcium alginate. *Engineering Letters* 17:4.

Algothmi, W. M., N. Badaru, Y. Yu, and J. G. Shapter. 2013. Alginate-graphene oxide hybrid gle beads: An efficient copper adsorbent material. *Journal of Colloid and Interface Science* 397:32–38.

Aliabadi, M., M. Irani, J. Ismaeili, and S. Najafzadeh. 2013. Design and evaluation of chitosan/hydroxyapatite composite nanofiber membrane for the removal of heavy metal ions from aqueous solution. *Journal of the Taiwan Institute of Chemical Engineers* 45(2):518–526.

Alka T., and P. Kathane. 2015. Adsorption of Cu^{2+} ions onto polyvinyl alcohol-alginate bound nano magnetite microspheres: A kinetic and thermodynamic study. *International Research Journal of Environment Sciences* 4(4):12–21.

Allcock, R. H., L. W. Frederick, and E. M. James. 2003. *Contemporary Polymer Chemistry* (3 Ed.) Prentice Hall, New Jersey: Pearson Education, p. 546.

Anirudhan, T. S., and S. Rijith. 2012. Synthesis and characterization of carboxyl terminated poly(methacrylic acid) grafted chitosan/bentonite composite and its application for the recovery of uranium(VI) from aqueous media. *Journal of Environmental Radioactivity* 106:8–19.

Aranaz, I., M. Mengíbar, R. Harris, I. Paños, B. Miralles, N. Acosta, G. Galed, and Á. Heras. 2009. Functional characterization of chitin and chitosan. *Current Chemical Biology* 3:203–230.

Auta, M., and B. H. Hameed. 2014. Chitosan–clay composite as highly effective and low-cost adsorbent for batch and fixed-bed adsorption of methylene blue. *Chemical Engineering Journal* 237:352–361.

Badawy, M. E. I., E. I. Rabea, T. M. Rogge, C. V. Stevens, G. Smagghe, W. Steurbaut, and M. Hofte. 2000. Synthesis and fungicidal activity of new N, O-acyl chitosan derivatives. *Biomacromolecules* 5(2):589–595.

Barrera-Díaz, C., M. I. López Meza, C. Fall, B. Bilyeu, and J. Cruz-Olivares. 2015. Lead(II) adsorption using allspice-alginate gel biocomposite beads. *Sustainable Environment Research* 25(2):83–92.

Barton, J., A., Niemczyk, K. Czaja, Ł. Korach, and B. Sacher-Majewska. 2014. Polymer composites, biocomposites and nanocomposites. Production, composition, properties and application fields. *Chemik* 68(4):280–287.

Batista, A. C. L., E. R. Villanueva, R. V. S. Amorim, M. T. Tavares, and G. M. Campos-Takaki. 2011. Chromium (VI) ion adsorption features of chitosan film and its chitosan/zeolite conjugate 13X film. *Molecules* 16:3569–3579.

Benito, Y., and M. Ruiz. 2002. Reverse osmosis applied to metal finishing wastewater. *Desalination* 142(3):229–234.

Bezbaruah, A. N., S. Krajangpan, B. J. Chisholm, E. Khan, and J. J. E. Bermudez. 2009. Entrapment of iron nanoparticles in calcium alginate beads for groundwater remediation applications. *Journal of Hazardous Materials* 166:1339–1343.

Bhuvaneshwari, S., V. Sivasubramanian, and S. Senthilrani. 2011. Biosorption of chromium from aqueous waste water using chitosan and desorption of chromium from biosorbent for effective reuse. *Research Journal of Chemistry and Environment* 15(2):187–195.

Bishop, P. L. 2002. *Pollution Prevention Fundamentals and Practice*. Tsinghua University Press, Beijing.

Boddu, V. M., K. Abburi, A. J. Randolph, and E. D. Smith. 2008a. Removal of copper(II) and nickel (II) ions from aqueous solutions by a composite chitosan biosorbent. *Separation Science and Technology* 43:1365–1381.

Boddu, V. M., K. Abburi, J. L. Talbott, E. D. Smith, and R. Haasch. 2008b. Removal of arsenic (III) and arsenic (V) from aqueous medium using chitosan-coated biosorbent. *Water Research* 42:633–642.

Bordes, P., E. Pollet, and L. Avérous. 2009. Nano-biocomposites: Biodegradable polyester/nanoclay systems. *Progress Polymer Science* 34:125–155.

Brinza, L., M. J. Dring, and M. Gavrilescu. 2007. Marine micro-and macro-algal species as biosorbents for heavy metals. *Environmental Engineering Management Journal* 6:237–51.

Budnyak, T., V. Tertykh, and E. Yanovska. 2014. Chitosan immobilized on silica surface for wastewater treatment. *Materials Science* 20(2):177–181.

Calagui, M. J. C., D. B. Senoro, C.-C. Kan, J. W. L. Salvacion, C. M. Futaland, and M.-W. Wane. 2014. Adsorption of indium(III) ions from aqueous solution usingchitosan-coated bentonite beads. *Journal of Hazardous Materials* 277:120–126.

Chanachai, A., R. Jiraratananon, D. Uttapap, G. Y. Moon, W. A. Anderson, and R. Y. M. Huang. 2000. Pervaporation with Chito-san/Hydroxyethylcellulose (CS/HEC) Blended Membranes. *Journal of Membrane Science* 166:271.

Chao, A. C., S. S. Shyu, Y. C. Lin, and F. L. Mi. 2004. Enzymatic grafting of carboxy groups on to chitosan to confer on chitosan the property of a cationic dye adsorbent. *Bioresource Technology* 91:157–162.

Chapman, A. R. O. 1987. The wild harvest and culture of Laminarialongicruris de la Pylaie in Eastern Canada.

Chatterjee S., S. Chatterjee, B. P. Chatterjee, A. K. Guha. 2007. Adsorption removal of congo red, carcinogenic textile dye by chitosan hydrogels; Binding mechanism, equilibrium and kinetics. *Colloids and Surfaces A: Physicochemical Engineering Aspect* 299:146–152.

Chen, C. Y., T. H. Chang, J. T. Kuo, Y. F. Chen, and Y. C. Chung. 2008. Characteristics of molybdate-impregnated chitosan beads (MICB) in terms of arsenic removal from water and the application of a MICB-packed column to remove arsenic from wastewater. *Bioresource Technology* 99:7487–7494.

Chen, J. H., G. P. Li, Q. L. Liu, J. C. Ni, W. B. Wu, and J. M. Lin. 2010. Cr(III) ionic imprinted polyvinyl alcohol/sodium alginate (PVA/SA) porous composite membranes for selective adsorption of Cr(III) ions. *Chemical Engineering Journal* 165:465–473.

Chen, J. H., H. T. Xing, H. X. Guo, G. P. Li, W. Weng, and S. R. Hu. 2013. Preparation, characterization and adsorption properties of a novel 3 aminopropyltriethoxysilane functionalized sodium alginate porous membrane adsorbent for Cr(III) ions. *Journal of Hazardous Materials* 248:285–294.

Cheraghali, R., H. Tavakoli, H. Sepehrian, and F. Scientia Iranica. 2013. Preparation, characterization and lead sorption performance of alginate-SBA-15 composite as a novel adsorbent. *Scientia Iranica* 20(3):1028–1034.

Cho, D. W., B. H. Jeon, C. M. Chon, Y. Kim, F. W. Schwartz, E. S. Lee, and H. Song. 2012. A novel chitosan/clay/magnetite composite for adsorption of Cu(II) and As(V). *Chemical Engineering Journal* 200–202:654–662.

Copello, G. J., F. Varela, R. Martínez Vivot, and L. E. Díaz. 2008. Immobilized chitosan as biosorbent for the removal of Cd(II), Cr(III) and Cr(VI) from aqueous solutions. *Bioresource Technology* 99:6538–6544.

Davis, T. A., B. Volesky, and A. Mucci. 2003. A review of the biochemistry of heavy metal biosorption by brown algae. *Water Research* 37:4311–4330.

de Moraes, M. A., D. S. Cocenza, F. da Cruz Vasconcellos, Leonardo F. Fraceto, and M. M. Beppu. 2013. Chitosan and alginate biopolymer membranes for remediation of contaminated water with herbicides. *Journal of Environmental Management* 131:222–227.

Deng, L., Y. Su, H. Su, X. Wang, and X. Zhu. 2007. Sorption and desorption of lead (II) from wastewater by green algae Cladophora fascicularis. *Journal of Hazardous Materials* 143:220–225.

Dutta, P. K., J. Dutta, and V. S. Tripathi. 2004. Chitin and chitosan: Chemistry, properties and applications. *Journal of Scientific and Industrial Research* 63:20–31.

Evans, J. R., W. G. Davids, J. D. MacRae, and A. Amirbahman. 2002. Kinetics of cadmium uptake by chitosan-based crab shells. *Water Research.* 36:3219–3226.

Florence, J. A. K., T. Gomathi, and P. N. Sudha. 2011. Equilibrium adsorption and kinetics study of chitosan-dust kenaf fiber composite. *Archives of Applied Science Research* 3(4):366–376.

Gadd, G. M. 2001. *Fungi in Bioremediation*. In G. M. Gadd Ed. Cambridge University Press, Cambridge, p. 481.

Gandhi, M. R., N. Viswanathan, and S. Meenakshi. 2010. Preparation and application of alumina/chitosan biocomposite. *International Journal of Biological Macromolecules* 47:146–154.

Gavhane Y. N., A. S. Gurav, and A. V. Yadav. 2013. Chitosan and its applications: A review of literature. *International Journal of Research in Pharmaceutical and Biomedical Sciences* 4(1):312–331.

Gonzalez-Davila, M., and F. J. Millero. 1989. The adsorption of copper to chitin in seawater. *Geochimica et Cosmochimica Acta* 54:761–768.

Gotoh, T., K. Matsushima, and K. Kikuchi. 2004. Preparation of alginate–chitosan hybrid gel beads and adsorption of divalent metal ions. *Chemosphere* 55:135–140.

Guibal, E. 2004. Interactions of metal ions with chitosan—Based sorbents: A review. *Separation and Purification Technology* 38:43–74.

Guibal, E., C. Milot, and J. Roussy. 1999. Molybdate sorption by cross-linked chitosanbeads: Dynamic studies. *Water Environment Resource* 71:10–17.

Gupta, V. K., A. Rastogi, V. K. Saini, and N. Jain. 2006. Biosorption of copper(II) from aqueous solutions by Spirogyra species. *Journal of Colloid and Interface Science* 296:59–63.

Hameed, B. H., M. Hasan, and A. L. Ahmad. 2008. Adsorption of reactive dye onto cross-linked chitosan/oil palm ash composite beads. *Chemical Engineering Journal* 136:164–172.

Han, X., Y. S. Wong, M. H. Wong, and N. F. Y. Tam. 2006. Biosorption and bioreduction of Cr(VI) by a microalgal isolate, *Chlorella miniata. Journal of Hazardous Materials* 146(1), 65–72.

Harrison, R. M. 1990. *Pollution: Causes, Effects of DCHB and Control.* Royal Society of Chemistry, Cambridge. pp. 63–83.

Hassan, A. F., A. M. Abdel-Mohsen, and H. Elhadidy. 2014a. Adsorption of arsenic by activated carbon, calcium alginate and their composite beads. *International Journal of Biological Macromolecules* 68:125–130.

Hassan, A. F., A. M. Abdel-Mohsen, and M. M. G. Fouda. 2014b. Comparative study of calcium alginate, activated carbon, and their composite beads on methylene blue adsorption. *Carbohydrate Polymers* 102:192–198.

He, X., H. Xu, and H. Li. 2015. Cr(VI) Removal from aqueous solution by chitosan/carboxyl-methyl cellulose/silica hybrid membrane. *World Journal of Engineering and Technology* 3:234–240.

Herrero, R., B. Cordero, P. Lodeiro, C. Rey-Castro, and M. E. S. D. Vicente. 2006. Interactions of cadmium(II) and protons with dead biomass of marine algae *Fucus* sp. *Marine Chemistry* 99:106–116.

Hritcu, D., G. Dodi, and M. I. Popa. 2012. Heavy metal ions adsorption on chitosan-magnetite microspheres. *International Review of Chemical Engineering* 4:364–368.

Hu, X.-J., J.-S. Wang, Y.-G. Liu, X. Li, G.-M. Zeng, Z.-L. Bao, X.-X. Zeng, A.-W. Chen, and F. Long. 2011. Adsorption of chromium (VI) by ethylenediamine-modified cross-linked magnetic chitosan resin: Isotherms, kinetics and thermodynamics. *Journal of Hazardous Materials* 185:306–314.

Huang, G. L., H. Y. Zhang, X. S. Jeffrey, and A. G. L. Tim. 2009. Adsorption of chromium(VI) from aqueous solutions using cross-linked magnetic chitosan beads. *Industrial & Engineering Chemistry Research* 48:2646–2651.

Ilankovan, P., S. Hein, C.-How Ng, T. S. Trung, and W. F. Stevens. 2006. Production of N-acetyl chitobiose from various chitin substrates using commercial enzymes. *Carbohydrate Polymers* 63:245–250.

Jassal, P. S., V. P. Raut, and N. Anand. 2010. Removal of chromium (VI) ions from aqueous solution onto chitosan and cross-linked chitosan beads. *Proceedings Indian National Science Academy* 76(1):1–6.

Jayakumar, R., M. Rajkumar, H. Freitas, N. Selvamurugan, S. V. Nair, T. Furuike, and H. Tamura. 2009. Preparation, characterization, bioactive and metal uptake studies of alginate/phosphorylated chitin blend films. *International Journal of Biological Macromolecules* 44:107–111.

Jodra, Y., and F. Mijangos. 2003. Cooperative biosorption of copper on calcium alginate enclosing iminodiacetic type resin. *Environmental Science Technology* 37:4362–4367.

Kalyani, S., B. Smitha, S. Sridhar, and A. Krishnaiah. 2008. Pervaporation separation of ethanol-water mixtures through sodium alginate membranes. *Desalination* 229:68–81.

Karthik, R., and S. Meenakshi. 2014. Removal of hexavalent chromium ions from aqueous solution using chitosan/polypyrrole composite. *Desalination and Water Treatment* 56(6):1–14.

Kathiravan, M. N., R. K. Rani, R. Karthick, and K. Muthukumar. 2010. Mass transfer studies on the reduction of Cr(VI) using calcium alginate immobilized *Bacillus* sp. in packed bed reactor. *Bioresource Technology* 101:853–858.

KFDA, 1995. Korea Food and Drug Administration. Food Additive Code.

Khairkar, S. R., and A. R. Raut. 2014. Adsorption studies for the removal heavy metal by Chitosan-G-Poly (acrylicacid-co-acrylamide) composite. *Science Journal of Analytical Chemistry* 2(6):67–70.

Khan, M. A., W. Jung, O.-H. Kwon, Y. M. Jung, K.-J. Paeng, S.-Y. Cho, and B.-H. Jeon. 2014. Sorption studies of manganese and cobalt from aqueous phase onto alginate beads and nano-graphite encapsulated alginate beads. *Journal of Industrial and Engineering Chemistry* 20(6):4353–4362.

Klimmek, S., and H. J. Stan. 2001. Comparative analysis of the biosorption of cadmium, lead, nickel, and zinc by algae. *Environmental Science Technology* 35:4283–4288.

Koide, S. S. 1998. Chitin-chitosan: Properties, benefits and risks. *Nutrition Research* 8(6):1091–1101.

Kramer, K. J., and D. Koga. 1986. Insect chitin: Physical state, synthesis, degradation and metabolic regulation. *Insect Biochemistry* 16:851–877.

Kuang S. P., Z. Z. Wang, J. Liu, and Z. C. Wu. 2013. Preparation of triethylene-tetramine grafted magnetic chitosan for adsorption of Pb(II) ion from aqueous solutions. *Journal of Hazardous Materials* 260:210–219.

Kumar, J. I. N., C. Oommen, and R. N. Kumar. 2009. Biosorption of heavy metals from aqueous solution by green marine macroalgae from Okha Port, Gulf of Kutch, India. *American-Eurasian Journal of Agricultural and Environmental Science* 6(3):317–323.

Kumar, Y. P., P. King, and V. S. R. K. Prasad. 2007. Adsorption of zinc from aqueous solution using marine green algae—*Ulva fasciata* sp. *Chemical Engineering Journal* 129:161–166.

Kusrini, E., N. Sofyan, D. M. Nurjaya, S. Santoso, and D. Tristantini. 2013. Removal of heavy metals from aqueous solution by hydroxyapatite/chitosan composite. *Advanced Materials Research* 789:176–179.

Lee, S. T., Mi, F. L., Shen, Y. J., and Shyu, S. S. 2001. Equilibrium and kinetic studies of copper (II) ion uptake by chitosan–Tripolyphosphate chelating resin. *Polymer* 42:1879–1892.

Lerivrey, J., B. Dubois, P. Decock, J. Micera, and H. Kozlowski. 1986. Formation of D-glucosamine complexes with Cu(II), Ni(II) and Co(II) ions. *Inorganica Chimica Acta* 125:187–190.

Li, X., Y. Li, S. Zhang, and Z. Ye. 2012. Preparation and characterization of new foam adsorbents of poly(vinyl alcohol)/chitosan composites and their removal for dye and heavy metal from aqueous solution. *Chemical Engineering Journal* 183:88–97.

Li, Y., B. Xia, Q. Zhao, F. Liu, P. Zhang, Q. Du, D. Wang, D. Li, Z. Wang, and Y. Xia. 2011. Removal of copper ions from aqueous solution by calcium alginate immobilized kaolin. *Journal of Environmental Sciences* 23(3):404–411.

Li, Z.-Y., S.-Y. Guo, and L. Li. 2006. Study on the process, thermodynamical isotherm and mechanism of Cr(III) uptake by *Spirulina platensis*. *Journal of Food Engineering* 75:129–136.

Liu, Q. B. Yang, L. Zhang, and R. Huang. 2015. Adsorption of an anionic azo dye by cross-linked chitosan/bentonite composite. *International Journal of Biological Macromolecules* 72:1129–1135.

Liu, X. W., Q. Y. Hu, Z. Fang, X. J. Zhang, and B. B. Zhang. 2009. Magnetic chitosan nanocomposites: A useful recyclable took for heavy metal ion removal. *Langmuir* 25:3–8.

Liu, Y., Z. Liu, W. Pan, and Q. Wu. 2008. Absorption behaviors and structure changes of chitin in alkali solution. *Carbohydrate Polymers* 72:235–239.

Liu, Y., Y. Zheng, and A. Wang. 2010. Enhanced adsorption of Methylene Blue from aqueous solution by chitosan-g-poly (acrylic acid)/vermiculite hydrogel composites. *Journal of Environmental Sciences* 22(4):486–493.

Ma, Z., N. Di, F. Zhang, P. Gu, S. Liu, and P. Liu. 2011. Kinetic and thermodynamic studies on the adsorption of Zn^{2+} onto chitosan-aluminium oxide composite material. *International Journal of Chemistry* 3(1):18.

Mahmood, Z., A. Amin, U. Zafar, M. A. Raza, I. Hafeez, and A. Akram. 2015. Adsorption studies of cadmium ions on alginate–calcium carbonate composite beads. *Applied Water Science* doi:10.1007/s13201-015-0302-2.

Mahmoud, G. A., and S. F. Mohamed. 2012. Removal of lead ions from aqueous solution using (Sodium alginate/itaconic acid) hydrogel prepared by gamma radiation. *Australian Journal of Basic and Applied Sciences* 6(6):262–273.

Mamta, T. 1999. *Quality Assessment of Water and Wastewater*. Lewis, Baca Roton.

McHugh, D. J. A. 2003. *Guide to the Seaweed Industry*. Food and Agriculture Organization of the United Nations, New York.

Muzzarelli, R. A. A. 1973. Natural chelating polymers. In R. Muzzarelli, Ed., *Chitosan*. Pergamon Press, New York, pp. 83–227.

Nadeem, U., and M. Datta. 2014. Adsorption studies of Zinc(II) ions on biopolymer composite beads of alginate-fly ash. *European Chemical Bulletin* 3(7):682–691.

Nekram, R., and J. Urmila. 2013. Removal of chromium (VI) ions from wastewaters by low cost adsorbent. *Research Journal of Chemistry and Environment* 17(9):1–99.

Ngah, W. S. W., and S. Fatinathan. 2008. Adsorption of Cu(II) ions in aqueous solution using chitosan beads, chitosan–GLA beads and chitosan–alginate beads. *Chemical Engineering Journal* 143:62–72.

Ngah, W. W. S., L. C. Teong, R. H. Toh, and M. A. K. M. Hanafiah. 2012. Utilization of chitosan–zeolite composite in the removal of Cu(II) from aqueous solution: Adsorption, desorption and fixed bed column studies. *Chemical Engineering Journal* 209:46–53.

Ngimhuang, J., J. Furukawa, T. Satoh, T. Furuike, and N. Sakairi. 2004. Synthesis of a novel polymeric surfactant by reductive N-alkylation of chitosan with 3-O-dodecyl-D-glucose. *Polymer* 45:837.

No, H. K., N. Y. Park, S. H. Lee, H. J. Hwang, and S. P. Meyers. 2002. Antibacterial activities of chitosans and chitosan oligomers with different molecular weights on spoilage bacteria isolated from tofu. *Journal of Food Science* 67:1511–1514.

Ozer, A., G. Gurbuz, A. C. Alimli, and B. K. Korabathi. 2009. Biosorption of copper (II) ions on Enteromorpha prolifera: Application of response surface methodology. *Chemical Engineering Journal* 146:377–387.

Pandey, S., and S. B. Mishra. 2011. Organic–Inorganic hybrid of chitosan/organoclay bionanocomposites for hexavalent chromium uptake. *Journal of Colloid and Interface Science* 361:509–520.

Park, H. G., T. W. Kim, M. Y. Chae, and I.-K. Yoo. 2007. Activated carbon-containing alginate adsorbent for the simultaneous removal of heavy metals and toxic organics. *Process Biochemistry* 42:1371–1377.

Peng, S., and H. Meng. 2014. Nanoporous magnetic cellulose—Chitosan composite microspheres: Preparation, characterization, and application for Cu (II) adsorption. *Industrial Engineering* 53(6):2106–2113.

Peng, S., H. Meng, Y. Ouyang, and J. Chang. 2014. Nanoporous magnetic cellulose–Chitosan composite microspheres: Preparation, characterization, and application for Cu(II) adsorption. *Industrial and Engineering Chemistry Research* 53(6):2106–2113.

Pereira, F. A. R., K. S. Sousa, G. R. S. Cavalcantia, M. G. Fonseca, Antonio G. de Souza, and A. P. M. Alves. 2013. Chitosan-montmorillonite biocomposite as an adsorbent for copper(II) cations from aqueous solutions. *International Journal of Biological Macromolecules* 61:471–478.

Pillai, C. K. S., W. Paul, and C. P. Sharma. 2009. Chitin and chitosan polymers: Chemistry, solubility and fiber formation. *Progress in Polymer Science* 34:641–678.

Pink, D. H. 2006. Investing in Tomorrow's Liquid Gold.Yahoo! http://finance.yahoo.com/columnist/article/trenddesk/3748.

Prescott, L. M., J. P. Harley, and D. A. Klein. 2002. *Microbiology*. McGraw-Hill Science/Engineering/Math, Boston edn. Fifth.

Priyabrata Pal, Fawzi Banat, Pal and Banat 2014. Contaminants in industrial lean amine solvent and their removal using biopolymers: A new aspect. *Journal of Physical Chemistry and Biophysics* 4:1.

Qin, Y., B. Shi, and J. Liu. 2006. Applications of chitosan and alginate in treating waste water containing heavy metal ions. *Indian Journal of Chemical Technology* 13: 464–469.

Raziyeh, S., A. Mokhate, M. Niyar, B. Hajir, and F. Shooka Khorram. 2010. Novel biocompatible composite (chitosan-zinc oxide nanopaticles): preparation, characterization and dye adsorption properties. *Colloids and Surfaces B. Bio interfaces* 1:86–93.

Rengaraj, S., K. H. Yeon, and S. H. Moon. 2001. Removal of chromium from water and wastewater by ion exchange resins. *Journal of Hazardous Material* 87:273–287.

Rinaudo, M. 2006. Chitin and chitosan: Properties and applications. *Progress in Polymer Science* 31:603–632.

Rincon, J., F. Gonzalez, A. Ballester, M. L. Blazquez, and J. A. Munoz. 2005. Biosorption of heavy metals by chemically-activated alga Fucus vesiculosus. *Journal of Chemical Technology and Biotechnology* 80:403–1407.

Romero-Gonzalez, M. E., C. J. Williams, and P. H. E. Gardiner. 2001. Study of the mechanisms of cadmium biosorption by dealginated seaweed waste. *Environmental Science Technology* 35:3025–3030.

Saravanan, D., T. Gomathi, and P. N. Sudha. 2013. Sorption studies on heavy metal removal using chitin/bentonite biocomposite. *International Journal of Biological Macromolecules* 53:67–71.

Saravanan, D., R. Hemalatha, and P. N. Sudha. 2011. Synthesis and characterization of cross linked chitin/bentonite polymer blend and adsorption studies of Cu (II) and Cr (VI) on chitin. *Der Pharma Chemica* 3:406–424.

Sashiwa, H., H. Yajima, and S. Aiba. 2003. Synthesis of a chitosan-dendimer hybrid and its biodegradation. *Biomacromolecules* 4:1244.

Sebastian, S., S. Mayadevi, B. S. Beevi, and S. Mandal. 2014. Layered clay-alginate composites for the adsorption of anionic dyes: A biocompatible solution for water/wastewater treatment. *Journal of Water Resource and Protection* 6:177–184.

Shawky, H. A. 2011. Improvement of water quality using alginate/montmorillonite composite beads. *Journal of Applied Polymer Science* 119(4):2371–2378.

Shilpa, A., S. S. Agrawal, and A. R. Ray. (2003). Controlled delivery of drugs from alginate matrix. *Journal of Macromolecular science part C Polymer Reviews* 43(2):187–221.

Sikder, M. T., Y. Mihara, M. S. Islam, T. Saito, S. Tanaka, and M. Kurasaki. 2014. Preparation and characterization of chitosan-carboxymethyl-β-cyclodextrin entrapped nanozerovalent iron composite for Cu(II) and Cr(IV) removal from wastewater. *Chemical Engineering Journal* 236:378–387.

Siraj, S., M. M. Islam, P. C. Das, S. M. Masum, I. A. Jahan, M. A. Ahsan, and M. Shajahan. 2012. Removal of chromium from tannery effluent using chitosan-charcoal composite. *Journal of Bangladesh Chemical Society* 25(1):53–61.

Smidsrod, O., and G. Skjak-Braek. 1990. Alginate as immobilization matrix for cells. *Trends in Biotechnology* 8:71–78.

Sowmya, A., and S. Meenakshi. 2014. A novel quaternized chitosan–melamine–glutaraldehyde resin for theremoval of nitrate and phosphate anions. *International Journal of Biological Macromolecules* 64:224–232.

Sudha, P. N., S. Celine, and S. Jayapriya. 2008. Removal of heavy metal cadmium from industrial wastewater using chitosan coated coconut charcoal. *Nature Environment and Pollution Technology* 6(3):421–424.

Sun, X. Q., B. Peng, Y. Jing, J. Chen, and D. Q. Li. 2009. Chitosan(chitin)/cellulose composite biosorbents prepared using ionic liquid for heavy metal ions adsorption. *Separations* 55:2062–2069.

Tang, X. H., S. Y. Tan, and Y. T. Wang. 2002. Study of the synthesis of chitosan derivatives containing benzo-21-crown-7 and their adsorption properties for metal ions. *Applied Journal of Polymer Science* 83:1886.

Tirtom, V. N., A. Dinçer, S. Becerik, T. Aydemir, and A. Çelik. 2012. Removal of lead (II) ions from aqueous solution by using crosslinked chitosan-clay beads. *Desalination and Water Treatment* 39:76–82.

Tran, H. V., L. D. Tran, and T. N. Nguyen. 2010. Preparation of chitosan/magnetite composite beads and their application for removal of Pb(II) and Ni(II) from aqueous solution. *Material Science and Engineering C* 30:304–310.

Tzu, T., T. Tsuritani, and K. Sato. 2013. Sorption of Pb(II), Cd(II), and Ni(II) toxic metal ions by alginate-bentonite. *Journal of Environmental Protection* 4:51–55.

Ulrich S., M. Sabine, K. Gunter, P. Wolfgang, and B. Horst. 2010. Algae-silica hybrid materials for biosorption of heavy metals. *Journal of Water Resource and Protection* 2:115–122.

Utracki, L. A. 1988. *Commercial Polymer Blends.* Chapran and Hall, London.

Vanamudan, A., K. Bandwala, and P. Pamidimukkala. 2014. Adsorption property of Rhodamine 6G onto chitosan-g-(N-vinylpyrrolidone)/montmorillonite composite. *International Journal of Biological Macromolecules* 69:506–513.

Varma, A. J., S. V. Deshpande, and J. F. Kennedy. 2004. Metal complexation by chitosan and its derivatives: A review. *Carbohydrate Polymers* 55:77–93.

Vieira, R. S., and M. M. Beppu. 2006. Dynamic and static adsorption and desorption of Hg (II) ions on chitosan membranes and spheres. *Water Research* 40:1726–1734.

Vilar, V. J., C. M. Botelho, J. M. Loureiro, and R. A. Boaventura. 2008. Biosorption of copper by marine algae Gelidium and algal composite material in a packed bed column. *Bioresource Technology* 99:5830–5838.

Vincent, T., and E. Guibal. 2000. Non-dispersive liquid extraction of Cr (VI) by TBP/aliquat 336 using chitosan-made hollow fibers. *Solvent Extraction and Ion Exchange* 18(6):1241–1260.

Wan, Y., K. A. M. Creber, B. Peppley, and V. T. Bui. 2003. Ionic conductivity of chitosan membranes. *Polymer* 44:1057–1065.

Wang, J., C. Chen. 2009. Biosorbents for heavy metals removal and their future. *Biotechnology Advances* 27:195–226.

Wang, X., L. Yang, J. Zhang, C. Wang, and Q. Li. 2014. Preparation and characterization of chitosan–poly(vinyl alcohol)/bentonite nanocomposites for adsorption of Hg(II) ions. *Chemical Engineering Journal* 251:404–412.

Weiner, M. L., 1992. An overview of the regulatory status and of the safety of chitin and chitosan as food and pharmaceutical ingredients. In C. J. Brine, P. A. Sandford, J. P. Zikakis, Ed., *Advances in Chitin and Chitosan.* Elsevier, London, pp. 663–670.

West, L. 2006. World water day: A billion people worldwide lack safe drinking water. http://environment. about. Com/od/environmental events/a/waterdayqa.htm. (Accessed date: March, 26)

Wu Jun, X., M. Yong-liang, S. Yang Gang, and G. Bai-ye Zhan. 2010. Preparation and performances of polysilicate aluminum ferric-chitosan. Bio Informatics and Biomedical Engineering (ICBBE), 4th International Conference, IEEE, China, pp. 1–4.

Wysokowski, M., Ł. Klapiszewski, D. Moszyński, P. Bartczak, T. Szatkowski, I. Majchrzak, K. Siwińska-Stefańska, V. V. Bazhenov, and T. Jesionowski. 2014. Modification of chitin with kraft lignin and development of new biosorbents for removal of cadmium(II) and nickel(II) ions. *Marine Drugs* 12(4):2245–2268.

Xiangliang, P., W. Jianlong, and Z. Daoyong. 2005. Biosorption of Pb(II) by Pleurotus ostreatus immobilized in calcium alginate gel. *Process Biochemistry* 40:2799–2803.

Yabur, R., Y. Bashan, and G. Hernández-Carmona. 2007. Alginate from the macroalgae Sargassum sinicola as a novel source for microbial immobilization material in wastewater treatment and plant growth promotion. *Journal of Applied Phycology* 19:43–53.

Yan, H., L. Yang, Z. Yang, H. Yang, A. Li, and R. Cheng. 2012. Preparation of chitosan/poly(acrylic acid) magnetic composite microspheres and applications in the removal of copper(II) ions from aqueous solutions. *Journal of Hazardous Materials* 229:371–380.

Yang, F., H. Liu, J. Qu, and J. P. Chen. 2011. Preparation and characterization of chitosan encapsulated *Sargassum* sp. biosorbent for nickel ions sorption. *Bioresource Technology* 102:2821–2828.

Yilmaz, E., and M. Bengisu. 2003. Preparation and characterization of physical gels and beads from chitin solutions. *Carbohydrate Polymers* 54:479–488.

Yoon, J., X. Cao, Q. Zhou, and L. Q. Ma. 2006. Accumulation of Pb, Cu and Zn in native plants growing on a contaminated Florida site. *Science of the Total Environment* 368:456–464.

Yu-Lin, S., L. Wei-Ying, and H. Zhang-Jun. 2010. Preparation of calcium alginate sorbent supporting the BaSO$_4$-APRB hybrid and application to clean dye waste. *Journal of Food, Agriculture & Environment* 8(2):956–961.

Yurlova, L., A. Kryvoruchko, and B. Kornilovich. 2002. Removal of Ni (II) ions from wastewater by micellar-enhanced ultra filtration. *Desalination* 144:255–260.

Zhang, S., F. Xu, Y. Wang, W. Zhang, X. Peng, and F. Pepe. 2013. Silica modified calcium alginate–Xanthan gum hybrid bead composites for the removal and recovery of Pb(II) from aqueous solution. *Chemical Engineering Journal* 234:33–42.

Zheng, Y. and A. Wang. 2009. Evaluation of ammonium removal using a chitosan-g-poly (acrylic acid)/rectorite hydrogel composite. *Journal of Hazardous Materials* 171:671–677.

Zhou, Y., S. Fu, L. Zhang, H. Zhan, and M. V. Levit. 2014. Use of carboxylated cellulose nanofibrils-filled magnetic chitosan hydrogel beads as adsorbents for Pb(II). *Carbohydrate Polymers* 101:75–82.

Zhu, L., L. Zhang, Y. Tang, and X. Kou. 2014a. Synthesis of sodium alginate graft poly (Acrylic acid-Co-2-acrylamido-2-methyl-1-propane sulfonic acid)/attapulgite hydrogel composite and the study of its adsorption. *Polymer-Plastics Technology and Engineering* 53(1):74–79.

Zhu, L., L. Zhang, Y. Tang, D. Ma, and J. Yang. 2014b. Synthesis of kaolin/sodium alginate-grafted poly(acrylic acid-*co*-2-acrylamido-2-methyl-1-propane sulfonic acid) hydrogel composite and its sorption of lead, cadmium, and zinc ions. *Journal of Elastomers and Plastics* 47(6):488–501.

20 Application of Marine Polymers in Membrane Technology

P. Angelin Vinodhini, R. Nithya,
P.N. Sudha, and Srinivasan Latha

CONTENTS

20.1 INTRODUCTION

Water, the most fabulous resource, has now become even more important than gold because of its depletion by natural and anthropogenic activities at an alarming rate round the world. Several countries are expected to face severe water crisis by the year 2025, and the problem will be worst where water shortage already exists (Bremere et al. 2001). This highlights the importance of adequate water management and treatment. To sustain the life of fast-growing global population, it is the responsibility of each and every individual across the globe to save water with utmost care. The impact of water scarcity and diminishing water quality can thus be prevented to certain level by treating it by various prevailing technologies. The most viable technology that is expected to be a critical solution for such problems is the membrane technology because of its potentiality to remove microorganisms such as bacteria and fungi, particulate material, and natural organic material and also because of its outstanding alignment with sustainable development and process intensification (Quist-Jensen et al. 2015).

20.1.1 Definition of Membrane

A membrane is defined as a thin layer of semipermeable material capable of separating substances when a driving force is applied across the membrane. The driving forces for the separation are hydrostatic pressure, concentration gradient, electrical potential, and pressure and concentration gradients (Agrawal et al. 2006). Hence, membranes are used to produce potable water, clean industrial effluents, and recover valuable constituents. Their intrinsic characteristics include efficiency, simplicity to operate, relatively high selectivity and permeability, and low energy requirements (Ahmad et al. 2015).

20.1.2 Membrane Processes

The four major pressure-driven membrane processes that have been studied for approximately 50 years are ultrafiltration (UF), nanofiltration (NF), microfiltration (MF), and reverse osmosis (RO). These membrane processes are the most viable ones in both water and wastewater treatments (Wang et al. 2014). Other pressure-driven membrane operations include gas separation and pervaporation. Besides these pressure-driven processes, there are also concentration driven operations (dialysis, osmosis, and forward osmosis), operations in electric potential gradient (electrodialysis, membrane electrolysis, and electrophoresis), and operations in temperature gradient (membrane distillation) (Sejal and Desai 2013). A bundle of membrane fibers or a multisheet set is assembled into a module for the application of filtration process. A module consists of a number of membrane elements. The typical membrane modules come in various configurations such as plate-and-frame, spiral wound, and tubular configurations. The latter can be in the form of a hollow fiber, (multi)tubular membrane, or capillary membrane, depending on the dimension of the tube (Bilad et al. 2014).

20.1.3 Antifouling Membranes

Fouling is a persistent problem that has to be considered in relation to the pretreatment system (Redondo and Lomax 2001), because it increases energy consumption and results in high operating cost (Zoua et al. 2011). It also shows decline in flux and hence the life span of a membrane. Pretreatment of surface water usually leads to membrane fouling by precipitation of sparingly soluble salts, by organic matter, or by the growth of a biofilm at the membrane surface. Deterioration of membrane performance is caused mostly by surface fouling and less so by inner fouling, because most cells are physically rejected and only tiny cells pass through the membranes (Hwang et al. 2013). Therefore, novel membrane types possessing inherent resistance against fouling need to be fabricated, which helps to solve this problem. In addition, surface modifications of existing membranes, resulting in a more hydrophilic polymer, may also lead to fouling resistant membranes (Belfer et al. 2001). Thus, hydrophilization of the membrane surface is generally opted in this scenario, so that there will be reduced interaction between the foulant and the barrier layer. It can be achieved by addition of some hydrophilic additives or by grafting of functional monomers on the membrane surface by some advanced techniques such as plasma treatment, redox reaction, and use of radiations (Mansourpanah and Momeni Habili 2013).

20.2   MARINE POLYMERS AS MEMBRANES

Most of the commercially available membranes are made from polymers that are either amorphous or semicrystalline. These polymeric membranes can be fabricated by a wide variety of methods, but the most versatile technique is the phase inversion, in which the polymer is transformed from a liquid or soluble state to a solid state (Mulder 2000). This technique is useful to obtain a variety of morphologies, ranging from microfiltration membranes with very porous structures to more dense reverse-osmosis membranes (Caneba and Soong 1985). Some of the marine polymers that find versatile application in the field of membrane technology are chitin, chitosan, alginate, and carrageenan.

20.2.1   CHITIN AND CHITOSAN

The second most naturally occurring biopolymer next to cellulose is chitin, which is a poly(β-(1→4)-N-acetyl-D-glucosamine) and is found in the exoskeleton of arthropods or in the cell walls of fungi and yeast, as well as in shells of crab and shrimp (Rinaudo 2006). Chitin is a nontoxic, biodegradable polymer (Kumar 2000) and is highly insoluble material that resembles cellulose in its insolubility and low chemical reactivity.

The most useful derivative of chitin is chitosan, which is obtained by alkaline deacetylation of chitin (Gibbs et al. 2004). It is a linear polysaccharide consisting of (1→4)-linked 2-amino-2-deoxy-β-D-glucopyranose and exhibits interesting properties such as biocompatibility and biodegradability and is nontoxic, nonimmunogenic, and noncarcinogenic (Kumar et al. 2004; Liu et al. 2012).

The highly basic polysaccharides, chitin and chitosan, have unique properties such as polyoxysalt formation, ability to form films, chelate metal ions, and optical structural characteristics (Hench 1998). Chitin is hydrophobic and is insoluble in water and in most of the organic solvents. It is soluble in hexafluoroisopropanol, hexafluoroacetone, and choloroalcohols in conjugation with aqueous solutions of mineral acids and dimethylamide containing 5% lithium chloride. Chitosan, on the other hand, is a hydrophilic polymer and its dissolution in water only takes place in dilute acidic solutions, in which organic acids (e.g., formic acid and acetic acid) or mineral acids (e.g., HCl and HNO_3) are utilized (Barros et al. 2011).

Chitosan finds numerous and extensive applications in biomedicine, wastewater treatment, food, cosmetics, and the fiber industry (Di Martino et al. 2005; Crini and Badot 2008; Shahidi et al. 1999; Dutta et al. 2009). This semicrystalline polymer being soluble in aqueous solutions is largely used in different applications in the form of solutions, gels, or films and fibers. There are many active groups in the molecular chains of chitosan, such as −OH and $−NH_2$, and therefore, it can be easily modified, and many derivatives have been prepared to meet different needs. Chitosan and its derivatives have been attracting more and more attention to the utilization in membrane materials due to the advantages of hydrophilicity, antibacterial, and environmental benignancy (Miao et al. 2008). Moreover, chitosan appears to be more useful as compared with chitin, since it has both amine and hydroxyl groups that can serve as chelating sites and can be chemically modified (Wan Ngah et al. 2002).

20.2.2 ALGINATE

Alginate, which is one of the polysaccharides extracted from seaweeds, is a linear copolymer composed of 1,4-linked β-D-mannuronic acid (M) and α-L-guluronic acid (G), which are combined into homopolymeric blocks (i.e., MM and GG blocks) and heteropolymeric block (i.e., MG blocks) (Draget et al. 2005). It was found that the combinations and sequences of these blocks in alginate affect their filtration behaviors (Meng and Liu 2013). Alginate beads have been extensively investigated for the uptake/separation toward various metal ions retained in water, which indicated high selectivity for water treatment. Alginates have been conventionally applied in the food industry as thickeners, suspending agents, emulsion stabilizers, gelling agents, and film-forming agents (Julian et al. 1988). Alginate was found to be a promising material for simultaneous removal of heavy metal ions and toxic organic pollutants (El-Tayieb et al. 2013).

Sodium alginate, the sodium salt of alginic acid, with an average molecular weight of 5,00,000 Da is a linear water-soluble anionic polymer (Wang et al. 2013). The physical properties such as viscosity and mean molecular weight of sodium alginate are very susceptible to physicochemical factors such as pH and total ionic strength. It rapidly forms a gel structure with the presence of divalent cations such as Ca^{2+}, resulting in a highly compacted gel network (Katsoufidou et al. 2007). Sodium alginate has been used as a membrane material recently, but because of its high-swelling character, it needs some modification such as crosslinking, blending, grafting, and addition of some inorganic filler (Kahya et al. 2010).

20.2.3 CARRAGEENAN

Carrageenans are large, highly flexible molecules that curl, forming helical structures. They are widely used in the food and other industries as thickening and stabilizing agents (Wu and Imai 2012). The polysaccharide chain consists of alternating 1,3-linked β-D-galactopyranosyl and 1,4-linked α-D-galactopyranosyl units (Xu et al. 2003). The main carrageenan types are kappa-, iota-, and lambda-carrageenans, and they can be prepared in pure forms by selective extraction techniques from specific seaweeds and plants within those species (Wu and Imai 2013). These isomers differ in the number and position of the ester sulfate groups on the repeating galactose units. Kappa- and iota-carrageenans form gels in the presence of potassium or calcium ions, whereas lambda-carrageenan does not form gel (Michel et al. 1997). Carrageenans form highly viscous aqueous solutions, and the viscosity depends on concentration, temperature, presence of other solutes, and the type of carrageenan and its molecular weight (Lai et al. 2000). They are well known for their gel-forming and thickening properties (Campo et al. 2009), and the gelling power of κ-carrageenans imparts excellent film-forming properties. The film formation includes a gelation mechanism during moderate drying, leading to a three-dimensional network formed by polysaccharide double helices and to a solid film after evaporation of the solvent (Karbowiak et al. 2006).

20.3 APPLICATIONS OF MARINE POLYMERS AS MEMBRANES

20.3.1 Chitin, Chitosan, and Their Derivatives

Miao et al. (2008) developed composite nanofiltration membranes by using N,O-carboxymethyl chitosan crosslinked by epichlorohydrin, using a method of coating and crosslinking. The structure and the morphology of the resulting membrane were characterized by attenuated total-reflection infrared spectroscopy and environmental scanning electron microscopy. The findings revealed that at 20°C and 0.40 MPa, the rejections of the resulting membrane to Na_2SO_4 and NaCl solutions (1000 mg/L) were 90.4% and 27.4% respectively. It was found that the rejections of the prepared composite nanofiltration membrane to the inorganic electrolyte solutions decreased in the order of Na_2SO_4, NaCl, $MgSO_4$, and $MgCl_2$.

Miao et al. (2013a) prepared a novel kind of amphoteric thin-film composite nanofiltration membrane by using sulfated chitosan/polysulfone ultrafiltration membrane, which acts as the base membrane, and epichlorohydrin as the active layer material, which is the crosslinking agent. It was found that at 0.40 MPa and ambient temperature, the rejections of the resultant membrane to Na_2SO_4 and NaCl solutions (1000 mg/L) were 90.8% and 32.5% respectively. The rejection performances suggested that the sulfated chitosan/polysulfone composite nanofiltration membranes crosslinked by epichlorohydrin have a potential for the separation of mono-/divalent inorganic electrolytes from low-molecular-weight organics.

In another study conducted by Miao and coworkers (2013b), a novel kind of amphoteric composite nanofiltration (NF) membrane was prepared via the method of coating and crosslinking, using an amphoteric derivative of chitosan, that is, sulfated chitosan (SCS), as the active layer material, poly(acrylonitrile) (PAN) ultrafiltration (UF) membrane as the support membrane, and hexamethylene diisocyanate (HDI) as the crosslinker. The membrane was characterized by attenuated total-reflection infrared spectroscopy, and the rejection properties were evaluated. The results suggested that the rejection performance to salt was dependent on the pH value of the feed solutions and reached the minimum, as the pH value of feed solution was equal to the isoeletric point (pI) of sulfated chitosan. The rejection to different inorganic salts was found to decrease in the order of K_2SO_4, Na_2SO_4, $MgSO_4$, KCl, NaCl, and MgC_{12}.

Composite nanofiltration membrane having chitosan as the active layer, supported on poly(1,4-phenylene ether-ether-sulfone) membrane, was synthesized by Shenvi et al. (2013). The chitosan layer was crosslinked by glutaraldehyde in two different concentrations and characterized using scanning electron microscopy and thermal analysis. The infrared spectroscopy results confirmed the crosslinking of the chitosan surface by glutaraldehyde. Contact angle measurement and water flux study were also done. From the results it was evident that poly(1,4-phenylene ether-ether-sulfone) has proved to be a good support membrane for preparation of composite membranes, and an increase in glutaraldehyde concentration increased the salt rejection of the membrane up to 34% for NaCl and 53% for $MgSO_4$.

In the work by Sidra Waheed et al. (2014), a number of cellulose acetate/polyethylene glycol-600 membranes with different ratios were prepared by two-stage phase-inversion protocol. The membranes were then modified using chitosan and were characterized for their compositional analysis, surface roughness, surface morphology, permeation properties, membrane hydraulic resistance, and antibacterial activity. The presence of functional group was determined by Fourier transform infrared (FTIR) spectra. It was clear from the observations that chitosan significantly enhanced the salt rejection and membrane hydraulic resistance and also exhibited remarkable antibacterial properties. Thus, the synthesis of cellulose acetate membrane doped with polyethylene glycol and modified with chitosan provided a convenient access toward the development of sustainable chemistry.

Chitosan (CS) was blended with copolymer PDMCHEA, made from 2-methacryloyloxy ethyl trimethylammonium chloride (DMC) and 2-hydroxyethyl acrylate (HEA), and the blend positively charged nanofiltration membranes (BPCNFMs) were prepared via chemical crosslinking method (Ji et al. 2015). The prepared membranes were then characterized by attenuated total-reflectance FTIR spectroscopy, wide-angle X-ray diffraction, differential scanning calorimetry, and field-emission scanning electron microscope. Mechanical properties were found to be greatly improved. The surface hydrophilicity and separation performances of BPCNFMs were examined by water contact angle and nanofiltration tests. High water permeability and salt selectivity were obtained from the results, and the stability and antifouling properties of BPCNFMs were significantly improved in the long-term nanofiltration process.

A novel positively charged composite nanofiltration membrane was prepared by coating aqueous quaternized chitosan onto a poly(acrylonitrile) UF membrane, subsequently crosslinked with epichlorohydrin (Huang et al. 2007). The effects of membrane preparation conditions on membrane properties and membrane characteristics were studied. At 25°C, the order of rejection to different model solutes was found to be $MgC_{12} \approx CaC_{12} > NaCl \approx KCl > MgSO_4 > Na_2SO_4$, revealing the characteristic of positively charged NF membranes. It was observed that the rejections to 1000 g/L MgC_{12} and CaC_{12} solutes were more than 0.96, so the membrane developed can be expected to be used in the hardness removal of wastewater.

In a study by Yoon et al. (2006), a new type of high-flux UF/NF medium based on an electrospun nanofibrous scaffold (e.g., polyacrylonitrile) coupled with a thin top layer of hydrophilic, water-resistant, but water-permeable coating (e.g., chitosan) was prepared. The study revealed that such nanofibrous composite membranes could replace the conventional porous membranes and exhibit a much higher flux rate for water filtration. The membrane containing an electrospun polyacrylonitrile scaffold with an average diameter of 124 to 720 nm and a porosity of about 70%, together with a chitosan top layer having a thickness of about 1 mm, exhibited a flux rate that is an order magnitude higher than commercial nanofiltration membranes in 24 h of operation, while maintaining the same rejection efficiency (>99.9%) for oily wastewater filtration.

Karima et al. (2014) fabricated fully bio-based composite membranes for water purification, with cellulose nanocrystals as functional entities in chitosan matrix via freeze-drying process followed by compacting. The chitosan bound the cellulose nanocrystals in a stable and nanoporous membrane structure, which was further stabilized by crosslinking with glutaraldehyde vapors. Scanning electron microscopy and Brunauer, Emmett, and Teller measurements were conducted and it was found that the membranes were nanoporous, with pores in the range of 13 to 10 nm. Based on the results, it was concluded that the membranes successfully removed 98%, 84%, and 70% of positively charged dyes Victoria Blue 2B, methyl violet 2B, and rhodamine 6G, respectively, after a contact time of 24 h.

Sun et al. (2007) prepared a novel composite nanofiltration membrane by overcoating the poly(acrylonitrile) ultrafiltration (UF) membrane with a glycol chitin thin layer. The composite NF membrane was characterized by scanning electron microscopy, infrared spectroscopy, and atomic force microscope. Rejections of Na_2SO_4, K_2SO_4, $MgSO_4$, NaCl, KCl, and MgC_{12} solutions (1.0 g/L) by the composite membrane were 95.2%, 91.5%, 41%, 31.1%, 31%, and 20.1%, respectively, at 25°C under 1.0 MPa, and permeation fluxes were 10.0, 10.1, 19.2, 19.7, 20.8, and 13.0 L/m² h, respectively. The results suggested that rejection performance is governed by solute–membrane and solute–solute electrostatic interactions.

In the work conducted by Boricha and Murthy (2009), new blend membranes with different compositions of acrylonitrile butadiene styrene and chitosan on polyether sulfone substrate membrane were prepared. The membranes were characterized by using FTIR spectroscopy–attenuated total reflectance (FTIR-ATR), X-ray diffraction (XRD), scanning electron microscopy (SEM), energy-dispersive X-ray analysis (EDXA), thermogravimetric analysis (TGA), and swelling behavior. These membranes were employed to separate mercury and sodium ions from aqueous solutions at different operating conditions, and the results showed that maximum rejections of mercury and sodium ions are 96.25% and 89.74%, respectively, for acrylonitrile butadiene styrene membrane. The results showed that chitosan membrane gave highest permeate volume flux among all the blended membranes.

An N,O-carboxymethyl chitosan/cellulose acetate blend nanofiltration membrane was prepared in acetone solvent (Boricha and Murthy 2010). The newly prepared blend membrane was characterized by using scanning electron microscopy (SEM), thermogravimetric analysis (TGA) and mechanical properties of membrane were also evaluated. The performance of the prepared NF membrane had been tested to separate chromium and copper from a common effluent-treatment-plant wastewater at different operating conditions. The results demonstrated that highest rejection for chromium and copper were observed to be 83.40% and 72.60%, respectively, at 1 MPa applied pressure and 16 L/min feed flow rate.

The surface of a base membrane made of chitosan/cellulose acetate blend was modified by reacting with heparin or quaternary ammonium or by being immobilized with silver ions by Liu et al. (2010). The modified membranes were then examined for their antibiofouling performance in terms of the antiadhesion and antibacteria effects with *Escherichia coli* pure culture and mixed-culture bacteria in a bioreactor that simulated the activated sludge wastewater treatment process. The results clearly showed that the antiadhesion approach that prevents the initial attachment of bacteria on a membrane surface is a more effective method than the antibacteria approach that aims at killing the bacteria already attached on the membrane surface.

The poly(acrylonitrile)/chitosan composite ultrafiltration membranes were prepared by filtration of chitosan solution through poly(acrylonitrile) base membrane and subsequent curing and treatment with NaOH (Musale et al. 1999). The membrane was characterized by different techniques such as FTIR–attenuated total reflectance, X-ray photoelectron spectroscopy, and scanning electron microscopy. Pure water permeation, pore size distribution, and molecular weight cutoff were determined. It was observed that these composite membranes had sharper molecular weight cutoff as well as narrower pore size distribution than the corresponding base membrane. From the results, it was obvious that the composite membranes were found to be stable in aqueous medium and showed reduction in pure water fluxes measured after filtration of aqueous acidic (pH 3.0) and basic (pH 11.0) solutions; this was attributed to the swelling of chitosan layer.

Jing et al. (2008) prepared composite nanofiltration membranes by using N,O-carboxymethyl chitosan and polysulfone by coating and crosslinking. The fermentation effluent from a wine factory was treated with the resulting composite NF membranes. The results suggested that the permeate flux and the removal efficiencies were found to increase with the increase of the driving pressure or the feed flow. It was concluded from the results that at 0.40 MPa and ambient temperature, the removal efficiencies were 95.5%, 70.7%, 72.6%, and 31.6% for color, chemical oxygen demand, total organic carbon, and conductivity, respectively. In addition, the membrane was found to be stable over a 10-h operation for the fermentation effluent treatment.

A novel composite nanofiltration membrane was prepared by using quaternized chitosan as a selective layer, poly(acrylonitrile) UF membrane as a support layer, and anhydride mixture as a crosslinking reagent (Huang et al. 2008a). These membranes were characterized by scanning electron microscope and were subjected to other characterizations such as pure water permeability, molecular weight cutoff, rejection, and swelling studies. With the increasing feed concentration, the rejection declined, whereas it was not affected by feed crossflow rate. From the results, they proposed that the rejections to $MgCl_2$ and $CaCl_2$ solutions reached up to 0.95, so the membranes developed could be used for the removal of hardness in water treatment process.

2-Hydroxypropyltrimethyl ammonium chloride chitosan/polyacrylonitrile positively charged composite nanofiltration (NF) membrane was prepared by using toluene diisocyanate as the crosslinking reagent (Huang et al. 2008b). It was characterized by using FTIR-ATR, and the permeability of pure water and the rejection performance to different salt solutions were evaluated. It was concluded that at 20°C and 30 L h^{-1} of cycling flow, the permeability of pure water through this membrane was 8.96 kgm^{-2} h^{-1} MPa^{-1}. It was also found that the rejection to different salt solutions increased in the order of Na_2SO_4, $MgSO_4$, NaCl, and $MgCl_2$.

The work by Jana et al. (2011) presented the fabrication of chitosan-based ceramic membranes by using dip-coating technique. Different ceramic membranes were prepared by varying chitosan concentration and dipping time and were characterized by using scanning electron microscope and air and hydraulic permeability tests. The results clearly showed that the chitosan-impregnated ceramic membranes were applicable for both microfiltration (MF) and ultrafiltration (UF) applications. The lowest-pore-size ultrafiltration membrane (pore size: 13 nm) was used for the removal of mercury and arsenic from wastewater by polymer-enhanced ultrafiltration (PEUF) technique using polyvinyl alcohol (PVA) as the chelating agent, and it was found that almost 100% removals were observed for both 500 μ g L^{-1} mercury and 1000 μ g L^{-1} arsenic.

El-Gendi et al. (2014) prepared novel polyamide-6/chitosan membranes for water desalting by using wet-phase inversion technique. The desalting performance of each prepared membrane was evaluated under different operating conditions. The results showed that the membrane flux was increased with the increase in operating pressure. The salt rejection and permeation flux have also found to be enhanced, which indicated that the addition of chitosan to the polyamide-6 membrane increased the membrane's hydrophilic property.

Novel thin-film composite (TFC) membrane was prepared by organoclay/chitosan nanocomposite coated on the commercial polyvinylidene fluoride (PVDF) microfiltration membrane (Daraei et al. 2013). Two different grades of organoclay (Cloisite 15A and 30B) were used in the study, and the membranes were examined with aqueous dye solution for its performance. From the results, it was obvious that methylene blue dye removal increased with applying organoclay particles in chitosan coating. The fabricated TFC membranes were analyzed using scanning electron microscopy, X-ray diffraction, and Fourier transform infrared spectroscopy.

Chitosan–glycerol (CSG) membranes were synthesized for microfiltration (MF) applications in wastewater treatment via the solution casting and solvent evaporation technique (Cadogan et al. 2015) and were crosslinked with phosphoric acid in the presence of ethanol. The membranes were characterized by tensile strength, swelling, Fourier transform infrared spectroscopy–attenuated total reflectance, and scanning electron microscopy studies to investigate their structural properties. Water permeation studies were conducted using a crossflow MF module, and the results indicated that 2:1 CSG membranes effectively removed more than 95% of bacteria, notably *E. coli*, from wastewater.

The high-performance polyethersulfone (PES) nanocomposite membranes were prepared by addition of synthesized Fe_3O_4/O-carboxymethyl chitosan (Fe_3O_4–OCMCS) nanoparticles in the casting solution at different amounts (Rahimi et al. 2014). The prepared blend membranes were characterized using FTIR, SEM, and permeation tests. The water flux was found to be improved by addition of nanoparticles, and the antifouling performance was studied, which revealed that 0.1 wt. % OCMCS–Fe_3O_4–PES membrane showed highest flux recovery ratio (FRR) value of 89%. Moreover, the addition of Fe_3O_4–OCMCS from 0 to 0.1 wt. % resulted in membranes with more number of finger-like channels from the SEM images.

Sudha et al. (2014) fabricated novel ultrafiltration membranes by blending chitosan with cellulose acetate and polyethylene glycol in N,N'-dimethylformamide by phase-inversion technique. The membranes were prepared in different ratios and characterized by using Fourier transform infrared spectroscopy, X-ray diffraction analysis, and scanning electron microscopy. The detection of water absorption capacity and the percentage rejection of chromium from industrial and artificial wastewater was carried out, and the results indicated that the blend with highest polyethylene glycol content showed maximum rejection of 48.46% and 54.96% in artificial and industrial wastewater, respectively.

Chitosan and poly(vinyl alcohol) blend membranes in various ratios were prepared and treated with formaldehyde (Yang et al. 2004). They were then characterized by using differential scanning calorimetry, dynamic mechanical analysis, and thermogravimetric analysis. The effects of chitosan content on water content and water vapor transmission rates on the blended hydrogel membrane were determined, and it was found that they were increased with an increase in chitosan content. The permeations of creatinine, 5-fluorouracil, uric acid, and vitamin B_{12} through the chitosan/poly(vinyl alcohol) blended hydrogel membranes were conducted. The results showed that the permeation of uric acid through the prepared hydrogel membranes is higher for the membranes with chitosan content higher than 80% in the blended hydrogel membranes.

Chitosan/poly(tetrafluoroethylene) composite membranes were prepared from casting a γ-(glycidyloxypropyl)trimethoxysilane (GPTMS)-containing chitosan solution on poly(styrene sulfuric acid)-grafted expended poly(tetrafluoroethylene) film surface (Liu et al. 2007). It was used in the pervaporation dehydration processes on isopropanol. This indicates the high performance of chitosan/poly(tetrafluoroethylene) composite membranes, which exhibited a permeation flux of 1730 g/m^2 h and a separation factor of 775 at 70°C on pervaporation dehydration of a 70 wt.% isopropanol aqueous solution. The studies also revealed that the membrane survived a long-term operation test of 45 days.

Chitosan composite membranes were prepared by casting solutions onto porous polyethersulfone ultrafiltration membranes with various surface-crosslinking densities (Lee et al. 1997). The surface-crosslinked chitosan composite membranes were subjected to pervaporation performance of water–alcohol mixtures, and it was found to exhibit a high selectivity value with a low permeation flux. By increasing feed ethanol concentration, permeate flux decreased. In addition, water concentration in the permeate decreased drastically at a feed ethanol concentration above 97 wt.%. From the study, it was known that the permeation rate of chitosan composite membranes is less temperature-dependent than that of polyvinyl alcohol.

Wang and coworkers (2010) prepared a novel composite membrane by ozone pretreatment, chitosan coating, and glutaraldehyde-crosslinking to resist the adsorption of proteins and the adhesion of bacteria. Experimental results demonstrated that the composite membrane had hydrophilicity and higher protein rejection. The results showed that the surface of composite membranes was found to be very effective in preventing biofilm formation, especially for the membrane with glutaraldehyde crosslink. Thus, they believed that this hydrophilization approach has great potential in industrial production to confer new properties on commercial hydrophobic membrane materials.

Wang and Spencer (1998) developed formed-in-place (FIP) ultrafiltration (UF) membranes from dilute solutions of chitosans with different molecular weights in 1% acetic acid on a macroporous titanium dioxide substrate. The ultrafiltration properties were characterized, and it was found that all the prepared membranes exhibited more than 90% bovine serum albumin (BSA) rejection at low ionic strength and there was very little dependence of the membrane formation capability on chitosan's molecular weight. The results concluded that pH had a marked effect on membrane surface properties, membrane stability, and membrane morphology.

A chitosan (CS) NF membrane was prepared with support of polyacrylonitrile (PAN) ultrafiltration membrane (Zhang et al. 2013) to retain γ-aminobutyric acid (GABA). Its acid resistance was dramatically improved by glutaraldehyde crosslink between hydroxyl groups, when its amine groups were protected by copper ion chelation in advance. The results indicated that the crosslinked CS/PAN composite membrane achieved 95% GABA rejection in pH 4.69 solution under the operation pressure of 0.2 MPa, whereas more than 90% of sodium acetate permeates the membrane.

Feng et al. (2014) successfully grafted chitosan onto the top surface of a bromomethylated poly(phenylene oxide) (BPPO) ultrafiltration membrane, without pretreating the membrane at harsh conditions and/or using other crosslinkers. Owing to grafting, the hydrophilicity of the membrane's top surface and the polar component of the total surface energy were found to be improved compared with the pristine BPPO membrane. The results suggested that the foulants adsorbed onto the top surface of chitosan/BPPO composite membranes were much easier to desorb during the cleaning process, which in turn results in higher flux recovery compared with the pristine BPPO membrane. It was also found that the antibacterial rate was improved by 70% in comparison with the pristine BPPO membrane.

Mixed-matrix membranes (MMMs) using chitosan (CS) and microporous titanosilicate (ETS-10) were prepared (Casado-Coterillo et al. 2014). The resulted membrane was characterized by using SEM and transmission electron microscopy (TEM), XRD, differential scanning calorimetry (DSC), and TGA. The pervaporation performance was also tested on the water–ethanol mixtures in the range 85 to 96 wt.% ethanol, and the results concluded that there was a good adhesion between ETS-10 nanoparticles and chitosan. The permeate flux was enhanced from 0.45 to 0.55 kg m^{-2} h^{-1} at 50°C for the ETS-10/CS MMM with respect to the pure CS membranes. The 5 wt.% loading of titanosilicate scarcely decreased the hydrophilic characteristic of the mixed-matrix membrane.

Silver metal nanoparticles were immobilized in chitosan/carboxymethylcellulose/BMI.BF4 (1-*n*-butyl-3-methylimidazolium tetrafluoroborate ionic liquid) (CS/CMC/IL) to form polymeric membrane with 20-μm thickness (Quadros et al. 2013) by using a simple solution-blending method. The results demonstrated that the CS/CMC/IL membrane containing Ag(0) showed increased antimicrobial activity against *E. coli* and *Staphylococcus aureus* when the Ag(0) concentration increased up to saturation at 10 mg. It was also found that the durability of the membrane was enhanced on addition of Ag(0) nanoparticles into the membrane.

Shiyan et al. (2014) prepared crosslinked chitosan membrane and hydroxymethylated lignin–chitosan crosslinked membrane by using glutaraldehyde as the crosslinking agent. They were characterized using FTIR and SEM, and the Cu(II) ion adsorption properties of both membranes were analyzed. The results indicated that crosslinked chitosan membrane was suitable for use only in aqueous solutions with pH values of 3.5 to 9.0, whereas hydroxymethylated lignin–chitosan crosslinked membrane maintained its shape even in concentrated HCl and NaOH solutions, which was proved to be worthy of further investigation.

Two different compositions of polysulfone in N-methylpyrrolidone (NMP) and chitosan in 1% acetic acid were blended to prepare polysulfone–chitosan (PSf–CS) ultrafiltration membranes by the diffusion-induced phase separation (DIPS) method

(Kumar et al. 2013). They were then characterized by FTIR-ATR, SEM, and contact angle measurements. From the results, it was shown that PSf–CS membrane has an enhanced hydrophilicity and improved flux compared with a PSf ultrafiltration membrane. An improved antifouling property was observed for PSf–CS blend membranes with an increase in chitosan composition.

20.3.2 ALGINATE

Alginate membranes for the pervaporation dehydration of ethanol–water and isopropanol–water mixtures were prepared and tested (Huang et al. 1999). The water-soluble sodium alginate membrane was mechanically weak, but it showed promising performance for the pervaporation dehydration. The sodium alginate membrane was crosslinked ionically by using various divalent and trivalent ions to control the water solubility. Among them, the alginate membrane crosslinked with Ca^{2+} ion showed the highest pervaporation performance in terms of flux and separation factors.

Novel two-ply dense composite membranes were prepared by Moon et al. (1999) by using successive castings of sodium alginate and chitosan solutions for the pervaporation dehydration of isopropanol and ethanol. The pervaporation performance of the two-ply membrane, with its sodium alginate layer facing the feed side and crosslinked or insolubilized in sulfuric acid solution, was compared with the pure sodium alginate and the chitosan membranes in terms of flux and separation factors. The results showed that for dehydration of 90 wt.% isopropanol–water mixtures, the performance of the two-ply membrane, which was moderately crosslinked in formaldehyde, was found to match the high performance of the pure sodium alginate membrane; also in addition, its mechanical properties were better than that of the pure sodium alginate membrane.

The polyion complex composite (PIC) membranes were prepared by using sodium alginate and chitosan (Kim et al. 2000), and the pervaporation characteristics were investigated for the separation of methyl *tert*-butyl ether (MTBE) and methanol mixtures. From the findings, it was evident that the prepared PIC membrane containing 2.0 wt.% sodium alginate solutions and 2.0 wt.% chitosan solution appeared to permeate only methanol from the feed, which showed excellent pervaporation performance. In addition, as the operating temperature was increased from 40°C to 55°C, the permeation rate of methanol was increased but that of MTBE decreased. These results were due to the physicochemical and structural properties of polyion complex membranes.

Alginate composite membrane crosslinked with 1,6-hexanediamine (HDM) or poly(vinyl alcohol) (PVA) was prepared by casting an aqueous solution of alginate and HDM (or PVA) on a hydrolyzed microporous polyacrylonitrile (PAN) membrane, and the crosslinked membranes were characterized by pervaporation separation of acetic acid/water mixtures (Wang 2000). From the results, it was shown that sodium alginate (SA) composite membrane crosslinked with HDM has a high separation factor of 161 and a good permeation rate of 262 g/m^2 h for pervaporation of 85 wt.% acetic acid aqueous solution at 70°C. However, the alginate composite membrane crosslinked with PVA has much lower separation properties.

Pervaporation (PV) membranes were prepared by blending hydrophilic polymers, poly(vinyl alcohol) (PVA), and sodium alginate (SA), which were then crosslinked with glutaraldehyde (GA) for the separation of acetic acid/water mixtures (Srinivasa Rao et al. 2006) and characterized by using XRD, FTIR, TGA, and tensile testing. Sorption studies and porosity measurements were carried out, and the results were compared with those of the commercial membrane (Sulzer pervap 2205). The prepared membrane appeared to have a good potential for dehydrating 90 wt.% acetic acid with a reasonably high selectivity of 21.5 and a substantial water flux of 0.24 $g/m^2/h/10$ μm.

In a study reported by Cahyaningrum et al. (2014), the viability of using ultrafiltration membranes was investigated, which was made by blending 85% deacetylated chitosan and sodium alginate biopolymers, with glutaraldehyde as the crosslinking agent for separation of uric acid. The membranes were characterized by FTIR and SEM. Mechanical stability was tested by using tensile testing. The findings showed that the membrane was able to filter out uric acid concentration of 90 mg/L, with the amount of uric acid filtered to be 48.23 mg/L.

Patil et al. (2009) investigated the development of hybrid composite membranes of sodium alginate loaded with hydrophilic alumina-containing Mobile Composition Matter-41 (Al-MCM-41) in different compositions, ranging from 3 to 10 wt.%, that are used for pervaporation (PV) dehydration of 1,4-dioxane and tetrahydrofuran (THF) from aqueous mixtures in compositions of 10 to 40 wt.% at 30°C. The prepared composite membranes were then characterized by Fourier transform spectroscopy, X-ray diffraction, and scanning electron microscopy. From the results, it was observed that flux and selectivity increased systematically with increasing amount of Al-MCM-41 particles in the sodium alginate matrix.

Nanofiltration composite membranes based on poly(vinyl alcohol) and sodium alginate were prepared by coating microporous polysulfone supports with dilute poly(vinyl alcohol)/sodium alginate (PVA/SA) blend solutions (Jegal et al. 2001). The concentration of the PVA/SA blend solutions ranged from 0.1 to 0.3 wt.%. The membranes were characterized with various methods such as SEM, FTIR, permeation tests, and z-potential measurements. Their chemical stabilities were tested by using three aqueous solutions with different pH, and the results were compared with that of a polyamide (PA) composite membrane prepared from piperazine (PIP) and trimesoyl chloride (TMC). It was found that the PVA/SA composite membranes prepared showed not only good chemical stabilities but also good permeation performances in the range of pH 1 to 13.

In a study conducted by Athanasekoua et al. (2010), the UF/NF membranes were functionalized with alginates to develop hybrid inorganic/organic materials for continuous, single-pass, wastewater treatment applications. The deposition and stabilization of alginates was carried out via physical (filtration/crosslinking) and chemical (grafting) procedures. The results have shown that the materials developed by means of the filtration process exhibited a 25% to 60% enhancement of their Cd^{2+}-binding capacity, depending on the amount of the filtered alginate solution, and the grafting process led to the development of alginate layers with adequate stability under acidic regeneration conditions.

Polyelectrolyte complex (PEC) membrane of cationic chitosan and anionic sodium alginate with fiber structure were prepared by freeze-drying method (Jiang et al. 2014). Freeze-dried fiber membranes were extensively characterized by using FTIR, XRD, z-potentials, SEM, and cytotoxicity assay. The study suggested that chitosan–sodium alginate samples showed better cell adhesion and proliferation than pure chitosan. The results indicated that two natural polyelectrolyte complex nanofibers were prepared by freeze-drying method and fitted for tissue engineering or as drug carriers.

Sodium alginate (SA) was used as the membrane material in the study carried out by Nigiz and Hilmioglu (2013). Pristine SA and zeolite 4A-filled SA mixed-matrix membranes (MMMs) have been prepared by solution-casting evaporation and cross-linking method. Phosphoric acid was used as the crosslinking agent. The membranes were analyzed by using scanning electron microscopy, thermogravimetric analysis, and Fourier transform infrared spectroscopy. Pervaporation performance of all membranes have been tested for dehydration of aqueous ethanol feed mixtures at 25°C, and it was found that with the addition of zeolite to the polymer, flux values increased. In addition, with increasing water content in the feed mixture, flux increased but selectivity decreased, as expected.

Sodium alginate (SA) hybrid membranes containing 6, 8, and 10 wt.% of Preyssler-type heteropolyacid $H_{14}[NaP_5W_{30}O_{110}]$ (HPA) were prepared and characterized by FTIR, SEM, TGA, DSC, and contact angle measurements (Magalad et al. 2010). Hybrid membranes exhibited increased pervaporation separation index (PSI) for selectively separating water from the azeotropic mixture (4 wt.% water + 96 wt.% ethanol) with ethanol. The highest separation factor of 59,976 with a flux of 0.043 kg/m^2 h was obtained for the hybrid membrane, that is, SA-6. It was reported that these membranes were highly water-selective. Activation energies for total permeation and permeation of water and ethanol were determined at various temperatures, and the negative heat of sorption indicated the predominance of Langmuir sorption mode for SA-6 hybrid membrane.

Chen et al. (2010) fabricated a novel composite nanofiltration (NF) membrane by overcoating the polysulfone ultrafiltration membrane with an alginate thin layer. The structure of the composite NF membrane was characterized by scanning electron microscopy and infrared spectroscopy. The results suggested that composite membrane with sodium alginate concentration of 2%, glutaraldehyde concentration of 0.9%, and the crosslinking time of 4 h at 30°C showed excellent performances. Results of salt rejections to Na_2SO_4, $MgSO_4$, NaCl, and $MgCl_2$ (1000 mg/L) were 87.2%, 21.5%, 32.0%, 12.2%, respectively.

In a recent study by Sajankumar ji Rao et al. (2015), mixed-matrix blend membranes (MMMs) of sodium alginate (SA)–hydroxy propyl cellulose (HPC) were prepared by incorporating with halloysite nanoclay (HNC) by solution-casting technique and characterized by using FTIR, SEM, and TGA. Pervaporation experiments of these membranes were investigated for the separation of isopropanol/water mixture at 30°C, and the results clearly showed that the flux of 0.3 wt.% HNC-loaded membrane of SA-HPCL-3 was higher than that of pristine SA–HPC blend membrane.

Calcium alginate membrane has a great potential for membrane-separation technology. The polymer frameworks of the membrane were successfully regulated by the mass fraction of homopolymeric blocks of α-L-guluronic acid (F_{GG}) in the entire molecular chain of alginate and the additive $CaCl_2$ as a crosslinker (Kashima and Imai 2012). The results suggested that the mechanical strength can be controlled by regulating the F_{GG} and $CaCl_2$ concentration, and the tortuosity increased linearly with increasing additive $CaCl_2$ concentration. It was also found that low-F_{GG} (0.18) membrane performed high permeability than high-F_{GG} (0.56) membrane.

In a recent study by Zhang et al. (2015), an antifouling, free-standing membrane was synthesized through the polymerization of acrylamide in the presence of sodium alginate by using N,N′-methylenebisacrylamide as the covalent crosslinker and $CaCl_2$ as the ionic crosslinker. The calcium alginate/polyacrylamide (CA/PAM) membranes were characterized using field-emission scanning electron microscopy (FESEM), Fourier transform infrared spectroscopy (FTIR), and thermal gravity (TG). The antifouling performance of the membrane was investigated, and it was found that the hydrogel filtration membrane showed limited adsorption and adhesion for bovine serum albumin (BSA) and yeast, and the rejection of BSA and yeast reached 98.53% and 99.64%, respectively. The results of this study indicated that the freestanding CA/PAM hydrogel nanofiltration membrane exhibited excellent antifouling properties and that it has promising application prospects in the fields of protein separation, microorganism filtration, and removal of dyes.

The changes in rheological and mechanical properties for some ionotropic crosslinked metal–alginate hydrogel complexes, in particular, copper–alginate membranes, in the presence of some organic solvents or buffer solutions have been investigated by Hassan et al. (2012). The experimental results showed that the hydrogels shrink in polar solvents but not in nonpolar solvents. Moreover, it was also observed that the gels were found to swell or shrink in buffer solutions, depending on the pH of the buffer used. The swelling extent for hydrogel spheres was found to decrease in the order $Cu > Ba \approx Ca > Zn > Pb$–alginates in universal buffers of pH = 5.33.

Sodium alginate (SA)/poly(vinyl pyrrolidone) (PVP) blend membranes were prepared and crosslinked with $CaCl_2$ for the separation of aqueous/dimethylformamide (DMF) mixtures (Solak and Şanlı 2011). Membranes were then characterized by FTIR and SEM, and their performance was examined by varying experimental parameters such as feed composition, operating temperature, and membrane thickness. The results obtained showed that blending SA with PVP decreased separation factor and increased the permeation rate as the permeation temperature was increased in vapor permeation (VP), whereas in the vapor permeation with temperature difference (TDVP) method, the separation factors increased and the permeation rates decreased as the temperature of the membrane's surrounding was decreased.

A sodium alginate dense membrane was prepared by crosslinking with phosphoric acid for the separation of ethanol–water mixtures at 30°C by the pervaporation method (Kalyani et al. 2008). The effects of experimental factors, such as the concentration of the feed solutions, membrane thickness, and the operating permeate pressure on sodium alginate membrane's performance were evaluated. Ion exchange capacity (IEC) studies were carried out for all crosslinked and uncrosslinked membranes to determine the total number of interacting groups present in the membranes. The results suggested that the crosslinked membranes were found to show promising performance for dehydration of ethanol containing smaller amounts of water. Furthermore, flux decreased with an increase in membrane thickness, and a reduction in both flux and selectivity was observed at higher permeate pressure.

20.3.3 CARRAGEENAN

Marine biopolymer κ-carrageenan–pullulan composite membrane was successfully prepared using casting method by Wu and Imai (2012). The water permeability of composite membrane was determined from the water mass flux throughput by an ultrafiltration apparatus. Results suggested that a higher-permeation mechanism of water results from higher water content in the composite membrane. For mass transfer examination through the composite membrane, five anionic organic chemicals of molecular weights ranging from 327 to 1017 Da were used. Molecular size recognition appeared outstanding based on the effective diffusion coefficient, and the membrane's molecular weight cutoff was established experimentally. Thus, it was stated that carrageenan–pullulan composite membrane possessing a crosslinked hydrophilic structure showed high selectivity and high water flux.

Pervaporation separation of water–ethanol was carried out with polyion complex membranes, which were prepared by the ion complex formation between κ-carrageenan and poly{1,3-bis[4-alkylpyridinium]propane bromide} with different numbers of methylene units between two ionic sites within a repeating unit (Jecal and Lee 1996). The membranes were characterized by FTIR and X-ray diffractometry. Dehydration of 90 wt.% aqueous ethanol solution was carried out at different temperatures (30°C, 40°C, 50°C, and 60°C), and the results showed permselectivity of 45,000 and permeability of 150 g/m² h at 30°C. From the results, it was concluded that with increasing operating temperature, permeability increased highly but selectivity decreased slightly.

Coelhoso et al. (2014) prepared membranes by using 67% κ-carrageenan and 33% pectin with different amounts of nanoclays (1%, 5%, and 10%) by the solution-intercalation method and casting. The films without nanoclay particles exhibited enhanced gas- and water-vapor-barrier properties. The results showed a positive effect on the films' barrier properties of the organic nanoclay particles inclusion. In addition, it was found that the permeability to carbon dioxide has been significantly reduced (50% reduction for 1% nanoclay content). On inclusion of nanoclay particles, the membranes have shown a decrease in their stiffness and an increase in elongation at break.

20.4 CONCLUSION AND FUTURE PROSPECTS

The main reason that has attracted the current researchers to study the use of biopolymers in membrane technology is the stringent environmental regulations. Since the biopolymers derived from natural raw materials are sustainable and renewable and can be disposed of easily into the environment, they are used for fabrication of a wide variety of membrane materials and are used for various applications such as water treatment, food industry, controlled drug delivery, bioseparation, chemical sensors, and tissue engineering. Their potential biocompatible properties make them an alternative to various artificial polymers. The biopolymer chitosan is an excellent boon to humans, which has already proved its strength in various fields, but still, its use is much anticipated. Chitosan membranes are very much utilized in membrane filtration processes such as ultrafiltration and nanofiltration in recent years. Alginate membranes, which are now viewed as an alternative to artificial polymer membranes, have been investigated in diverse ways such as pervaporation and ultrafiltration.

However, the formation of carrageenan membranes has been less investigated. In future, their use can be further explored by combining with other marine biological polymers to develop a new membrane material. Advanced membrane materials of marine origin should be developed for promising separation technology, which can be achieved by improving their chemical and mechanical properties.

ACKNOWLEDGMENT

The authors are grateful to the authorities of the D.K.M. College for Women and Thiruvalluvar University, Vellore, Tamil Nadu, India, for their support. They are also thankful to the editor for the opportunity to review such an innovating field.

REFERENCES

Agrawal, A., V. Kumar, and B. D. Pandey. 2006. Remediation options for the treatment of electroplating and leather tanning effluent containing chromium—A review. *Mineral Processing and Extractive Metallurgy Review* 27(2):99–130.

Ahmad, A., S. Waheed, S. M. Khan, S. E-Gul, M. Shafiq, M. Farooq, K. Sanaullah, and T. Jamil. 2015. Effect of silica on the properties of cellulose acetate/polyethylene glycol membranes for reverse osmosis. *Desalination* 355:1–10.

Athanasekoua, C. P., G. E. Romanosa, K. Kordatosb, V. Kasselouri-Rigopouloub, N. K. Kakizisa, and A. A. Sapalidis. 2010. Grafting of alginates on UF/NF ceramic membranes for wastewater treatment. *Journal of Hazardous Materials* 182:611–623.

Barros, J. A. G., A. J. C. Brant, and L. H. Catalina. 2011. Hydrogels from chitosan and a novel copolymer poly (N-Vinyl-2- Pyrollidone-Co-Acrolein). *Materials Sciences and Applications* 2:1058–1069.

Belfer, S., J. Gilron, Y. Purinson, R. Fainshtein, N. Daltrophe, M. Priel, B. Tenzer, and A. Thoma. 2001. Effect of surface modification in preventing fouling of commercial SWRO membrane at the Eilat seawater desalination pilot plant. *Desalination* 139:169–176.

Bilad, M. R., Hassan A. Arafat, and I. F. J. Vankelecom. 2014. Membrane technology in micro-algae cultivation and harvesting: A review. *Biotechnology Advances* 32:1283–1300.

Boricha, A. G. and Z. V. P. Murthy. 2009. Acrylonitrile butadiene styrene/chitosan blend membranes: Preparation, characterization and performance for the separation of heavy metals. *Journal of Membrane Science* 339:239–249.

Boricha, A. G. and Z. V. P. Murthy. 2010. Preparation of N, O-carboxymethyl chitosan/cellulose acetate blend nanofiltration membrane and testing its performance in treating industrial wastewater. *Chemical Engineering Journal* 157:393–400.

Bremere, I., M. Kennedy, A. Stikker, and J. Schipper. 2001. How water scarcity will effect the growth in the desalination market in the coming 25 years. *Desalination* 138:7–9.

Cadogan, E. I., C.-H. Lee, S. R. Popuri, and H.-Y. Lin. 2015. Characterization, fouling, and performance of synthesized chitosan–glycerol membranes in bacterial removal from municipal wastewater. *Desalination and Water Treatment* 1–13. doi: 10.1080/19443994.2015.1089192

Cahyaningrum, S. E., N. Widyastuti, and N. Qomariah. 2014. Filtration of uric acid using ultra filtration membrane chitosan-glutaraldehyde-alginate. *Research Journal of Pharmaceutical, Biological and Chemical Sciences* 5(3):999–1005.

Campo, V. L., D. F. Kawano, D. B. Da Silva Jr., and I. Carvalho. 2009. Carrageenans: Biological properties, chemical modifications and structural analysis—A review. *Carbohydrate Polymers* 77:167–180.

Caneba, G. T., and D. S. Soong. 1985. Polymermembrane formation through the thermal-inversion process. 1. Experimental study ofmembrane structure formation. *Macromolecules* 18:2538–2545.

Casado-Coterillo, C., F. Andrés, C. Téllez, J. Coronas, and Á. Irabien. 2014. Synthesis and characterization of ETS-10/chitosan nanocomposite membranes for pervaporation. *Separation Science and Technology* 49:1903–1909.

Chen, X., X. Gao, W. Wang, D. Wang, and C. Gao. 2010. Study of sodium alginate/polysulfone composite nanofiltration membrane. *Desalination and Water Treatment* 18:198–205.

Coelhoso, I. M., A. R. V. Ferreira, and V. D. Alves. 2014. Biodegradable barrier membranes based on nanoclays and carrageenan/pectin blends. *International Journal of Membrane Science and Technology* 1:23–30.

Crini, G., and P. M. Badot. 2008. Application of chitosan, a natural aminopolysaccharide, for dye removal from aqueous solutions by adsorption processes using batch studies: A review of recent literature. *Progress in Polymer Science* 33:399–447.

Daraei, P., S. S. Madaeni, E. Salehi, N. Ghaemi, H. S. Ghari, M. A. Khadivi, and E. Rostami. 2013. Novel thin film composite membrane fabricated by mixed matrix nanoclay/chitosan on PVDF microfiltration support: Preparation, characterization and performance in dye removal. *Journal of Membrane Science* 436:97–108.

Di Martino, A., M. Sittinger, and M. V. Risbud. 2005. Chitosan: A versatile biopolymer for orthopaedic tissue-engineering. *Biomaterials* 26:5983–5990.

Draget, K. I., O. Smidsrød, and G. Skjåk-Bræk. 2005. *Biopolymers Online*. Weinheim: Wiley-VCH Verlag GmbH & Co. KGaA, Alginates from Algae, pp. 1–30.

Dutta, P. K., S. Tripathi, G. K. Mehrotra, and J. Dutta. 2009. Perspectives for chitosan based antimicrobial films in food applications. *Food Chemistry* 114:1173–1182.

El-Gendi, A., A. Deratani, S. A. Ahmed, and S. S. Ali. 2014. Development of polyamide-6/chitosan membranes for desalination. *Egyptian Journal of Petroleum* 23:169–173.

EL-Tayieb, M. M., M. M. El-Shafei, and M. S. Mahmoud. 2013. The role of alginate as polymeric material in treatment of tannery wastewater. *International Journal of Science and Technology* 2(2):218–224.

Feng, Y., X. Lin, H. Li, L. He, T. Sridhar, A. K. Suresh, J. Bellare, and H. Wang. 2014. Synthesis and characterization of chitosan-grafted BPPO ultrafiltration composite membranes with enhanced antifouling and antibacterial properties. *Industrial and Engineering Chemistry Research* 53:14974–14981.

Gibbs, G., J. M. Tobin, and E. Guibal. 2004. Influence of chitosan preprotonation on reactive black 5 sorption isotherms and kinetics. *Industrial and Engineering Chemistry Research.* 43:1–11.

Hassan, R., F. Tirkistani, I. Zaafarany, A. Fawzy, M. Khairy, and S. Iqbal. 2012. Polymeric biomaterial hydrogels. I. Behavior of some ionotropic cross-linked metal-alginate hydrogels especially copper-alginate membranes in some organic solvents and buffer solutions. *Advances in Bioscience and Biotechnology* 3:845–854.

Hench, L. L. 1998. Biomaterials: A forecast for the future. *Biomaterials* 19:1419.

Huang, R. Y. M., R. Pal, and G. Y. Moon. 1999. Characteristics of sodium alginate membranes for the pervaporation dehydration of ethanol-water and isopropanol-water mixtures. *Journal of Membrane Science* 160:101–113.

Huang, R., G. Chen, B. Yang, and C. Gao. 2008b. Positively charged composite nanofiltration membrane from quaternized chitosan by toluene diisocyanate cross-linking. *Separation and Purification Technology* 61:424–429.

Huang, R., G. Chen, M. Sun, and C. Gao. 2008a. Preparation and characterization of quaternized chitosan/poly(acrylonitrile) composite nanofiltration membrane from anhydride mixture cross-linking. *Separation and Purification Technology* 58:393–399.

Huang, R.-H., G.-H. Chen, M.-K. Sun, Y.-M. Hu, and C.-J. Gao. 2007. Preparation and characteristics of quaternized chitosan/poly(acrylonitrile) composite nanofiltration membrane from epichlorohydrin cross-linking. *Carbohydrate Polymers* 70:318–323.

Hwang, T., S.-J. Park, Y.-K. Oh, N. Rashid, and J.-I. Han. 2013. Harvesting of *Chlorella* sp. KR-1 using a cross-flow membrane filtration system equipped with an anti-fouling membrane. *Bioresource Technology* 139:379–382.

Jana, S., A. Saikia, M. K. Purkait, and K. Mohanty. 2011. Chitosan based ceramic ultrafiltration membrane: Preparation, characterization and application to remove Hg(II) and As(III) using polymer enhanced ultrafiltration. *Chemical Engineering Journal* 170:209–219.

Jecal, J. and K.-H. Lee. 1996. Development of polyion complex membranes for the separation of water-alcohol mixtures. III. Preparation of polyion complex membranes based on the k-carrageenan for the pervaporation separation of water-ethanol. *Journal of Applied Polymer Science* 60:1177–1183.

Jegal, J. N.-W. Oh, D.-S. Park, and K.-H. Lee. 2001. Characteristics of the nanofiltration composite membranes based on PVA and sodium alginate. *Journal of Applied Polymer Science* 79:2471–2479.

Ji, Y.-L., Q.-F. An, F.-Y. Zhao, and C.-J. Gao. 2015. Fabrication of chitosan/PDMCHEA blend positively charged membranes with improved mechanical properties and high nanofiltration performances. *Desalination* 357:8–15.

Jiang, C., Z. Wang, X. Zhang, X. Zhu, J. Nie and G. Ma. 2014. Crosslinked polyelectrolyte complex fiber membrane based on chitosan–sodium alginate by freeze-drying. *RSC Advances* 4:41551–41560.

Jing, M., L. Lingling, C. Guohua, G. Congjie, and D. Shengxiong. 2008. Preparation of N,O-carboxymethyl chitosan composite nanofiltration membrane and its rejection performance for the fermentation effluent from a wine factory. *Chinese Journal of Chemical Engineering* 16(2):209–213.

Julian, T. N., G. W. Radebaugh, and S. J. Wisniewski. 1988. Permeability characteristics of calcium alginate films. *Journal of Controlled Release* 7:165–169.

Kahya, S., E. K. Solak, and O. Sanlı. 2010. Sodium alginate/poly(vinyl alcohol) alloy membranes for the pervaporation, vapour permeation and vapour permeation with temperature difference separation of dimethylformamide/water mixtures: A comparative study. *Vacuum* 84:1092–1102.

Kalyani, S., B. Smitha, S. Sridhar, and A. Krishnaiah. 2008. Pervaporation separation of ethanol–water mixtures through sodium alginate membranes. *Desalination* 229:68–81.

Karbowiak, T., F. Debeaufort, D. Champion, and A. Voilley. 2006. Wetting properties at the surface of iota-carrageenan-based edible films. *Journal of Colloid and Interface Science* 294(2):400–410.

Karima, Z., A. P. Mathewa, M. Grahn, J. Mouzon, and K. Oksman. 2014. Nanoporous membranes with cellulose nanocrystals as functional entity in chitosan: Removal of dyes from water. *Carbohydrate Polymers* 112:668–676.

Kashima, K. and M. Imai. 2012. Impact factors to regulate mass transfer characteristics of stable alginate membrane performed superior sensitivity on various organic chemicals. *Procedia Engineering* 42:964–977.

Katsoufidou, K., S. G. Yiantsios, and A. J. Karabelas. 2007. Experimental study of ultrafiltration membrane fouling by sodium alginate and flux recovery by backwashing. *Journal of Membrane Science* 300:137–146.

Kim, S.-G., G.-T. Lim, J. Jegal, and K.-H. Lee. 2000. Pervaporation separation of MTBE (methyl tert-butyl ether) and methanol mixtures through polyion complex composite membranes consisting of sodium alginate/chitosan. *Journal of Membrane Science* 174:1–15.

Kumar, M. N. V. R. 2000. A review of chitin and chitosan applications. *Reactive and Functional Polymers* 46:1–27.

Kumar, M. N. V. R., R. A. A. Muzzarelli, C. H. Muzzeralli, and A. J. Sashiwa. 2004. Chitosan chemistry and pharmaceutical perspectives. *Chemical Reviews* 104:6017–6084.

Lai, V. M. F., P. A. L. Wong, and C. Y. Lii. 2000. Effects of cation properties on sol-gel transition and gel properties of κ-carrageenan. *Journal of Food Science* 65:1332–1337.

Lee, Y. M., S. Y. Nam, and D. J. Woo. 1997. Pervaporation of ionically surface crosslinked chitosan composite membranes for water-alcohol mixtures. *Journal of Membrane Science* 133:103–110.

Liu, C. X., D. R. Zhanga, Y. Hea, X. S. Zhaob, and R. Bai. 2010. Modification of membrane surface for anti-biofouling performance: Effect of anti-adhesion and anti-bacteria approaches. *Journal of Membrane Science* 346:121–130.

Liu, Y.-L., C.-H. Yu, K.-R. Lee, and J.-Y. Lai. 2007. Chitosan/poly(tetrafluoroethylene) composite membranes using in pervaporation dehydration processes. *Journal of Membrane Science* 287:230–236.

Liu, Z., X. Ge, Y. Lu, S. Dong, Y. Zhao, and M. Zeng. 2012. Effects of chitosan molecular weight and degree of deacetylation on the properties of gelatine-based films. *Food Hydrocolloids* 26:311–317.

Magalad, V. T. A. R. Supale, S. P. Maradur, G. S. Gokavi, and T. M. Aminabhavi. 2010. Preyssler type heteropolyacid-incorporated highly water-selective sodium alginate-based inorganic–organic hybrid membranes for pervaporation dehydration of ethanol. *Chemical Engineering Journal* 159:75–83.

Mansourpanah, Y., and E. Momeni Habili. 2013. Preparation and modification of thin film PA membranes with improved antifouling property using acrylic acid and UV irradiation. *Journal of Membrane Science* 430:158–166.

Meng, S., and Liu, Y. 2013. Alginate block fraction and their effects on membrane fouling. *Water Research*. 47(17):6618–6627.

Miao, J. L.-C. Zhang, and H. Lin. 2013a. A novel kind of thin film composite nanofiltration membrane with sulfated chitosan as the active layer material. *Chemical Engineering Science* 87:152–159.

Miao, J., G. Chen, C. Gao, and S. Dong. 2008. Preparation and characterization of N, O-carboxymethyl chitosan/Polysulfone composite nanofiltration membrane crosslinked with epichlorohydrin. *Desalination* 233:147–156.

Miao, J., H. Lin, W. Wang, and L.-C. Zhang. 2013b. Amphoteric composite membranes for nanofiltration prepared from sulfated chitosan crosslinked with hexamethylene diisocyanate. *Chemical Engineering Journal* 234:132–139.

Michel, A. S., M. M. Mestdagh, and M. A. V. Axelos. 1997. Physico-chemical properties of carrageenan gels in presence of various cations. *International Journal of Biological Macromolecules* 21:195–200.

Moon, G. Y., R. Pal, and R. Y. M. Huang. 1999. Novel two-ply composite membranes of chitosan and sodium alginate for the pervaporation dehydration of isopropanol and ethanol. *Journal of Membrane Science* 156:17–27.

Mulder, M. 2000. Phase inversion membranes. In: *Membrane Preparation, University of Twente, Enschede*, pp. 3331–3346. The Netherlands: Academic Press.

Musale, D. A., A. Kumar, and G. Pleizier. 1999. Formation and characterization of poly(acrylonitrile)/chitosan composite ultrafiltration membranes. *Journal of Membrane Science* 154:163–173.

Nigiz, F. U. and N. D. Hilmioglu. 2013. Pervaporation of ethanol/water mixtures by zeolite filled sodium alginate membrane. *Desalination and Water Treatment* 51:637–643.

Patil, M. B., R. S. Veerapura, S. D. Bhata, C. D. Madhusoodanab, and T. M. Aminabhavi. 2009. Hybrid composite membranes of sodium alginate for pervaporation dehydration of 1,4-dioxane and tetrahydrofuran. *Desalination and Water Treatment* 3:11–20.

Quadros, C., V. W. Faria, M. P. Klein, P. F. Hertz, and C. W. Scheeren. 2013. Chitosan/carboxymethylcellulose/ionic liquid/Ag(0) nanoparticles form a membrane with antimicrobial activity. *Journal of Nanotechnology* 2013:1–9.

Quist-Jensen, C. A., F. Macedonio, and E. Drioli. 2015. Membrane technology for water production in agriculture: Desalination and wastewater reuse. *Desalination* 364:17–32.

Rahimi, Z., A. A. Zinatizadeh, and S. Zinadini. 2014. Preparation and characterization of a high antibiofouling ultrafiltration PES membrane using OCMCS-Fe3O4 for application in MBR treating wastewater. *Journal of Applied Research in Water and Wastewater* 1:13–17.

Kumar, R., A. M. Isloor, A. F. Ismail, S. A. Rashid and T. Matsuura. 2013. Polysulfone–chitosan blend ultrafiltration membranes: Preparation, characterization, permeation and antifouling properties. *RSC Advances* 3:7855–7861.

Redondo, J. A., and I. Lomax. 2001. Y2K generation FILMTEC RO membranes combined with new pretreatment techniques to treat raw water with high fouling potential: Summary of experience. *Desalination* 136:287–306.

Rinaudo, M. 2006. Chitin and chitosan: Properties and applications. *Progress in Polymer Science* 31(7):603–632.

Sajankumar ji Rao, U., K. V. Sekharnath, Y. Maruthi, P. KumaraBabu, K. Chowdoji Rao and M. C. S. Subha. 2015. Mixed matrix blend membranes of sodium alginate—Hydroxy propyl cellulose loaded with halloysite nano clay used in pervaporation technique for dehydration of isopropanol Mixture at 30°C. *International Journal of Engineering Sciences & Research Technology* 4(1):653–662.

Sejal, S. J., and R. N. Desai. 2013. Polymer membrane technology. *International Journal of Engineering Science and Innovative Technology* 2(2):400–403.

Shahidi, F., J. K. V. Arachchi, and Y-J. Jeon. 1999. Food applications of chitin and chitosans. *Trends in Food Science Technology* 10:37–51.

Shenvi, S. S., S. A. Rashid, A. F. Ismail, M. A. Kassim, and A. M. Isloor. 2013. Preparation and characterization of PPEES/chitosan composite nanofiltration membrane. *Desalination* 315:135–141.

Shiyan H., G. Fang, S. Li, G. Liu and G. Jiang. 2014. Cu(II) ion adsorption onto hydroxymethylated lignin-chitosan crosslinked membrane. *BioResources* 9(3):4971–4980.

Solak, E. K. and O. Şanlı. 2011. Separation performance of sodium alginate/poly(vinyl pyrrolidone) membranes for aqueous/dimethylformamide mixtures by vapor permeation and vapor permeation with temperature difference methods. *Advances in Chemical Engineering and Science* 1:305–312.

Srinivasa Rao, P., A. Krishnaiah, B. Smitha, and S. Sridhar. 2006. Separation of acetic acid/water mixtures by pervaporation through poly(vinyl alcohol)–sodium alginate blend membranes. *Separation Science and Technology* 41:979–999.

Sudha, P. N., P. A. Vinodhini, K. Sangeetha, S. Latha, T. Gomathi, J. Venkatesan, and S. K. Kim. 2014. Fabrication of cellulose acetate-chitosan-polyethylene glycol ultrafiltration membrane for chromium removal. *Der Pharmacia Lettre* 6(1):37–46.

Sun, H., G. Chen, R. Huang, and C. Gao. 2007. A novel composite nanofiltration (NF) membrane prepared from glycolchitin/poly(acrylonitrile) (PAN) by epichlorohydrin crosslinking. *Journal of Membrane Science* 297:51–58.

Waheed, S., A. Ahmad, S. M. Khan, Sabad-e- Gul, T. Jamil, A. Islam, and T. Hussain. 2014. Synthesis, characterization, permeation and antibacterial properties of cellulose acetate/polyethylene glycol membranes modified with chitosan. *Desalination* 351:59–69.

Wan Ngah, W. S., S. A. Ghani, and L. L. Hoon. 2002. Comparative adsorption of lead(II) on flake and bead-types of chitosan. *Journal of the Chinese Chemical Society* 49:625–628.

Wang, C., F. Yang, and H. Zhang. 2010. Fabrication of non-woven composite membrane by chitosan coating for resisting the adsorption of proteins and the adhesion of bacteria. *Separation and Purification Technology* 75:358–365.

Wang, W., Y. Zhang, M. Esparra-Alvarado, X. Wang, H. Yang, and Y. Xie. 2014. Effects of pH and temperature on forward osmosis membrane flux using rainwater as the makeup for cooling water dilution. *Desalination* 351:70–76.

Wang, X., and H. G. Spencer. 1998. Formation and characterization of chitosan formed-in-place ultrafiltration membranes. *Journal of Applied Polymer Science* 67:513–519.

Wang, X.-P. 2000. Modified alginate composite membranes for the dehydration of acetic acid. *Journal of Membrane Science* 170:71–79.

Wang, Y., F. Zhang, Y. Chu, B. Gao and Q. Yue. 2013. The dye or humic acid water treatment and membrane fouling by polyaluminum chloride composited with sodium alginate in coagulation–ultrafiltration process. *Water Science & Technology* 67(10):2202–2209.

Wu, P. and M. Imai. 2013. Excellent dyes removal and remarkable molecular size rejection of novel biopolymer composite membrane. *Desalination and Water Treatment* 51:5237–5247.

Wu, P., and M. Imai. 2012. Outstanding molecular size recognition and regulation of water permeability on κ-carrageenan-pullulan membrane involved in synergistic design of composite polysaccharides structure. *Procedia Engineering* 42:1313–1325.

Xu, J. B., J. P. Bartley, and R. A. Johnson. 2003. Preparation and characterization of alginate–carrageenan hydrogel films crosslinked using a water-soluble carbodiimide (WSC). *Journal of Membrane Science* 218:131–146.

Yang, J. M., W. Y. Su, T. L. Leu, and M. C. Yang. 2004. Evaluation of chitosan/PVA blended hydrogel membranes. *Journal of Membrane Science* 236:39–51.

Yoon, K., K. Kim, X. Wang, D. Fang, B. S. Hsiao, and B. Chu. 2006. High flux ultrafiltration membranes based on electrospun nanofibrous PAN scaffolds and chitosan coating. *Polymer* 47:2434–2441.

Zhang, X., B. Lin, K. Zhao, J.Wei, J. Guo, W. Cui, S. Jiang, D. Liu, and J. Li. 2015. A freestanding calciumalginate/polyacrylamide hydrogel nanofiltration membrane with high anti-fouling performance: Preparation and characterization. *Desalination* 365:234–241.

Zhang, X., X. Jin, C. Xu, and X. Shen. 2013. Preparation and characterization of glutaraldehyde crosslinked chitosan nanofiltration membrane. *Journal of Applied Polymer Science* 128:3665–3671.

Zoua, L., I. Vidalis, D. Steele, A. Michelmore, S. P. Low, and J. Q. J. C. Verberk. 2011. Surface hydrophilic modification of RO membranes by plasma polymerization for low organic fouling. *Journal of Membrane Science* 369:420–428.

21 Chitin and Its Derivatives in the Remediation of Industrial Effluent

M. Saranya, T. Gomathi, G. Saraswathi, and P.N. Sudha

CONTENTS

21.1   INTRODUCTION

It has been more than two centuries since chitin was discovered formally and considered very important from the scientific and industrial point of view, as it has much utilization in many different areas.

The development of mercantile applications for chitin has progressed. The first known use of chitosan was as a durable, flexible film used as a component in the varnish applied to Stradivarius violins; however, new efforts are changing its vision in the market. The emphasis on environmentally friendly technology has stimulated interest in biopolymers, which are more versatile and far more biodegradable than their synthetic counterparts. This chapter highlights the basic brainwave of chemistry and the application of this polysaccharide that is gaining much interest due to the properties it presents and the many applications in various fields. Thousands of scientific articles have been reported in the last 20 years, where companies appeared to engage and exploit this material worldwide. Through investigation, many questions have arisen but those have not yet been answered; however, this polysaccharide has been very successful in many operations.

Chitin is a naturally occurring nitrogen-containing polysaccharide related chemically to cellulose poly-β-(1$\rightarrow$4)-N-acetyl-D-glucosamine (Austin et al. 1981). Chitin and its derivatives find applications in various fields, mainly paper making, textiles printing and sizing, flocculation, ion-exchange chromatography, removal of metal ions from industrial effluents, manufacture of pharmaceuticals and cosmetics, and as an additive in the food industry (Ramachandran Nair 1994).

Chitin occurs in three polymorphic forms, which differ in the arrangement of molecular chains within the crystal cell. α-Chitin is the tightly compacted, most crystalline polymorphic form, in which the chains are arranged in an antiparallel fashion. β-Chitin is the form in which the chains are parallel, and γ-chitin is the form in which two chains are "up" to everyone "down" (Vaaje-Kolstad et al. 2005). The unique properties of chitin and its derivative chitosan include solubility behavior in various media, that is, solution viscosity; polyelectrolyte behavior; polyoxysalt formation; ability to form films and chelate metal ions; and optical and structural characteristics (Madhavan 1992). Chitin and its derivatives hold great economic value because of their versatile biological activities and chemical applications (Andrade et al. 2003).

Industries such as paper and pulp mills, dyestuff, distilleries, and tanneries are also producing highly colored wastewaters. It is in the textile industry that the largest quantities of aqueous wastes and dye effluents are discharged from the dyeing process, with both strong persistent color and a high biochemical oxygen demand (BOD), both of which are aesthetically and environmentally unacceptable (Wang et al. 2007). Industrial revolution accelerated developments in all fields such as technology, automobile, and textile. As a result, large amounts of metal ions are being released into the environment on a daily basis. Mining operations, metal-plating facilities, power generation facilities, electronic device manufacturing units, and tanneries release toxic metal ions into waste streams. Among the current pollution control technologies, biodegradation of synthetic dyes by various microbes is emerging as an effective and promising approach. The bioremediation potential of microbes and their enzymes acting on synthetic dyes has been demonstrated, with others needing to be explored in the future as alternatives to conventional physicochemical approaches (Husain 2006; Ali 2010). It is obvious that each process has its own constraints in terms of cost, feasibility, practicability, reliability, stability, environmental impact, sludge production, operational difficulty, pretreatment requirements, the extent of the organic removal, and potential toxic by-products. In addition, the use of a single process may not completely decolorize the wastewater and degrade the dye molecules.

Recently, numerous approaches have been studied for the development of cheaper and more effective adsorbents containing natural polymer. Among these biopolymers, chitosan is particularly an excellent adsorbent. Properties of chitin and its derivatives deserve particular attention and are used for the treatment of tannery wastewater due to its particular structure, physicochemical characteristics, chemical stability, high reactivity, and excellent selectivity toward metal and aromatic compounds, resulting from the presence of chemical reactive groups in polymer chains. Moreover, it is well known that polysaccharides that are renewable, abundant, and biodegradable have a capacity to associate physical and chemical interactions with a wide variety of molecules.

Furthermore, this chapter aims to convince young readers to further research on the possible technology that tends to care for the environment and remediation of industrial effluent.

21.2   WHY IS REMEDIATION OF INDUSTRIAL EFFLUENT NECESSARY?

Huge industrial establishments and their indiscriminate discharges pose a great threat to our environment. Industrial wastewater not only deteriorates the quality of soil, crop, and environment but also is directly harmful to the human, animal, and aquatic lives. Unplanned discharges of wastewater from industries degrade the quality of food crops. The total land irrigated with raw or partially diluted wastewater has been estimated to be about 20 million hectares in 50 countries, which is approximately 10% of the total irrigated land (FAO 2003).

Heavy metal toxicity can cause chronic and degenerative conditions. General symptoms include headache, short-term memory loss, mental confusion, sense of unreality, distorted perception, pain in muscles and joints, and gastrointestinal upsets, food intolerances, allergies, vision problems, chronic fatigue, and fungal infections. Sometimes, the symptoms are vague and difficult to diagnose (Sahni 2011). In order to provide a remedy, techniques such as solvent extraction, ion-exchange process, membrane filtration, electrodeposition, and solid-phase extraction based on adsorption are important for preconcentration and separation of trace metal ions (Peñaranda and Sabino 2010) that are present in the industrial effluents.

The presence of heavy metal ions in various water resources has stirred great concern because of their high toxicity and nonbiodegradability (Monier 2012). They leach out from waste dumps and pollute soils, thereby entering the food chain. Bioaccumulation, a phenomenon by which metals increase in concentration at every level of the food chain and are passed onto the next higher level, may also result (Monier and Abdel-Latif 2013). It is well known that heavy metals can damage the nerves, liver, and bones, and they block functional groups of essential enzymes (Hadi 2012).

21.2.1 THE EFFECTS OF INDUSTRIAL DISCHARGE ON FRESHWATER

The industrial discharge carries various types of contaminants to the river, lake, and groundwater. The quality of freshwater is very important, as it is highly consumed by humans for drinking, bathing, irrigation, and so on.

River is a system that includes the main course and its tributaries. The water chemistry of a river is affected by the lithology of the reservoir, atmospheric, and anthropogenic inputs. Furthermore, the transport of natural and anthropogenic sources to the oceans and their state during land–sea interaction can be determined by the quality of water from rivers and estuaries. The studies conducted by Jonathan et al. (2008) noted that there is relationship between the water particle interactions and solution chemistry, such as flocculation, organic and inorganic complexation, adsorption, and sediment resuspension.

21.2.2 THE EFFECTS OF INDUSTRIAL DISCHARGE ON GROUNDWATER

Groundwater is regarded as the largest reservoir of drinkable water for mankind. To many countries, groundwater is one of the major sources of water supply for domestic, industrial, and agricultural sectors. In India, groundwater supplies more than 50% for irrigation and 80% for drinking water (Singh et al. 2009).

21.2.3 THE EFFECTS OF INDUSTRIAL DISCHARGE ON LAND

Kisku et al. (2000) noted that for soil contaminated by industrial discharge could accumulate toxic metals such as iron (Fe), zinc (Zn), copper (Cu), and manganese (Mn) these are the trace elements essential to plant life, whereas lead (Pb), chromium (Cr), nickel (Ni), and cadmium (Cd) are toxic even at a very low concentration.

21.2.4 THE EFFECTS OF INDUSTRIAL DISCHARGE ON SEAWATER

Metals that have altered biogeochemically along the flows from river to estuaries and coastal area are transported to the ocean, and the original composition of seawater and sediments is altered (Jonathan et al. 2008).

21.2.5 THE IMPACT ON HUMAN HEALTH

High concentrations of Al can cause hazard to brain function such as memory damage and convulsions. In addition, there are studies suggesting that Al is linked to Alzheimer disease (Jordao et al. 2002). Cadmium is harmful to both human health and aquatic ecosystems. It is carcinogenic, embryotoxic, teratogenic, and mutagenic and may cause hyperglycemia, reduced immunopotency, and anemia, as it interferences with iron metabolism (Rehman and Anjum 2010). Furthermore, in the body, Cd has been shown to result in kidney and liver damages and deformation of bone structures (Alkarkhi et al. 2008). Iron is an essential element in several biochemical and enzymatic processes. It is involved in the transport of oxygen to cells. However, at high concentration, it can increase the production of free radicals, which are responsible for degenerative diseases and ageing (Jordao et al. 2002). High potassium concentration may cause nervous and digestive disorders (Purushotham et al. 2011), kidney heart disease, coronary artery disease, hypertension, diabetes, adrenal insufficiency, and preexisting hyperkalemia. Infants may also experience renal reserve and immature kidney function (WHO 2009). High concentration of fluoride can cause dental and skeletal fluorosis such as mottling of teeth, deformation of ligaments, and bending of the spinal cord (Raju et al. 2009).

21.3 WASTEWATER TREATMENT

In Japan, chitin was first used for wastewater treatment because of its metal-binding properties. It is also good for cleaning up toxic organic compounds.

21.3.1 TYPES OF INDUSTRIAL WASTEWATER

There are many types of industrial wastewater based on the different industries and the contaminants; each sector produces its own particular combination of pollutants (see Table 21.1).

TABLE 21.1
Types of Sectors and Pollutants

Sector	Pollutant
Iron and steel	biochemical oxygen demand (BOD), chemical oxygen demand (COD), oil, metals, acids, phenols, and cyanide
Textiles and leather	BOD, solids, sulfates, and chromium
Pulp and paper	BOD, COD, solids, and chlorinated organic compounds
Petrochemicals and refineries	BOD, COD, mineral oils, phenols, and chromium
Chemicals	COD, organic chemicals, heavy metals, SS, and cyanide
Nonferrous metals	Fluorine and suspended solids (SS)
Microelectronics	COD and organic chemicals
Mining	SS, metals, acids, and salts

The pulp and paper industry relies heavily on chlorine-based substances, and as a result, pulp and paper mill effluents contain chloride organics and dioxins, as well as suspended solids and organic wastes. Chlorinated organic compounds, produced during the chlorination bleaching phase, are made soluble in dilute alkali and are extracted from pulp in the subsequent eraction phase (Prasad and Joyce 1991). Photoprocessing shops produce silver, dry cleaning and car repair shops generate solvent waste, and printing plants release inks and dyes The metal-working industries discharge chromium, nickel, zinc, cadmium, lead, iron, and titanium compounds; among them, the electroplating industry is an important pollution distributor.

The wastewater produced from pharmaceutical industry has a very bad quality for wastewater treatment. Usually, the concentration of chemical oxygen demand (COD) is around 5000 to 1500 mg/L, the concentration of BOD_5 is relative low, and the ratio of BOD_5/COD is lower than 30%, which means that the wastewater has a poor biodegradability. Such wastewater has bad color and high (or low) pH value, and it needs a strong, permanent method, followed by a biological treatment process with a long reaction time.

The petrochemical industry discharges a lot of phenols and mineral oils. Moreover, wastewater from food-processing plants is high in suspended solids and organic material. Like the various characteristics of industrial wastewater, the treatment of industrial wastewater must be designed specifically for the particular type of effluent produced.

21.4   CHITIN

Chitin with $(C_8H_{13}O_5N)_n$ is a long-chain polymer of N-acetylglucosamine, a derivative of glucose, and is found in many places throughout the natural world. It is a characteristic component of the cell walls of fungi, the exoskeletons of arthropods such as crustaceans (e.g., crabs, lobsters, and shrimps) and insects, the radulae of mollusks, and the beaks and internal shells of cephalopods, including squid and octopuses. The structure of chitin is comparable to the polysaccharide cellulose, forming crystalline nanofibrils or whiskers. In terms of function, it may be compared to the protein keratin. Chitin has also proven to be useful for several medical and industrial purposes.

In butterfly wing scales, chitin is often organized into stacks of nanolayers or nanosticks made of chitin nanocrystals that produce various iridescent colors by thin-film interference: similar, analogous structures made of keratin are found in iridescent bird plumage.

21.4.1   PROPERTIES AND STRUCTURE OF CHITIN

Chitin is highly hydrophobic and is insoluble in water and most organic solvents. It is soluble in hexafluoroisopropanol, hexafluoroacetone, and chloroalcohols, in conjunction with aqueous solutions of mineral acids and dimethylacetamide (DMAc) containing 5% lithium chloride (LiCl) (Dutta et al. 2003).

Chitin is a white, hard, inelastic, nitrogenous polysaccharide found in the exoskeleton as well as in the internal structure of invertebrates. The waste of these natural polymers is a major source of surface pollution in coastal areas.

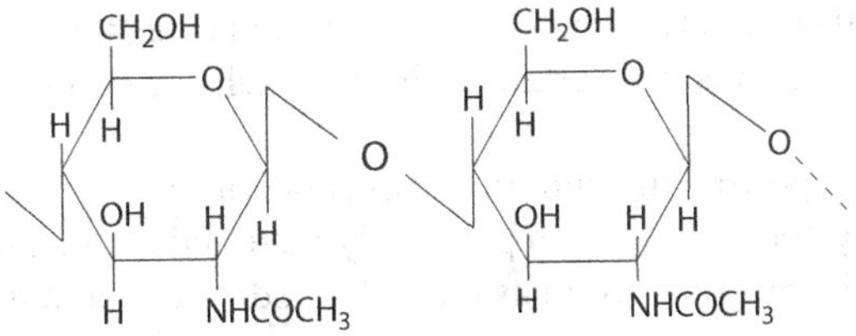

FIGURE 21.1 Structure of chitin.

Chitin is structurally similar to cellulose, but it has acetamide groups at the C-2 positions instead of hydroxyl groups. Therefore, it is a nitrogen (amido/amino)-containing polysaccharide, with repeating units of 2-acetamido/amino-2-deoxy-(1 4)-β-D-glucopyranose (Figure 21.1). In addition to its unique polysaccharide architecture, the presence of little amino groups (5%–15%) in chitin (Van Luyen et al. 1996; Peter 2002) is highly advantageous for providing distinctive biological functions and for conducting modification reactions.

21.4.2 DERIVATIVES OF CHITIN

Chitin can be either partially or completely hydrolyzed via chemical or enzymatic methods. Partial hydrolysis produces chitooligosaccharides. N-acetyl-glucosamine and glucosamine monomers are obtained on complete hydrolysis. Glycol chitin, a partially o-hydroxyethylated chitin, was the first derivative of practical importance.

Derivatives of chitin may be classified into two categories; in each case, the N-acetyl groups are removed, and the exposed amino function then reacts either with acyl chlorides or anhydrides to give the group NHCOR or is modified by reductive amination to NHCH$_2$COOH of greatest potential importance are derivatives of both types formed by reaction with bi- or polyfunctional reagents, thus carrying sites for further chemical reaction. Special attention has been given to chemical modification chitin, since it has the greatest potential to be fully exploited. With pure form of chitin, reactions are carried out mostly in the solid state, owing to the lack of solubility in ordinary solvents. A 50% deacetylated chitin has been found to be soluble in water (Peter et al. 2000; Dutta et al. 2002).

For smooth modification, water-soluble form of chitin is a useful starting material through various reactions in the solution phase. Some of the very recently reported chitin derivatives are enumerated as follows.

21.5 MULTIPLE MODIFICATION OF CHITIN

There are some cases in which:

1. The reactivity of chitin is insufficient to participate in the desired reaction.
2. The modified chitin does not possess the desired properties.
3. Some site(s) of chitin must be protected (and finally deprotected) to sustain during the modification reaction(s).

In such instants, there are two general approaches via chemical modification when the graft polymerization is in a certain pathway to achieve desired characteristics:

1. *In situ* and/or posttreatment of the graft copolymer.
2. Graft copolymerization onto a previously modified chitin. So, the products may generally be preferred to as multiply modified materials.

21.5.1 Carboxymethyl Chitin (CM-Chitin)

The preparation of carboxymethyl chitin (CM-chitin) is also an extension from the preparation of carboxymethyl cellulose (CM cellulose). Similar to the preparation of CM cellulose, chitin was activated by alkaline treatment. The typical procedure of preparing CM-chitin involves two stages:

1. Preparation of the alkali-chitin slurry.
2. Reaction of the alkali-chitin with chloroacetic acid.
3. The use of isopropanol improved the carboxymethylation reaction; however, partial N-deacetylation was an unavoidable consequence. The biodegradability of CM-chitin was significantly greater than chitin and was attributed to the high degree of substitution.

Traditional methods to generate a variety of derivatized chitins have mainly used strong bases or acids under heterogeneous conditions. Treatment of chitin with concentrated base, typically NaOH, gives alkali-chitin, which can act as a nucleophile in SN2 reactions with various electrophilic reagents. A good example is the preparation of 6-O-CM-chitin.

21.5.2 6-Deoxy-Di(Carboxy)Methyl Chitin

A total of 0.33 g of tert-butoxide (3 mmol) was dissolved in 10 mL anhydrous dimethyl sulfoxide (DMSO) and added to 6-deoxy-diethylmalonate-chitin, with a substitution degree of 0.62 (0.30 g, ~1 mmol)/30 ml DMSO solution. Deionized water (0.4 mL) was added to catalyze the reaction carried out at ambient temperature for 16 h. The reaction mixture was dialyzed against water for 72 h and acidified to a pH value of 2. The precipitate was filtered and dried at 50°C to give 0.12 g of a brown-colored product. The yield was 75%.

21.5.3 6-O-Carboxyphenyl Chitin

Potassium tert-butoxide (0.43 g, 3.9 mmol) was dissolved in 10 mL of anhydrous dimethyl sulfoxide (DMSO) and added to 20 mL of 6-O-ethylbenzoate chitin (Degree of substitution DS = 0.66, 0.40 g, ~1.3 mmol)/DMSO 53 solution. Deionized (0.4 mL) water was added to catalyze the reaction performed at ambient temperature for 8 h. The reaction mixture was dialyzed against water for 72 h, acidified to a pH value of 2, and filtered. The precipitate was freeze-dried to give 0.28 g of product. The yield was 80%.

21.5.4 6-O-Sulfated Chitin

A quantity of 0.4 g of purified chitin (c.a. 2 mmol) was stirred in 30 mL of 5% LiCl/DMAc until dissolution was complete. Then, 2.0 g of sulfur trioxide–pyridine complex (c.a. 12 mmol) was predissolved in 10 mL of 5% LiCl/DMAc and transferred into chitin solution by syringe. The reaction proceeded at room temperature for the given reaction time. After reaction, the reaction mixture was poured into 250 mL of acetone, and the white fibrous precipitate was filtered out and redissolved into 80 mL water. The obtained solution was adjusted to pH $\approx$ 10 with 5% NaOH solution and dialyzed against water for 72 h. The dialyzed solution was filtered and concentrated to 30 mL by rotary evaporation. To the concentrated solution, 100 mL of acetone was added, and the precipitate was collected either by direct filtration or by centrifugation, depending on the molecular weight. The obtained precipitate was dried at 50°C overnight, ground as powder, and stored in a desiccator until used.

21.5.5 Dibutyryl Chitin

Shrimp shell's chitin powder with particle size of 200 mesh and viscosity average molar mass $M_v = 454{,}6 \times 10^3$ g/mol was delivered by FRANCE CHITIN, Marseille, France. The synthesis of dibutyryl chitin (DBC) was carried out under heterogeneous conditions by using chitin, butyric anhydride, and 72% perchloric acid in approximate proportion equal to 10:50:6.8 (g/g). The intrinsic viscosity value of DBC determined in DMAc solutions at 25°C was 1.70 dL/g and the weight average molar mass, determined by size-exclusion chromatography (SEC) method coupled with light scattering and viscometry, was $M_w = 132 \times 10^3$ g/mol.

Another possible reaction to produce DBC is the so-called homogeneous reaction in methane sulfonic acid. Intrinsic viscosity value of the obtained DBC by the homogeneous reaction determined in DMAc solutions with DBC was 5.70 dL/g and the corresponding weight average molar mass was 456 10^3 g/mol.

A DBC with a higher molecular weight was obtained by the homogeneous reaction in methane sulfonic acid. The starting chitin has a mean amount of 2800 monomers in the polymer chain. The mean amount of monomers for the DBC obtained by the homogeneous reaction is 1340, and for the DBC obtained from the heterogeneous reaction, it is 450. The water-soluble chitin derivative has less degradation of the polymer chains for the homogeneous reaction than for the heterogeneous reaction with confirmed biological properties.

Dibutyryl chitin is obtained in the reaction of shrimp chitin with butyric anhydride, under heterogeneous condition, in which perchloric acid was used as a catalyst (Szumilewicz and Szosland 2000).

21.5.6 Hydroxymethyl Chitin

Modification of chitin is also often affected via water-soluble derivatives of chitin (mainly CM-chitin). The same type of chemical modifications (etherification and esterification) as for cellulose can be performed on the available C-6 and C-3 –OH groups of chitin (Rinaudo and Reguant 2000).

21.5.7 Hydroxyethyl Chitin

Hydroxyethylation (or glycolation) of chitin is affected by treating alkali chitin with ethylene oxide to give hydroxyethyl chitins or glycol chitins. However, the reaction is carried out under strongly alkaline conditions; N-deacetylation also takes place at the same time (Kurita et al. 1999).

21.5.8 Phosphoryl Chitin

Chitin was phosphorylated according to the method of Lehrfeld (1997). Five grams of oven-dried chitin was suspended in 40 mL of pyridine and cooled to 8°C. A total of 20 mL of dichloromethane containing 5 mL of phosphorus oxychloride was added to the previous mixture and heated at 115°C for 2 h. The mixture was filtered, and the phosphorylated material was washed with 0.1N HCl, distilled water, and methanol and was air-dried.

21.5.9 Tosyl Chitin

The synthesis of tosyl chitin was first reported by Kurita et al. (1991). The degree of substitution of the tosylation reaction was closely correlated with the concentration of tosyl chloride, and complete substitution was obtained with 20 folds of tosyl chloride. Tosyl chitin was found to be hydrophilic when the degree of substitution (DS) was less than 0.3 but became hydrophobic and soluble in polar organic solvents when the DS was more than 0.4. N-deacetylation was observed during the reaction due to the use of strong base.

21.5.10 6-Deoxy Chitin

Deoxy chitin is synthesized by using sodium borohydride with tosyl chitin. Complete reduction of tosyl chitin to 6-deo xychitin was accomplished at a temperature less than 80°C for 5 h; this was confirmed by the absence of sulfur (Kurita et al. 1991).

21.5.11 O-Acetyl Chitin

O-Acetyl chitin was synthesized and subjected to graft copolymerization with MMA via a photo-induced grafting by Morita et al. (1997). They conducted the noncatalytic reaction in a rotary photochemical reactor irradiating UV light with a 160 W low-pressure mercury lamp at distance of 75 mm. A grafting percentage ~490% was achieved under optimized conditions: O-acetyl-chitin (DS, 0.81) 0.15 g, H_2O 10 mL, MMA-2 mL, temperature 50°C, and irradiation time 4 h.

21.5.12 Mercapto Chitin

Mercapto chitin was prepared in a two-step reaction. Tosyl chitin was first converted to thioacetyl chitin using potassium thioacetate, and the S-acetyl group was removed with alkali treatment to yield mercapto chitin. Similar to iodochitin, mercapto chitin was graft-copolymerized with styrene (Ruiz et al. 2000), and the grafting percentage could reach 1000%.

21.5.13   IODO CHITIN

Iodination of tosyl chitin was achieved by sodium iodide in DMSO. Although replacement was not complete at 60°C, reaction at less than 80°C for 24 h showed little residue of sulfur. The resulting iodo chitin was further graft-polymerized with styrene either via cationic or radical activation, and the resulting graft polymers based on chitin showed good solubility or swellability (Kurita et al. 1992).

21.5.14   CHITOSAN

Chitosan is one of the most important derivatives of chitin obtained after partial deacetylation of chitin, which has been employed for a variety of applications in diverse fields for its various appealing applications. The positive aspects of chitosan include its biocompatibility, biodegradability, and nontoxicity. Chitin is soluble in aqueous acidic media (pH < 6.0) at about 50% degree of deacetylation (DDA) and is called chitosan. Chitosan is produced from chitin by deacetylation with highly concentrated (40%–50%) solutions of sodium hydroxide at high temperatures (100°C–1500°C), exclusive of air, for about an hour (Johnson and Peniston 1982).

21.5.15   CARBOXYMETHYL CHITOSAN

Carboxymethylation was carried out by stirring chitosan (5 g) in 20% NaOH (w/v, 100 mL) for 15 minutes, and then, monochloroacetic acid (15 g) was added dropwise to the reaction mixture and the reaction was continued for 2 h at 40°C $\pm$ 2°C with stirring. Then, the reaction mixture was neutralized with 10% acetic acid and poured into an excess of 70% methanol. The produced carboxymethyl chitosan (CMCh) was filtered using a G2 sintered funnel and was washed with methanol. The product was dried in vacuum at 55°C for 8 h to give 6.5 g of dried CMCh. The degree of substitution of CMCh was determined to be 0.75 according to the method described in literature (Wu et al. 2003).

21.5.16   N-TRIMETHYLENE CHLORIDE CHITOSAN

N-trimethylene chloride (TMC) is a quaternary derivative of chitosan (CS), and it has a superior aqueous solubility, intestinal permeability, and higher absorption over a wide pH range. The TMC polymers are designated according to their degree of methylation such as TMC-20%, TMC-40%, and TMC-60%. The trimethylene chloride (TMC) solubility decreases with high degrees of substitution, (Hamman et al. 2002) demonstrated that quaternization of TMC decreases the transepithelial electrical resistance and thereby influences its drug absorption-enhancing properties.

21.5.17   DICHLOROACETYL CHITOSAN

Chitosan solution was prepared by dissolving 1.0 g chitosan in 2% dilute acetic acid (100 mL), with constant stirring at room temperature. Dichloroacetyl chitosan (DCAC) (5 mL) was added dropwise to the homogenous mixture, with continuous stirring at the same temperature. The reaction was carried out for 15, 30, and 45 minutes in separate batches. The reaction was ceased by adding the mixture to MeOH to precipitate out the derivatives. The excess acid was neutralized by sodium bicarbonate, followed by filtration.

21.5.18 LAUROYLCHITOSAN

1 gram of chitosan was dissolved in methane sulfonic acid (100 mL) for 1 h at room temperature. To this solution, lauroyl chloride (3 equi./sugar unit of CS) was added, followed by addition of triethanolamine (TEA). After this, the mixture was stirred at room temperature for 5 h; 30 g of crushed ice was added to stop the reaction. The acidic mixture was dialyzed for 1 h to remove most of the acids, followed by neutralizing the remaining acids by TEA in CS with sodium bicarbonate. Finally, the mixture was again lyophilized for more than three days. The above reaction was also carried out under the same conditions, without the addition of TEA.

Table 21.2 shows various applications of chitin and its derivatives. Among these applications, chitin and its derivatives have major utilization in wastewater treatment from industries, which cause hazards in the environment; these have been briefly discussed in this chapter.

21.6 DIFFERENT TECHNIQUES FOR TREATMENT OF INDUSTRIAL EFFLUENTS

Chemical, biological, and physical processes for wastewater treatment are currently the most commonly used methods of treating aqueous hazardous waste. Chemical treatment converted waste into less hazardous substance by using various techniques such as flocculation, oxidation or reduction, flotation, electroflotation, membrane filtration, ion exchange, irradiation, precipitation, ozonation, adsorption, and chemical precipitation. Biological treatment uses microorganisms to degrade organic compounds in the waste stream. Processes of physical treatment include gravity separation; phase-change system, such as air and stream stripping of volatiles from liquid waste; and various filtration operations, including adsorption.

21.7 APPLICATIONS IN REMEDIATION OF EFFLUENT

Unplanned industrialization, urbanization, and rapid growth of population affect the aquatic environment. The heavy metals render the water unsuitable for drinking and are also highly toxic to human beings. In order to remove copper from wastewater by using natural biopolymers, Saravanan and Sudha (2014) had examined adsorption using chitin–bentonite composite. It was also observed that the chitin–bentonite composite always had greater adsorption capacities.

The potential use of chitin, prepared from shrimp shells, is for the removal of Reactive Black 5 (RB5), an anionic dye from simulated wastewater. The technique used to remove RB5 is the adsorption method. The adsorption increases with the increment of the initial concentration of RB5 solution. The amount of adsorption

TABLE 21.2
Field of Application of Chitin and Its Derivatives

Field of Application	Applications
Water treatment	Chelation of metal ions, pesticides, phenols, dyes, DTT, PCBs, proteins, and amino acids; detoxifying water from oil and greases; and determination of lead in water samples
Textile industry	Wool finishing, dyeing improvement, textile preservative, and deodorant agent; textile printing and antimicrobial finishing; flocculants; and dye removal from textile wastewater
Wood industry	Wood adhesive, preservative, protector, fungicide, improvement of wood quality, and remediation of waste wood
Cement industry	Water proofing and water repellent
Miscellaneous industries	Leather, plastics, cigarettes, and solid-state batteries
Paper manufacture and photography	Filter for water purification, biodegradable packaging for food and agricultural products, surface treatment, paper sizing and finishing, water-resistant paper, wrapping and toilet paper, card board, hard sheets, paper improvement agent, chromatography paper, printing, fixing agent for color photography, filling agent, and color film
Environment pollution control	Ecofriendly; treatment of industrial, nuclear, and food-processing wastes; flocculation, precipitation, and capturing of pollutants from sewage; and decontamination and removal of hazardous pollutants from marine environment
Food industry and feed additives	Food preservative, antioxidant, emulsifier, thickener, stabilizer, cryoprotectant, clarifier, viscosifier, gelling agent, flavor extender, livestock, and fish-feed additive
Genetic engineering	Gene carrier and DNA vaccine delivery, and protects DNA from DNAase degradation
Agriculture	Seed and fruit coating, fertilizer, biopesticide and fungicide, growth enhancers, stimulator for plant hormones responsible for root formation, stem growth, and fruit development
Cosmetics/toiletries	Hydrating agent, moisturizer; bath lotion; face, hand, and body creams; skin and hair products (skin creams, shampoos, lacquers, varnishes, soap, and so on); oral care; fragrances; and men's toiletries
Dietetique	Antifats, hypocholesterolemic, dietary fiber, weight loss, no caloric value
Pharmacology and para-pharmaceuticals	Drug delivery, excipient, decrease toxicity, sustained drug release, cottons, sponges, bandages, plasters, films, fibers, and wetting agent
Dentistry	Dental surgery and therapy, dental materials, dental creams, and dental plague inhibitor
Medicine/veterinary	Artificial skin and blood vessels; surgical sutures; orthopedics; contact lenses; hemodialysis; treatment of renal failure, tumors, leukemia, and hypoinsulinemia; wound healing; bone regeneration accelerator; control of AIDS virus; and treatment of burns
Biotechnology	Immobilization of cells and enzymes, matrix for affinity and gel permeation chromatography, cell culture, substrates for enzymes, biosensor construction, membranes' permeability control, and reverse osmosis

of RB5 increases with the increase in temperature. Therefore, it may be concluded that chitin is a potential biosorbent for the removal of dyes from aqueous solution (Begum et al. 2012).

Chitin and chitosan were comparatively employed for remediation of chromated copper arsenate (CCA) preservative-treated wood in recent years becasue of the release of chromium, copper, and arsenic elements from waste wood during land filling, burning, composting, and other disposal methods (Kartal and Imamura 2005).

In a recent study by Sun et al. (2009), it was observed that sulfur atoms also have a strong affinity for arsenic. Hence, the authors synthesized polyaspartate and chitosan blends derivatized with -SH functionalities. Blends were reacted with mercaptoacetic (thioglycolic) acid affording the –SH derivative. This polymer showed better arsenic-removal behavior (As removal > 22%) than other adsorbents, leading to a lower arsenic equilibrium concentration.

Cationic polymers were more effective than nonionic polymers as coagulants of lignin from wastewater of pulp and paper industry . The use of both polyethyleneimine (PEI) and hexamethylene diamine epichlorohydrin (HE) resulted in color removal of about 80%, but only 30% total organic carbon (TOC) was eliminated from alkaline black liquor wastewater after 30 minutes of settling under gravity. Therefore, chitosan, a natural coagulant, removed up to 90% of color and 70% of TOC. Chitosan was more effective at a pH of 7.0, whereas other coagulants performed better at pH 6.0. Greater amounts of alum (between 900 ppm and 1200 ppm) and chitosan (between 1200 ppm and 1800 ppm) were needed compared with the levels of HE (between 300 ppm and 400 ppm) and PEI (between 400 ppm and 500 ppm) to effect maximum removal efficiencies (Ganjidoust et al. 1997).

Filipkowska et al. (2014) found that phosphates may be successively removed from aqueous solutions as a result of their adsorption onto crosslinked chitosan, especially chitosan crosslinked with epichlorohydrin (ECH), which is a beneficial crosslinking agent, as it does not block active centers of chitosan that are responsible for phosphates adsorption.

Hema et al. (2012) reported that chitin/poly vinyl alcohol (PVA)/silk fibron (SF) (1:1:1) ternary blend can be synthesized through solution blending for the removal of heavy metal ions from the electroplating industrial effluents. The study concluded that the use of chitin/PVA/SF (1:1:1) ternary blend for heavy metals' removal appears to be technically feasible, ecofriendly, and highly efficacious.

The removal of heavy metals from electroplating wastewater is a matter of paramount importance due to their high toxicity, which causes major environmental pollution problems (Liu et al. 2013). The result revealed that ethylene glycol diglycidyl ether–chitosan, nanoscale zero-valent iron beads prepared had the capacity to remediate actual electroplating wastewater and could become an effective and promising technology for in situ remediation of heavy metals.

The adsorption of Remazol black 13 (reactive) dye onto chitosan in aqueous solutions was investigated by Annadurai et al. (2008). Therefore, review is done on the current available technologies for wastewater treatment. Remazol black 13 (reactive) dye removal using chitosan as adsorbent is an effective, cheaper methods and also applicable on large scale (Robinson et al. 2001).

Chitosan-coated calcium alginate and chitosan-coated silica were developed as biosorbents. These biomaterials are effective adsorbents for the removal of Ni(II) from aquatic medium (Vijaya et al. 2007).

Sudha (2010) reported on the heavy metal removal such as cadmium and chromium from industrial wastewater by using chitosan-coated coconut charcoal and chitosan-impregnated polyurethane foam, respectively. Adsorption and determination of metal ions such as zinc(II) and vanadium (II) onto chitosan from sea water have been studied.

Khairkar and Raut (2014) observed chitosan-g-poly(acrylic acid-co-acryl amide), a new sorbent material, and gave information about its pore size, good chemical stability and good thermal stability, which reveal its applicability toward metal extraction. This low-cost adsorbents are effective for the removal of metal ions from aqueous solutions. Various metal ions removal % is in the order of, $Cu^{2+}>Cd^{2+}>Ni^{2+}>Pb^{2+}$ ions. These metal ions were adsorbed onto the adsorbents very rapidly within the first 120 min have been reported.

Zhu et al. (2012) investigated in single and ternary metal system the competitive adsorption of Pb(II), Cu(II), and Zn(II) onto a novel xanthate-modified magnetic chitosan (XMCS). In a single system, equilibrium studies showed that the adsorption of Pb(II), Cu(II), and Zn(II) followed the Langmuir model, and they found that the maximum adsorption capacities were 76.9, 34.5, and 20.8 mg/g, respectively. In a ternary system, they found the combined action of the metals to be antagonistic and that the metal sorption followed the order of Pb(II) > Cu(II) > Zn(II). The Langmuir isotherm fitted the data of Pb(II) and Cu(II) well, whereas the equilibrium data of Zn(II) was well fitted in the Freundlich model.

Chitosan with nylon-6 membranes was used as an adsorbent to remove copper and cadmium ions from synthetic wastewater. Characterization of the synthesized membrane has been done with Fourier transform infrared (FTIR), X-ray diffraction (XRD), thermogravimetric analysis (TGA), and scanning electron microscopy (SEM). The optimum pH for removal of Cd(II) and Cu(II) was found to be 5, using chitosan with nylon-6. The removal efficiency of copper increased in the pH range from 3 to 5. The optimum pH for copper was found to be 5. The removal efficiency of Cu^{+2} ions onto chitosan increased rapidly with an increase in contact time from 0 to 360 minutes and then reached equilibrium after 360 minutes (Prakash et al. 2012).

The novel chitin/polyethylene glycol binary blend as a new biosorbent for cadmium was studied. It removes cadmium ions from aqueous solutions, and the sorption capacity was strongly effective. These results can be helpful in designing a wastewater system for the removal of metal ions (Mohan and Syed Shafi 2013).

The graft copolymerizations of chitosan with acrylamide have been done in the presence of cerium ammonium nitrate (CAN) as a redox initiator and by novel technique ultraviolet irradiation. This showed that the grafted copolymer has improved porosity and fractured structure, which can be responsible for adsorption of molecules. Significant results have been found for the industrial application. Hence, chitosang-polyacrylamide can be used for wastewater treatment at industrial level (Ali et al. 2011).

The high cost of activated carbon limits its use in adsorption. Many varieties of low-cost adsorbents have been developed and tested to remove heavy metal. Karthikeyan et al. (2004) examined the removal of Zn(II) by using chitosan. They found that an optimum contact period of 6 minutes was required for the maximum removal of zinc(II) by chitosan. The adsorption mechanism also depends on the particle size of the adsorbent, pH of the medium, and the presence of other anions such as chlorides and nitrates. The optimum pH was found to be 7, and the equilibrium data were well fitted in the Langmuir isotherm. Thermodynamic and equilibrium parameters showed that the adsorption process was endothermic and spontaneous in nature.

Vold et al. (2003) studied the selective adsorption of copper, zinc, cadmium, and nickel on further deacetylated commercial chitosan and observed a higher selectivity to copper than to zinc, cadmium, and nickel, between pH of 5 and 6.

Schmuhl et al. (2001) studied the ability of chitosan as an adsorbent for Cu(II) ions in aqueous solution. The experiments were done as batch processes. Equilibrium studies were conducted on both crosslinked and non-crosslinked chitosan for both metals. They found the optimum pH was 3 to 5 for the removal of Cu(II). From the experimental data, it was observed that the metal concentration for copper can be lowered from 10 mg/L to 2.4 mg/L by means of the batch process.

Removal of arsenic from contaminated drinking water was also studied on a chitosan–chitin mixture. It showed a capacity of 0.13 microequivalents As/g (pH = 7.0) (Elson et al. 1980).

A chitosan–charcoal composite was prepared. The composite was used to remove Cr from aqueous solution, and an optimum condition was found for maximum removal, which was used later for the treatment of tannery effluents. The Cr removal efficiency of the composite was more than 90% (Siraj et al. 2012).

Nadeem (2013) indicated that chitosan is a good adsorbent for removal of chromium (VI) from aqueous solutions. The kinetics of the adsorption data showed that the applicability of removal of metal was rapid and effective.

Mishra and Tripathy (1993) have reported that anionic (direct, acid, and reactive dyes), cationic (basic) dyes, and nonionic (disperse) dyes can be removed from dye-containing effluent this way. Wastewater is passed over the ion exchange resin until the available exchange sites are saturated: anionic (direct, acid, and reactive dyes), cationic (basic) dyes, and nonionic (disperse) dyes. Advantages of this method include no loss of adsorbent on regeneration, Organic solvents are expensive, and the ion exchange method is not very effective for disperse dyes. Together, they represent about 90% of all organic colorants. It is important to note that dye molecules have many different and complicated structures, and their adsorption behavior is directly related to the chemical structure, the dimensions of the dye's organic chains, and the number and positioning of the functional groups of the dye. This is one of the most important factors influencing adsorption. However, the way in which adsorption is affected by the chemical structure of the dyes is not clearly identified.

Shanmugapriya et al. (2013) reported that the chitosan-g-polyacrylonitrile (PAN) copolymer was prepared successfully. The copolymer was chosen for the batch adsorption studies by varying adsorbent dose, pH, and contact time under optimized conditions, and metal analyses were carried. The results showed that the copolymer was an excellent adsorbent.

The wastewater from the textile industry is contaminated with a complex set of oxygen-demanding materials and poses a great problem to the natural environment. The conventional aluminum-based coagulants have a possible link to Alzheimer's disease, but chitosan is more favorable in wastewater treatment due to its environment friendly characteristic. As a result, the wastewater from textile industry was treated with chitosan via coagulation and flocculation processes.

On account of its good adsorption properties, chitin-based materials had been used for the removal of industrial pollutants and adsorption of silver thiosulfate complexes and actinides (Songkroah et al. 2004).

21.8 CONCLUSION

Scientific databases reveal thousands of articles and patents related to chitin and its derivatives and increasingly open up new possibilities to produce new derivatives and new applications. In addition, through the study of this biopolymer and due to the great demand of chitin, it is very important to direct all efforts to seek methods of production through environment-friendly processes and, on the other hand, through genetic engineering methods, thus finding the way to produce a more uniform material. As discussed in this chapter, chitin's behavior in various applications within diverse areas is governed by its molecular weight, degree of deacetylation, degree of polymerization, and source of obtention.

The characteristic of wastewater discharged from textile industrial activities was strictly controlled by the Department of Environment. This was because the wastewater from the textile industry was contaminated with a complex set of oxygen-demanding materials and posed a great problem to the natural environment. The management of textile industrial effluents is a complicated task, taking into consideration the complexity of the waste compounds that may be present, in addition to the dyes, and the numerous established options for the treatment and reuse of water. Wide ranges of water pH, temperature, salt concentration, and variations in the chemical structure of numerous dyes in use today add to the complication. Economical removal of color from effluents remains an important problem, even though a number of successful systems employing various physicochemical and biological processes have been successfully implemented. Regulatory agencies are increasingly interested in new, efficient, and improved decolorization technologies.

Solid and evolving scientific knowledge and research are of the utmost relevance for the effective response to current needs. In view of the requirement for a technically and economically satisfactory treatment, a flurry of emerging technologies is being proposed; these novel technologies are at different stages of being tested for commercialization. A broader validation of these new technologies and the integration of different methods in the current treatment schemes will be most likely take place in the near future, rendering them both efficient and economically viable.

The treatment of industrial dyeing effluent that contains a large number of organic dyes by adsorption process, using easily available low-cost adsorbents, is an interesting alternative to the traditionally available aqueous waste-processing techniques (chemical coagulation/flocculation, ozonation, oxidation, photodegradation, and so on). The distribution of size, shape, and volume of voids species in the porous materials is directly related to the ability to perform the adsorption. Undoubtedly, chitin, a low-cost adsorbent, offers many promising benefits for commercial purposes in the future.

REFERENCES

Ali, A. Z., J. Venkatesan, S. K. Kim, and P. N. Sudha. 2011. Beneficial effect of chitosang-polyacrylamide copolymer in removal of heavy metals from industrial dye effluents. *International Journal of Environmental Sciences* 1(5):820.

Ali, H. 2010. Biodegradation of synthetic dyes-a review. *Water Air Soil Pollution* doi:.1 007/s 11270-010-0382-4.

Alkarkhi, F. A., N. Ismail, and A. M. Easa. 2008. Assessment of arsenic and heavy metal contents in cockles (Anadaragranosa) using multivariate statistical techniques. *Journal of Hazardous Materials* 150(3):783–789.

Andrade, V. S., N. B. de Barros, K. Fukushima, and G. M. T. de Campos. 2003. Effect of medium components and time of cultivation on chitin production by Mucorcircinelloides(Mucorja vanicus IFO 4570) A factorial study. *Revista Iberoamericana De Micologia* 20:149–153.

Annadurai, G., L. Y. Ling, and J.-F. Lee. 2008. Adsorption of reactive dye from an aqueous solution by chitosan: Isotherm, kinetic and thermodynamic analysis. *Journal of Hazardous Materials* 152:337–346.

Austin, P. R., C. J. Brine, J. E. Castle, and J. P. Zikakis. 1981. Chitin: New facets of research. *Science* 212:749–753.

Begum, H. A., A. K. Mondal and T. Muslim. 2012. Muslim Bangladesh. *Pharmaceutical Journal* 15(2):145–152.

Dutta, P. K., M. K. Khatua, J. Dutta, and R. Prasad. 2003. Use of chitosan-DMAc/LiCl gel as drug carriers. *International Journal of Chemical Science* 1:93–102.

Dutta, P. K., M. N. V. Ravikumar, and J. Dutta. 2002. Chitin and chitosan for versatile applications. *Journal of Macromolecular Science Part C:Polymer Reviews* C4:2307.

Elson, C. M., D. H. Davies, and E. R. Hayes. 1980. Removal of arsenic from contaminated drinking water by a chitosan/chitin mixture. *Water Research* 14:1307–1311.

FAO. 2003. Food and Agriculture Organization of the United Nation, World Water Development Report, Natural Resources and Environment Department, Water Development and Management Unit. http://www.fao.org/nr/water/, Accessed July 21, 2010.

Filipkowska, U., T. Jóźwiak, and P. Szymczyk. 2014. Application of cross-linked chitosan for phosphate removal from aqueous solutions. *Progress on Chemistry and Application of Chitin and Its Derivatives*, Volume XIX, doi:10.15259/PCACD.19.01.

Ganjidoust, H., K. Tatsumi, T. Yamagishi, and R. N. Gholian. 1997. Effect of synthetic and natural coagulation on lignin removal from pulp and paper wastewater. *Water Science Technology* 35:291–296.

Hadi, A. G. 2012. Adsorption of nickel ions by synthesized chitosan. *British Journal of Science* 6:109.

Hamman, J. H., M. Stander, and A. F. Kotze. 2002. Effect of the degree of quaternisation of N-trimethyl chitosan chloride on absorption enhancement: In vivo evaluation in rat nasal epithelia. *International Journal of Pharmaceutics* 232:235–42.

Hema, S., R. Ramya, and Sudha, P. N. 2012. Preparation of chitin/PVA/SF ternary blend for heavy metal ion removal from electroplating industrial effluent. *Elixir Applied Chemistry* 46:8273–8278.

Husain, Q. 2006. Potential applications of the oxidoreductive enzymes in the decolourisation and detoxification of textile and other synthetic dyes from polluted water: A review. *Critical Reviews in Bio-Technology* 26:201–221.

Johnson, E. L., and Q. P. Peniston. 1982. Utilkation of shellfish waste for chitin and chitosan production. In: Martin, R. E., G. J. Flick, C. E. Hebard, and D. R. Ward, eds. *Chemistry and Biochemistry of Marine Food Products*. Westport, CT:AVI Pub. Co., pp. 415–422.

Jonathan, M., S. Srinivasalu, N. Thangadurai, T. Ayyamperumal, J. Armstrong-Altrin, and V. Ram-Mohan. 2008. Contamination of Uppanar River and coastal waters off Cuddalore, Southeast coast of India. *Environmental Geology* 53(7):1391–1404.

Jordao, C., M. Pereira, and J. Pereira. 2002. Metal contamination of river waters and sediments from effluents of kaolin processing in Brazil. *Water, Air, & Soil Pollution* 140(1):119–138.

Kartal, S. N., and Y. Imamura. 2005. Removal of copper, chromium, and arsenic from CCA-treated wood onto chitin and chitosan. *Bioresource Technology* 96:389–392.

Karthikeyan, G., K. Anbalagan, and N. Muthulakshmi Andal. 2004. Adsorption dynamics and equilibrium studies of Zn (II) onto chitosan. *Journal of chemical Science* 116:119–127.

Khairkar, S. R., and R. A. Raut. 2014. Adsorption studies for the removal heavy metal by chitosan-g-poly (acrylicacid-co-acrylamide) composite. *Science Journal of Analytical Chemistry* 2(6):67–70.

Kisku, G., S. Barman, and S. Bhargava. 2000. Contamination of soil and plants with potentially toxic elements irrigated with mixed industrial effluent and its impact on the environment. *Water, Air, & Soil Pollution* 120(1):121–137.

Kurita, K., J. Amemiya, T. Mori, and Y. Nishiyama. 1999. Comb-shaped chitosan derivatives having oligo(ethylene glycol) side chains. *Polymer Bulletin* 42(4):387–393.

Kurita, K., S. Inoue, and S. Nishimura. 1991. Preparation of soluble chitin derivatives as reactive precursors for controlled modifications: Tosyl- and iodo-chitin. *Journal of Polymer Science Part A: Polymer Chemistry* 29:937.

Kurita, K., S. Inoue, K. Yamamura, H. Yoshino, S. Ishii, and S. Nishimura. 1992. Cationic and radical graft copolymerization of styrene onto iodochitin. *Macromolecules* 25:3791–3794.

Lehrfeld, J. 1997. Conversion of agricultural residues into cation exchange materials. *Journal of Applied Polymer Science* 61:2099–2105.

Liu, T., X. Yang, Z.-L. Wang, and X. Yan. 2013. Enhanced chitosan beads—Supported Fe^0 nanoparticles for removal of heavy metals from electroplating wastewater in permeable reactive barriers. *Water Research* 47(17):6691–6700, www.elsevier.com/locate/waters.

Madhavan, P. 1992. Chitin and chitosan and their novel applications. In: *Popular Science Lecture Series, Central Institute of Fisheries Technology,* CIFT, Matsyapuri Cochin, India, pp. 6–7.

Mishra, G., and M. Tripathy. 1993. A critical review of the treatment for decolourization of textile effluent. *Colourage* 40:35–38.

Mohan, K., and S. Syed Shafi. 2013. Removal of cadmium from the aqueous solution using chitin/polyethylene glycol binary blend. *Der Pharmacia Lettre* 5(4):62–69.

Monier, M. 2012. Adsorption of Hg(II), Cu(II) and Zn(II) ions from aqueous solution using formaldehyde cross-linked modified chitosan-thioglyceraldehyde Schiff's base. *International Journal of Biological Macromolecules* 50:773.

Monier, M., and D. A. Abdel-Latif. 2013. Modification and characterization of PET fibers for fast removal of Hg(II), Cu(II) and Co(II) metal ions from aqueous solutions. *Journal of Hazardous Materials* 250:122.

Morita, Y., Y. Sugahara, A. Takahashi, and M. Ibonai. 1997. Non-catalytic photo-induced graft copolymerization of methylmethacrylate onto O-acetyl-chitin. *European Polymer Journal* 33:1505–1509.

Nadeem, U. 2013. Chromium adsorption kinetics from aqueous metal solutions using chitosan. *European Chemical Bulletin* 2(10):706–708.

Peñaranda, A. J. E., and M. A. Sabino. 2010. Effect of the presence of lignin or peat in IPN hydrogels on the sorption of heavy metals. *Polymer Bulletin* 65:495.

Peter, M. G. 2002. Chitin and chitosan from animal sources, In: *Biopolymers,(Polysaccharides II),* De Baets, S., E. J. Van-damme, and A. Steinbuchel eds., Weinheim: Wiley VCH, 2 Ch. 15.

Peter, M. G., A. Domard, and R. A. A. Muzzarelli, (ed.). 2000. In: *Advances in Chitin Science.* Potsdam Germany: Universitat Potsdam.

Prakash, N., P. N. Sudha, and N. G. Rengnathan. 2012. Copper and cadmium removal from synthetic industrial wastewater using chitosan and Nylon 6. *Environmental Science and Pollution Research* 19:2930–2941.

Prasad, D. W., and T. W. Joyce. 1991. Colour removal from kraft bleach plant effluents by trichodermasp. *Tappi Journal* 74:165–169.

Purushotham, D., A. Narsing Rao, M. Ravi Prakash, S. Ahmed, and G. Ashok Babu. 2011. Environmental impact on groundwater of Maheshwaram Watershed, Ranga Reddy district, Andhra Pradesh. *Journal of the Geological Society of India* 77(6):539–548.

Raju, J., N., P. Ram, and S. Dey. 2009. Groundwater quality in the lower Varuna River basin, Varanasi district, Uttar Pradesh. *Journal of the Geological Society of India* 73(2):178–192.

Ramachandran Nair, K. G. 1994. Life saving drugs and growth promoters from shrimp. *Fish World* 3, 21–23.

Rehman, A. and M. S. Anjum. 2010. Cadmium uptake by yeast, candida tropicalis, isolated from industrial effluents and its potential use in wastewater clean-up operations. *Water, Air, and Soil Pollution* 205(1):149–159.

Rinaudo, M. and J. Reguant. 2000. Polysaccharide derivatives. In: Frollini, E., A. L. Leao, and L. H. C. Mattoso, eds. *Natural Polymers and Agro Fibers Composites.* Sao Carlos, Bresil: CIP-BRASIL, pp. 15–39.

Robinson, T., G. McMullan, R. Marchant, and P. Nigam. 2001. Remediation of dyes in textile effluent: A critical review on current treatment technologies with a proposed alternative. *Bioresource Technology* 77:247–255.

Ruiz, M., A. M. Sastre, and E. Guibal. 2000. Palladium sorption on glutaraldehyde-cross-linked chitosan. *Reactive & Functional Polymers* 45:155–173.

Sahni, S. K. 2011. Hazardous metals and minerals pollution in India, *Position Paper Published on Behalf of Indian National Science Academy*, Bahadurshah Zafar Marg, August, 2011, New Delhi.

Saravanan, D., and P. N. Sudha. 2014. Batch adsorption studies for the removal of copper from wastewater using natural biopolymer. *International Journal of Chem Tech Research* 6(7):3496–3508.

Schmuhl, R., H. M. Krieg, and K. Keizer. 2001. Adsorption of Cu(II) and Cr(II) ions by chitosan: Kinetics and equilibrium studies. *Water SA* 27(1):1–8.

Shanmugapriya, A., M. Hemalatha, B. Scholastica, and T. Augustine Arul Prasad. 2013. Adsorption studies of lead (II) and nickel (II) ions on chitosan-G-polyacrylonitrile. *Der Pharma Chemica* 5(3):141–155.

Singh, R., B. Sengupta, R. Bali, B. Shukla, V. V. S. Gurunadharao, and R. Srivatstava. 2009. Identification and mapping of chromium (VI) plume in groundwater for remediation: A case study at Kanpur, Uttar Pradesh. *Journal of the Geological Society of India* 74(1):49–57.

Siraj, S., M. D. M. Islam, P. C. Das, M. D. S. Masum, I. A. Jahan, M. D. A. Ahsan, and M. D. Shajahan. 2012. Removal of chromium from tannery effluent using chitosan-charcoal composite. *Journal of Bangladesh Chemical Society* 25(1):53–61.

Songkroah, C., W. Nakbanpote, and P. Thiravetyan. 2004. Recovery of silver–thiosulfate complexes with chitin. *Process Biochem* 39:1553–1559.

Sudha, P. N. 2010. Chitin, chitosan and derivatives for waste water treatment. In: S.-K. Kim ed., *Chitin, Chitosan, Oligosaccharides and their Derivatives* London:CRC Press, 561–585.

Sun, B., Z. Mi, G. An, G. Liu, and J.-J. Zou. 2009. Preparation of biomimetic materials made from polyaspartyl polymer and chitosan for heavy-metal removal. *Industrial and Engineering Chemistry Research* 48:9823–9829.

Szumilewicz, J., and L. Szosland. 2000. Determination of the absolute molar mass of chitin and dibutyrylchitin by means of size exclusion chromatography coupled with light scattering and viscometry. In: Uragami, T., K. Kurita, and T. Fukamizo, eds. *Chitin and Chitosan*. Tokyo: Ko- dansha Scientific Ltd, pp. 99–102.

Vaaje-Kolstad, G., D. R. Houston, A. H. K. Riemen, Eijsink, and V. G. H. van Aalten. 2005. Crystal structure and binding properties of the serratiamarcescens chitin-binding protein CBP21. *Journal of Biological Chemistry* 280:11313–11319.

Van Luyen, D., and D. M. Huong. 1996. Chitin and derivatives, In: Salamone J. C. ed. *Polymeric Materials Encyclopedia*, Boca Raton (Florida):CRC, Volume 2, pp. 1208–1217.

Vijaya, Y., R. Srinivasapopuri, M. Veera Boddu, and A. Krishnaiah. 2007. Modified chitosan and calcium alginate niopolymer sorbents for removal of nickel (II) through adsorption. *Carbohydrate Polymers* 72:261–271.

Vold, I. M. N., K. M. Vårum, E. Guibal, and O. Smidsrød. 2003. Binding of ions to chitosan— Selectivity studies. *Carbohydrate Polymers* 54:471–477.

Wang, X. J., X. Y. Gu, D. X. Lin, F. Dong, and X. F. Wan. 2007. Treatment of acid rose dye containing waste-water by ozonizing-biological aerated filter. *Dyes Pigments* 74(3):736.

WHO. 2009. Potassium in drinking-water. Background Document for Preparation of WHO Guidelines for Drinking-Water Quality, WHO/HSE/WSH/09.01/7, Geneva, Switzerland.

Wu, G. Y., L. W. Chan, and S. Y. Szeto. 2003. Preparation of O-carboxymethylchitosans and their effect on color yield of acid dyes on silk. *Journal of Applied Polymer Science* 90:2500–2502.

Zhu, Y., J. Hu, and J. Wang. 2012. Competitive adsorption of Pb(II), Cu(II), Zn(II) onto xanthate-modified magnetic chitosan. *Journal of Hazardous Materials* 221–222:155–161.

22 Industrial Applications of Alginate

K. Vijayalakshmi, Srinivasan Latha,
Maximas H. Rose, and P.N. Sudha

CONTENTS

22.1   INTRODUCTION

Polysaccharides are the most abundant industrial raw materials that have been the subject of intensive research nowadays due to their sustainable, biodegradable, and biosafety nature. In recent years, significant progress has been made in discovering and developing new algal polymers that possess novel and highly functional properties. Alginates are established among the most versatile biopolymers and are used in a wide range of applications; they are quite abundant in nature, since they occur both as a structural component in marine brown algae (Phaeophyceae), comprising up to 40% of the dry matter, and as capsular polysaccharides in soil bacteria. On account of their physicochemical characteristics, chemical stability, particular structure, and high reactivity, the alginate biopolymers also have an excellent selectivity and a high ability to form complexes with various heavy metals (Aravindhan et al. 2007; Ngomsik et al. 2009). The industrial applications of alginates were mainly linked to their water-retaining ability, gelling, viscosifying, and stabilizing properties. Owing to the mature industrial sector in many developed countries, the market for alginates and derivatives is observed to be growing at a modest rate. Among the various industries, the textile and food and beverage industries are still the major consumers for alginates, and this consumption is expected to grow at a healthy rate. For various reasons, researchers are exploring the possible applications of modified forms of alginates, having various structures, functions, and properties, which are synthesized via chemical and physical reactions.

22.2   OVERVIEW OF ALGINATES

Biomaterials are the materials derived from the natural sources; these have been traditionally designed to be inert and not to interact with biological systems in the host. These materials intended to interface with biological systems to evaluate, treat, augment, or replace any tissue, organ, or function of the body (Williams 2009). Among the various biomaterials, alginate is of particular interest for a broad range of applications due to its outstanding properties in terms of biocompatibility, biodegradability, nonantigenicity, and chelating ability (Su and Tan 2013). The generic term alginate means the various derivatives of alginic acid that can either occur naturally in certain brown seaweeds (alginophyter) or can be produced from natural derivatives (Viswanathan and Nallamuthu 2014). In 2013, the North American region formed the largest market for alginates and derivatives and was valued at 120.3 million dollar. In general, alginates, such as polysaccharides, are polydisperse with respect to molecular weight, which is widely used as a stabilizer, viscosifier, and gelling agent in the food and beverage industries (Li et al. 2011). In addition, specifically, the alginate matrices containing aqueous internal environments were found to be ideal for the encapsulation of proteins, small molecules, and under normal physiological conditions. Since the alginate matrices are very biodegradable, they can be readily broken down (Gombotz and Wee 1998). In order to overcome the drawbacks of alginates such as the mechanical weakness and poor cell adhesion, alginates can be mixed with other materials. In the literature, certain attempts have been worked out by various researchers to overcome this limitation, which includes blending with other biopolymers (Iwasaki et al. 2004; Rinaudo 2008), chemical grafting with oligopeptides (Rowley et al. 1999; Alsberg et al. 2001), and addition of hydroxyapatite.

22.2.1 GENERAL STRUCTURES AND TERMINOLOGY

Algins are salts of alginic acid, a natural polymer found in the cell wall of brown algae (Phaeophyceae) as part of a wide family of glycans that compose this group of organisms. These glycans are laminaran, cellulose, sulfated hexouronoxylofucans, fucoidan, and alginate (Silva et al. 2012). The anionic polysaccharide alginates derived from brown algae belong to the family of unbranched true block copolymers composed of interdispersed homopolymeric regions of alternating structures of (1–4) linked-D-mannuronic acid (M) and L-guluronic acid (G) with widely varying composition and sequence, respectively (Figure 22.1). The monomeric units of mannuronic acid (M) and guluronic acid (G) present in alginates do not occur randomly but rather in a block-like fashion, where G blocks are responsible for specific ion binding and hence also the gelling properties of alginates (Draget and Taylor 2011). The primary structure of alginates is mainly composed of homogeneous M–M segments (M blocks), homogeneous G–G segments (G blocks), and alternating M–G segments (MG blocks).

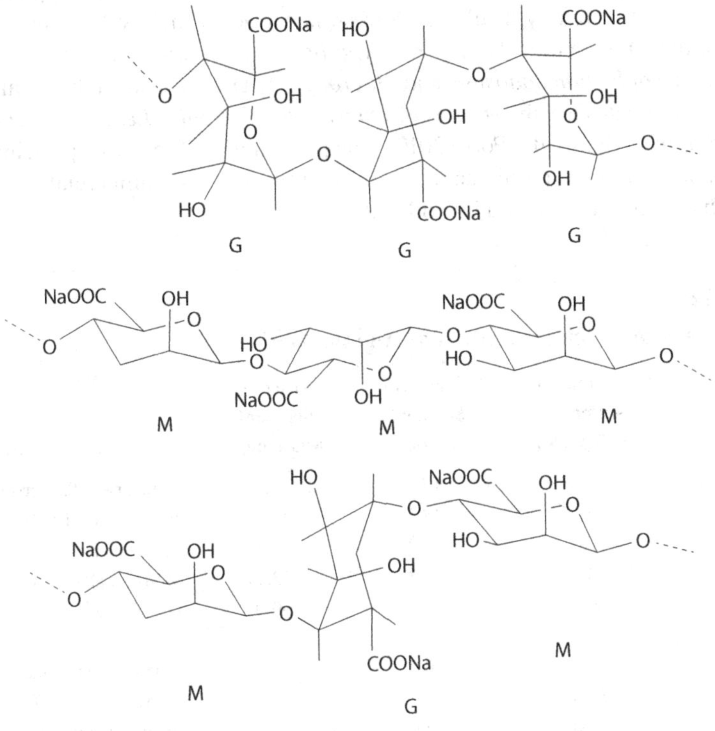

FIGURE 22.1 Structure of sodium alginate.

The sequential distribution and relative amount of mannuronic acid and guluronic acid blocks in sodium alginate depend on the marine sources, producing species and seasonal and geographical variations (D'Ayala et al. 2008). Until Fischer and Dorfel identified the L-guluronate residue, D-mannuronate was regarded as the major component of alginate (Fischer and Dorfel 1955). Alginate possessing more number of mannuronic acid groups has flat ribbon-like molecular appearance, whereas the presence of more number of guluronic acid groups has buckled chain-like appearance. The length of each block of mannuronic acid and guluronic acid residues depends on the various sources, and more than 200 different alginates are currently being manufactured (Tonnesen and Karlsen 2002). Mainly, alginates occur naturally in seaweed in the form of calcium, magnesium, and sodium salts. In order to transform seaweeds into products such as protanal alginates and protoacid alginic acid, alginates were extracted thoroughly by removing all biological and inorganic impurities.

22.2.2 SOURCES OF ALGINATES

Marine plant resources are attracting more and more attention as a raw material for the production of alginic acid. Seaweeds are the main primary sources for the production of alginates. By treatment with aqueous alkali solutions, typically with NaOH, the commercially available alginate is extracted mainly from brown algae (Phaeophyceae), including *Laminaria hyperborea*, *Laminaria digitata*, *Laminaria japonica*, *Ascophyllum nodosum*, and *Macrocystis pyrifera*. Some other commercial sources of alginates are the species of *Durvillaea*, *Ecklonia*, *Lessonia*, *Sargassum*, and *Turbinaria* (Bixler and Porse 2010). The percentages of the three principal types of block structures in alginic acid, prepared from various commercial brown seaweeds, have been represented in Table 22.1.

TABLE 22.1
Percentages of Block Structures of Alginic Acid

Alginate from	Polymannuronic Segments (M Type, %)	Polyguluronic Segments (G Type, %)	Mixed Segments (MG Type, %)	References
Macrocystis	40.6	17.7	41.7	Penman and Sanderson (1972)
pyrifera	36.5	18.5	45.0	Morris et al. (1980)
Laminaria	20.3	49.3	30.4	Pennman and Sanderson (1972)
hyperborea	23.1	43.3	33.7	Morris et al. (1980)
Laminaria japonica	36.0	14.0	50.0	Ji et al. (1984)
Ascophyllum	38.4	20.7	41.0	Pennman and Sanderson (1972)
nodosum	37.8	21.4	40.8	Morris et al. (1980)
	35.0	13.0	52.0	Haug et al. (1974)
Laminaria	49.0	25.0	26.0	Grasdalen et al. (1981)
digitata	43.0	23.0	34.0	Haug et al. (1974)

A wide range of grades of sodium alginate produced from the cold sea weeds such as *Laminaria, Macrocystis,* and *Ascophyllum* may be categorized as low (20–50 mPa.s* or cps**), medium (400–500 mPa.s), and high (800–900 mPa.s) viscosity. Around 35% of moisture content were present in the air-dried *L. hyperborea* samples, whereas in case of the air-dried samples of *Lessonia, Durvillaea,* and *L. japonica,* the moisture content can vary from 15% to 20%. *Macrocystis* was harvested on the east coast of Tasmania, Australia, from 1964 to 1973, but due to the insufficient available quantity for sustaining an alginate industry, it was also harvested on the west coast of North America, from the Monterey Peninsula in central California to the middle of the west coast of Baja California. It has been estimated that the United States harvests about 150,000 t (wet) and Mexico harvests about 40,000 t (wet) per year (ITC 1981).

An expensive raw material used for the production of alginate was *Laminaria* species, which was harvested principally in Scotland, Ireland, Norway, France, China, Japan, and Korea. Some examples of *Laminaria* species used for the production of alginate are given as follows: *L. japonica, L. hyperborea,* and *L. digitata.* In the Asian countries, *Laminaria* is very popularly used as a food. Especially in China, for alginate extraction process, the *Laminaria* material that is unsuitable for food is used. The cultivation of *L. japonica* has been very successful in china, reaching about one million tons of wet seaweed annually. From the one million tones, about two-thirds are used as food and the surplus is available for alginate production.

Ascophyllum nodosum, one of the sources of alginate grown in the intertidal zone, has been harvested in the southern parts of Nova Scotia, and it was also harvested by hand in Scotland, Ireland, for more than a century. The United Kingdom and the United States have utilized *Durvillaea antarctica* from Chile and *Durvillaea potatorum* from Australia for alginate production. In the year 1985, the export of alginates from Chile were about 390 t, but recently, the current exports from Australia are about 3000 t per annum. *Lessonia* is also one of the primary raw materials used for the production of alginates collected from Chile. In 1978, Chile exported about 2045 t of alginates, and among those, around 1,313 t were exported to Japan and the remainder was exported to the United States and Canada (ITC 1981).

The total export had increased to 5810 t by the year of 1985. *Ecklonia cava,* which grows in deep water up to 20 m, was harvested by divers in both Japan and Koreaand was utilized by local alginate producers. The alginate production yield was found to be about 140 kg from a dried ton of *Lessonia,* and for the other seaweeds such as *Ascophyllum, L. japonica,* and *Durvillaea,* the production yield was found to be about 120 kg, 170 kg, and 240 kg, respectively. Reports on the structure of alginates (Shyamali et al. 1984; Wedlock et al. 1986) from *Sargassum* and *Turbinaria* indicate that they could be very useful in applications requiring the formation of strong gels. The sodium alginate produced from *Sargassum* and *Turbinaria* generally has a viscosity of 20 to 50 mPa.s (equivalent to around 1,200 mPa.s at 3% concentration). Some examples of freight on board (f.o.b.) prices for air-dried seaweed per ton were found to be given as follows: Chilean *Lessonia,* US$150; South African *Ecklonia,* US$250; Australian *Durvillaea,* US$400; Chinese *L. japonica,* US$500–US$700; and UK *Ascophyllum,* US$350.

These prices can show considerable variation from year to year with the fluctuation of the exchange rate of US dollars versus the currency of the country of origin of the seaweed. In addition, the alginates were also especially extracted from brown seaweeds and from bacteria belonging to the genera *Pseudomonas* and *Azotobacter* (Rehm 2002). The bacterial alginate produced from *Azotobacter* has a high concentration of G blocks, and its gels have a relatively high stiffness (Hay et al. 2010).

22.2.3 EXTRACTION OF ALGINATES

The British chemist Stanford first described alginate (the preparation of "alginic acid" from brown algae) with a patent dated January 12, 1881 (Stanford 1881). At the end of the nineteenth century, British chemist E.C. Stanford carried out scientific studies on the extraction of alginates from brown seaweed, and after 50 years, the large-scale production of alginate was introduced. The global production of alginate is 26,500 tons and is valued at US$318 million annually. Alginates were mainly extracted from seaweeds and bacteria. When compared with the extraction of alginates from seaweeds, the alginates extracted through the bacterial biosynthesis (*Azotobacter* and *Pseudomonas*) route have more defined chemical structures and physical properties. The various steps involved in the alginate biosynthesis were given as follows: (i) precursor substrate synthesis, (ii) polymerization and cytoplasmic membrane transfer, (iii) periplasmic transfer and modification, and (iv) the export through the outer membrane (Remminghorst and Rehm 2006). The recent progress in regulation of alginate biosynthesis from bacteria and the relative ease of modification of bacteria enable the production of alginate with tailor-made features and wide applications in biomedical field.

The industry extraction protocol for alginate from seaweed is mainly divided into five steps: acidification, alkaline extraction, solid/liquid separation, precipitation, and drying (Pérez et al. 1992). Through the alkali digestion process, precipitation by acidification, centrifugation, and drying, the algin is manufactured as sodium alginate at the cottage industry level. The general processing scheme for the production of alginates from seaweed is represented in Figure 22.2.

The initial steps involved in the production of sodium alginate from seaweed are cleaning, chemical pretreatment, and separation of the extract, followed by acidification/precipitation of alginic acid. Depending on the seaweed species concerned, higher quantities of reactant and water are required in the alkali extraction step, and several hours are required to attain the optimum extraction yield. Depending on the alkaline extraction time, the rheological properties of alginates become varied: the reaction conditions seem to favor bacterial development and endogenous alginate lyase activity, the likely cause of alginate degradation (Moen et al. 1997).

Alginate is extracted for commercial purposes from various species of kelp, or brown algae, including *L. hyperborea*, *A. nodosum*, and *M. pyrifera*. The evaluation of reactive extrusion as a new process for the alkaline extraction of alginates from *L. digitata* was carried out by Peggy Vauche and his coworkers (Peggy Vauche et al. 2008). The obtained results suggest that when compared with the batch process, the reactive extrusion process appeared to be more efficient for the alkaline extraction of alginates from *L. digitata* in several key ways. Time demand is reduced from about

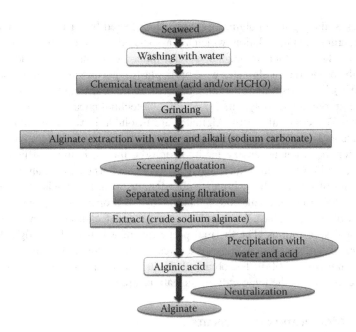

FIGURE 22.2 Extraction process of alginate.

an hour to only a few minutes, water and reactant requirements are divided by more than a factor 2, extraction yield is 15% higher (relative enhancement), and the rheological properties of the product are enhanced.

In order to suit alginate for various applications, it can be prepared with a wide range of average molecular weights (50–100,000 residues). The ratio of mannuronic acid and guluronic acid varies based on weed source and the growing conditions. By the addition of a variety of different chemicals, the viscosity of alginates can be modified and enhanced. The viscosity of 1% solution of alginate in water is a measure of its effectiveness as a thickening agent (Coppen and Nambiar 1991).

22.2.4 PROPERTIES OF ALGINATES

Alginates extracted from different species of brown seaweed often have variations in their chemical structure, resulting in different physical properties. Knowledge of the monomer ring conformations is necessary to understand the polymeric properties of alginates. Highly developed harvesting techniques and stringent processing give us the ability to control alginate properties such as gel strength, particle size, and viscosity. Certain critical factors that affect the physical properties of alginate and its resultant hydrogels are the composition (i.e., M/G ratio), sequence, G-block length, and molecular weight (George and Abraham 2006). Among the various units, the G blocks provide gel-forming capacity and the MM and MG units provide flexibility to the uronic acid chains, with flexibility increasing in the order GG < MM < MG. By increasing the length of G block and the molecular weight, the mechanical properties of alginate gels are typically enhanced. The physicochemical and rheological properties of the alginate polymer were greatly affected by variability in monomer block structures and acetylation, which are associated with the source of alginate.

With the help of their molecular weight, monomer composition, and sequence pattern, the properties of alginates were particularly determined (Remminghorst and Rehm 2006). The possibility of manipulating the molecular weight of alginate would allow the production of polymers for specific biotechnological/biomedical applications (Diaz-Barrera et al. 2010). Alginates are insoluble in water-miscible solvents such as alcohols and ketones. If certain compounds present in water compete with alginate for the water necessary for its hydration, then it is more difficult to dissolve alginate in water. Certain typical approaches such as chemical and/or physical crosslinking of hydrophilic polymers were done to form hydrogels (Varghese and Elisseeff 2006; Lee and Yuk 2007). The biological properties of polysaccharides, especially of alginates, have been explored since many decades in countless medical and surgical applications. The thermal properties of water-insoluble alginate films containing di- and trivalent cations were investigated by Nakamura and his coworkers (Nakamura et al. 2000). The obtained results indicated that alginates form compact structures when the ionic radii of the cations are lower.

22.2.5 MODIFICATION OF ALGINATES

Alginate has an abundance of free hydroxyl and carboxyl groups, two types of functional groups distributed along the polymer chain backbone, and hence, it can be readily modified to alter the characteristics in comparison with the parent compounds. The performance of sodium alginate in all fields has been improved by modifying alginate in the form of hydrogels, beads, films, membranes, and so on, with different methods such as blending (Kurkuri et al. 2002), grafting (Toti et al. 2002), and crosslinking (Wang 2000). Alginate can also be processed as capsules, beads, and fibers, modified with other natural and synthetic polymers or films. Alginate-based hydrogels can be prepared by various crosslinking methods, and especially, the modified forms of alginates were utilized as adsorbents for the treatment of industrial effluents. In order to improve the chemical stability, currently, alternative modifications have been performed in sodium alginate.

Recent studies on the formation of calcium alginate gel reveal three distinct and successive steps of calcium binding to alginate, with increasing calcium concentration: (1) interaction of calcium with a single G monomer, (2) formation of egg-box dimers, and (3) lateral association of dimers to form multimers (Fang et al. 2007). Continuous research on the utilization of suitable materials in many newer applications was carried out by various researchers, and consequently, the modified products obtained from alginic acid and alginates are being successfully used in a variety of applications. Sodium alginate alone (Chan and Heng 2002) or aldehyde-crosslinked sodium alginate along with ovalbumin or gelatin (Kulkarni et al. 2000) and their microparticles and beads have been prepared for various applications.

22.2.5.1 Physical Modification

The physical modification of alginates was done by mixing or blending the parent polysaccharides with suitable substrates such as the monomer or oligomer or even a polysaccharide/polymer. The characteristic changes observed in the physically modified alginates are brought about by charge-transfer complexes imparting supramolecular structural orientations and by virtue of association of compounds facilitated by weak forces (Van der Waals force) and by hydrogen bonds, but not by breaking and/or forming chemical bonds. The physical modification phenomenon can give rise to improved properties in the parent polysaccharides, which may be used for newer applications. By solution-casting method, a series of polyethylene oxide/sodium alginate blended films were prepared, and the observed results of these prepared blends have mechanical properties superior to those of poly(ethylene oxide) films alone (Caykara et al. 2005). In addition, reports from the authors' laboratory also reveal that the physical modified forms of the robust hydrogel systems based on agar/sodium alginate blend (Meena et al. 2008) as well as grafted blend of sodium alginate and agar (Chhatbar et al. 2009) have excellent applications in various fields.

22.2.5.2 Chemical Modification

Needs for chemical modification concern the improvement of mechanical properties, solubility, biocompatibility, control of biodegradability, and manufacturing and shaping. The main sites that are ideal for chemical functionalization in alginate are the free hydroxyl and carboxyl groups along its molecule chain. Properties such as degradability, hydrophobicity, and biological characteristics can be altered by functionalizing available hydroxyl and/or carboxyl groups or by interfering with carbon–carbon bonds. Chemical modification mainly concerns the improvement of mechanical properties, control of biodegradability, shaping, manufacturing, biocompatibility, and solubility. Different approaches were followed for the modification of alginates, and this can be given as follows: by blending or chemical linkages with synthetic biopolymers; by physical and chemical crosslinking process; by surface coating of micro- or nanospheres with biocompatible synthetic polymers; by hydrophobization through alkylation reactions; and by the modulation of guluronic/mannuronic acid ratio or of deacetylation degree.

By covalent attachment of cysteine onto sodium alginate, the mucoadhesive properties of alginate can be improved, and this was reported by Schnürch and his coworkers (Schnürch et al. 2001). Strong hydrogels of amphiphilic derivatives of sodium alginate in aqueous solution were prepared by the chemical covalent binding of long alkyl chains onto the polysaccharide backbone via ester functions (Leonard et al. 2004). By dispersion in sodium chloride solution, the microparticles were prepared from this hydrophobic alginate. A selected approach utilized to activate the polysaccharide for the successive chemical modifications was the introduction of aldehydic groups, which are more reactive than hydroxyl or carboxylic ones, onto sodium alginate via periodate oxidation (Balakrishnan and Jayakrishnan 2005). One more chemical modification process is the grafting process, which provides the addition of certain desirable properties to a polysaccharide, without greatly disturbing the strength and other mechanical properties of the polysaccharide. Graft copolymerization is usually accomplished by generating radical sites on the first polymer backbone, onto which the monomer of the second polymer is copolymerized.

The graft copolymerization of vinyl monomers onto alginate substrates initiated by ceric ammonium nitrate had been extensively used for their property modification (Fares 2003). A superadsorbent hydrogel was prepared by the grafting of poly (acrylic acid) onto an alginate (Pourjavadi et al. 2008). Sodium alginate-graft-poly (N-vinyl-2-pyrrolidone) hydrogel was utilized for the controlled oral delivery of indomethacin drugs (Isıklan et al. 2008). Pourjavadi and his coworkers reported about the pH-responsive properties of the partially hydrolyzed crosslinked alginate-graft-polymethacrylamide, a novel biopolymer-based superabsorbent hydrogel (Pourjavadi et al. 2005). With the help of thermogravimetric analysis, the thermal stability of sodium alginate (SA) and its graft copolymers of acrylonitrile (AN), methyl acrylate (MA), ethyl acrylate (EA), and methyl methacrylate (MMA) has been examined in air atmosphere, and from the characteristic decomposition temperatures, it was identified that the order of decreasing stability was found to be as follows: SA-g-polyacrylonitrile (PAN) > SA-g-polymethyl acrylate(PMA) > SA-g-polyethyl acrylate(PEA) > SA-g-polymethyl methacrylate(PMMA) (Shah et al. 1996). Crosslinking of alginates with aldehydes has also been done successfully, resulting in the modified properties. Yang and his coworkers reported about the successful preparation of cellulose/alginate blend membranes crosslinked by Ca^{2+} bridge in 5 wt.% $CaCl_2$. The observed results reveal that strong hydrogen-bonding interaction between cellulose and alginate exists in the cellulose/alginate blend membranes (Yang et al. 2001).

22.3 APPLICATIONS OF ALGINATES

Alginates find many applications such as the manufacturing of paper and cardboard, pharmaceutical, cosmetic creams, and processed foods (Chapman 1987). In addition, alginates also found numerous applications in biomedical science, engineering, food, printing, dyeing, papermaking, and other industries due to their favorable properties, including stabilizing properties, high viscosity in aqueous solutions, biocompatibility, and ease of gelation (Becker et al. 2001; Martins et al. 2007; Huang et al. 2012). Alginate is typically used in the form of a hydrogel (three-dimensionally crosslinked networks composed of hydrophilic polymers with high water content) in some formulations preventing gastric reflux (Kuo and Ma 2001; Stevens et al. 2004); drug delivery; and biomedicine, including wound healing, tissue engineering, and environmental applications.

Alginates can be effectively used as adsorbents for the removal of heavy metals from wastewater. Alginates play an important role in wastewater treatment, especially in the removal heavy metal ions, due to their advantages such as facile obtaining procedure and being biodegradable, biocompatible, economical, and environmental friendly. When mixed with calcium ions, alginate produces a gel structure, and hence it acts as a potential coagulant and flocculant in water treatment. Industrially, alginates are widely used as thickening, gelling, or stabilizing agents (McHugh 1987; Perez et al. 1992), and in some cases, they act as immunostimulatory agents (Gopinathan and Panigrahy 1983).

22.3.1 FOOD AND AGRICULTURAL FIELD

The food-grade microparticles were created by utilizing biopolymers such as proteins and polysaccharides as building blocks. Many studies have shown that the shelf life of foods and the quality of fish were prolonged and preserved with the help of the edible coatings made up of protein, polysaccharide, and oil-containing materials (Artharn et al. 2009; Fan et al. 2009). In the food industry, alginate has been used as one of the polysaccharide materials in the preparation of edible coatings. These biopolymer-based films can help keep good quality and prolong the shelf life of foods by maintaining the flavor, retarding fat oxidation, increasing water barrier, reducing the degree of shrinkage distortion, and preventing microbe contamination. In addition to glycemic control, sodium alginate appears to have a particular value in appetite and food-intake regulation.

Based on unique and excellent properties, alginate is now added to numerous kinds of food, such as ice cream, jelly, lactic drinks, dressings, instant noodle, and beer. Alginate has excellent functions as a gelling agent, thickening agent, texture improver (for noodles), emulsifier, and colloidal stabilizer to improve the quality of food. Alginate's thickening property was mainly utilized in sauces, syrups, and toppings for ice cream. Safety of alginate for food applications is certified by the Food and Agriculture Organization (FAO)/World Health Organization (WHO) as one of the safest food additives. In order to maintain higher concentrations of preservatives on the surface of foods, the coatings present in the food may also serve as carriers for antimicrobial compounds and antioxidant.

The coating of pork, fish, shrimp, and scallop with sodium alginate can prolong their shelf life, reducing thawing loss and cooking loss, helping in weight loss, and maintaining the functional properties during frozen storage (Wang et al. 1994; Zeng and Xu 1997; Wanstedt et al. 1981; Yu et al. 2008). Alginate has unique colloidal properties and can form strong gels or insoluble polymers through crosslinking with Ca^{2+} by posttreatment of $CaCl_2$ solution, and this gelling property was utilized in the formation of jellies in the food industry. The edible dessert jellies formed by simply mixing alginate and calcium in water or milk are often promoted as instant jellies or desserts.

Devi and Kakati (2013) prepared the porous microparticles of different sizes by polyelectrolyte complexation of biopolymers gelatine A and sodium alginate for microencapsulation of food bioactives. The observed results revealed that the optimum conditions for maximum complexation between gelatine and sodium alginate were observed at the ratio of 1.9:3.5 by weight and pH 3.7. The porous and pH-responsive gelatine–sodium alginate microparticles are likely to have potential applications in food encapsulation, smart drug delivery, separation of biomolecules, enzyme immobilization, and so on. In order to preserve frozen fish, the calcium alginate films and coatings have been used. The oils in oily fish such as herring and mackerel can become rancid through oxidation, even when quick-frozen and stored at low temperatures. If the fish is frozen in a calcium alginate jelly, the fish is protected from air, and rancidity from oxidation is very limited. Yongling Song and his coworkers studied about the effect of sodium alginate-based edible coating containing different antioxidants on the quality and shelf life of refrigerated bream (*Megalobrama amblycephala*). The obtained results indicated that coating treatments retarded the decay of fish compared with uncoated bream (Song et al. 2011).

22.3.2 Cell and Enzyme Immobilization

The technique of combining biocatalyst in an insoluble support matrix is termed immobilization. When compared with their free cell counterparts, the immobilized cells entrapped within a polymer matrix or attached onto the surface of a solid support have advantages such as the easier harvesting of the biomass, enhanced wastewater treatment, and enriched bioproduct generation, since they are resistant to harsh environments such as salinity, metal toxicity, and pH. The immobilized cells recover the cells in a less-destructive way, protect the aging cultures against the harmful effects of photoinhibition, yield higher biomass concentrations, and enhance the cost-effectiveness of the process by reusing the regenerated biomass. Immobilized microalgae have been used for a diverse number of bioprocesses, including gaining access to high-value products (biohydrogen, biodiesel, and photopigments), in removal of nutrients (nitrate, phosphate, and ammonium ions), in removal of heavy metal ions, as biosensors, and in stock culture management. The immobilized cells occupy less space, are easier to handle, and can be used repeatedly for product generation (Mallick 2002).

Alginate is one of the most widely used polymers employed in immobilization and microencapsulation technologies (Taqieddin and Amiji 2004). The immobilization of biomaterials or living cells in alginate gels is a well-established technology used in an increasing number of biomedical and industrial applications. The temperature-independent sol/gel transition in the presence of multivalent cations (e.g., Ca^{2+}) and the specific biological effect of sodium alginate make it highly suitable as an immobilization matrix for living cells. The high-molecular-weight polymers such as polyacrylamide, starch, and cellulose were used as matrix in the immobilization process. The most common polymeric matrix used to immobilize microorganisms for many uses is the biodegradable alginate (Bashan and De Bashan 2010). The entrapment within calcium alginate is the most widely used technique for immobilizing cells and enzymes. The lower microorganisms (bacteria, yeasts, and fungi) and cells can be easily immobilized with a number of methods: entrapment, ion-exchange adsorption, porous ceramics, and even covalent bonding (Souza 2002). The advantage of immobilizing enzymes or cells over free cells is to increase their stability and efficiency. The successful encapsulation of glucose oxidase (GOX) into calcium alginate–chitosan microspheres (CACM) using an emulsification–internal gelation–enzyme adsorption–coating by chitosan method with high residual activity had been established by Xia Wang and his coworkers (Wang et al. 2011). The reported results herein indicate that the CACM–GOX has a great potential as a flour improver.

The metal cations can readily be exchanged with sodium alginate and then be coordinated with the −OH of the carboxylate groups to generate the ion-crosslinked alginates (Yan Chun et al. 2014). The instability of alginate occurs when the gels are in contact with cations that serve as chelating agents and anti-gelling cations, such as dissolved phosphorus, ethylenediaminetetraacetic acid (EDTA) citrates, sodium bicarbonate, and several more (Kierstan and Coughlan 1985; Dainty et al. 1986; Martinsen et al. 1989). The damage to the polymeric alginate spheres increases *in situ* experiments, mainly because of the elimination or replacement of the common solidifying cation Ca^{2+} with other cations or anions, such as P-3 and Na^+, which causes alginate to have a lower mechanical strength and makes it more susceptible to leakage of entrapped cells (Moreira et al. 2006). Hence, the joint immobilization (also known as coimmobilization) of bacteria and microalgae in alginate beads was proposed and demonstrated in most of the cases for wastewater treatment. Proposals for materials used for hardening of alginate beads involve adding polyvinyl alcohol (Chen and Lin 1994; Wang et al. 1995), polyvinylpyrrolidone (Doria-Serrano et al. 2001), carboxymethylcellulose (Joo et al. 2001), and so on.

In order to lessen the environmental problems arising due to wastewater, the methods of cell entrapment and cell immobilization in a porous polymeric matrix have been applied (Hill and Khan 2008; Siripattanakul-Ratpukdi 2012). The cell entrapment technique was successfully applied to both municipal and industrial wastewater treatment (Siripattanakul and Khan 2010). Typical polymers used as an entrapment matrix, including calcium alginate, carrageenan, polyvinyl alcohol, and cellulose triacetate, were reported. The potential of using immobilized cells for bioremediation of heavy metal pollutants in industrial processes is regarded as a valuable application. Laboratory experiments were performed to study the nutrient removal of phosphate, nitrate, and ammonia uptake of free and immobilized cells of marine microalgae, *Chlorella salina*. The cell immobilization was carried out in sodium alginate matrix, and the cells were found to be highly efficient in the removal of excess nutrients in untreated tannery effluent. This was reported by Jayasudha and Sampathkumar (2014).

Silica-immobilized *Medicago sativa* (alfalfa) was utilized as an adsorbent for removing copper ions from aqueous solutions by Gardea-Torresdey et al. (2002). The reported results indicate that the immobilized biomass appears to have a greater potential than raw biomass in packed bed or fluidized bed reactors due to the benefits such as better capabilities of regeneration, control of particle size, reuse, and recovery, without destruction of biomass beads (Shah et al. 1996). Immobilization with different polymeric materials is studied for enzyme encapsulation, along with their application in the treatment of various pollutants (Zille et al. 2003). *Candida xylopsoci* (Z-HS 51) was immobilized in sodium alginate, and its potential for the bioremediation of mercury was evaluated by Amin and Latif (2013). The reported results herein indicate that the immobilization does not affect the shelf life of microbes but provides favorable microenvironmental conditions for organisms, protects against harsh environment, improves genetic stability, and can be transferred easily and safely at any time and place.

Most of the principles involved in enzyme immobilization are directly applicable to cell immobilization. Applications of this versatile method include immobilization of hybridomas for the production of monoclonal antibodies, immobilization of cells in bioreactors, entrapment of plant protoplasts and plant embryos ("artificial seeds") for micropropagation, and the entrapment of enzymes and drugs (Dean Madden 2007). When they were in separate solutions, nearly complete removal of copper and nickel metals by alginate-entrapped *Chlorella vulgaris* cells was observed by Mehta and Gaur (Mehta and Gaur 2001). On the other hand, the presence of copper in the nickel solution inhibited the biosorption of both metals either by immobilized or free cells, due to the competition of different metal ions on the same active sites of microalgae. The removal of cadmium and zinc metals using alginate-immobilized *Chlorella homosphaera* was done by Da Costa and Leite (1991). They also observed that the biosorption of Cd(II) and Zn(II) alone was much higher than the biosorption when these two metal ions were combined.

The cell immobilization was carried out in sodium alginate matrix, and the cells were found to be highly efficient in the removal of excess nutrients in untreated tannery effluent. Crude L-amino acid oxidase (L-AAO) of *Aspergillus fumigatus* immobilized in various solid supports, namely entrapment in calcium alginate gel and gelatin gel and then the adsorption in nylon membrane by crosslinking with glutaraldehyde, was investigated by Susmita Singh and her cowokers (Singh et al. 2012). The obtained results indicate that the immobilization of *A. fumigatus* L-AAO in calcium alginate gel was found to be the most favorable, since the percentage entrapped activity was maximal in calcium alginate beads (31.77%) when compared with the adsorption in nylon membrane (26.88%).

Arpana Hemraj Jobanputra and her coworkers reported about the use of inert solid matrix calcium alginate as a supporting material for the immobilization of rifamycin oxidase from *Chryseobacterium* species. Rifamycin oxidase from *Chryseobacterium* species was found to be involved in the transformation of rifamycin B to S, the starting antibiotic derivative for the synthesis of several semisynthetic rifamycins. The investigation was done on the catalytic properties of immobilized rifamycin oxidase. The obtained results reveal that 3% sodium alginate and 0.2 M calcium chloride ($CaCl_2$) were found to be the optimum concentrations for maximal biotransformation. The optimum temperature was found to be 45°C, and the enzyme was usable up to four cycles (Jobanputra et al. 2011).

22.3.3 BIOMEDICAL FIELD

Natural biodegradable polymers have received much more attention in the last decades due to various applications in the fields related to environmental protection and the maintenance of physical health. Polysaccharide-based biomaterials are an emerging class in several biomedical fields such as drug-delivery devices and tissue regeneration, particularly for cartilage and gel entrapment systems for the immobilization of cells. Biopolymers have received attention as tissue engineering (TE) substrates, with several studies examining materials such as gelatin, alginate, and chitosan as cell scaffolds for both two-dimensional (2D) and three-dimensional (3D) cell cultures (Pan et al. 2005; Park et al. 2005; Barralet et al. 2005; Zhang et al. 2006).

Among the various biopolymers, alginate has found numerous applications in biomedical science and engineering due to its favorable properties, including biocompatibility and ease of gelation. It is extensively used in pharmaceutical industries as a suspending and emulsifying agent (Reilly et al. 2000). The alginate hydrogels have been particularly attractive in drug delivery, tissue engineering, and wound healing, as these gels retain structural similarity to the extracellular matrices in tissues and can be manipulated to play several critical roles (Lee and Mooney 2012). In recent years, the reason for an increased interest of alginates in specific biomedical applications was due to the enhancement of efficient treatment of esophageal reflux as well as due to the creativity of multiquality calcium fibers for dermatology and wound healing. They are also used for high- and low-gel-strength dental impression materials. The use of alginate polymer as a surfactant in the emulsion drug-delivery investigations was identified as a promising research avenue.

22.3.3.1   Wound Healing

Local wound infection has been a great challenge for wound care clinicians, with few management options. The adoption of alginate dressings was effectively halted in the early 1970s, and the use of alginate dressings as hemostatic agents was reported both in vitro and in clinical studies after the Second World War (Thomas 2010). The forcing of sodium alginate under pressure through the fine apertures into the calcium salt solution produces alginate fibers, and this provides the foundation for alginate wound dressings. The major reason behind the selection of alginate as a dressing material is that it will manage wound exudate, as it is claimed that alginate can absorb 15 to 20 times its own weight in wound fluid. In a wide range of presentations, alginate dressings were manufactured in a variety of forms, such as from flat sheets to rope and ribbons (MA healthcare Ltd, *Wound Care Handbook 2011–2012, London*).

Rope and ribbon versions were mainly used to lightly pack cavity wounds, and the flat sheets tend to be utilized for the superficial wounds. Each year, large quantities of alginate dressings were utilized to treat exuding wounds, such as infected surgical wounds, leg ulcers, and pressure sores. Originally, these dressings were a loose fleece formed primarily from calcium alginate fibers (Thomas 2000). Moreover, the evaluation of silver alginate powder as a dressing material proved to be compatible, which assisted with infection-free healing with the release of silver over a sustained period of time. This silver alginate powder was well suited for abnormal-contouring wounds, making it very versatile for use. Alginate-based dressings are indicated for bleeding wounds, since calcium alginate is a natural hemostat (Paul and Sharma 2004).

The gel-forming property of alginate helps in removing the dressing without much trauma. In the future, it may be feasible to achieve increased fluid-handling capacities in alginate dressings, with additional benefits such as antimicrobial capability. Glutaraldehyde-crosslinked sodium alginate/gelatin hydrogels were utilized in wound-dressing applications. The reported results indicate that the SA/G-50/50 hydrogel crosslinked via Ca^{2+} ions was found to be a potential nontoxic wound-dressing material capable of adequate provision of moist environment for comfortable wound healing. Mennini et al. (2011) developed chitosan–Ca–alginate microspheres for colon delivery of celecoxib–hydroxypropylbeta–cyclodextrin–PVP complex. Chitin–calcium alginate composite fibers were evaluated for wound care dressings by Shamshina et al. (2014). Wound healing studies (rat models and histological evaluation) indicated that chitin–calcium alginate-covered wound sites underwent normal wound healing with reepithelialization and that coverage of dermal fibrosis with hyperplastic epidermis was consistently complete after only 7 days of treatment.

22.3.3.2   Tissue Engineering

An important therapeutic strategy utilized for the present and future medicine is the tissue engineering, which involves the development of temporary or, in some cases, permanent biological substitutes for failing tissues and organs. Alginate is readily processable for applicable 3D scaffolding materials such as hydrogels, microspheres, microcapsules, sponges, foams, and fibers (Su and Tan 2013). Sodium alginate has applications as a material for the encapsulation and immobilization of a variety of cell types for immunoisolatory and biochemical processing applications. Sodium alginate forms a biodegradable gel when crosslinked with calcium ions, and this has been exploited in cartilage tissue engineering, since chondrocytes do not dedifferentiate when immobilized in it.

Mosahebi et al. (2001) showed that alginate gels promoted the viability and function of Schwann cells for neural applications. The evaluation of sodium alginate for bone marrow cell tissue engineering was done by Wang and his coworkers. From the obtained results, it was evident that depending on composition, calcium-crosslinked alginate can act as a substrate for rat marrow cell proliferation and has the potential for use as a 3D degradable scaffold (Wang et al. 2003). Tissue engineering with 3D biomaterials represents a promising approach for developing hepatic tissue to replace the function of a failing liver. The results highlight the importance of cell density on the hepatocellular functions of 3D hepatocyte constructs as well as the advantages of alginate matrices as scaffoldings (Dvir-Ginzberg et al. 2004). Archana and her coworkers reported about the use of chitosan–pectin, chitosan–alginate, and chitosan–pectin alginate scaffolds for tissue engineering applications. The observed results showed that when compared with chitosan–pectin and chitosan–alginate, the ternary chitosan–pectin alginate scaffolds has excellent antibacterial activity and cell viability (Archana et al. 2013).

Immobilized cells or tissue in alginate gels can also be used as bioartificial organs in tissue engineering applications, since alginate functions as a protective barrier toward physical stress and also to avoid immunological reactions with the host. Porous hydroxyapatite (HAp)/chitosan–alginate composite scaffolds are prepared through *in situ* coprecipitation and freeze-drying for bone tissue engineering, and the reported results indicate that HAp/chitosan–alginate composite scaffold was shown to be more effective for new bone generation than chitosan–alginate scaffold (Jin et al. 2012). Novel hybrid hydrogels based on alginate and keratin were successfully produced for the first time by Raquel Silva and his coworkers. The obtained results demonstrated that the alginate/keratin hybrid biomaterials supported proliferation, cell attachment, and spreading, and this proved that such novel hybrid hydrogels might find applications as scaffolds for soft tissue regeneration (Silva et al. 2014). Alginate scaffold has been used for preparation of soft or hard tissue engineering, and the obtained results suggest that the highly porous crosslinked alginate membrane lay a foundation for the construction of skin tissue engineering scaffold (Gong et al. 2015).

22.3.3.3 Drug Delivery

An important part of the pharmaceutical aspect of chemical engineering is the controlled drug delivery, which is dedicated to the release of therapeutically active agents into the body. The main goal of controlled drug delivery is to dispense the drug at a predetermined rate, either constant or in intervals, to the optimum target area for absorption, in order to control the drug concentration in these regions. As naturally derived polymers, due to their nonimmunogenicity nature, the alginate polymers are currently under investigation for drug-delivery application (Gombotz and Wee 1998). Alginate material is a promising candidate for site-specific mucosal delivery, and this was due to its very strong bioadhesive ability. Hydrogel-forming polymers (e.g., alginates and poloxamers) were used as encapsulation materials for controlled drug delivery to mucosal tissue by Moebus and his coworkers (Moebus et al. 2009).

In vitro evaluation of alginate beads of ibuprofen for oral sustained drug delivery was done by Jharana Mallick and his coworkers (Mallick et al. 2013). The obtained result implies that the microspheres produced with 2.5% (W/V) sodium alginate had the optimum prolonged-release pattern, whereas the microspheres produced with 2% (W/V) sodium alginate had the highest-delay release of the incorporated drug, and this indicates that the formulations of ibuprofen–sodium alginate microspheres are likely to offer a reliable means of delivering ibuprofen by the oral route. Demiroz et al. (2007) prepared alginate-based mesalazine tablets for intestinal drug delivery. Alginate-based drug-delivery system was developed by Ciofani and his coworkers, specifically for neurological applications, by considering the neuroprotection and the target application of neural regeneration (Ciofani et al. 2008).

Davidovich Pinhas et al. (2009) prepared mucoadhesive drug-delivery systems by utilizing hydrated thiolated alginate. The extensive studies have shown that dry, uncrosslinked, compressed tablets made from thiolated polymers adhere better to the mucus layer compared with the native polymers. Chitosan–Ca–alginate microspheres were developed for colon delivery of celecoxib–hydroxypropylbeta-cyclodextrin–PVP complex by Menini and his coworkers (Mennini et al. 2011). Vijay Kumart Malesu and his coworkers reported about the use of novel nanocomposite of chitosan and alginate blended with Cloisite 30B as a drug-delivery system for anticancer drug curcumin (Malesu et al. 2011).

Synthesis and swelling behavior of a superabsorbent hydrogel based on alginate and polyacrylamide (PAAm) was investigated by Sadeghi and his coworkers (2014). The results reported herein indicate that the alginate–polyacrylamide hydrogel exhibited a pH-responsive swelling–deswelling behavior at pHs 3 and 9, respectively, and this on–off switching behavior provides the hydrogel with the potential to control the delivery of bioactive agents. The potential of alginate fibers incorporated with drug-loaded nanocapsules as drug delivery systems was evaluated by Liu and his coworkers (2014). The drug-release tests show that the cumulative release amount increased with an increase in the proportion of nanocapsules present in the fiber, and this work suggests that the addition of nanocapsules-containing drugs into the spinning dopes is a promising strategy to fabricate novel drug-loaded fibers for immediate drug delivery for wound dressing.

22.4   TREATMENT OF INDUSTRIAL EFFLUENTS

Effective effluent treatment is an important step toward conserving our water resources (Mugdha and Usha 2012). In general, especially in small-scale industries, the removal of fine particles can allow discharges below the target standard limits, leading to the improvement in effluent quality. The result is a clear, apparently clean effluent, which is discharged into natural water bodies. Sodium alginate plays an important role in removing toxic heavy metal ions (wastewater treatment) because of its advantages, such as facile obtaining procedure and biocompatible, biodegradable, economical, and environmental friendly nature.

The strong chelating properties of alginic acid and alginate salts for metal ions were mainly due to the abundance of various functional groups such as carboxylic, hydroxyl, and oxo groups. Alginate gel with significantly structural strength was formed by crosslinking alginic acid with polyvalent ions such as calcium ions (Nestle and Kimmich 1996). The crosslinking process is usually caused by the binding of polyvalent ion with two or more carboxylic groups on adjacent polymer chains, which is also accompanied by chelation of the ion by the hydroxyl and carboxyl groups of the polymer chains (Shimizu and Takada 1997).

Calcium alginate may be prepared in various forms such as powder and fibers and can be used as cell immobilization support. In order to increase the properties of alginate prepared in the form of bead, it may be protonated, crosslinked, or doped with another metallic ion. In order to increase the metal-uptake capacities, various chemical treatments such as carboxylation, phosphorylation, and sulfonation may be applied on alginic acid; however, these treatments tend to increase the cost of the resulting product (Fiset et al. 2008). The use of sodium alginate in effluent treatment has been under exploration for the past two decades. Several studies on metal sorption using alginate products have been represented in Table 22.2.

22.4.1 FROM TEXTILE INDUSTRIES

By virtue of its contribution to overall industrial output and employment generation, the textile industries have great economic significance. In terms of pollution, the textile industry has been condemned as one of the world's worst offenders, and this is due to the fact that about 10% to 15% of all the dyes used in the industry are lost with wastewater during processing (Harikumar et al. 2013). In textile dyeing process, a large amount of chemically different dyes are used. A significant proportion of these dyes enter the environment via wastewater, which poses a threat to the environment (Dayaram and Dasgupta 2008). The presence of even very low concentrations of dyes in effluent is highly visible, and degradation products of these textile dyes are often carcinogenic (Kim et al. 2003). Nowadays, in many parts of the world, the treatment of textile dyeing industries has been a challenging task.

When compared with other industries, the textile industries rank first in usage of dyes for coloration of fibers (Maynard 1983; Zollinger 1987; Grag et al. 2004; Arunachalam and Annadurai 2011), and hence, the wastewater produced from the tanning and textile industries contains large amount of exhausted dyes and pigments, leading to the polluted environment. Previously, it has been estimated that about 10,000 dyes and pigments were produced and about 7×10^5 tons were used in different industries, such as textile, rubber, paper, and cosmetic. Colored wastewater from the textile industries is rated as the most polluted in almost all industrial sectors (Andleeb et al. 2010). Attempts have been made by several researchers to develop an inexpensive and efficient method for the treatment of disperses dyes that are potentially toxic and even carcinogenic. Due to their toxic and aesthetical impacts on receiving waters, the textile effluent treatment is of interest nowadays.

A promising alternative to replace or supplement the present processes of dye removal from dye wastewaters is the biosorption process (Fu and Viraraghavan 2003). Calcium alginate has been investigated as a possible coagulant due to its

TABLE 22.2
List of Utilization of Alginates in Metal Ion Removal

Removal of Metals	Sorbents	Studied Parameters	References
Ni(II)	Alginate beads	Sorption desorption cycle, effect of alginate beads, pH, initial metal ion concentration, the Langmuir model	Al-Rub et al. (2004)
Cu(II), Mn(II)	Alginate gel beads	Fourier transform infra red (FTIR) and scanning electron microscopy (SEM) characterization, doped alginate beads with cyanogens bromide and 1,6-diaminohexane	Gotoh et al. (2004)
Co(II), Cr(III), Cu(II), Ni(II), Zn(II)	Protonated alginate beads	Effect of metal uptake, ionic strength, pH, protonation, beads' morphology	Ibanez and Umetsu (2004)
Cr(III)	Protonated dry alginate beads	Batch tests, effect of pH, mechanism, electron probe X-ray micro analysis-energy dispersive X-ray micro analysis (EPMA-EDX) analysis	Ibanez and Umetsu (2004)
Cu(II), Pb(II)	Carboxylated alginic acid	Desorption, effect of ionic strength, and organic material effect	Jeon et al. (2005)
Pb(II)	Carboxylated alginic acid	Desorption; carboxylated alginic acid using $KMnO_4$, FTIR, and ^{13}C nuclear magnetic resonance ($^{13}CNMR$) characterization; elemental analysis	Jeon et al. (2002)
Cu(II), Cd(II), Pb(II)	Alginate beads, alginate extracted from *Laminaria digitata*	Alginate beads' characterization; batch metal uptake; Langmuir, Freundlich, and Sips models; kinetic model; batch kinetic model	Papageorgiou et al. (2006)
Cu(II)	Chitosan/sodium alginate beads	Effect of treatment time, chitosan and alginate concentration, temperature	Qin et al. (2006)
Pb(II), Cd(II)	Calcium alginate microparticles	Influence of the heavy metal initial concentration on adsorption kinetics	Nita et al. (2007)
Cr(VI), Ca(II), Cd(II), Cu((II), Pb(II), Ni(II), Fe(II), Mn(II)	Calcium-crosslinked alginate beads	Characterization, tannery wastewater treatment	EL-Tayieb et al. (2013)
As(V)	Iron-crosslinked alginate nanoparticles	Column studies—effect of bed height, flow rate, and metal ion concentration; bed depth service time (BDST) plot	Singh et al. (2014)
Cu(II)	Nanochitosan/ sodium alginate/ microcrystalline cellulose beads	Characterization, batch metal uptake, Langmuir and Freundlich models, kinetic model	Vijayalakshmi et al. (2016)

gelling abilities. The development and application of horseradish peroxidase (HRP) immobilized on calcium alginate gel beads has been reported for successful and effective decolorization of textile industrial effluent (Gholami-Borujeni et al. 2011). Biological treatment of bacterium with saw dust seems to be a viable option for the treatment of effluents from dye-based industries, which pose a major problem. The effective removal of methylene blue (MB) from aqueous solution in a batch-stirred tank reactor was done by using alginate/polyvinyl alcohol–kaolin clay composite material by El-Latif et al. (2010).

Boucherit and his coworkers reported the use of cucurbita peroxidase (C-peroxidase) extracted from courgette in decolorization of disperse dye in free and immobilized forms by using calcium alginate gel entrapment process (Boucherit et al. 2012). Calcium alginate used as a green support for TiO_2 immobilization can be used for developing a new environmentally friendly immobilization system for large-scale water treatment. Sodium alginate, extracted from the brown marine alga *Turbinaria decurrens*-based hydrogel, graft polymerized with poly(itaconic acid), NaAlg/IA, was employed in studies on the adsorption kinetic of Pb^{2+} in aqueous solution (Mahmoud and Mohamed 2012).

22.4.2 FROM PAPERMAKING INDUSTRIES

The manufacture of paper generates significant quantities of wastewater, as high as 60 m^3/ton of paper produced. The raw wastewaters from paper and board mills can be potentially very polluting. In the papermaking process, the paper sludge is a solid residue that is currently disposed in land fields or burned, which consequently pollutes the environment. Papermaking wastewater contains some difficult degradation substances such as lignin, cellulose, and many tiny colloidal materials (Matsushita et al. 2004; Srivastava et al. 2005; Wang et al. 2006). Flocculation process is widely used for papermaking wastewater pretreatment or advanced treatment (Yang et al. 2010). Sodium alginate is used as a flocculation-reinforcing agent in papermaking wastewater treatment, and it acts as a framework material in flocculation. It will accelerate the forming of flocculation particles and shorten the time of flocculation.

Defang Zeng and his coworkers reported about the use of composite consisting of sodium alginate, polyaluminum ferric chloride, and cationic polyacrylamide as flocculants in treating wastewater from papermaking industries (Zheng et al. 2011). The observed results indicated that it achieved the best flocculation performance when the raw material mass ratio was 2:1:1 and the optimum dosage of the composite flocculant was found to be 20 mg/L. The removal efficiencies of chemical oxygen demand (COD) and turbidity with this composite flocculant reached 89.6% and 99.2%, respectively. The decolorization of paper mill effluent by sodium alginate-immobilized cells of *Phanerochaete chrysosporium* was investigated by Gomathi and her coworkers. The obtained results indicate that the combination of calcium alginate-immobilized *P. chrysosporium* with the addition of C and N sources helped achieve high treatment efficiency in color removal. When the immobilized culture was used under aerobic conditions, it was found that biological oxygen demand (BOD) and COD and other characteristics of the effluent were also reduced and high transparency of the effluent was obtained (Gomathi et al. 2012).

22.4.3 FROM TANNERIES

Typically, the tanneries are characterized as pollution-intensive industrial complexes, which generate widely varying and high-strength wastewater. Tannery waste is actually a complex mixture that makes the design of effluent treatment challenging. Wattle extract (vegetable-based tanning dye), chrome tannin (residual tanning broth containing chromium), and chemical dye compounds were found to be the three significant pollutants in the tannery effluent (Kanagaraj and Mandal 2012). Proper elimination of pollutants from the tannery effluents is essential in industrialized countries and is becoming increasingly important from an environmental and human health point of view in the developing and emerging countries (Breisha 2010).

By utilizing sodium alginate, the chemical coagulants such as sodium citrate, ammonium aluminum sulfate, aluminum sulfate, and calcium carbonate were immobilized in the bead form to treat tannery wastewater samples. After immobilization, chemical coagulants were found more effective in the reduction in electrical conductivity (EC), total dissolved solids (TDS), phenolphthalein, total phenolphthalein, COD, and chromium amounts in comparison with their native forms. The observed results clearly demonstrate that the immobilized ammonium aluminum sulfate was found to be more effective for chromium removal from the tannery industry's wastewater. The immobilization of chemical coagulants can enhance their effectiveness in pollution-removal processes (Imran et al. 2012).

Biomass/polymer matrices beads (BPMB) prepared by the immobilization of Baker's yeast strain (*Saccharomyces cerevisiae*) biomass in alginate extract (3%) were investigated for chromium biosorption from aqueous solution. The obtained results reveal that the prepared BPMB beads offer excellent potential for chromium removal from contaminated sites, with concentrations ranging between 200 mg L^{-1} and 1000 mg L^{-1}. Biosorbent can remove chromium up to 77% for synthetic solution and 85% for raw tannery wastewater (Mahmoud et al. 2015). Literature reports indicate that biodegradation involving microorganism is a suitable process for wastewater treatment. The use of microalgae in effluent treatment has been under exploration in recent decades. The cells of marine microalgae *C. salina* immobilized using sodium alginate are a promising biological remediator compared with the free cells for nutrient removal of phosphate, nitrate, and ammonia from the tannery industrial effluent and can improve the quality of water to their discharging limits.

A total of six species of bacteria—*Pseudomonas putida*, *P. fluorescens*, *Klebsiella pneumoniae*, *Escherichia coli*, *Staphylococcus aureus*, and *Bacillus subtilis*—were isolated from the effluent initially by Srinivas Gidhamaari and his coworkers. These isolated bacteria were immobilized using sodium alginate, and this was then utilized for the effluent treatment. The obtained results reveal that due to the immobilization of bacteria on sodium alginate, the BOD and COD levels were reduced nearly 75% and 65%, respectively. From the above observation, it was concluded that the immobilized bacterium *P. putida* could be used to treat various industrial effluents effectively (Gidhamaari et al. 2012).

22.4.4 FROM DAIRY INDUSTRIES

One of the major causes of pollution is the wastewater generated from the dairy industries. The generated wastewater is highly degradable and hence requires specialized treatment to minimize environmental problems. Primarily, the dairy industry wastewater was generated from the cleaning and washing operations in the milk-processing plants. The generation of dairy wastewater was estimated to be 2.5 times the volume of the milk processed (Kadu et al. 2013). The wastewater resulting from cheese production is the most polluting among all types of dairy wastewaters, since it contains a huge quantity of organic biodegradable matters, which can disrupt aquatic and terrestrial ecosystems, and hence, it requires specialized treatment to minimize environmental problems (Kaur et al. 2014).

Since the bulk of the pollution load from a typical diary is the organic material from whole milk, which is biodegradable in nature, the diary wastewater should most appropriately be treated by the biological means. In fluidized bed bioreactor, experiment was conducted by Ravichandra and his coworkers to test the biological conversion of sulfides using calcium alginate-immobilized cells of *Thiobacillus* sp., which was isolated from aerobic sludge of distillery and dairy effluent treatment plant. The batch-fluidized bed bioreactor is operated for 168 hours, with an initial sulfide concentration of 150 mg/L. The observed results revealed that at the end of 168 hours, 100% sulfide oxidation is achieved by the continuous supply of sterile air as an oxidant (Ravichandra et al. 2006).

The potential of free and immobilized fungal isolates to treat the dairy wastewater at different concentrations of dairy effluent was investigated by Amanpreet and Chaman (2014). Five fungal sp. D1W and D4S (*Alternaria* sp.), D3S (*Fusarium* sp.), and D2W and D5S (*Aspergillus sp.*) were isolated from dairy effluent in two different seasons. The fungal isolates were efficiently immobilized on sodium alginate beads. This study revealed that when compared with the immobilized fungal cells, the free fungal cells showed better removal of organic pollutants in dairy effluent. Results concluded that free cells of D1W (*Alternaria* sp.) is competent to treat dairy wastewater and have the potential to reduce the physicochemical parameters at different concentrations of dairy effluent.

22.5 FUTURE DIRECTIONS FOR RESEARCH

In the future, efforts should be made to improve the alginate biomaterial for further enhancement in its application results. The alginate dressings have been used clinically since the mid-1940s and in commercial production for almost 30 years. In future, it may be feasible to achieve increased fluid-handling capacities in alginate dressings, with additional benefits such as antimicrobial capability. Alginate and its derivatives have a very great potential in treatment of wastewater. Moreover, designing of new biosorbents by modification of alginate with various other materials explore their innovative properties against environmental pollution.

22.6 CONCLUSION

A new generation of biodegradable natural biomaterials is emerging due to the significant progress of regenerative medicine and wastewater treatment with the development of modern science and technology. A brief review on the promising marine sources of sodium alginate and on the use of alginates in biomedical, food, and agricultural fields and in the treatment of wastewater from various industries has been reported. Further investigations with a multidisciplinary approach are imperative in order to develop alginates as useful in many fields. We expect that this chapter provides insights on the use of sodium alginate for researchers working to discover new materials with new properties for the valuable applications of these materials.

REFERENCES

Al-Rub, F. A. A., M. H. El-Naas, F. Benyahia, and I. Ashour. 2004. Biosorption of nickel on blank alginate beads, free and immobilized algal cells. *Process Biochem.* 39:1767–1773.

Alsberg, E., K. W. Anderson, A. Albeiruti, R. T. Franceschi, and D. J. Mooney. 2001. Cell-interactive alginate hydrogels for bone tissue engineering. *J. Dent. Res.* 80:2025–2029.

Amanpreet, K. and S. Chaman. 2012. Dairy wastewater treatment by free and immobilized fungal isolates. *J. Microbiol. Biotech. Res.* 4:31–37.

Amin, A. and Z. Latif. 2013. Detoxification of mercury pollutant by immobilized yeast strain candida xylopsoci. *Pak. J. Bot.* 45:1437–1442.

Andleeb, S., N. Atiq, M. I. Ali, R. Razi-UL-Hussain, M. Shafique, B. Ahmed, P. B. Ghumro, M. Hussain, A. Hameed, and S. Ahmed. 2010. Biological treatment of textile effluent in stirred tank bioreactor. *Int. J. Agric. Biol.* 12:256–260.

Aravindhan, N., N. Fathima, J. R. Rao, and B. U. Nair. 2007. Equilibrium and thermodynamic studies on the removal of basic black dye using calcium alginate beads. *Colloid. Surf. A Phys. Chem. Eng. Asp.* 299:232–238.

Archana, D., L. Upadhay, R. P. Tewari, J. Dutta, Y. B. Huang, and P. K. Dutta. 2013. Chitosan-Pectin-Alginate as a novel scallfold for tissue engineering applications. *Ind. J. Biotech.* 12:475–482.

Artharn, A., T. Prodpran, and S. Benjakul. 2009. Round scad protein-based film: Storage stability and its effectiveness for shelf-life extension of dried fish powder. *Food Sci. Technol.* 42:1238–1244.

Arunachalam, R. and G. Annadurai. 2011. Optimized response surface methodology for adsorption of dyestuff from aqueous solution. *J. Environ. Sci. Technol.* 4:65–72.

Balakrishnan, B. and A. Jayakrishnan. 2005. Self-cross-linking biopolymers as injectable in situ forming biodegradable scaffolds. *Biomaterials* 26:3941–3951.

Barralet, J. E, L. Wang, M. Lawson, J. T. Triffitt, P. R. Cooper, and R. M. Shelton. 2005. Comparison of bone marrow cell growth on 2D and 3D alginate hydrogels. *J. Mater Sci-Mater Med.* 16:515–519.

Bashan, Y. and L. E. De-Bashan. 2010. How the plant growth-promoting bacterium Azospirillum promotes plant growth-a critical assessment. *Adv. Agron.* 108:77–136.

Becker, T. A., D. R. Kipke, and T. Brandon. 2001. Calcium alginate gel: A biocompatible and mechanically stable polymer for endovascular embolization. *J. Biomed. Mater. Res.* 54:76–86.

Bixler, H. J. and H. Porse. 2010. A decade of change in the seaweed hydrocolloids industry. *J. Appl. Phycol.* 23:321–335.

Boucherit, N., M. Abouseoud, and L. Adoura. 2012. Degradation of disperse dye from textile effluent by free and immobilized Cucurbita pepo peroxidase. *EPJ Web of Conferences.* 29:00008.

Breisha, G. Z. 2010. Bio-removal of nitrogen from wastewaters—A review. *Nat. Sci.* 8:210–228.

Caykara, T., S. Demirci, M. S. Eroglu, and O. Guven. 2005. Poly(ethylene oxide) and its blends with sodium alginate. *Polymer* 46:10750–10757.

Chan, L. W. and P. W. S. Heng. 2002. Effects of aldehydes and methods of cross-linking on properties of calcium alginate microspheres prepared by emulsification. *Biomaterials* 23:1319–1326.

Chapman, A. R. O. 1987. The wild harvest and culture of Laminaria longicruris de laPylaie in Eastern Canada. In M. S. Doty, T. F. Caddy, & B. Santelices (Eds.), FAO Fisheries Technical Paper, 181. *Case Studies of Seven Commercial Seaweed Resources.* Food and agriculture organization of the United Nations, Rome, pp. 193–238.

Chen, K. C. and Y. F. Lin. 1994. Immobilization of microorganisms with phosphorylated polyvinyl alcohol (PVA) gel. *Enzyme. Microb. Technol.* 16:79–83.

Chhatbar, M. U., R. Meena, K. Prasad, and A. K. Siddhanta. 2009. Agar/sodium alginate graft polyacrylonitrile a stable Hydrogel system. *Ind. J. Chem.* 48A:1085–1090.

Ciofani, G., V. Raffa, T. Pizzorusso, A. Menciassi, and P. Dario. 2008. Characterization of an alginate-based drug delivery system for neurological applications. *Med. Eng. Phys.* 30:848–855.

Coppen, J. J. W. and P. Nambiar. 1991. Agar and Alginate Production from Seaweed in India Bay of Bengal Programme BOBP/WP/69 Post-Harvest Fisheries.

d'Ayala, G. G., M. Malinconico, and P. Laurienzo. 2008. Marine derived polysaccharides for biomedical applications: Chemical modification approaches. *Molecules* 13:2069–2106.

Da Costa, A. C. A. and S. G. F. Leite. 1991. Metals biosorption by sodium alginate immobilized *Chlorella homosphaera* cells. *Biotechnol. Lett.* 13:559–562.

Dainty, A. L., K. H. Goulding, P. K. Robinson, H. Simpkins, and M. D. Trevan. 1986. Stability of alginate-immobilized algal cells. *Biotechnol. Bioeng.* 28:210–216.

Davidovich-Pinhas, M., O. Harari, and H. Bianco-Peled. 2009. Evaluating the mucoadhesive properties of drug delivery systems based on hydrated thiolated alginate. *J Control Rel.* 136:38–44.

Dayaram, P., and D. Dasgupta. 2008. Decolorisation of synthetic dyes and textile wastewater using Polyporus rubidus. *J. Environ. Biol.* 29:831–836.

Dean Madden. 2007. Immobilised yeast Immobilisation of yeast in calcium alginate beads, National Centre for Biotechnology Education, University of Reading Science and Technology Centre, Reading RG6 6BZ UK, 1–5.

Demiroz, F. T., F. Acarturk, S. Takka, and K. O. Boyunaga. 2007. Evaluation of alginate based mesalazine tablets for intestinal drug delivery. *Eur. J. Pharma. and Biopharm.* 67:491–497.

Devi, N. and D. K. Kakati. 2013. Smart porous microparticles based on gelatin/sodium alginate polyelectrolyte complex. *J. Food. Eng.* 117:193–204.

Diaz-Barrera, A., P. Silva, J. Berrios, and F. Acevedo. 2010. Manipulating the molecular weight of alginate produced by *Azotobacter vinelandii* in continuous cultures. *Bioresour. Technol.* 101:9405–9408.

Doria-Serrano, M. C., F. A. Ruiz-Treviño, C. Rios-Arciga, M. Hernández Esparza, and P. Santiago. 2001. Physical characteristics of poly (vinyl alcohol) and calcium alginate hydrogels for the immobilization of activated sludge. *Biomacromol.* 2:568–574.

Draget, K. and C. Taylor. 2011. Chemical, physical and biological properties of alginates and their biomedical implications. *Food Hydrocoll.* 25:251–256.

Dvir-Ginzberg, M., I. Gamlieli-Bonshtein, R. Agbaria, and S. Cohen. 2004. Liver tissue engineering within alginate scaffolds: Effects of cell-seeding density on hepatocyte viability, morphology, and function. *Tissue Eng.* 9:757–766.

El-Latif, M. A. M., M. F. El-Kady, A. M. Ibrahim, and M. E. Ossman. 2010. Alginate/polyvinyl alcohol—Kaolin composite for removal of methylene blue from aqueous solution in a batch stirred tank reactor. *J. Am. Sci.* 6:280–292.

EL-Tayieb, M. M., M. M. El-Shafei, and M. S. Mahmoud. 2013. The role of alginate as polymeric material in treatment of tannery wastewater. *Int. J. Sci. Technol.* 2:218–224.

Fan, W. J., J. X. Sun, and Y. C. Chen. 2009. Effects of chitosan coating on quality and shelf life of silver carp during frozen storage. *Food Chem.* 115:66–70.

Fang, Y., S. Al-Assaf, G. O. Phillips, K. Nishinari, T. Funami, P. A. Williams et al. 2007. Multiple steps and critical behaviors of the binding of calcium to alginate. *J. Phys. Chem. B.* 111:2456–62.

Fares, M. M. 2003. Graft copolymerization onto chitosan-II. Grafting of acrylic acid and hydrogel formation. *J. Polym. Mater.* 20:75–82.

Fischer, F. G. and H. Dorfel. 1955. Die polyuronsauren der braunalgen-(kohlenhydrate der algen-I). *Z Physiol. Chem.* 302:186–203.

Fiset, J.-F., J.-F. Blaiset, and P. A Riveros. 2008. Review on the removal of metal ions from effluents using seaweeds, alginate derivatives and other sorbents. *Revue des Sciences de l'Eau.* 21:283–308.

Gardea-Torresdey, J., M. Hejazi, K. Tiemann, J. G. Parsons, M. Duarte-Gardea, and J. Henning. 2002. Use of hop (Humulus lupulus) agricultural by-products for the reduction of aqueous lead(II) environmental health hazards. *J. Hazard. Mater.* 91:95–112.

George, M. and T. E. Abraham. 2006. Polyionic hydrocolloids for the intestinal delivery of protein drugs. *J. Contr. Rel.* 114:1–14.

Gholami-Borujeni, F., A. H. Mahvi, S. Naseri, M. A. Faramarzi, R. Nabizadeh, and M. Alimohammadi. 2011. Application of immobilized horseradish peroxidase for removal and detoxification of azo dye from aqueous solution. *Res. J. Chem. Environ.* 15:217–222.

Gidhamaari, S. M. E. Boominathan, and E. Mamidala. 2012. Studies of efficiency of immobilizedbacteria in tannery effluent treatment. *J. Bio. Innov.* 2:33–42.

Gomathi, V. Cibichakravarthy, B. Ramanathan, A. Sivaramaiah Nallapeta, V. Ramanjaneya, R. Mula, and D. Jayasimha Rayalu. 2012. Decolourization of paper mill effluent by immobilized cells of phanerochaete chrysosporium. *Int. J. Plant. Animal Environ. Sci.* 2:141–146.

Gombotz, W. R. and S. F. Wee. 1998. Protein release from algiante matrices. *Adv. Drug. Reviews.* 31:267–285.

Gong, Y., G. T. Han, Y. M. Zhang, J. F. Zhang, W. Jiang, X. W. Tao, and S. C. Gao. 2015. Preparation of alginate membrane for tissue engineering. *J. Polym. Eng.* 36(4), 363–370.

Gopinathan, C. P. and R. Panigrahy. 1983. Seaweed resources. *CMFRI Bull.* 34:47–51.

Gotoh, T., K. Matsushima, and K. Kikuchi. 2004. Preparation of alginate-chitosan hybrid gel beads and adsorption of divalent metal ions. *Chemosphere* 55:135–40.

Grag, V. K., R. Kumar, and R. Gupta. 2004. Removal of malachite green dye from aqueous solution by adsorption using agro-industries waste: A case study of Phosopis ceneraria. *Dyes Pigments* 62:1–10.

Harikumar, P. S., Litty Joseph, and A. Dhanya. 2013. Photocatalytic degradation of textile dyes by hydrogel supported titanium dioxide nanoparticles. *J. Environ. Eng. Ecol. Sci.* 1–9 doi: 10.7243/2050-1323-2-2.

Haug, A., B. Larsen, and O. Smidsrod. 1974. Uronic acid sequence in alginate from different sources. *Carbohydr. Res.* 32:217–25.

Hay, I. D., Z. U. Rehman, A. Ghafoor, and B. H. A. Rehm. 2010. Bacterial biosynthesis of alginates. *J. Chem. Technol. Biotechnol.* 85:752–759.

Hill, C. B. and E. Khan. 2008. A Comparative study of immobilized nitrifying and co-immobilized nitrifying and denitrifying bacteria for ammonia removal of sludge digester supernatant. *Water Air Soil Pollu.* 195:23–33.

Huang, X. J., Y. Xiao, and M. D. Lang. 2012. Micelles/sodium alginate composite gel beads: A new matrix for oral drug delivery of indomethacin. *Carbohydr. Polym.* 87:790–798.

Ibanez, J. P. and Y. Umetsu. 2004. Uptake of trivalent chromium from aqueous solutions using protonated dry alginate beads. *Hydrometallurgy* 72:327–334.

Imran, Q., M. A. Hanif, M. S. Riaz, S. Noureen, T. M. Ansari, and H. N. Bhatti. 2012. Coagulation/flocculation of tannery wastewater using immobilized chemical coagulants. *J. Appl. Res. Technol.* 10:79–86.

Isıklan, N., M. Inal, and M. Yigitoglu. 2008. Synthesis and characterization of poly(N-vinyl-2-pyrrolidone) grafted sodium alginate hydrogel beads for the controlled release of indomethacin. *J. Appl. Polym. Sci.* 110:481–493.

ITC (International Trade Centre), 1981. *Pilot Survey of the World Seaweed Industry and Trade.* Geneva, International Trade Centre UNCTAD/GATT, p. 111.

Iwasaki, N., S. T. Yamane, T. Majima, Y. Kasahara, A. Minami, and K. Harada. 2004. Feasibility of polysaccharide hybrid materials for scaffolds in cartilage tissue engineering: Evaluation of chondrocyte adhesion to polyion complex fibers prepared from alginate and chitosan. *Biomacromol.* 5:828–833.

Jayasudha, S. and P. Sampathkumar. 2014. Nutrient removal from tannery effluent by free and immobilized cells of marine microalgae *chlorella salina*. *Int. J. Environ. Biol.* 4:21–26.

Jeon, C., J. Y. Park, and Y. J. Yoo. 2002. Characteristics of metal removal using carboxylated alginic acid. *Water Res.* 36:1814–1824.

Jeon C., Y. J. Yoo, and W. H. Hoell. 2005. Environmental effects and desorption characteristics on heavy metal removal using carboxylated alginic acid. *Bioresour. Technol.* 96:15–19.

Ji, M. H., et al. 1984. Studies on the M:G ratios in alginate. *Hydrobiologia* 116/117:554–6.

Jin, H. H., D. H. Kim, T. W. Kim, K. K. Shin, J. S. Jung, H. C. Park, and S. Y. Yoon. 2012. In vivo evaluation of porous hydroxyapatite/chitosan-alginate composite scaffolds for bone tissue engineering. *Int. J. Biol. Macromol.* 51:1079–85.

Jobanputra, A. H., B. A. Karode, and S. B. Chincholkar. 2011. Calcium alginate as supporting material for the immobilization of rifamycin oxidase from Chryseobacterium species. *Biotechnol. Bioinf. Bioeng.* 1:529–535.

Joo, D. S., M. G. Cho, J. S. Lee, J. H. Park, J. K. Kwak, Y. H. Han, and R. Bucholz. 2001. New strategy for the cultivation of microalgae using microencapsulation. *J. Microencapsul.* 18:567–576.

Kadu, P. A., R. B. Landge, and Y. R. M. Rao. 2013. Treatment of dairy wastewater using rotating biological contactors. *Eur. J. Exp. Biol.* 3:257–260.

Kanagaraj, J. and A. B. Mandal. 2012. Combined biodegradation and ozonation for removal of tannins and dyes. *Newsletter of the Council of Scientific and Industrial Research* 62:148–170.

Kaur, V., M. B. Bera, P. S. Panesar, H. Kumar, and J. F. Kennedy. 2014. Welan gum: Microbial production, characterization, and applications. *Int. J. Biol. Macromol.* 65:454–461.

Kierstan, M. P. J. and M. P. Coughlan. 1985. Immobilisation of cells and enzymes by gel entrapment. In Woodward J. (Ed.) *Immobilised Cells and Enzymes: A Practical Approach.* IRL Press, Oxford, pp. 39–48.

Kim, S., C. Park, T. H. Kim, J. Lee, and S. W. Kim. 2003. COD reduction and decolorization of textile effluents using a combined process. *J. Biosci. Bioeng.* 95:102–105.

Kulkarni, A. R., K. S. Soppimath, T. M. Aminabhavi, and W. E. Rudzinski. 2000. Glutaraldehyde crosslinked sodium alginate beads containing liquid pesticide for soil application. *Eur. J. Pharm. Biopharm.* 63:97–105.

Kuo, C. K. and P. X. Ma. 2001. Ionically crosslinked alginate hydrogels as scaffolds for tissue engineering: Part 1. Structure, gelation rate and mechanical properties. *Biomater.* 22:511–521.

Kurkuri, M. D., U. S. Toti, and T. M. Aminabhavi. 2002. Synthesis and characteization of blend membranes of sodium alginate and poly (vinyl alcohol) (PVA) for the pervaporation separation of water—Iso propanol mixtures. *J. Appl. Polym. Sci.* 86:3642–3651.

Lee, K. Y. and D. J. Mooney. 2012. Alginate: Properties and biomedical applications. *Prog. Polym. Sci.* 37:106–126.

Lee, K. Y. and S. H. Yuk. 2007. Polymeric protein delivery systems. *Progr Polym Sci.* 32:669–697.

Leonard, M., M. R. Boisseson De, P. Hubert, F. Dalencon, and E. Dellacherie. 2004. Hydrophobically modified alginate hydrogels as protein carriers with specific controlled release properties. *J. Contr. Rel.* 98:395–405.

Li, J.-W., S. Dong, J. Song, C.-B. Li, X.-L. Chen, B.-B. Xie, and Y.-Z. Zhang. 2011. Purification and characterization of a bifunctional alginate lyase from *pseudoalteromonas* sp. *Mar. Drugs.* 9:109–123.

Liu, L., L. Jiang, G. K. Xu, C. Ma, X. G. Yang, and J. M. Yao. 2014. Potential of alginate fibers incorporated with drug-loaded nanocapsules as drug delivery systems. *J. Mater. Chem. B.* 2:7596–7604.

MA Healthcare Ltd. *Wound Care Handbook 2011–2012.* MA Healthcare Ltd, London.

Mahmoud, G. A. and S. F. Mohamed. 2012. Removal of lead ions from aqueous solution using (sodium alginate/itaconic acid) hydrogel prepared by gamma radiation. *Aust. J. Basic Appl. Sci.* 6:262–273.

Mahmoud, M. S. and S. A. Mohamed. 2015. Calcium alginate as an eco-friendly supporting material for Baker's yeast strain in chromium bioremediation. *HBRC Journal.* doi: http://dx.doi.org/10.1016/j.hbrcj.2015.06.003.

Malesu, V. K., D. Sahoo, and P. L. Nayak. 2011. Chitosan–sodium alginate nanocomposites blended with cloisite 30b as a novel drug delivery system for anticancer drug curcumin. *Int. J. Appl. Biol. Pharm. Technol.* 2:402–411.

Mallick, J., D. Sahoo, D. M. Kar, and J. Makwana. 2013. Alginate beads of ibuprofen for oral sustained drug delivery: An in vitro evaluation. *Int. J. Pharm. Chem. Biol. Sci.* 3:595–602.

Mallick, N. 2002. Biotechnological potential of immobilized algae for wastewater N, P and metal removal: A review. *Biometals* 15:377–390.

Martins, S., B. Sarmento, E. B. Souto, and D. C. Ferreira. 2007. Insulin-loaded alginate microspheres for oral delivery effect of polysaccharide reinforcement on physicochemical properties and release profile. *Carbohydr. Polym.* 69:725–731.

Martinsen, A., G. Skjak-Bræk, and O. Smidsrød. 1989. Alginate as immobilization material. I. Correlation between chemical and physical properties of alginate gel beads. *Biotechnol. Bioeng.* 33:79–89.

Matsushita, Y., A. Iwatsuki, and S. Yasuda. 2004. Application of cationic polymer prepared from sulfuric acid lignin as a retention aid for usual rosin sizes to neutral papermaking. *The Japan Wood Research Society* 50:540–544.

Maynard, C. W. 1983. Dye application, manufacture of dye intermediates and dyes. In Kent J. A. (Ed.). *Riegel's Handbook of Industrial Chemistry.* Van Nostrand Reinhold, New York, pp. 809–861.

McHugh, D. J. 1987. Production, properties and uses of alginates. *FAO Fish Technol.* 288:58–115.

Meena, A. K., K. Kadirvelu, G. K. Mishra, C. Rajagopal, and P. N. Nagar. 2008. Adsorptive removal of heavy metals from aqueous solution by treated sawdust (Acacia arabica). *J. Hazard. Mater.* 150:604–611.

Mehta, S. K. and J. P. Gaur. 2001. Removal of Ni and Cu from single and binary metal solutions by free and immobilized *Chlorella vulgaris*. *Eur. J. Protistol.* 37:261–271.

Mennini N., S. Furlanetto, M. Cirri, and P. Mura. 2011. Quality by design approach for developing chitosan-Ca-alginate microspheres for colon delivery of celecoxib-hydroxypropyl-b-cyclodextrin-PVP complex. *Euro. J. Pharm. Biopharm.* 80(1):67–75.

Moebus, K., J. Siepmann, and R. Bodmeier. 2009. Alginate–poloxamer microparticles for controlled drug delivery to mucosal tissue. *Euro. J. Pharm. Biopharm.* 72:42–53.

Moen, E., B. Larsen, and K. Ostgaard. 1997. Aerobic microbial degradation of alginate in Laminaria hyperborea stipes containing different levels of polyphenols. *J. Appl. Phycol.* 9:45–54.

Moreira, S. M., M. Moreira-Santos, L. Guilhermino, and R. Ribeiro. 2006. Immobilization of the marine microalga Phaeodactylum tricornutum in alginate for in situ experiments: Bead stability and suitability. *Enzyme Microb. Technol.* 38:135–141.

Morris, E. R., D. A. Rees, and D. Thom. 1980. Characteristics of alginate composition and block-structure by circular dichroism. *Carbohydr. Res.* 81:305–14.

Mosahebi, A., M. Simon, M. Wiberg, and G. Terenghi. 2001. A novel use of alginate hydrogel as Schwann cell matrix. *Tissue Eng.* 7:525–534.

Mugdha, A. and M. Usha. 2012. Enzymatic treatment of wastewater containing dyestuffs using different delivery systems. *Sci. Revs. Chem. Commun.* 2:31–40.

Nakamura, K., E. Kinoshita, T. Hatakeyama, H. Hatakeyama, and Thermochim. 2000. TMA measurement of swelling behavior of polysaccharide hydrogels. *Thermochim. Acta* 352:171–176.

Nestle, N. and R. Kimmich. 1996. NMR Microscopy of heavy metal absorption in calcium alginate beads. *Appl. Biochem. Biotechnol.* 56:9–17.

Ngomsik, A. F., A. Bee, J. M. Siaugue, D. Talbot, V. Cabuil, and G. Cote. 2009. Co(II) removal by magnetic alginate beads containing Cyanex. *J. Hazard. Mater.* 166:1043–1049.

Nita, I., M. Iorgulescu, M. F. Spiroiu, M. Ghiurea, C. Petcu, and O. Cinteza. 2007. The adsorption of heavy metal ions on porous calcium alginate microparticles. *Analele Universitäńii din Bucuresti* 1:59–67.

Pan, J. L., Z. M. Bao, J. L. Li, L. G. Zhang, C. Wu, and Y. T. Yu. 2005. Chitosan-based scaffolds for hepatocyte culture. In X. Zhang, J. Tanaka, Y.Yu and Y. Tabata (Eds.) ASBM6: *Advanced Biomaterials* VI, 288-289:91–94.

Papageorgiou, S. K., F. K. Katsaros, E. P. Kouvelos, J. W. Nolan, H. Le Deit, and N. K. Kanellopoulos. 2006. Heavy metal sorption by calcium alginate beads from *Laminaria digitata*. *J. Hazard. Mater.* 137:1765–1772.

Park Y., M. Sugimoto, A. Watrin, M. Chiquet, and E. B. Hunziker. 2005. BMP-2 induces the expression of chondrocyte-specific genes in bovine synovium-derived progenitor cells cultured in three-dimensional alginate hydrogel. *Osteoarthr. Cartilage.* 13:527–536.

Paul, W. and C. P. Sharma. 2004. Chitosan and alginate wound dressings: A short review. *Trends Biomater. Artif. Organs.* 18:18–23.

Penman, A. and G. R. Sanderson. 1972. A method for the determination of uronic acid sequence in alginates. *Carbohydr. Res.* 25:280.

Perez. R., R. Kaas, F. Campello, S. Arbault, and O. Barbaroux. 1992. *La Culture Des Algues Marines Dans Le Monde*. IFREMER, Plouzane, France, pp. 614.

Pourjavadi, A., M. S. Amini-Fazl, and H. Hosseinzadeh. 2005. Partially hydrolyzed cross-linked alginate-*graft*-polymethacrylamide as a novel biopolymer-based superabsorbent hydrogel having pH-responsive Properties. *Macromol. Res.* 13:45–53.

Pourjavadi, A., B. Farhadpour, and F. Seidi. 2008. Synthesis and investigation of swelling behavior of grafted alginate/alumina superabsorbent composite. *Starch/Stärke.* 60:457–466.

Qin, Y., B. Shi, and J. Liu. 2006. Applications of chitosan and alginate in treating wastewater containing heavy metal ions. *Ind. J. Chem. Technol.* 13:464–469.

Ravichandra P., M. Ramakrishna, A. Gangagni Rao, and Annapurna Jetty. 2006. Sulfide oxidation in a batch fluidized bed bioreactor using immobilized cells of isolated *thiobacillus* sp. (iict-sobdairy-201) as biocatalyst. *J. Eng. Sci.Technol.* 1:21–30.

Rehm, B. H. A. 2002. Alginates from bacteria. *Biopolymers* 8:179–212.

Reilly, W. J. (Jr). 2000. In J.P. Remington and A. R. Gennaro (Eds.) *Remington the Science and Practice of Pharmacy*, Lipin Cott Williams & Wilkins, Philadelphia, p. 1030.

Remminghorst, U. and B. H. A. Rehm. 2006. Bacterial alginates: From biosynthesis to applications. *Biotechnol Lett.* 28:1701–1712.

Rinaudo, M. 2008. Main properties and current applications of some polysaccharides as biomaterials. *Polym. Int.* 57:397–430.

Rowley, J. A., G. Madlambayan, and D. J. Mooney. 1999. Alginate hydrogels as synthetic extracellular matrix materials. *Biomater.* 20:45–53.

Sadeghi, M., F. Shafiei, E. Mohammadinasab, L. Mansouri, and M. J. Khodabakhshi. 2014. Biodegradable hydrogels based on alginate for control drug delivery systems. *Current World Environ.* 9(1):109–113.

Schnurch, A. B., C. E. Kast, and M. F. Richter. 2001. Improvement in the mucoadhesive properties of alginate by the covalent attachment of cysteine. *J. Control. Release.* 71:277–285.

Shah, S. B., C. P. Patel, and H. C. Trivedi. 1996. Thermal behavior of graft copolymers of sodium alginate. *Die Angewandte Makromolekulare Chemie.* 235:1–13.

Shamshina, J. L. G. Gurau, L. E. Block, L. K. Hansen, C. Dingee, A. Walters, and R. D. Rogers. 2014. Chitin–calcium alginate composite fibers for wound care dressings spun from ionic liquid solution. *J. Mater. Chem. B.* 2:3924–3936.

Shimizu, T. and A. Takada. 1997. Preparation of Bibased superconducting fiber by metal biosorption of NaAlginate. *Polymer Gels Networks* 5:267–283.

Shyamali, S., M. De Silva, and N. Savitri Kumar. 1984. Carbohydrate constituents of the marine algae of Sri Lanka. 2. Composition and sequence of uronate residues in alginates from some brown seaweeds. *J. Nat. Sci. Counc.* 12:161–6.

Silva, R., R. Singh, B. Sarker, D. G. Papageorgiou, J. A. Juhasz, J. A Roether, I. Cicha, J. Kaschta, D. W Schubert, K. Chrissafis, R. Detsch, and A. R. Boccaccini. 2014. Hybrid hydrogels based on keratin and alginate for tissue engineering. *J. Mater. Chem. B.* 2:5441–5451.

Silva, T. H., A. Alves, B. M. Ferreira, J. M. Oliveira, L. L. Reys, R. J. F. Ferreira, R. A. Sousa, S. S. Silva, J. F. Mano, and R. L. Reis. 2012. Materials of marine origin: A review on polymers and ceramics of biomedical interest. *Int. Mater. Rev.* 57: 276–306.

Singh, P., S. K. Singh, J. Bajpai, A. K. Bajpai, and R. B. Shrivastava. 2014. Iron crosslinked alginate as novel nanosorbents for removal of arsenic ions and bacteriological contamination from water. *J. Mater. Res. Technol.* 3:195–202.

Singh, S., B. K. Gogoi, and R. L. bezbaruah. 2012. Calcium alginate as a support material for immobilization of l-amino acid oxidase isolated from aspergillus fumigates. *IIOAB J* 3:7–11.

Siripattanakul-Ratpukdi, S. 2012. Ethanol production potential from fermented rice noodle wastewater treatment using entrapped yeast cell sequencing batch reactor. *Appl. Water Sci.* 2:47–53.

Siripattanakul, S. and E. Khan. 2010. Fundamentals and applications of entrapped cell bioaugmentation for contaminant removal. In Shah V (Ed.) *Emerging Environmental Technologies*, Vol 2. Springer, Berlin, pp. 147–169.

Song, Y., L. Liu, H. Shen, J. You, and Y. Luo. 2011. Effect of sodium alginate-based edible coating containing different anti-oxidants on quality and shelf life of refrigerated bream (*Megalobrama amblycephala*). *Food Control.* 22:608–615.

Souza, S. F. D. 2002. Trends in immobilized enzyme and cell technology. *Ind. J. Biotechnol.* 1:321–338.

Srivastava, V. C., I. D. Mall, and I. M. Mishra. 2005. Treatment of pulp and paper mill waste-water with polyaluminium chloride and bagasse fly ash. *Coll. Surf A Physicochem. Eng. Asp.* 260:17–28.

Stanford, E. C. C. 1881. Improvements in the manufacture of useful products from seaweeds, British patent 142.

Stevens, M. M., H. F. Qanadilo, R. Langer, and V. P. Shastri. 2004. A rapid-curing alginate gel system: Utility in periosteum-derived cartilage tissue engineering. *Biomater.* 25:887–894.

Su, J., S. H. Tan. 2013. Alginate-based biomaterials for regenerative medicine applications. *Materials* 6:1285–1309.

Taqieddin, E. and M. Amiji. 2004. Enzyme immobilization in novel alginate-chitosan core-shell microcapsules. *Biomater.* 25:1937–1945.

Thomas, S. 2000. Alginate dressings-Do they influence wound healing. *J. Wound Care.* 2000:1–10.

Thomas, S. 2010. *Surgical Dressings and Wound Management.* Medetec Publications, Cardiff.

Tonnesen, H. H. and J. Karlsen. 2002. Alginate in drug delivery systems. *Drug Dev. Ind. Pharm.* 28:621–30.

Toti, U. S., M. Y. Kariduraganavar, K. S. Soppimath, and T. M. Aminabhavi. 2002. Sorption, diffusion and pervaporation separation of water–acetic acid mixtures through the blend membranes of sodium alginate and guargum-grafted-polyacrylamide. *J. Appl. Polym. Sci.* 83:259–272.

Varghese, S. and J. H. Elisseeff. 2006. Hydrogels for musculoskeletal tissue engineering. *Adv. Polym. Sci.* 203:95–144.

Vauche, P., R. Kaas, A. Arhaliass, R. Baron, and J. Legrand. 2008. A new process for extract-ing alginates from *laminaria digitata*: Reactive extrusion. *Food. Bioproc. Technol.* 1:297–300.

Vijayalakshmi, K., T. Gomathi, S. Latha, T. Hajeeth, and P. N. Sudha. 2016. Removal of copper(II) from aqueous solution using nanochitosan/sodium alginate/microcrystalline cellulose beads. *Int. J. Biol. Macromol.* 82:440–452.

Viswanathan, S. and T. Nallamuthu. 2014. Extraction of sodium alginate from selected sea-weeds and their physiochemical and biochemical properties. *Int. J. Innov. Res. Sci. Eng. Technol.* 3:10999–11003.

Wang, H. L., G. S. Liu, P. Li, and F. Pan. 2006. The effect of bioaugmentation on the perfor-mance of sequencing batch reactor and sludge characteristics in the treatment process of papermaking wastewater. *Bioprocess Biosyst. Eng.* 29:283–289.

Wang, J., W. Hou, and Y. Qian. 1995. Immobilization of microbial cells using polyvinyl alco-hol (PVA)–polyacrylamide gels. *Biotechnol Tech.* 3:203–208.

Wang, J. X., Q. H. Liu, and Y. Teng. 1994. Research on coatings of frozen mussel flesh. *Food Sci.* 2:70–72.

Wang, L., R. M. Sheltona, P. R. Coopera, M. Lawsonb, J. T. Triffittb, and J. E. Barraleta. 2003. Evaluation of sodium alginate for bone marrow cell tissue engineering. *Biomater.* 24:3475–3481.

Wang, X. K.-X. Zhu, and H.-M. Zhou. 2011. Immobilization of glucose oxidase in alginate-chitosan microcapsules. *Int. J. Mol. Sci.* 12:3042–3054.

Wang, X. P. 2000. Modified alginate composite membranes for the dehydration of acetic acid. *J. Membr. Sci.* 170:71–79.

Wanstedt, K. G., S. C. Seideman, and L. S. Donnelly. 1981. Sensory attributes of precooked, calcium alginate-coated pork patties. *J. Food. Protect.* 44:732–735.

Wedlock, D. J., B. A. Fasihuddin, and G. O. Phillips. 1986. Characterization of alginates from Malaysia. In G. O. Phillips, D. J. Wedlock and P. A. Williams (Eds.) *Gums and Stabilizers for the Food Industry.* Elsevier, London, Vol. 3, pp. 47–67.

Williams, D. F. 2009. On the nature of biomaterials. *Biomaterials* 30:5897–5909.

Yan Chun, H. C. Chun Xia, and C. Chen. 2014. Sodium alginate intercalated zinc-containing layered double hydroxides for the catalytic α-Pinene oxidation. *J. Res. Develop. Chem.* 2014:1–9.

Yang, X. J., A. G. Fane, and S. MacNaughton. 2001. Removal and recovery of heavy metals from wastewater by supported liquid membranes. *Water Sci. Technol.* 43:341–348.

Yang, X. W., Y. D. Shen, and P. Z. Li. 2010. Intrinsic viscosity, surface activity, and flocculation of cationic polyacrylamide modified with fluorinated acrylate. *Polym. Bull.* 65:111–122.

Yu. X. L., X. B. Li, and X. L. Xu. 2008. Coating with sodium alginate and its effect on the functional properties and structure of frozen pork. *J. Muscle Foods* 19:333–351.

Yuzhu Fu, and T. Viraraghavan. 2003. Column studies for biosorption of dyes from aqueous solutions on immobilised *Aspergillus niger* fungal biomass. *Water SA.* 29:465–472.

Zeng, D., D. Hu, and J. Cheng. 2011. Preparation and study of a composite flocculant for papermaking wastewater treatment. *J. Environ. Protect.* 2:1370–1374.

Zeng, Q. and Q. Xu. 1997. Study on preservation techniques of fish, shrimp, scallop of edible coating. *J. Dalian Fish* 12:37–42.

Zhang, L., Q. Ao, A. J. Wang, G. Y. Lu, L. J. Kong, Y. D. Gong, and N. A. Zhao. 2006. Sandwich tubular scaffold derived from chitosan for blood vessel tissue engineering. *J Biomed Mater Res A.* 77:277–284.

Zille, A., T. Tzanov, G. M. Gubitz, and A. Cavaco-Paulo. 2003. Immobilized laccase for decolourization of reactive black 5 dyeing effluent. *Biotechnol. Lett.* 25:1473–1477.

Zollinger, H. 1987. *Color Chemistry-Synthesis, Properties and Applications of Organic Dyes and Pigments.* VCH Publishers, New York, pp. 92–102.

23 Application of Marine Polymers in Dye and Textile Industries

P. Sivaperumal, K. Kamala, and R. Rajaram

CONTENTS

23.1 INTRODUCTION

Water is one of the basic necessary natural resources, unfortunately exploited the most nowadays. Rapid urbanization and industrialization with textile industries are posing a hazard to the water bodies with the release of various harmful and toxic dye effluents. In this context, synthetic dyes' pollution is a great environmental concern due to the widespread use and low removal rate of synthetic dyes during aerobic wastewater treatment. More than 10,000 different dyes are used worldwide, and about 8×10^5 tons of synthetic dyes are expended globally by textile industries (Walker and Weatherley 1997). Moreover, effluent water from textile, which contains load of dyes, can induce color to water, along with organic content, leading to severe hazard or imbalance in ecological system (Hassani et al. 2015). Particularly, 93% of intake water after processing comes out as colored wastewater from textile industries because of dyes (Wijannarong et al. 2013). Moreover, the nonbiodegradable dye-colored wastewater is an unpleasant and severe damage to the aquatic ecosystem and food chain (Forgacsa et al. 2004; Aksu and Tezer 2005). These pollutants may cause profuse sweating, severe headache, and mental confusion to humans and other ecological issues (Bhattacharyya and Sharma 2005). Therefore, effluent treatment is most desirable before enter into nearby water bodies.

Different methods have been applied for dyes' removal such as activated sludge (Pala and Tokat 2002), oxidation using chemicals (Kartik and Mehta 2014), photodegradation

(Seshadri et al. 1994), and adsorption methods (Yeh et al. 1993; Mahmoud et al. 2007). The methods of adsorption have been recognized as one of the most significant techniques (Rio et al. 2005). Most of the inorganic and organic adsorbents of activated carbon (Malik 2004), Zeolites (Syafalni et al. 2012) and Chitosan, modified starch (Delval et al. 2005) respectively are involved in absorption studies. Many organic adsorbents have been applied for treatment of heavy metals in polluted water by producing metal complexes. Recent studies have found that some metal complexes are practical adsorbents for separation and removal of dyes (Jang et al. 2007).

In the context of treatment of textile industry's effluent water for degradation of dyes, there are different research works going on, based on the physical, chemical, and biological removal techniques such as coagulation, flocculation, membrane filtration, electrochemical, ozonation, bioaccumulation, and oxidation processes (Ince and Tezcanh 1999; Rai et al. 2005; Wojnarovits and Takacs 2008; Solmaz et al. 2009). In addition to all the above-mentioned techniques, adsorption method has been widely utilized for the dye removal, and it is applicable in real time for water treatment (Danis et al. 1998; Imamura et al. 2002). Nowadays, research attention mainly focus on cost-effective and *in situ* methods for the treatment of effluents (Tyagi and Yadav 2001). Textile effluent comprise a mixture of dyes; hence, its review by Gupta et al. (2015) is important to promote the existing techniques as well as to study new techniques to decolorize a mixture of dyes rather than a single dye solution. Further, all such methods had some problems due to limitations, and none of them were successfully implemented for the removal of color from wastewater. Therefore, adsorption techniques have been used very efficiently in dyes' removal from aqueous solutions and have been utilized in water treatment (Namasivayam et al. 1996; Blackburn 2004). Nevertheless, adsorption and the formation of inclusion complexes quiet seem to be the most effective and cheapest methods for the purification of industrial effluents. Native adsorbents such as biopolymers are a good alternative to expensive and unselective purification techniques. For example, marine biopolymer such as polysaccharide-based materials, chitin and chitosan, could be cheapest and effective alternatives to commonly used systems (Babel and Kurniawan 2003; Crini 2005). They exhibit a high binding capacity and specificity while being nontoxic, stable, and renewable.

23.2 INDUSTRIAL WASTE AROUND AQUATIC ENVIRONMENT

The quantity of industrial waste is closely linked to the level of economic activity in a country. The lack of land areas and resources used for the harmless disposal of wastes, the growing tourism industry, the growing population, and significance increase in the polluting and harmful substances combine to make pollution prevention and waste management a challenging task. The presence of color in industrial effluents is aesthetically undesirable. The main sources of colored organic effluents are textile, plastic, leather, paper, mineral, and food processing industries. Generally, the dyes are having multiple properties, and they are resistant to breakdown on long-term exposure to sunlight and water and in other atrocious conditions. Therefore, the treatment of dyes from wastewater is getting more difficult. In the overall category of textile synthetic dyes, majorly azo dyes constitute 70% of worldwide production (700,000 ton/year), and during industrial operation processes, about 25% of dyes come out in wastewaters.

These dyes are known as hazardous pollutants, as they cause environmental and health problems to earth and aquatic living organisms (Dos Santos et al. 2005; Crini 2006). Therefore, it is very much essential to treat the dyes from effluents before they are discharged into the environmental matrices.

There are a huge variety of hazardous soil contaminants, with different effects on the environment and human health, depending on their possible characteristics of scattering, solubility in water or oil, carcinogenicity, and others. Mineral oils constitute the key class of organic soil contaminants. In addition, the harmful effects of accidental spills on the environment depend on the category of oil as well as on the additives, which are significantly involved in the toxicity of the spill (Aluyor and Ori-Jesu 2009). Chlorinated hydrocarbons used for solvents, preservative agents, pesticides, pharmaceuticals, and dyes are widely distributed pollutants. These chemicals are associated with an excessive variety of cancers (Badawi et al. 2000). Another group of concern comprises polycyclic aromatic hydrocarbons (PAHs), which are feast into the environment through the waste disposal; combustion of fossil fuels; and accidental spills of petroleum, coal, and wood-preserving products. Moreover, PAHs are known to have acute toxic effects and/or possess mutagenic, teratogenic, and carcinogenic properties (Cerniglia 1993). In addition, BTEX compounds (benzene; toluene; ethylbenzene; and o-, m-, and p-xylenes) are widely used in industrial synthesis and also lead carcinogenic and neurotoxic diseases (Levin et al. 2003). Organophosphorus compounds used as petroleum additives, pesticides, and band plasticizers are involved in many degenerative syndromes of the nervous system and are strong mutagens, causing carcinogenesis and chromosomal aberrations (Singh 2009; Sirotkina et al. 2012).

23.3 ROLE OF MARINE POLYMERS IN WASTEWATER TREATMENT

For bioremediation purposes, the marine polymers actually gained overwhelming importance only during the early part of the twentieth century, when it became evident that the polymers could replace almost all the conventionally used materials with cheap cost. The main advantages of these polymers in remediation over conventional treatment methods include low price, high effectiveness, minimization of chemicals, restoration of biosorbent, biological mud, and possibility of metal recovery (Gupta et al. 2009; Saha and Orvig 2010). Some of the natural biopolymer biosorbents include chitosan and modified chitosan. Biopolymer of polyaminosaccharide chitosan, synthesized from the deacetylation of chitin, consists of unbranched chains of 2-acetoamido-2-deoxy-D-glucose. The major biopolymer of chitosan is more beneficial than chitin, since it has more number of accelerating amino groups and can be chemically modified (Jayakumar et al. 2010). Chitosan is biocompatible, environment friendly, and biodegradable material and has excessive potential for sorption of metal ions due to the presence of amino and hydroxyl groups in its chemical structure (Jayakumar et al. 2007, 2010; Maya et al. 2012; Sankar et al. 2012). A notable example is represented by calix[4]arenes, which have high removal ability for selected water-soluble azo dyes (Yilmaz et al. 2007). Furthermore, biopolymers of chitin and starch are abundant and also flexible to produce selective and biodegradable compounds such as cyclodextrin and chitosan. Further, compound like linear polycation with high similarity to reactive dyes of anthraquinone and azo derivatives of reactive blue and reactive red are commonly used in textile dyeing and chemical research. Crosslinking of these biopolymers results in the development of beads, which improve their handling. Current crosslinking agents for starch, cyclodextrin, and chitosan are ethylene glycol diglycidyl ether, glutaraldehyde, and epichlorohydrin, respectively. Several publications on starch, epichlorohydrin-crosslinked cyclodextrin, and glutaraldehyde-crosslinked chitosan showed an extraordinary affinity, selectivity, and capability toward anthraquinone and azo dye pollutants in wastewater treatment (Delval et al. 2002; Chiou and Li 2002; Crini 2003).

For instance, chitosan has chelating and complexing properties contributing to interactions with dyes. Moreover, the presence of reactive groups in chitosan allows for the generation of intermolecular hydrogen bonds, chemical activation, and crosslinkage. However, the disadvantages of using chitosan are the variability in its characteristics, its pH sensitivity, and that the dispersal of the acetyl groups along the support cannot be controlled (Crini et al. 2009). Therefore, it is not suitable for cationic dyes if not modified. Crini (2005) also reported different industrial dyes and other textile pollutants in wastewater as well as a suitable adsorbent with the associated adsorption capacities. Polymers are not only used in wastewater purification methods for dye and textile industrial pollutants, but, due to dyes' attraction to polymers and several low-molecular compounds or somewhat-metal ions, dye-containing polymers could also be used for the exposure and determination of metal pollutants in the industrial wastewaters. The cumulative use of lead materials in the industry causes high levels of contamination of effluent and hazards to human health. Early studied revealed the great selectivity of specific anthraquinone derivatives to lead ions (Tavakkoli et al. 1998; Reza et al. 1998). Correspondingly, anthraquinone-based polyvinyl chloride (PVC) membranes in which anthraquinone is covalently attached to the polymer are of ample value for lead determination in wastewater.

23.4 BIOREMEDIATION OF DYE AND TEXTILE INDUSTRIAL WASTE BY USING MARINE POLYMERS

A dye is defined as a colored organic compound, which when applied to fabrics or any other substance imparts a permanent desired color and the color is not degraded by washings, biological effects, and exposure to sunlight (Rachakornkij et al. 2004). Most of the colored textiles, leather, and plastic articles are treated for color by azo dyes and pigments (Pankaj et al. 2012). Dyes are classified based on property and usage as follows: acid, cationic (basic), disperse, direct, reactive, sulfur, and vat dyes. Moreover, these dyes come out as a mixture of dyes from industry in full load of organic content. There are different types of techniques that have been employed for dye removal bearing industrial effluents. These techniques include precipitation, electrochemical technologies, and ion-exchange membrane. According to the literature, these technologies are very expensive because preliminary investment as well as operational and maintenance costs are so high, not ecofriendly, and usually suitable for only one kind of concentration of dye (Nevine 2008; Ismail et al. 2012). To overcome these different forces, water treatment has been initiated and taken as a challenging task for scientific field (Aksu 2005).

Marine biopolymers have potential applications in the bioremediation of dye and textile industry-polluted waters. The process of bioremediation was mainly influenced by microorganisms and their polymeric substances, which enzymatically attack the pollutants and change them to innocuous products. As bioremediation can be active only where environmental conditions permit microbial growth and activity, its application often involves the influence of environmental parameters to allow microbial growth and degradation to ensue at a faster rate. The process of bioremediation is a very gentle process (Karigar and Rao 2011). Only certain species of bacteria and fungi have confirmed their ability as effective pollutant degraders. Many strains are known to be effective as bioremediation agents but only under laboratory conditions (Kumar et al. 2011). The limitation of bacterial growth is under the influence of temperature, oxygen, pH, moisture, soil structure and suitable level of nutrients, poor bioavailability of contaminants, and occurrence of supplementary toxic compounds. Although microorganisms can exist in extreme environment, most of them favor conditions that are difficult to achieve outside the laboratory (Bernhard-Reversat and Schwartz 1997; Vidali 2001; Dana and Bauder 2011).

Earlier, wastes were conventionally disposed by burrowing a hole and filling it with waste material. This method of waste disposal was difficult to tolerate, owing to the lack of new place for dumping every time. New tools for waste disposal that practice high-temperature incineration and chemical decomposition have been evolved. Although they can be very active at decreasing a wide range of contaminants, at the same time, they have a number of drawbacks. These methods are difficult, uneconomical, and lack public recognition. The associated scarcities in these methods have motivated researchers toward harnessing modern-day bioremediation technology as an appropriate alternative. The ancestries and sources of pollution are different: industrial activities include metal processing and mining, industry effluents, petrochemical and industrial complexes, pulp and paper industries, dye industries, chemical weapons production, and industrial manufacturing and man-made activities include agricultural practices and traffic. Particularly, dye remains in industrial wastewaters have contaminated an important source of water pollution. Approximately 10% to 15% of unused dyes pass in wastewater after dyeing and after the subsequent washing processes (Rajamohan and Karthikeyan 2006).

For several years, the colored wastewater was treated by using many physical and chemical processes. These skills are unsuccessful in removing dyes in addition to the high cost of the treatments. Biosorption was later recognized as the preferred skill for bleaching of colored wastewater (Rana and Samir 2014). Ultimately, the efficient treatments for color removal from colored effluents composed of combined approaches using combinations of physical, chemical, and biological decolorization techniques (Galindo and Kalt 1999; Robinson et al. 2001; Azbar et al. 2004). Physical and chemical methods for treatment of dye wastewater are not commonly applied to textile industries due to the high costs and discarding problems. Green technologies to combat with this problem comprise adsorption of dyestuffs on bacterial and fungal biomass (Yang et al. 2009; Fu and Viraraghavan 2002) and low-cost nonconventional adsorbents (Crini 2006; Ferrero 2007). Later on, Tony et al. (2013) reported the microbial decolorization of azo dye (Reactive Black 5) using white-rot fungus *Pleurotus eryngii* F032. Similarly, Abedin (Abedin 2008) also stated the decolorization of crystal violet and malachite green by the fungus *Fusarium solani*. In addition, Tak et al. (2004) found that at high pH values, reactive dye solutions are highly negatively charged and dye removal efficiency by white rot fungi was readily decreased. This might be the reason for the adverse effect of alkaline range of pH on fungal enzymes involved in dye biodegradation.

23.5   MARINE POLYMERS: DECOLORING AGENTS

Dyes have two major components: chromophores (unsaturated group) and auxo chromophores (improve absorbance to substrate). Most of the dyes are aromatic compounds, which are applied by various processes of printing surface coating on substrates (Rangnekar and Singh 1980). All colored compounds are not a dye and it might be not suitable for coloured substrate, for example, chemical copper sulphate will not use in any substrate for leathers, textile fibers, food stuffs, and oils (Rangnekar and Singh 1980). In contrast, when azo dyes are applied to textile fibers at suitable condition, the azo dyes can hang on fiber due to compatibility nature and this product called as a dyestuff (Rangnekar and Singh 1980). After processing, the dyes are directly released into the environment from the textile, plastic, cosmetics, and medicine industries. This causes toxic effects on animals and humans (Azmi et al. 1998; Robinson et al. 2001). Therefore, various physicochemical and biological methods were tried for decolorization, including membrane filtration, activated carbon usage, fungal discoloration, and electrochemical techniques (Do and Chen 1994; Alinsafi et al. 2005). However, highly stable dyes' degradation will be slowed down due to their aromatic structure (Fleischmann et al. 2015). Biopolymers are natural absorbents, which have effective chelating ability. This facilitates their use as alternative cost-effective techniques for discoloration (Babel and Kurniawan 2003; Crini 2006). Furthermore, biopolymers are selective biodegradable compounds, such as cyclodextrin and chitosan from starch and chitin, respectively (Delval et al. 2002; Chiou and Li 2002; Crini 2003). Most frequently used dyes in textile industries are reactive blue and red dyes; these are decolorized by biopolymer of starch and chitin, which has been reported as epichlorohydrin. It showed a significant selectivity and affinity to the azo dyes in the environment (Delval et al. 2002; Chiou and Li 2002). Biopolymers are used to detect metal pollution in the environment and industrial wastewater by their affinity for low-molecular-weight compounds and dye (Tavakkoli et al. 1998; Reza et al. 1998).

In recent years, biopolymer wastewater treatments have received more attention because of their efficient removal of pollutants from the environments (Ruthven 1984). Biopolymers are most available in nature, for example, chitosan, which is highly available in crustacean shells (Rinaudo 2006). Chitosan is a low-cost material and is composed of b-(1-4)-linked N-acetylglucosamine. It structurally resembles cellulose, but its acetamide groups are located at C-2 position, which is advantageous for biosorption and modification reactions. However, it is insoluble in water, which was the main difficulty and the reason behind the initiation of the process of developing the chitin derivative chitosan (Rinaudo 2006).

23.6 ADVANCED BIOREMEDIATION TECHNOLOGY BY USING MARINE POLYMERS

Industrialization has led to an increase in the release of toxic effluents, including toxic chemicals such as heavy metals. Particularly, most common heavy metals such as copper, mercury, chromium, lead, nickel, cadmium, and arsenic are being discharged by textile, tanning, paper, electroplating, and pulp industries (Volesky 2001). These heavy metals create serious environmental problems by entering into the food chain, thus leading to several health disorders in humans (Kortenkamp et al. 1996). Therefore, there is an urgent need to safeguard water and food resources from heavy metal contamination by dye and textile industries. It has also become vital to purify water contaminated by heavy metal ions and other organic pollutants. The advanced technology was developed in the bioremediation research by using nanocomposite polymers. New functional nanocomposite materials with infused nanoparticles are in the leads to nanobased dye and textile water treatment methods. More vision can be consequent from recent research work on chitosan-based nanocomposites, which are one of the cheapest, less expensive nanoproducts. The synergistic action of distinct polymers such as chitosan nanoparticles is being used as biosorption for heavy metal removal.

Recent research has concentrated on heavy metal removal by chitosan nanoparticles with clays such as kaolinite, bentonite. and montmorillonite. Clays have natural capability to remove heavy metals, similar to chitin and chitosan polymers. Recently, investigations on nanochitosan– clay complex for heavy metal ion removal have been reported. Khedr et al. (2012) have reported the removal of lead ion by modified chitosan–montmorillonite nanocomposite. Later on, Futalan et al. (2011) have evaluated Nickel(II) ion removal by chitosan-coated bentonite of up to 88% in fixed-bed column. Similarly, Pandey and Mishra (2011) also studied the removal of hexavalent chromium from aqueous solution by using by chitosan–montmorillonite nanocomposite. Chitosan–magnetite nanocomposites are reported for the removal of Fe(III) ions from industrial aqueous solution (Namdeo and Bajpai 2008). Chitin/chitosan nanohydroxyapatite composites could remove Cu(II) ions from industrial wastewater (Rajiv Gandhi et al. 2011). It has been stated that the sorption capacity of chitosan nanohydroxyapatite is quite better than chitin nanohydroxyapatite. In addition, ethylenediamine-modified magnetic chitosan particles were also reported to adsorb radioactive uranyl ions (Wang et al. 2011). Similarly, Hritcu et al. (2012) have also reported the adsorption of uranyl ions and thorium radioactive by unmodified magnetic chitosan particles.

Chitosan is a great biopolymer obtained from chitin by deacetylation, which is extensively available in nature sources. To improve heavy metal adsorption properties, recently, chitosan are modified into nanoparticles. Universally, chitin is available in nature in abundance, and after cellulose, it is the second most available biopolymer. It is found as a major essential component of algae, fungi, insects, mollusks, crustaceans, and marine invertebrates such as shrimp, crab, krill, and shellfish as well as their waste (Deshpande 1986; Chen and Chang 1994). Owing to its usual origin, chitosan is biocompatible and biodegradable (Srinivasa et al. 2009), which makes it the most appropriate candidate for use as an adsorbent.

Current water treatment technologies have many disadvantages such as being expensive, creating secondary pollutants in sludge, and being unsuccessful in treating effluents with low metal concentrations (Han et al. 2006). Commercially available adsorbents such as activated carbon are extremely efficient but are more expensive (Cybelle et al. 2011). Worldwide, the solid waste from the processing of crustaceans' shells and shellfish constitutes large amount of chitinaceous waste (Nomanbhay and Palanisamy 2005), which can be renewed to chitosan by partial deacetylation as a low-cost adsorbent. Moreover, chitosan has the maximum sorption capacity for several heavy metal ions among the various biopolymers, due to the presence of primary amine at C-2 position of the glucosamine residues (Yi et al. 2005). However, it has disadvantages such as tendency to agglomerate or form gels, softness, and nonavailability of reactive binding sites (Nomanbhay and Palanisamy 2005). Yet, the addition of advanced nanoparticles increases the usability of chitosan-based biopolymer.

23.7   CONCLUSION

Bioremediation technology for wastewater treatment is gaining momentum globally. In different fields, marine biopolymers can be applied for industrial waste treatment. The scope of bioremediation is to decrease the concentration of industrial waste pollutants at undetectable levels or lower than the limits established as safe by regulatory agencies. On the basis of our study, we have concluded that the impact and application of marine biopolymer are quite addressing for treatment of dye and textile industrial waste. Some of the biopolymers are already on the market, and other biopolymers require significant research before they can be considered for full-scale wastewater application. Their future development and commercialization face different types of challenges, including technical hurdles, cost-effectiveness, and potential environment and human health risk. Marine polymers are perhaps more appropriate tools for use in the removal of dye and textile industrial contamination from the aquatic environment.

ACKNOWLEDGMENTS

The authors are grateful to SRM University, India, for providing necessary facilities and are thankful to Dr. A. K. Pal, Former Joint-Director, ICAR-CIFE, India, for giving valuable suggestion and moral support.

The coAuthor Dr. K. Kamala is thankful to SERB-DST for financial support through N-PDF (File No:PDF/2015/000680) scheme.

REFERENCES

Abedin, R.M.A. 2008. Decolorization and biodegradation of crystal violet and malachite green by *Fusarium solani* (martius) saccardo. A comparative study on biosorption of dyes by the dead fungal biomass. *American Journal of Botany* 1: 17–31.

Aksu, Z., and S. Tezer. 2005. Biosorption of reactive dyes on the green alga *Chlorella vulgaris*. *Process Biochemistry* 40(3–4): 1347–1361.

Alinsafi, A., M. Khemis, M. Pons, J. Leclerc, A. Yaacoubi, A. Benhammou, and A. Nejmeddine. 2005. Electro coagulation of reactive textiles dyes and textiles waste water. *Chemical Engineering and Processing* 44: 461–470.

Aluyor, E.O., and M. Ori-Jesu. 2009. Biodegradation of mineral oils a review. *African Journal of Biotechnology* 8: 915–920.

Azbar, N., A. Bayram, A. Filibeli, A. Muezzinoglu, F. Sengul, and Ozer. 2004. A review of waste management options in olive production. *Critical Review of Environmental Science and Technology* 34: 209–247.

Azmi, W., R.K. Sani, U.C. Banerijee. 1998. Biodegradation of triphenylmethane dyes in solid and liquid media. *Enzyme Microbial Technology* 22: 185–191.

Babel, S., and T.A. Kurniawan. 2003. Low cost adsorbents for heavy metals uptake from contaminated water: A review. *Journal of Hazardous Materials* 97: 219–243.

Badawi, A.F., E.L. Cavalieri, and E.G. Rogan. 2000. Effect of chlorinated hydrocarbons on expression of cytochrome P450 1A1, 1A2 and 1B1 and 2- and 4-hydroxylation of 17β-estradiol in female Sprague–Dawleyrats. *Carcinogenesis* 21: 1593–1599.

Bernhard-Reversat, F., and D. Schwartz. 1997. Change in lignin content during litter decomposition in tropical forest soils (Congo) comparison of exotic plantations and native stands, *Earth and Planetary Science Letter* 325: 427–432.

Bhattacharyya, K.G., and A. Sharma. 2005. Kinetics and thermodynamics of methylene blue adsorption on neem (Azadiracta indica) leaf powder. *Dyes and Pigments* 65: 51–59.

Blackburn, R.S. 2004. Natural polysaccharides and their interactions with dye molecules: applications in effluent treatment. *Environmental Science and Technology* 38: 4905–4909.

Cerniglia, C.E. 1993. Biodegradation of polycyclic aromatic hydrocarbons. *Current Opinion in Biotechnology* 4: 331–338.

Chen, J.P., and K.C. Chang. 1994. Immobilization of chitinase on a reversibly soluble-insoluble polymer for chitin hydrolysis. *Journal of Chemical Technology Biotechnology* 60: 133–140.

Chiou, G., and H. Li. 2002. Adsorbtion behavior of reactive dye in aqueous solution on chemical cross-linked chitosan beads. *Chemophere* 50: 1095–1105.

Crini, G. 2003. Recent developments in polysaccharide based materials used as adsorbents in waste water treatment. *Progresses Polymeric Science* 30: 38–70.

Crini, G. 2005. Recent developments in polysaccharide-based materials used as adsorbents in wastewater treatment. *Progress in Polymer Science* 30: 38–70.

Crini, G. 2006. Non-conventional low-cost adsorbents for dye removal: A review. *Bioresource Technology* 97: 1061–1085.

Crini, G., E. Guibal, M. Morcellet, G. Torri, and P.M. Badot. 2009. Chitin and chitosan preparation, properties and main applications. In *Chitin and Chitosan: Application of Some Biopolymers*, Besancon, France: University press of Franche-Comte. p. 307.

Cybelle, M.F., C.C. Kan, M.L. Dalida, C. Pascua, and M.W. Wan. 2011. Comparative and competitive adsorption of copper, lead, and nickel using chitosan immobilized on bentonite. *Carbohydrate Polymers* 83: 697–704.

Dana, L.D., and J.W. Bauder. 2011. *A General Essay on Bioremediation of Contaminated Soil*. Bozeman, Mont: Montana State University.

Danis, T.G., T.A. Albanis, D.E. Petrakis, and P.J. Pomonis. 1998. Removal of chlorinated phenols from aqueous solutions by adsorption on alumina pillared clays and mesoporous alumina aluminum phosphates. *Water Research* 32(2): 295–302.

Delval, F., G. Crini, S. Bertini, C. Filiatre, and G. Torri. 2005. Preparation, Characterization and sorption properties of cross-linked starch-based exchangers. *Carbohydrate Polymers* 60: 67–75.

Delval, S., G. Crini, N. Morin, J. Vebrel, S. Bertini, and G. Torri, G. Delval. 2002. The sorption of several types of dye on crosslinked polysaccharide derivatives. *Dyes and Pigments* 53: 79–92, 57.

Deshpande, M.V. 1986. Enzymatic degradation of chitin and its biological application. *Journal of Scientific & Industrial Research* 45: 277–281.

Do, J.S., and M.L. Chen. 1994. Decolourization of dye containing solutions by electrocoagulation. *Journal of Applied Electro Chemistry* 24: 785–790.

Dos Santos, A.B., M.P. Madrid, A.J.M. Starns, J.B. Van Lier, and F.J. Cervantes. 2005. Azo dye reduction by mesophilic and thermophilic anaerobic consortia. *Biotechnology Progress* 21: 1140–1145.

Ferrero, F. 2007. Dye removal by low cost adsorbents: Hazelnut shells in comparison with wood sawdust. *Journal of Hazardous Materials* 142: 144–152.

Fleischmann, C., M. Lievenbruck, and H. Ritter. 2015. Polymers and dyes: Developments and applications. *Polymers* 7: 717–746.

Forgacsa, E., C. Tibor, O. Gyula, and D. Aim. 2004. Removal of synthetic dyes from waste-waters: A review. *Environmental International* 30: 953–971.

Fu, Y., and T. Viraraghavan. 2002. Removal of congo red from an aqueous solution by fungus Aspergillus niger. *Advances in Environmental Research* 7: 239–247.

Futalan, C.M., C.C. Kan, M.L. Dalida, C. Pascua, and M.W. Wan. 2011. Fixed-bed column studies on the removal of copper using chitosan immobilized on bentonite. *Carbohydrate Polymers* 83: 697–704.

Galindo, C., and T. Kalt. 1999. UV/H2O oxidation of azo dyes in aqueous media: Evidence of a structure—Degradability relationship. *Dyes and Pigments* 42: 199–207.

Gupta, V., P. Carrott, M.M.L.R. Carrott, and Suhas. 2009. Low-cost adsorbents: Growing approach to wastewater treatment: A review. *Critical Reviews in Environmental Science and Technology* 39: 783–842.

Gupta, V.K., S. Khamparia, I. Tyagi, D. Jaspal, and A. Malviya. 2015. Decolorization of mixture of dyes: A critical review. *Global Journal of Environmental Science and Management* 1: 71–94

Han, R., W. Zou, H. Li, Y. Li, and J. Shi. 2006. Copper (II) and lead (II) removal from aqueous solution in fixed-bed columns by manganese oxide coated zeolite. *Journal of Hazardous Materials* 137: 934–942.

Hassani, S., M.R. Sepand, A. Jafari, J. Jaafari, R. Rezaee, and M. Zeinali. 2015. Protective effects of curcumin and vitamin E against chlorpyrifos-induced lung oxidative damage. *Human and Experimental Toxicology* 34(6): 668–676.

Hritcu, D., D. Humelnicu, G. Dodi, and M.L. Popa. 2012. Magnetic chitosan composite particles: Evaluation of thorium and Uranyl ion. *Carbohydrate Polymers* 87: 1185–1191.

Imamura, K., E. Ikeda, T. Nagayasu, T. Sakiyama, and K. Nakanishi. 2002. Adsorption behaviours of methhylene blue and its congeners on a stainless steel surface. *Journal of Colloid and Interface Science* 245: 50–57.

Ince, N.H., and G. Tezcanh. 1999. Treatability of textile dye bath effluents by advanced oxidation: Preparation for reuse. *Water Science and Technology* 40: 183–190.

Ismail, M., M. Loganathan, and P.A. Gastian Theodar. 2012. Effect of bio adsorbents in removal of colour and toxicity of textile and leather dyes. *Journal of Eco Biotechnology* 4: 1–10.

Jang, M., S.H. Min, J.K. Park, and E.J. Tlachac. 2007. Hydrous ferric oxide incorporated diatomite for remediation of arsenic contaminated groundwater. *Environmental Science and Technology* 41: 3322.

Jayakumar, R., N. Nwe, S. Tokura, and H. Tamura. 2007. Sulfated chitin and chitosan as novel biomaterials. *International Journal of Biological Macromolecules* 40: 175–181.

Jayakumar, R., M. Prabaharan, S. Nair, S. Tokura, H. Tamura, and N. Selvamurugan. 2010. Novel carboxymethyl derivatives of chitin and chitosan materials and their biomedical applications. *Progress in Materials Science* 55: 675–709.

Karigar, C.S., and S.S. Rao. 2011. Role of microbial enzyme in bioremediation of pollutants: A review. *Enzyme Research* 11: 1–11.

Kartik H.G. and Mehali J.M. 2014. Removal of color from different dye wastewater by using ferric oxide as an adsorbent. *International Journal of Engineering Research and Applications* 4(5): 102–109.

Khedr, M.A., A.I. Waly, A.I. Hafez, and Hanaa Ali. 2012. Synthesis of modified chitosan—Montmorillonite nanocomposite. *Australian Journal of Basic and Applied Sciences* 6(6): 216–226.

Kortenkamp, A., M. Casadevall, S.P. Faux, A. Jennar, R.O.J. Shayer, N. Woodbridge, and P. A. Obrien. 1996. Role for molecular oxygen in the formation of DNA damage during the reduction carcinogen of the chromium (VI) by glutathione. *Archives of Biochemistry Biophysics* 329: 199–207.

Kumar, A., B.S. Bisht, V.D. Joshi, and T. Dhewa. 2011. Review on bioremediation of polluted environment: A management tool. *International Journal of Environmental Science* 1: 1079–1093.

Levin, L., A. Viale, and A. Forchiassin. 2003. Degradation of organic pollutants by the white rot basidiomycete trametestrogii. *International Biodeterioration & Biodegradation* 52: 1–5.

Mahmoud, A.S., A.E. Ghaly, and S.L. Brooks. 2007. Influence of temperature and pH on the stability and colorimetric measurement of textile dyes. *American Journal of Biotechnology and Biochemistry* 3(1): 33–41.

Malik, P.K. 2004. Dye removal from wastewater using activated carbon developed from sawdust: Adsorption equilibrium and kinetics. *Journal of Hazardous Materials* B 113: 81–88.

Maya, S., S. Indulekha, V. Sukhithasree, K. Smitha, S.V. Nair, R. Jayakumar, and R. Biswas. 2012. Efficacy of tetracycline encapsulated O-carboxymethyl chitosan nanoparticles against intracellular infections of *Staphylococcus aureus*. *International Journal of Biological Macromolecules* 51: 392–399.

Namasivayam, C., N. Muniasamy, K. Gayatri, M. Rani, and K. Ranganathan. 1996. Removal of dyes from aqueous solutions by cellulosic waste orange peel. *Bioresource Technology* 57: 37–43.

Namdeo, M. and S.K. Bajpai. 2008. Chitosan-magnetite nanocomposites (CMNs) as magnetic carrier particles for removal of Fe (III) from aqueous solutions. *Colloids and Surfaces A. Physicochemical Engineering Aspects* 320: 161–168.

Nevine, K.A. 2008. Removal of reactive dye from aqueous solutions by adsorption onto activated carbon prepared from sugarcane bagasse pith. *Desalination* 223: 152–161.

Nomanbhay, S.M., and K. Palanisamy. 2005. Removal of heavy metal from industrial wastewater using chitosan-coated oil palm shell charcoal. *Electronic Journal of Biotechnology* 8: 44–53.

Pala, A., and E. Tokat. 2002. Color removal from cotton textile industry wastewater in an activated sludge system with various additives. *Water Research* 36: 2920–2925.

Pandey, S. and S.B. Mishra. 2011. Organic-inorganic hybrid of chitosan/organo clay bionanocomposites for hexavalent chromium uptake. *Journal of Colloid and Interface Science* 361: 509–520.

Pankaj, T., G. Bhawna, G. Goyal, and P.K. Prem. 2012. A comparative study of sonosorption of reactive red 141 Dye on TiO2, banana peel, orange peel and hardwood saw dust. *Journal of Applicable Chemistry* 14: 505–511.

Rachakornkij, M., S. Rungchuay, and S. Teachakulwiroj, 2004. Removal of reactive dye from aqueous solution using bagasse fly ash. *Songklanakarin Journal of Science and Technology* 26 (1): 13–24.

Rai, H.S., M.S. Bhattacharyya, J. Singh, T.K. Bansal, P. Vats and U.C. Banerjee. 2005. Removal of dyes from the effluent of textile and dyestuff manufacturing industry: A review of emerging techniques with reference to biological treatment. *Critical Reviews in Environmental ScienceTechnology* 35: 219–238.

Rajamohan, N. and C. Karthikeyan. 2006. Kinetic studies of dye effluent degradation by *Pseudomonas Stutzeri*. *Asian Journal of Microbiology* 8(1): 39–43.

Rajiv Gandhi, M., G.N. Kousalya and S. Meenakshi. 2011. Removal of copper (II) using chitin/chitosan nano-hydroxyapatite composite. *International Journal of Biological Macromolecules* 48: 119–124.

Rana, K., and T. Samir. 2014. Biodecolourization of textile dye effluent by biosorption of fungal biomass materials. *Physicsprocedia* 55: 437–444.

Rangnekar, D.W., and P.P. Singh, 1980. *An Introduction to Synthetic Dyes.* Bombay: Himalaya. p. 240.

Reza, P.H., A. Forghaniha, H. Sharghi, and M. Shamsipur. 1998. Lead selective membrane potentiometric sensor based on a recently synthesized bis(anthraquinone) sulfide derivative. *Analytical Letter* 31: 2591–2605.

Rinaudo, M. 2006. Chitin and chitosan prosperities and applications. *Progress Polymer Science* 31: 603–632.

Rio, S., C. Faur-Brasquet, L. Le Coq, and P. Le Cloirec. 2005. Structure Characterization and Adsorption Properties of Pyrolyzed Sewage Sludge, *Environmental Science and Technology* 39: 4249–4257.

Robinson, T., G. McMullan, R. Marchant, and P. Nigam. 2001. Remediation of dyes in textile effluent: A critical review on current treatment technologies with a proposed alternative. *Bioresource Technology* 77: 247–255.

Ruthven, D.M. 1984. *Principles of Adsorption and Adsorption Processes.* New York: Wiley-Interscience, p 464.

Saha, B., and C. Orvig. 2010. Biosorbents for hexavalent chromium elimination from industrial and municipal effluents. *Coordination Chemistry Reviews* 254: 2959–2972.

Sankar, D., K. Chennazhi, S.V. Nair, and R. Jayakumar. 2012. Fabrication of chitin/poly (3-hydroxybutyrate-co-3-hydroxyvalerate) hydrogel scaffold. *Carbohydrate Polymers* 90: 725–729.

Seshadri, S., P.L. Bishop, and A.M. Agha. 1994. Anaerobic/aerobic treatment of selected azo dyes in wastewater. *Waste Management* 14: 127–137.

Singh, B. K. 2009. Organo phosphorus-degrading bacteria: Ecology and industrial applications. *Nature Reviews Microbiology* 7(2): 156–164.

Sirotkina, M., I. Lyagin, and E. Efremenko. 2012. Hydrolysis of organo phosphorus pesticides in soil: New opportunities with eco-compatible immobilized His6-OPH. *International Biodeterioration & Biodegradation* 68: 18–23.

Solmaz, A., S.K. Ustun, G.E. Birgul, and A. Yonar, 2009. Advanced oxidation of textile dyeing effluents: comparison of Fe+2/H2O2,Fe+3/H2O2, O3 and chemical coagulation processes. *Fresenius Environmental Bulletin* 18: 1424–1433.

Srinivasa, R.P., Y. Vijaya, M.B. Veera, and A. Krishnaiah. 2009. Adsorptive removal of copper and nickel ions from water using chitosan coated PVC beads. *Bioresource Technology* 100: 194–199.

Syafalni, S., I. Abustan, S.N.F. Zakaria, and M.H. Zawawi. 2012. Raw water treatment using bentonite-chitosan as a coagulant. *Water Science and Technology: Water Supply* 12(4): 480–488.

Tak, H.K., Y. Lee, J. Yang, B. Lee, C. Park, and S. Kim. 2004. Decolorization of dye solutions by a membrane bioreactor (MBR) using white-rot fungi. *Desalination* 168: 287–293.

Tavakkoli, N., Z. Khojasteh, H. Sharghi, and M. Shamsipur, 1998. Lead ion selective membrane electrodes based on the some recently synthesized 9, 10-anthraquinone derivatives. *Analytica Chimica Acta* 360: 203–208.

Tony, H., L. Adnan, A.R. Mohd Yusoff, A. Yuniarto, M. Rubiyatno, A. Ahmad Zubir, Z.C. BadrKhudhair, and M. Abu Naser. 2013. Microbial decolorization of an azo dye reactive black 5 using white-rot fungus pleurotuseryngii F032. *Water Air and Soil Pollution* 224: 1595.

Tyagi, O.D. and M. Yadav. 2001. A textbook of synthetic dye. Anmol Publications PVT Ltd. New Delhi, India.

Vidali, M., 2001. Bioremediation: An overview. *Pure Applied Chemistry* 73: 1163–1172.

Volesky, B. 2001. Detoxification of metal-bearing effluents: Biosorption for the next century. *Hydrometallurgy* 59: 203–216.

Walker, G.M. and L.R. Weatherley. 1997. A simplified predictive model for biologically activated carbon fixed beds. *Process Biochemistry* 32: 327–335.

Wang, J.S., R.T. Peng, J.H. Yang, Y.C. Liu, and X.J. Hu. 2011. Preparation of ethylenediamine-modified magnetic chitosan complex for adsorption of uranyl ions. *Carbohydrate Polymers* 84: 1169–1175.

Wijannarong, S., S. Aroonsrimorakot, P. Thavipoke, and S. Sangjan. 2013. Removal of reactive dyes from textile dyeing industrial effluent by ozonation process. *APCBEE Procedia* 5: 279–282.

Wojnarovits, L., and E. Takacs. 2008. Irradiation treatment of azo-dye containing wastewater: An overview. *Radiation Physics and Chemistry* 77: 225–244.

Yang, X.Q., X.X. Zhao, C.Y. Liu, Y. Zheng, and S.J. Qian. 2009. Decolorization of azo, triphenylmethane and anthraquinone dyes by a newly isolated *Trametes* sp. SQ01 and its laccase. *Process of Biochemistry* 4: 1185–1189.

Yeh, R.L., R. Liu, H.M. Chiu, and Y.T. Hung. 1993. Comparative study of adsorption capacity of various adsorbents for treating dye wastewaters. *International Journal of Environmental Studies, Section B: Environmental Science and Technology* 44: 259.

Yi, H., L. Wu, W.E. Bentley, R. Ghodssi, C.W. Rubloff, J.N. Culver, and G.F. Payne. 2005. Bio fabrication with chitosan. *Biomacromolecules* 9: 2881–2894.

Yilmaz, A., E. Yilmaz, M. Yilmaz, R.A. Bartsch. 2007. Removal of azo dyes from aqueous solutions using calix [4] arene and β-cyclodextrin. *Dyes and Pigments* 74: 54–59.

Index

Note: Page numbers followed by f and t refer to figures and tables, respectively.

9781032339597